Design Data Handbook
for Mechanical Engineers
in SI and Metric Units

Fourth Edition

Compiled by

K. Mahadevan
Former Principal
Karnataka Regional Engineering College (NIT-K),
Surathkal, Karnataka

K. Balaveera Reddy
Former Vice Chancellor
Visvesvaraya Technological University
Belgaum, Karnataka
Ex-Professor, Department of Mechanical Engineering
Karnataka Regional Engineering College, Surathkal

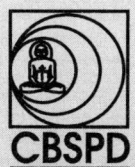

CBSPD

W0235505

CBS Publishers & Distributors Pvt Ltd

New Delhi ⊙ Bengaluru ⊙ Chennai ⊙ Kochi ⊙ Kolkata ⊙ Lucknow ⊙ Mumbai
Hyderabad ⊙ Jharkhand ⊙ Nagpur ⊙ Patna ⊙ Pune ⊙ Uttarakhand

Design Data Handbook
for Mechanical Engineers

ISBN: 978-81-239-2315-4

Copyright © Authors and Publisher

Fourth Edition: 2013
    Reprint: 2014, 2015, 2016, 2017, 2018, 2019, 2020, 2021, 2022, 2023, **2024**
Third Edition: 1987 Reprint: 1989, 1993, 1998, 1999, 2000, 2001, 2002, 2003, 2004, 2005, 2006, 2007, 2008, 2009, 2010, 2011, 2012

Published by **Satish Kumar Jain** and produced by **Varun Jain** for

CBS Publishers & Distributors Pvt Ltd

4819/XI Prahlad Street, 24 Ansari Road, Daryaganj, New Delhi 110 002, India.
Ph: 011-23266838, 23289259   Website: www.cbspd.com
                                  e-mail: delhi@cbspd.com

Corporate Office: 204 FIE, Industrial Area, Patparganj, Delhi 110 092
Ph: 011-4934 4934   Fax: 011-4934 4935
                 e-mail: publishing@cbspd.com; publicity@cbspd.com

Branches

- **Bengaluru:** Seema House 2975, 17th Cross, KR Road, Banasankari 2nd Stage, Bengaluru 560 070, Karnataka, India
  Ph: +91-80-26771678/79   Fax: +91-80-26771680   e-mail: bangalore@cbspd.com
- **Chennai:** 7, Subbaraya Street, Shenoy Nagar, Chennai 600 030, Tamil Nadu, India
  Ph: +91-44-26680620, 26681266   Fax: +91-44-42032115   e-mail: chennai@cbspd.com
- **Kochi:** 42/1325, 1326, Power House Road, Opp KSEB, Power House, Ernakulum Kochi 682 018, Kerala, India
  Ph: +91-484-4059061-65,67   Fax: +91-484-4059065   e-mail: kochi@cbspd.com
- **Kolkata:** 147, Hind Ceramics Compound, 1st Floor, Nilgunj Road, Belghoria, Kolkata-700056, West Bengal, India
  Ph: +033-25633055, 033-25633056   e-mail: kolkata@cbspd.com
- **Lucknow:** Basement, Khushnuma Complex, 7 Meerabai Marg (Behind Jawahar Bhawan), Lucknow-226001, UP, India
  Ph: +0522-4000032   e-mail: tiwari.lucknow@cbspd.com
- **Mumbai:** PWD Shed, Gala no 25/26, Ramchandra Bhatt Marg, Next to JJ Hospital Gate no. 2, Opp. Union Bank of India, Noorbaug, Mumbai-400009, Maharashtra, India
  Ph: 022-66661880/89   e-mail: mumbai@cbspd.com

Representatives

- Hyderabad   0-9885175004
- Patna   0-9334159340
- Jharkhand   0-9811541605
- Pune   0-9664372571
- Nagpur   0-8692091830
- Uttarakhand   0-9716462459

Printed at Glorious Printers, Jhilmil Industrial Area, Delhi, India

Foreword

It gives me great pleasure to write the 'Foreword' to 'Design Data Handbook' by Prof. K. Mahadevan and Shri K. Balaveera Reddy of Karnataka Regional Engineering College, Surathkal, Karnataka. The principal feature of this Handbook is the introduction of SI Units and perhaps this is the first Handbook so written in India.

Brilliant developments in the field of Engineering Design are taking place at a rapid rate, but most of them are based on firm ground of existing and proven data and ideas. Hence, any competent and successful design engineer should, apart from being a creator and analyst, be familiar with current design data, design codes and practices, etc. The authors, with their long teaching experience, have presented all the important mechanical design data in an orderly way in the form of charts, formulae and tables, enabling calculation of dimensions of various machine elements required for the preparation of working drawings. **References** have been included at the end of each chapter enabling the user to get further information on the respective topics. Further, the data and the **nomenclature** contained in this Handbook conform to **IS specifications** wherever applicable.

I am confident that the Handbook will be very useful to practicing design engineers for their day-to-day work and thus be a welcome addition to design offices. It will also be useful to **teachers** and **students** of Mechanical Engineering Design of Technical Universities and Colleges, as this meets their syllabi and provides an useful addition to their Libraries.

I would like to congratulate the authors for their efforts to bring out this useful Handbook.

Prof. R. G. Narayanamurthy
Director
Indian Institute of Technology
MADRAS

Preface to the Fourth Edition

In the preparation of this fourth edition, most of the topics/chapters have been upgraded and improved by adding additional information on current design. Some changes have been made to refine the presentation and to enhance the coverage of every topic. Every effort has been made to eliminate errors. We hope the present edition will be appreciated by all design engineers.

The authors are greatly indebted to M/s. Sriranga Digital Software Technologies Pvt. Ltd., Srirangapatna, Karnataka and M/s. CBS Publishers & Distributors Pvt. Ltd., New Delhi in getting the book printed in an excellent manner.

February 2013
                                                          K. Balaveera Reddy

Preface to the Third Edition

While preparing this third edition, the authors have carefully gone through the syllabus Machine Design Course of many other Universities, so that the presentation could be of more use to the students studying the course in Machine Design. In this edition the notes on "Designation, Properties and Uses of Materials" has been brought up-to-date taking into consideration the I.S.I. Standards. Many chapters have been revised. A chapter on "Rotation Discs" has been included, Every attempt has been made to make this book a good reference hand book for Mechanical Engineering students and also Machine Designers.

May 1986
                                                          K. Mahadevan
                                                          K. Balaveera Reddy

Preface to the Second Edition

In the light of several requests from various sections of people who have been using the Design Data Hand Book, it was decided to have the Metric Units along with S.I. Units, for better utilization of the hand book.

While revising the Data Hand Book in the above manner, steps have been taken to remove certain minor errors which had crept in the earlier edition; further some additional information also have been added. We do hope the Design Data Hand Book will continue to receive the same patronage as before.

May 1983
                                                          K. Mahadevan
                                                          K. Balaveera Reddy

Preface to the First Edition

Machine Design is one of the basic subjects of Mechanical Engineering and a thorough knowledge of the design aspects of machine elements is essential for both engineering students and practising engineers. Working out the design of a machine as a whole, or its components, usually involves the use of several formulae, equations and other relevant data and the availability of all such information in one single hand book will not only remove the unnecessary task of remembering the required formulae and equations but will also aid the students and practising engineers to solve the problems in Machine Design in quicker time.

This Design Data Hand Book has been prepared keeping the above views in mind. The Data compiled in this Hand Book have been presented in SI (System International) Units since the adoption of SI Units has already been accepted in our country. It may be mentioned that several other countries have been using the SI Units for science and engineering subjects in recent years. The symbols used in the hand book are also those pertaining to SI Units. As far as possible, data available in ISI Standards have been used, at the appropriate places, after converting the information to SI Units. Reference has been made to several standard text-books on machine design while compiling the data for the hand book and a list of references is included at the end of each chapter so that the readers can refer to the relevant books for obtaining further information on the topic.

Care has been taken to include data on almost all the important topics embracing machine design and it is thus hoped that the hand-book will be quite useful to the engineering students of all the Universities in our Country. Further, necessary conversion factors and tables have also been presented in Appendix V, so that design problems can be solved even when the data given are in FPS or Metric units.

In a hand book of this nature containing large amount of data in the form of equations, tables, etc., it is realised that errors might have crept in, in spite of the care taken in reading the proofs. The authors will feel grateful to the readers if they could bring to our attention, the errors if any, noticed by them.

We are very grateful to Prof. R. G. Narayanamurthy, Director, Indian Institute of Technology, Madras, for writting the foreward.

We express our sincere appreciation to M/s. Sharada Press, Mangalore, for having taken infinite pains in getting the book printed in an excellent manner.

We do hope the hand book will be useful not only to students and teachers but also to practising engineers.

K. Mahadevan
K. Balaveera Reddy

Acknowledgements

The authors wish to place on record their gratefulness to the publishers of the following books for having permitted us to use the material, as indicated below, from their books.

McGraw-Hill Book Company, New York, U.S.A.

(a) Shigley–Machine Design

figs. 2.24, 2.25, 7.15, 9.13, 9.14, 9.15, 9.16, 9.17, 11.3, 11.4, 12.7, 12.10

tables. 7.2, 9.3, 10.9, 12.1 and A-2

(b) Vallance and Doughtie–Design of Machine Members

figs. 25, 49, 54, 150, 202

tables. 16, 17, 19, 29, 43, 55, 84, 85

(c) Black–Machine Design

figs. 4.16, 17.10, x-1 to x-16

tables. 4.1

(d) Roark–Formulas for Stress and Strain

pp. 100-109–table III

pp. 148-149–table VII

Intext Educational Publishers, Pennsylvania, U.S.A.
Siegel, Maleev and Hartman–Mechanical Design of Machines

figs. 4.30, 5.11, 5.12, 5.21, 5.28, 5.29, 6.2, 6.3, 6.7, 9.24, 9.25, 10.2, 10.5, 10.7, 10.10, 10.13, 10.14, 11.8, 11.9, 11.10, 12.1, 12.2, 13.4, 15.14, 15.17, 15.18, 15.19, 15.22, 17.11, 17.14, 17.28.

tables. 4.1, 4.3, 4.4, 5.3, 6.1, 12.1, 13.1, 13.2, 13.3, 13.4, 15.3, 15.4, 15.7, 15.8, 17.2

John Wiley and Sons, Inc., Publishers, New York, U.S.A.
Peterson–Stress Concentration Design Factors

figs. 10, 16, 24, 28, 32, 38, 42, 46, 57, 58, 59, 60, 66, 67, 69, 86, 88, 100, 101, 102, 109, 110.

Finally we wish to acknowledge our particular indebtedness to Indian Standards Institution for the several Indian Standards incorporated in our Data Hand Book and to the authors and publishers of various books consulted by us in the compilation of the Data Hand Book.

Note regarding the usage of the Design Data Hand Book for S.I. and Metric Units

The Design Data Hand Book has been compiled in both Metric and International System (SI) of Units. The following few illustrations regarding the use of the hand book in both the units have been given for better utilization of the hand book.

(a) Symbols:

For each symbol (which is same in both the cases), the relevant units used are indicated against each symbol: For example:

$$F_r \text{ is the Radiat force acting on the tooth, N (kgf).}$$

The units in SI system for F_r is N, and in metric system, kgf. The units in *Metric system* for each symbol has been indicated *within the brackets*, whereas in SI system is written prior to the Metric Unit.

$$A \text{ is the cross-sectional area, } mm^2.$$

The unit for the cross-sectional area, A in both the systems is same, i.e., mm^2.

(b) Formulae:

In flat belts, the relation between the stress σ and elongation, e. $\quad \sigma = C_1^2 \, e^2$ Eq. 14.11.

$$\text{where} \quad \sigma \text{ is the stress in belt, } MN/m^2 \, (kgf/mm^2).$$
$$e \text{ is the elongation, mm/mm.}$$
$$C_1 = \text{a constant}$$
$$= 70(22.35) \text{ for leather belts.}$$

The value of the constant C_1 in SI system is 70 and in *metric system* it is 22.35, which has been indicated *within the brackets*.

(c) Tables:

Table 12.7. Allowable static stress σ_d to use in Lewis formulae

Material	Allowable static stress, MN/m^2 (kgf/mm^2)	BHN
Cast Iron Grade 20	47.1 (4.80)	200
Cast Iron Grade 25	56.4 (5.75)	220

The allowable stress value for Cast Iron grade 20 material in SI system is 47.1 MN/m^2 and in Metric system it is 4.80 kgf/mm^2. The values, corresponding to *metric system* have been indicated *within the brackets* and for SI system is written prior to the values given in Metric system.

Contents

1   Stress Analysis   **1**

Simple Stresses and Strains-General bending and torsion equations. Combined Stresses-Maximum normal stress and shear stress theories. Compound Stresses-Uniaxial, Biaxial and Plane stress system-Mohr's circle diagram. Superposition (Eccentric loading). Biaxial and Triaxial deformations-stresses in terms of strains. Hertz contact stresses-Spherical and cylindrical surfaces. Thermal stresses. Columns-Euler's, Parabolic, Straight line, Rankine and Ritter's column formulae.

2   Working Stresses   **19**

Stress concentration-Direct, Bending and Torsional stresses, notch sensitivity index. Theories of failure-Maximum normal stress (Rankine), Maximum strain (Saint-Vanant's), Maximum shear stress (Guest's), Shear energy (Henky-Von mises) and Total strain energy (Haigh's) theories. Design for strength-Size factor, Reliability factor, static and fatigue loads, Relation between tensile strength and endurance limit, static plus alternating simple loads. Fatigue failure equations-Gerber's, good man's and Soderberg relations-equivalent stresses. Inertia stresses and centrifugal loads. Impact Energy-General equations for the stress and deformation (deflection) under impact. Resilience-without impact and with impact.

3   Design of Shafts   **49**

Torsion of Circular Shafts-Solid and hollow shafts, Torque transmitted. ASME code for design of transmission shafting-maximum normal and shear stress theories, Fluctuating loads, Axial load in addition to torsional and bending loads. Crank Shafts-over hung crank shafts, forged and cast iron crank shafts, Torsion of rectangular bars.

4   Keys, Pins, Cotter and Knuckle Joints   **61**

Square and Rectangular keys-Strength of keys. Taper keys and keyways-Forces acting on taper key cross-section and length of key. Feather keys-one and two feather keys, Forces acting on feather keys. Round taper pin keys-Mean diameter. Parallel side splines/straight sided splines-Torque transmitted. Involute Splines-Torque capacity. Cotter Joint-Design of rod, socket and cotter. Knucklet Joint-Design of eye and forked end and pin.

deflection, initial gap with pre-stress load on clip bolts. Disc springs or Belleville Springs-Relation between load and axial deflection, stress at the inner and outer edge. Rubber Springs-Rubber in compression, shear, torsional shear and deflection.

centre distance, pitch length, tensions and power ratings. Strength of Manila rope-diameter, maximum and effective tension and power transmitted. Hoisting Tackle-Single sheave, Effort and load, Two Blocks and efficiency of the hoist. Differential Chain Block-Effort and load, efficiency. Wire Rope-Bending stress and load, service load, construction of wire ropes. Hoisting and power chains-working load, sheve diameter, speed of chain, pitch, allowable working load, number of strands, centre distance, chain length and check for actual factor of safety. Precision Roller chains, Bush chains, and Leaf chains-proportionate dimensions.

Viscosity, specific gravity, shearing stress, force and torque, Petroff's relation, coefficient of friction, bearing modulus, bearing pressure, sommerfeld number, friction variable, power loss, minimum film thickness variable, flow variable and temperatures. Pressure-fed Bearings-oil flow, coefficient of friction. Heat Dissipation of Bearings-Heat generated, heat dissipating capacity and temperature rise of the bearing wall. Bearing Shells-Thickness of bearing shells and bearing caps.

Tooth load, shaft load in a belt drive. Radial Ball Bearings, Radial Roller Bearings and Taper Roller Bearings-Relation between load and life, rating life in millions of revolutions and working hours, basic load rating, radial and Trust loads, equivalent load, fluctuating bearing load, static load rating of rolling bearings, life factors.

Kinetic energy, change in (excess) Energy, weight of flywheel rim, flywheel effect. Engine Flywheels- Average energy, change in energy, weight of flywheel rim, stresses in fly-wheel rim and arms, proportionate dimensions, check for maximum tensile stress in the arms and cross-section of arms.

Steam engine cylinder, thickness of cylinder (Lame's, Grashof's and Clavarino's equation). Internal combustion engine cylinder-Diameter, thickness, water space, thickness of cylinder heads and bolts. Steam engine pistons-proportionate dimensions of cast iron and cast steel pistons, diameter of piston rod, inertia forces. Trunk Pistons-Thicknesses, length, stroke, diameter of piston pin, check the strength of piston pin, proportionate dimensions of piston rings.

Inertia force, bending moment, bending stress, stress due to axial load (Rankine-Gordon formula), connecting rod sections, Reciprocating motion, Inertia force, small and big end proportionate dimensions and cap thickness. Common strap and fixed strap end connecting rods, solid or Box end type, Marine type of connecting rod end-proportionate dimensions.

Undamped free vibrations - rectilinear and torsional systems, equations of motion, natural frequency, Rayleigh's method and beam vibrations. Damped free vibrations - viscous damping, equations of motion, damping ratio, critical damping, logarithmic decrement. Forced vibration - Harmonic excitation-Steady state solution with viscous damping, equations of motion, magnification factor and phase angle. Recriprocating and rotating unbalance - equations of motion.

Base Excitation-Equation of motion, amplitude ratio and phase angle. Vibration Isolation-Force through springs and damper, transmissibility. Whirling of Rotating Shafts-dynamic deflection, critical speed of multi-rotor shaft system (Dunkerley's equation). Trosional Vibrations-Two disc semi definite system, principle mode of vibration, equations of motion and frequency equations. Three-disk semi definite system-Equations of motion, frequency equations, natural frequencies and amplitude ratios. Geared systems-Equivalent system, equivalent inertia, equivalent spring constant and natural frequencies.

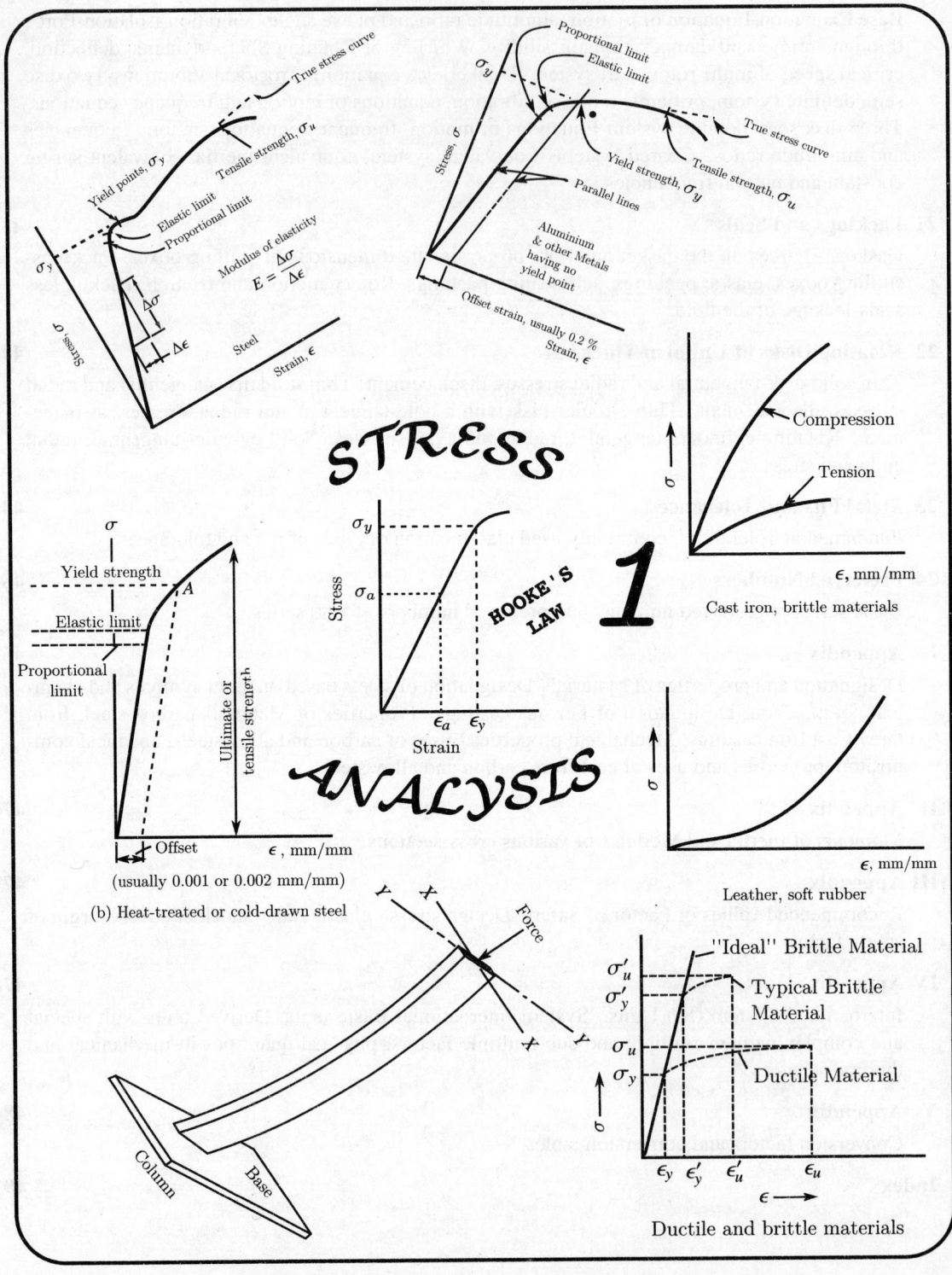

STRESS

ANALYSIS

HOOKE'S LAW

1

True stress curve

Yield points, σ_y
Tensile strength, σ_u
Elastic limit
Proportional limit
Modulus of elasticity $E = \dfrac{\Delta\sigma}{\Delta\epsilon}$
σ_y
$\Delta\sigma$
$\Delta\epsilon$
Steel
Strain, ϵ
Stress σ

Proportional limit
Elastic limit
σ_y
True stress curve
Yield strength, σ_y
Tensile strength, σ_u
Parallel lines
Aluminium & other Metals having no yield point
Offset strain, usually 0.2 %
Strain, ϵ
Stress, σ

Yield strength
Elastic limit
Proportional limit
A
Ultimate or tensile strength
Offset
ϵ, mm/mm
(usually 0.001 or 0.002 mm/mm)
(b) Heat-treated or cold-drawn steel
σ

σ_y
σ_a
Stress
Strain
ϵ_a ϵ_y

Compression
Tension
ϵ, mm/mm
σ
Cast iron, brittle materials

σ
ϵ, mm/mm
Leather, soft rubber

Y X
Force
Y
X Y
Column
Base

"Ideal" Brittle Material
σ'_u
σ'_y
Typical Brittle Material
σ_u
σ_y
Ductile Material
σ
ϵ_y ϵ'_y ϵ'_u ϵ_u
$\epsilon \longrightarrow$
Ductile and brittle materials

Stress Analysis

Symbols	Description and Units
A	cross sectional area, mm^2
A_s	area under shear, mm^2
c	distance from neutral axis to the extreme fibre, mm
E	modulus of elasticity or young's modulus, $MN/m^2(kgf/mm^2)$
e	eccentricity, as of force application, mm
F	force, N(kgf)
F_s	direct shear force, N(kgf)
F_{cr}	critical load that will cause rupture, N(kgf)
G	modulus of rigidity, $MN/m^2(kgf/mm^2)$
I, J	rectangular and polar moment of inertia respectively, mm^4
k	radius of gyration of cross-section, mm
M	bending moment, N-mm(kgf-mm)
R	radius of curvature, mm
T	torque or torsional moment, N-mm(kgf-mm)
Z, Z_p	rectangular and polar section modulus respectively, mm^3
α	the coefficient of linear expansion, mm/mm/K(mm/mm/°C)
γ	shearing Strain, rad/mm
δ	axial deformation or total elongation, mm
δ_s	angular deformation, rad
ϵ	strain or deformation per unit length, mm/mm
$\epsilon_x, \epsilon_y, \epsilon_z$	strain due only to stresses in the x, y, z directions respectively, mm/mm
μ	poisson's ratio
σ_D	stress, direct or normal, tensile or compression, $MN/m^2 (kgf/mm^2)$
σ	stress, $MN/m^2 (kgf/mm^2)$
$\sigma_x, \sigma_y, \sigma_z$	normal stresses in x, y, z directions respectively, $MN/m^2 (kgf/mm^2)$
σ_1, σ_2	maximum and minimum normal stresses respectively, $MN/m^2(kgf/mm^2)$

Symbols   Description and Units

Symbols	Description and Units
σ_{yp}	tensile stress at yield point, MN/m^2(kgf/mm^2)
σ_e	stress at the elastic limit, MN/m^2(kgf/mm^2)
τ	shear stress, MN/m^2(kgf/mm^2)
τ_{xy}	shear stress, x and y direction, MN/m^2(kgf/mm^2)
τ_{yp}	shear stress at yield point, MN/m^2 (kgf/mm^2)
τ_D	direct shear stress, MN/m^2 (kgf/mm^2)

Particular	Equation	Eqn. No.
Simple Stresses and Strains:		
The direct stress in simple tension or compression. Fig. 1.1(a)	$\sigma_D = \sigma = \pm \dfrac{F}{A}$	1.1(a)
Maximum Bending stress at point P. Fig. 1.1(b)	$\sigma_b = \sigma = \dfrac{Mc}{I} = \dfrac{M}{Z} = \dfrac{32M}{\pi d^3} = \dfrac{32FL}{\pi d^3}$	1.1(b)
Direct shear stress. Fig. 1.1(c)	$\tau_D = \tau = \dfrac{F_s}{A_s}$	1.1(c)
Maximum Torsional shear stress. Fig. 1.1(d)	$\tau = \dfrac{Tr}{J} = \dfrac{T}{Z_p} = \dfrac{16T}{\pi d^3}$	1.1(d)
Strain or deformation per unit length due to direct axial load	$\epsilon = \dfrac{\sigma}{E} = \dfrac{F}{AE}$	1.2(a)

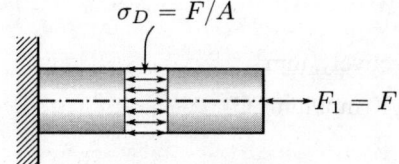

Fig. 1.1(a): *Direct stress*

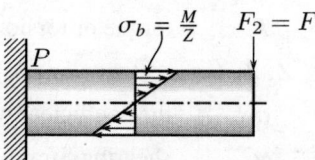

Fig. 1.1(b): *Bending stress*

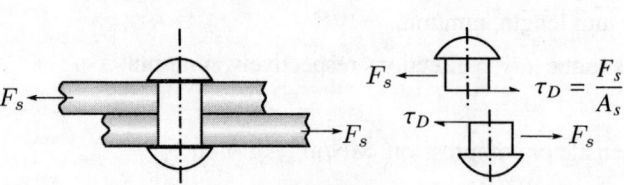

Fig. 1.1(c): *Direct shear stress*

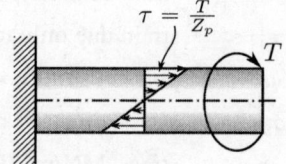

Fig. 1.1(d): *Torsional shear stress*

Particular	Equation	Eqn. No.
Deformation or Total elongation of a member due to direct axial load	$\delta = \dfrac{\sigma L}{E} = \dfrac{FL}{AE}$ where 'L' is the length of the bar, mm	1.2(b)
Shear strain due to direct shear force (radians)	$r = \dfrac{\tau}{G}$	1.2(c)
The general bending equation	$\dfrac{M}{I} = \dfrac{E}{R} = \dfrac{\sigma}{C}$	1.3(a)
The general torsion equation	$\dfrac{T}{J} = \dfrac{G\theta}{L} = \dfrac{\tau}{r}$	1.3(b)
The angle of twist in a shaft subjected to a torque (radians)	$\theta = \dfrac{TL}{JG}$	1.3(c)

Combined Stresses:

(i) Combined axial and Bending loads [Fig. 1.2(a)]

The maximum normal stress due to combined axial and bending loads (super position)	$\sigma_{max} = \sigma_D + \sigma_b = \sigma = \dfrac{F}{A} + \dfrac{M}{Z}$	1.4

(ii) Combined axial, bending and torsional loads [Fig. 1.2(b), 1.2(c) and 1.2(d)]

According to maximum normal stress theory	$\sigma_{max} = \dfrac{\sigma}{2} + \sqrt{\left(\dfrac{\sigma}{2}\right)^2 + \tau^2}$	1.5(a)
According to maximum shear stress theory	$\tau_{max} = \sqrt{\left(\dfrac{\sigma}{2}\right)^2 + \tau^2}$	1.5(b)

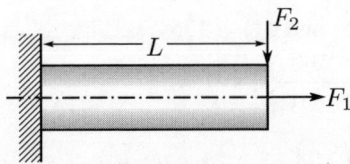

Fig. 1.2(a): *Combined axial and bending loads (T = 0)*

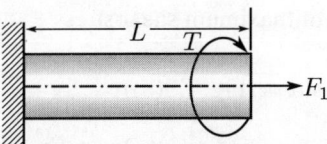

Fig. 1.2(b): *Combined axial and torsional loads (F_2 = 0)*

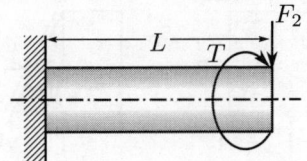

Fig. 1.2(c): *Combined torsional and bending loads (F_1 = 0)*

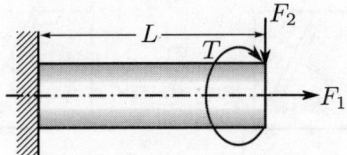

Fig. 1.2(d): *Combined axial, bending and torsional loads*

Particular	Equation	Eqn. No.
Compound Stresses:		
(i) *Uniaxial stress system* [Fig. 1.3(a)]		
The normal stress in the plane at any desired angle ϕ	$\sigma_n = \sigma_x \cos^2 \phi = \sigma_1 \cos^2 \phi$	1.6(a)
The shear stress at any desired angle ϕ	$\tau = \dfrac{\sigma_x}{2} \sin 2\phi = \dfrac{\sigma_1}{2} \sin 2\phi$	1.6(b)
The principal stresses	$(\sigma_1 = \sigma_x)$ and $(\sigma_2 = 0)$	1.6(c)
Direction of principal stresses	$\phi_1 = 0°$	1.6(d)
Maximum shear stress at 45°	$\tau_{\max} = \dfrac{\sigma_x}{2} = \dfrac{\sigma_1}{2}$	1.6(e)
Direction of maximum shear stress	$\phi_{S_1} = 45°$	1.6(f)
(ii) *Biaxial stress system* [Fig. 1.3(b)]		
The normal stress in the plane at any desired angle ϕ	$\sigma_n = \left(\dfrac{\sigma_x + \sigma_y}{2}\right) + \left(\dfrac{\sigma_x - \sigma_y}{2}\right)\cos 2\phi$	1.7(a)
The shear stress at any desired angle ϕ	$\tau_n = \left(\dfrac{\sigma_x - \sigma_y}{2}\right)\sin 2\phi$	1.7(b)
The principal stresses	$(\sigma_1 = \sigma_x)$ and $(\sigma_2 = \sigma_y)$	1.7(c)
Direction of principal stresses	$(\phi_1 = 0°)$ and $(\phi_2 = 90°)$	1.7(d)
Maximum shear stress at $\phi = 45°$	$\tau_{\max} = \left(\dfrac{\sigma_x - \sigma_y}{2}\right) = \left(\dfrac{\sigma_1 - \sigma_2}{2}\right)$	1.7(e)
Direction of maximum shear stress	$\phi_{s_1} = 45°$ and $\phi_{S_2} = 135°$	1.7(f)
Resultant stress (Fig. 1.3(b))	$\sigma = \sqrt{\sigma_n^2 + \tau^2}$	1.7(g)
Direction of resultant stress (Fig. 1.3(b))	$\tan \theta = \left(\dfrac{\sigma_n}{\tau}\right)$	1.7(h)

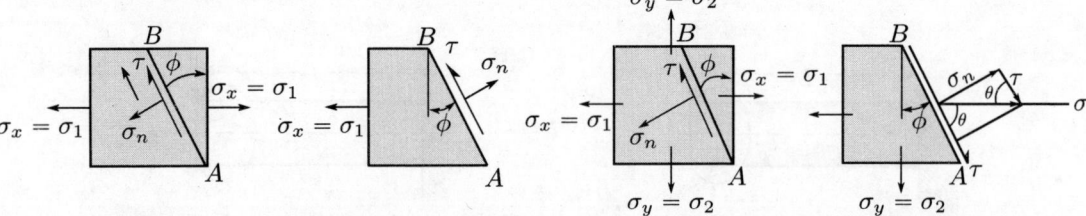

Fig. 1.3(a): *Uniaxial stress system*   **Fig. 1.3(b): *Biaxial stress system***

Particular	Equation	Eqn. No.
(iii) *Plane stress system* [Fig. 1.4(a)] The normal stress in the plane at any desired angle ϕ	$\sigma_n = \left(\dfrac{\sigma_x + \sigma_y}{2}\right) + \left(\dfrac{\sigma_x - \sigma_y}{2}\right)\cos 2\phi$ $\qquad + \tau_{xy}\sin 2\phi$	1.8(a)
The shear stress at any desired angle ϕ	$\tau_n = \left(\dfrac{\sigma_x - \sigma_y}{2}\right)\sin 2\phi - \tau_{xy}\cos 2\phi$	1.8(b)
Maximum principal stress	$\sigma_1 = \left(\dfrac{\sigma_x + \sigma_y}{2}\right) + \sqrt{\left(\dfrac{\sigma_x - \sigma_y}{2}\right)^2 + \tau_{xy}^2}$	1.8(c)
Minimum principal stress	$\sigma_2 = \left(\dfrac{\sigma_x + \sigma_y}{2}\right) - \sqrt{\left(\dfrac{\sigma_x - \sigma_y}{2}\right)^2 + \tau_{xy}^2}$	1.8(d)
Direction of principal stress [Fig. 1.4(b)]	$\tan 2\phi_1 = \left(\dfrac{2\tau_{xy}}{\sigma_x - \sigma_y}\right)$ where ϕ_1 and ϕ_2 are 90° apart.	1.8(e)
Maximum shear stress	$\tau_{\max} = \pm\sqrt{\left(\dfrac{\sigma_x - \sigma_y}{2}\right)^2 + \tau_{xy}^2} = \dfrac{\sigma_1 - \sigma_2}{2}$	1.8(f)
Direction of shear stress [Fig. 1.4(c)]	$\tan(2\phi_s) = \left(\dfrac{\sigma_x - \sigma_y}{2\tau_{xy}}\right)$	1.8(g)

Direction of maximum shear stress $\phi_{s\,\max} = \phi_1 + 45°$

Direction of minimum shear stress $\phi_{s\,\min} = \phi_1 + 135°$

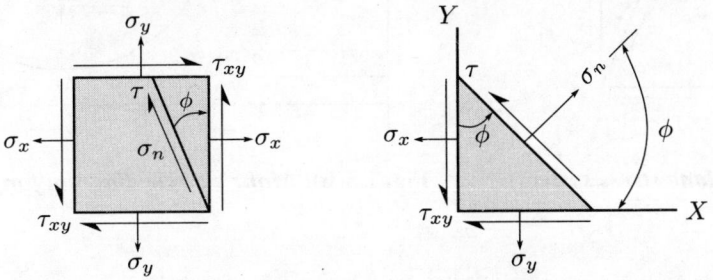

Fig. 1.4(a): *Plane stress system*

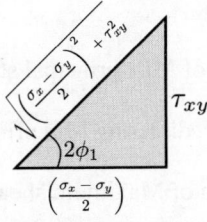

Fig. 1.4(b): *Direction of principal stress*

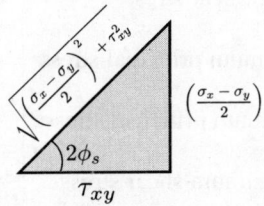

Fig. 1.4(c): *Direction of shear stress*

Particular	Equation	Eqn. No.
Mohr's circle diagram: Fig. 1.5(a) and 1.5(b)		
Equation for the Mohr's circle diagram	$\left(\sigma_n - \dfrac{\sigma_x + \sigma_y}{2}\right)^2 + \tau^2 = \left(\dfrac{\sigma_x - \sigma_y}{2}\right)^2 + (\tau_{xy})^2$	1.9(a)
Equation for the Mohr's circle diagram	$(\sigma_n - C)^2 + \tau^2 = R_1^2$	1.9(b)
	which is the equation of a circle	
	Where $C = \dfrac{\sigma_x + \sigma_y}{2}$	1.9(c)
	and $R_1^2 = \left(\dfrac{\sigma_x - \sigma_y}{2}\right)^2 + (\tau_{xy})^2$	1.9(d)

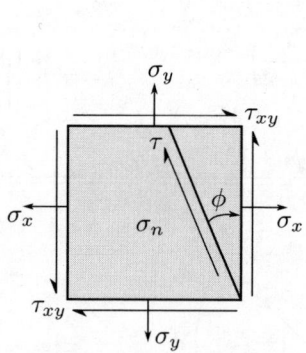

Fig. 1.5(a): *Plane stress system*

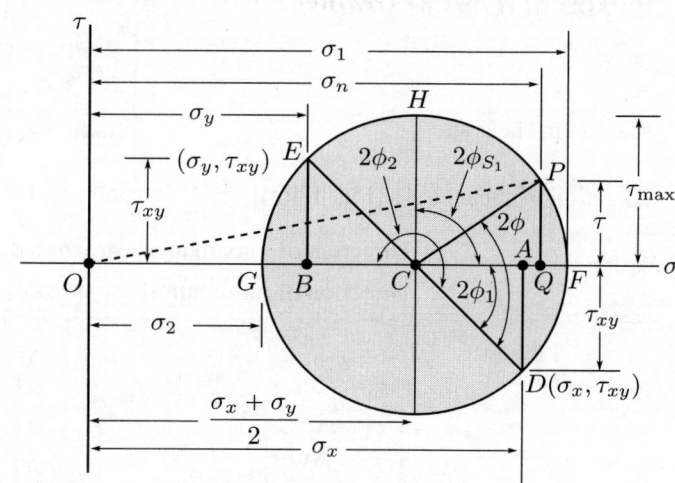

Fig. 1.5(b): *Mohr's circle diagram for plane stress*

$OA = \sigma_x$, Stress in x-direction	$OQ = \sigma_n$, Normal stress
$OB = \sigma_y$, Stress in y-direction	$PQ = \tau$, Tangential stress
$AD = BE = \tau_{xy}$, Shear stress	$OP = \sigma$, Resultant Stress
$OF = \sigma_1$, Maximum principal stress	$\frac{1}{2}\angle DCF = \phi_1$, Direction of Max principal stress
$OG = \sigma_2$, Minimum principal stress	$\frac{1}{2}\angle DCB = \phi_2 = \phi_1 + 90°$, directing Min principal stress
$CH = \tau_{\max}$, Maximum shear stress	$\frac{1}{2}\angle HCF = \phi_{S_1}$, Direction of Maximum shear stress

Particular	Equation	Eqn. No.
Superposition: *(Eccentric loading)* (Fig. 1.6)		
Maximum normal stress due to direct tension or compression combined with bending	$\sigma = \dfrac{F}{A} \pm \dfrac{M}{Z} = \dfrac{F}{A} \pm \dfrac{Fe}{Z}$	1.10
Biaxial deformation:– (Fig. 1.3(b))		
Poisson's ratio	$\mu = \dfrac{-\epsilon_y}{\epsilon_x} = \dfrac{-\epsilon_z}{\epsilon_x}$	1.11(a)
Resultant unit deformation or strain in the X-direction	$\epsilon_x = \dfrac{\sigma_x}{E} - \mu\dfrac{\sigma_y}{E}$	1.11(b)
Resultant unit deformation or strain in the Y-direction	$\epsilon_y = \dfrac{\sigma_y}{E} - \mu\dfrac{\sigma_x}{E}$	1.11(c)
Stresses in terms of strains:		
The normal stress in the X-direction	$\sigma_x = \dfrac{(\epsilon_x + \mu\epsilon_y)E}{1 - \mu^2}$	1.11(d)
The normal stress in the Y-direction	$\sigma_y = \dfrac{(\epsilon_y + \mu\epsilon_x)E}{1 - \mu^2}$	1.11(e)
Triaxial deformations: (Fig. 1.7(b))		
Resultant unit deformation or strain in the X-direction	$\epsilon_x = \dfrac{1}{E}\left[\sigma_x - \mu(\sigma_y + \sigma_z)\right]$	1.12(a)
Resultant strain in the Y-direction	$\epsilon_y = \dfrac{1}{E}\left[\sigma_y - \mu(\sigma_z + \sigma_x)\right]$	1.12(b)
Resultant strain in the Z-direction	$\epsilon_z = \dfrac{1}{E}\left[\sigma_z - \mu(\sigma_x + \sigma_y)\right]$	1.12(c)
Relation between the constants E, G and μ for a given material	$G = \dfrac{E}{2(1 + \mu)}$	1.12(d)

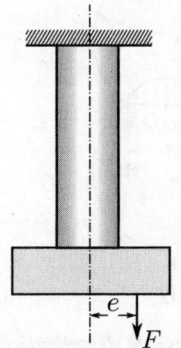

Fig. 1.6: *Eccentric load*

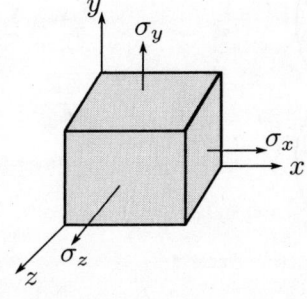

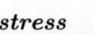

(a) *With no shear stress*

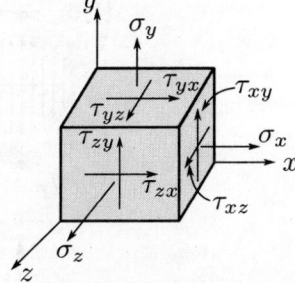

(b) *With shear stress*

Fig. 1.7: *Triaxial stress system*

Particular	Equation	Eqn. No.
Hertz contact stresses:		
a) Spherical surfaces:		
When two solid spheres are pressed together with a force, the radius of the area of contact (Fig. 1.8(a))	$a = \left[\dfrac{3F}{8} \dfrac{(1 - \mu^2)(1/E_1 + 1/E_2)}{(1/d_1 + 1/d_2)} \right]^{\frac{1}{3}}$	1.13(a)
When a solid sphere of diameter d_1 and a plane surface are pressed together with a force, the radius of the area of contact	$a = \left[\dfrac{3F}{8} \dfrac{(1 - \mu^2)(1/E_1 + 1/E_2)}{(1/d_1)} \right]^{\frac{1}{3}}$	1.13(b)
When a solid sphere of diameter d_1 is pressed against an internal spherical surface of diameter d_2, the radius of the area of contact	$a = \left[\dfrac{3F}{8} \dfrac{(1 - \mu^2)(1/E_1 + 1/E_2)}{(1/d_1 - 1/d_2)} \right]^{\frac{1}{3}}$	1.13(c)
The maximum pressure at the centre of contact area	$p_{\max} = \dfrac{3F}{2\pi a^2}$	1.13(d)
	where a is the radius of the contact area	
b) Cylindrical surfaces:		
When two cylinders are pressed together the half width of the rectangular area of contact (Fig. 1.8(b))	$b = \left[\dfrac{2F}{\pi L} \dfrac{(1 - \mu^2)(1/E_1 + 1/E_2)}{(1/d_1 + 1/d_2)} \right]^{\frac{1}{2}}$	1.14(a)
	where L is the length of the contacting surfaces	

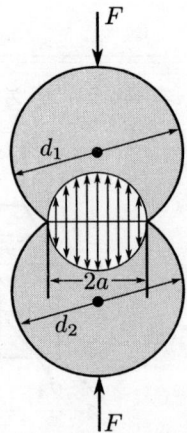

Fig. 1.8(a): *Pressure distribution between two Spheres*

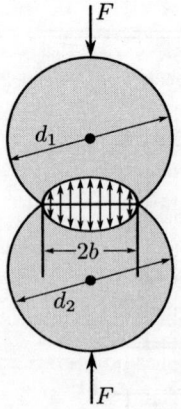

Fig. 1.8(b): *Pressure distribution between two Cylinders*

Particular	Equation	Eqn. No.
When a cylinder of diameter d_1 is pressed against a plane surface, the half width of the rectangular area of contact	$b = \left[\dfrac{2F}{\pi L}\dfrac{(1-\mu^2)(1/E_1 + 1/E_2)}{(1/d_1)}\right]^{\frac{1}{2}}$	1.14(b)
When a cylinder of diameter d_1 is pressed against an internal cylinder surface of diameter d_2 the half width of the rectangular area of contact	$b = \left[\dfrac{2F}{\pi L}\dfrac{(1-\mu^2)(1/E_1 + 1/E_2)}{(1/d_1 - 1/d_2)}\right]^{\frac{1}{2}}$	1.14(c)
The maximum pressure at the centre of contact area	$p_{max} = \dfrac{2F}{\pi b L}$ where b is the half width of the rectangular area of contact	1.14(d)

Thermal stresses:

Thermal expansion	$\delta_t = \alpha L_0(t - t_0)$ where L_0 is the length of the bar at the initial temperature t_0, K($^\circ$C) $(t - t_0)$ = change in temp, K. ($^\circ$C)	1.15(a)
The total length at a temperature t, K($^\circ$C)	$L = L_0[1 + \alpha(t - t_0)]$	1.15(b)
Stress set up in the bar due to change in the temperature	$\sigma = E\alpha(t - t_0)$	1.15(c)

Columns:

Euler's column formula for the critical load

$$F_{cr} = \frac{n\pi^2 EI}{L^2} = \frac{n\pi^2 EAk^2}{L^2} = \frac{n\pi^2 EA}{(L/k)^2}$$ 1.16(a)

where L is the length of the column, mm

n = constant depending on the condition of the restraint of column ends (coefficient of end conditions) (Fig. 1.9)

= 0.25 for one fixed end and one free end

= 1.00 for both ends free, i.e. both ends are guided or hinged

= 4 for both ends fixed rigidly

= 1 to 4 for both ends flat

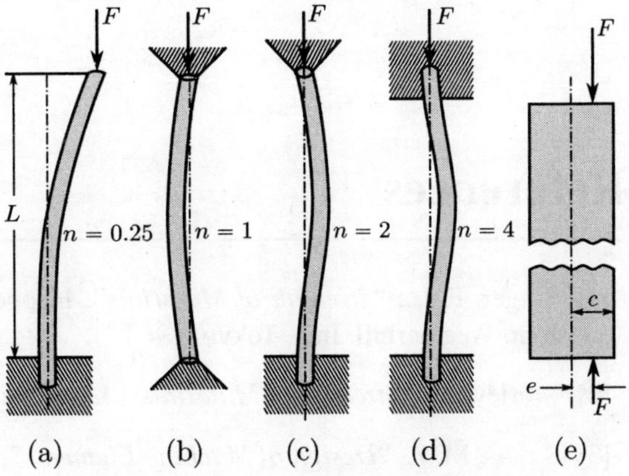

Fig. 1.9: *End conditions of columns*

Particular	Equation	Eqn. No.
Parabolic column formula to determine the critical load	$F_{cr} = A\sigma_{yp}\left[1 - \dfrac{\sigma_{vp}}{4n\pi^2 E}(L/k)^2\right]$	1.16(b)
Straight line column formula to determine the critical load	$F_{cr} = A\left(\sigma_{yp} - C\dfrac{L}{k}\right)$ where $C = (2\sigma_{yp}/3\pi)\sqrt{\sigma_{yp}/3nE}$ $\quad\quad = $ a constant	1.16(c)
Rankine formula to determine the induced stress in a column	$\sigma_c = \dfrac{F}{A}\left[1 + a(L/k)^2\right]$	1.16(d)

where F is the external force on the column, N(kgf)

a is the constant in Rankine formula from Table 1.2

Ritter's formula, which is a modification of the Gordon-Rankine formula, for determining the induced stress, σ_c in a short column	$\sigma_c = \dfrac{F}{A}\left[1 + (L/k)^2\dfrac{\sigma_e}{\pi^2 nE}\right]$	1.16(e)

***Eccentrically loaded columns* (Fig. 1.9(e))**

To determine the maximum combined stress by Ritter's formula	$\sigma_c = \dfrac{F}{A}\left[\left(1 + (L/k)^2\dfrac{\sigma_e}{\pi^2 nE} + \dfrac{ce}{k^2}\right)\right]$	1.16(f)

where e is the distance between the load and the centroid and

c is the distance from the centre of gravity to the outer most fiber

References

[1] Singer, F. L., "*Strength of Materials*", Happer and Rom, New York, Evanston and London and John Weatherhill, Inc., Tokyo, 1962.

[2] Morley, A., "*Strength of Materials*", Longmans, Green and Co. Ltd., London, 1953.

[3] Spotts, M. F., "*Design of Machine Elements*", 3rd edition, Prentice Hall, Inc., Maruzen Co. Ltd.

[4] Shigley, J. E., "Machine Design", 9th edition, McGraw Hill Education Private Ltd., New Delhi, 2011.

Table 1.1 *Physical constants of some common materials*

Material	Modulus of Elasticity, $E \times 10^{-3}$ MN/m^2 (kgf/mm^2)	Modulus of rigidity, $G \times 10^{-3}$ MN/m^2 (kgf/mm^2)	Poisson's ratio, μ	Density, kg/m^3
Aluminium (alloys)	71.0 (7.24)	26.2 (2.67)	0.334	2730
Beryllium	287.1(29.28)	–	–	1820
Beryllium copper	124.2(12.66)	48.3 (4.92)	0.285	8230
Brass	95.1 (9.70)	34.3 (3.50)	0.30-0.40	8450
Bronze	109.0(11.10)	–	–	8730
Carbon steel	202.0(20.60)	78.5 (8.00)	0.292	7820
Cast Iron, gray	100.0(10.20)	41.4 (4.22)	0.211	7200
Copper	120.6(12.30)	38.3 (3.90)	0.260	8960
Inconel	214.0(21.80)	76.0 (7.75)	0.290	8960
Lead	15.7 (1.60)	7.5 (0.76)	0.450	11340
Megnesium	44.8 (4.57)	16.6 (1.69)	0.350	1800
Molybdenum	331.0(33.75)	117.2(11.95)	0.307	10200
Monel metal	179.3(18.28)	65.6 (6.68)	0.320	8830
Nickel steel	196.1(20.00)	75.6 (7.80)	0.291	7750
Phosphor bronze	111.0(11.32)	41.4 (4.22)	0.349	8160
Stainless steel (18-8)	190.3(19.40)	73.1 (7.45)	0.305	7750
Titanium	103.5(10.55)	–	–	4480
Tungsten	437.3(41.53)	173.6(17.70)	0.170	19300
Zirconium	68.4 (6.97)	–	–	6500

Table 1.2 *The Values of Constant 'a' in equation 1.16(d)*

	Both ends round	Both ends fixed	One end round, one fixed
Steel	$\dfrac{1}{6250}$	$\dfrac{1}{25000}$	$\dfrac{1.95}{25000}$
Cast Iron	$\dfrac{1}{1250}$	$\dfrac{1}{5000}$	$\dfrac{1.95}{5000}$
Wrought Iron	$\dfrac{1}{900}$	$\dfrac{1}{36000}$	$\dfrac{1.95}{36000}$
Timber	$\dfrac{1}{750}$	$\dfrac{1}{3000}$	$\dfrac{1.95}{3000}$

Table 1.3 (a) Properties of Various Cross Sections

Type (1)	Section (2)	Moment of Inertia I (3)	Distance to Farthest Point c (4)	Section Modulus $Z = \dfrac{I}{c}$ (5)	Radius of Gyration $k = \sqrt{\dfrac{I}{A}}$ (6)
a		$\dfrac{bh^3}{12}$	$\dfrac{h}{2}$	$\dfrac{bh^2}{6}$	$0.289h$
b		$\dfrac{b}{12}(H^3 - h^3)$	$\dfrac{H}{2}$	$\dfrac{b(H^3 - h^3)}{6H}$	$\sqrt{\dfrac{H^3 - h^3}{12(H - h)}}$
c		$\dfrac{BH^3 - bh^3}{12}$	$\dfrac{H}{2}$	$\dfrac{BH^3 - bh^3}{6H}$	$\sqrt{\dfrac{BH^3 - bh^3}{12(BH - bh)}}$
d		$\dfrac{Bc_1^3 - bh^3 + ac_2^3}{3}$ $h = c_1 - d$	$c_1 = \dfrac{aH^2 + bd^2}{2(aH + bd)}$ $c_2 = H - c_1$	$\dfrac{I}{c_1}$ and $\dfrac{I}{c_2}$	$\sqrt{\dfrac{I}{Bd + a(H - d)}}$

Table 1.3 (a) Properties of Various Cross Sections–(Contd.)

(1)	(2)	(3)	(4)	(5)	(6)
e		$\dfrac{BH^3 + bh^3}{12}$	$\dfrac{H}{2}$	$\dfrac{BH^3 + bh^3}{6H}$	$\sqrt{\dfrac{BH^3 + bh^3}{12(BH + bh)}}$
f		$\dfrac{(6b^2 + 6bb_0 + b_0^2)h^3}{36(2b + b_0)}$	$\dfrac{(3b + 2b_0)h}{3(2b + b_0)}$	$\dfrac{(6b^2 + 6bb_0 + b_0^2)h^2}{12(3b + b_0)}$	$\sqrt{\dfrac{I}{A}}$
g		$\dfrac{\pi D^4}{64} = \dfrac{\pi R^4}{4}$	$\dfrac{D}{2} = R$	$\dfrac{\pi D^3}{32} = 0.0982D^3$	$\dfrac{D}{4} = \dfrac{R}{2}$
h		$\dfrac{\pi}{64}(D_1^4 - D_2^4)$ $= \dfrac{\pi}{4}(R_1^4 - R_2^4)$	$\dfrac{D_1}{2} = R_1$	$\dfrac{\pi(D_1^4 - D_2^4)}{32D_1}$	$\sqrt{\dfrac{D_1^2 + D_2^2}{4}}$ $\sqrt{\dfrac{R_1^2 + R_2^2}{2}}$
i		$\dfrac{\pi bh^3}{64}$	$\dfrac{h}{2}$	$\dfrac{\pi bh^2}{32}$	$\dfrac{h}{4}$

Table 1.3 (b) Properties of Various Cross Sections

Type	Section	Polar Moment of Inertia (J)	$Z_p = J/R$ Polar Section Modules	k_p Polar radius of gyratress
a		$\dfrac{\pi D^4}{32}$	$\dfrac{\pi D^3}{16}$	$\dfrac{D}{\sqrt{8}} = 0.354D$
		$\dfrac{\pi}{32}(D_1^4 - D_2^4)$	$\dfrac{\pi}{16}\dfrac{(D_1^4 - D_2^4)}{D_1}$	$\sqrt{\dfrac{D_1^2 + D_2^2}{8}} = 0.354\sqrt{D_1^2 + D_2^2}$
		$\dfrac{\pi hb}{4}(h^2 + b^2)$	$\dfrac{\pi hb^2}{16}$ $h > b$	$\dfrac{1}{4}\sqrt{h^2 + b^2}$
		$\dfrac{bh}{12}(b^2 + h^2)$	$\dfrac{2b^2h}{9}$ $h > b$	$\sqrt{\dfrac{b^2 + h^2}{12}} = 0.289\sqrt{b^2 + h^2}$

Table 1.4 Shear, Moment and Deflection Formulas for Beams*

Loading, support, and reference number	Reactions R_1 and R_2, vertical shear V	Bending moment M, maximum bending moment	Deflection y and maximum deflection
1. Cantilever, end load	$R_2 = +F$ $V = -F$	$M = -Fx$ Max $M = -FL$ at B	$y = -\dfrac{1}{6}\dfrac{F}{EI}(x^3 - 3L^2x + 2L^3)$ Max $y = -\dfrac{1}{3}\dfrac{FL^3}{EI}$ at A
2. Cantilever, intermediate load	$R_2 = +F$ A to B: $V = 0$ B to C: $V = -F$	A to B: $M = 0$ B to C: $M = -F(x - b)$ Max $M = -Fa$ at C	A to B: $y = -\dfrac{1}{6}\dfrac{F}{EI}(-a^3 + 3a^2L - 3a^2x)$ B to C: $y - \dfrac{1}{6}\dfrac{F}{EI}$ $[(x - b)^3 - 3a^2(x - b) + 2a^3]$ Max $y = -\dfrac{1}{6}\dfrac{F}{EI}(3a^2L - a^3)$
3. Cantilever, uniform load $W = wl$	$R_2 = +W$ $V = -\dfrac{W}{L}x$	$M = -\dfrac{1}{2}\dfrac{W}{L}x^2$ Max $M = -\dfrac{1}{2}WL$ at B	$y = -\dfrac{1}{24}\dfrac{W}{EIL}(x^4 - 4L^3x + 3L^4)$ Max $y = -\dfrac{1}{8}\dfrac{WL^3}{EI}$
4. End supports, center load	$R_1 = +\dfrac{1}{2}F, R_2 = +\dfrac{1}{2}F$ A to B: $V = +\dfrac{1}{2}F$ B to C: $V = -\dfrac{1}{2}F$	A to B: $M = +\dfrac{1}{2}Fx$ B to C: $M = +\dfrac{1}{2}F(L - x)$ Max $M = +\dfrac{1}{4}FL$ at B	A to B: $y = -\dfrac{1}{48}\dfrac{F}{EI}(3L^2x - 4x^3)$ Max $y = -\dfrac{1}{48}\dfrac{FL^3}{EI}$ at B

Table 1.4 Shear, Moment and Deflection Formulas for Beams* (Contd.)

5. End supports, intermediate

$R_1 = +F\dfrac{b}{L}; R_2 = +F\dfrac{a}{L}$

A to B : $V = +F\dfrac{b}{L}$

B to C : $V = -F\dfrac{a}{L}$

A to B : $M = +F\dfrac{x}{L}$

B to C : $M = +F\dfrac{a}{L}(L-x)$

Max $M = +F\dfrac{ab}{L}$ at B

A to B : $y = -\dfrac{Fbx}{6EL}$

$[2L(L-x) - b^2 - (L-x)^2]$

B to C : $y = -\dfrac{Fa(L-x)}{6EL}$

$[2Lb - b^2 - (L-x)^2]$

Max $y = -\dfrac{Fab}{27EL}(a+2b)\sqrt{3a(a+2b)}$ at

$x = \sqrt{\dfrac{1}{3}a(a+2b)}$ when $a > b$

6. End supports, uniform load

$W = wl$

$R_1 = +\dfrac{1}{2}W; R_2 = +\dfrac{1}{2}W$

$V = \dfrac{1}{2}W\left(1 - \dfrac{2x}{L}\right)$

$M = \dfrac{1}{2}W\left(x - \dfrac{x^2}{L}\right)$

Max $M = +\dfrac{1}{8}WL$ at $x = \left(\dfrac{L}{2}\right)$

$y = -\dfrac{1}{24}\dfrac{Wx}{EL}(L^3 - 2Lx^2 + x^3)$

Max $y = -\dfrac{5}{384}\dfrac{WL^3}{EI}$ at $x = \left(\dfrac{L}{2}\right)$

7. One end fixed, one end supported, centre load

$R_1 = \dfrac{5}{16}F; R_2 = \dfrac{11}{16}F$

$M_2 = \dfrac{3}{16}F$

A to B : $V = \dfrac{5}{16}F$

B to C : $V = \dfrac{11}{16}F$

A to B : $M = \dfrac{5}{16}Fx$

B to C : $M = F\left(\dfrac{1}{2}L - \dfrac{11}{16}x\right)$

Max + M = $\dfrac{5}{32}FL$ at B

Max − M = $-\dfrac{5}{16}FL$ at C

A to B : $y = \dfrac{1}{96}\dfrac{F}{EI}(5x^3 - 3L^2x)$

B to C : $y = \dfrac{1}{96}\dfrac{F}{EI}$

$\left[5x^3 - 16\left(x - \dfrac{1}{2}\right)^3 - 3L^2x\right]$

Max $y = -0.00932\dfrac{FL^3}{EI}$ at $x = 0.4472L$

8. One end fixed, one end supported, uniform load

$W = wl$

$R_1 = \dfrac{3}{8}W; R_2 = \dfrac{5}{8}W$

$M_2 = \dfrac{1}{8}WL$

$V = W\left(\dfrac{3}{8} - \dfrac{x}{L}\right)$

$M = W\left(\dfrac{3}{8}x - \dfrac{1}{2}\dfrac{x^2}{L}\right)$

Max + M = $\dfrac{9}{128}WL$ at $x = \dfrac{3}{8}L$

Max − M = $-\dfrac{1}{8}WL$ at B

$y = \dfrac{1}{48}\dfrac{W}{EIL}(3Lx^3 - 2x^4 - L^3x)$

Max $y = -0.0054\dfrac{WL^3}{EI}$ at $x = 0.4215L$

Table 1.4 Shear, Moment and Deflection Formulas for Beams* (Contd.)

9. Both ends fixed, center load

$$R_1 = \frac{1}{2}F; \quad R_2 = \frac{1}{2}F$$
$$M_1 = \frac{1}{8}FL; \quad M_2 = \frac{1}{8}FL$$

A to B : $V = +\frac{1}{2}F$

B to C : $V = -\frac{1}{2}F$

A to B : $M = \frac{1}{8}F(4x - L)$

B to C : $M = \frac{1}{8}F(3L - 4x)$

Max $+ M = \frac{1}{8}FL$ at B

Max $- M = \frac{1}{8}FL$ at A and C

A to B : $y = -\frac{1}{48}\frac{F}{EI}(3Lx^2 - 4x^3)$

Max $y = -\frac{1}{192}\frac{FL^3}{EI}$ at E

---

10. Both ends fixed, intermediate load

$$R_1 = \frac{Fb^2}{L^3}(3a+b)$$
$$R_2 = \frac{Fa^2}{L^3}(3b-a)$$
$$M_1 = F\frac{ab^2}{L^2}; \quad M_2 = F\frac{a^2b}{L^2}$$

A to B : $V = R_1$

B to C : $V = R_1 - F$

A to B : $M = -F\frac{ab^2}{L^2} + R_1 x$

B to C : $M = -F\frac{ab^2}{L^2} + R_1 x$

Max $+ M = -F\frac{ab^2}{L^2} + R_1 a$ at B

Max $- M = -M_1$ when $a < b$

Max $- M = -M_2$ when $a > b$

A to B : $y = -\frac{1}{6}\frac{Fb^2x^2}{EIL^3}(3ax + bx - 3aL)$

B to C : $y = -\frac{1}{6}\frac{Fa^2(L-x)^2}{EIL^3}$
$[(3b+a)(L-x) - 3bL]$

Max $y = -\frac{2}{3}\frac{F}{EI}\frac{a^3b^2}{(3a+b)^2}$ if $a > b$

at $x = \frac{2aL}{3a+b}$

Max $y = -\frac{2}{3}\frac{F}{EI}\frac{a^2b^3}{(3b+a)^2}$

at $x = L - \frac{2bL}{3b+a}$ if $a < b$

---

11. Both ends fixed, uniform load

$$R_1 = \frac{1}{2}W; \quad R_2 = \frac{1}{2}W$$
$$M_1 = \frac{1}{12}WL, \quad M_2 = \frac{1}{12}WL$$
$$V = \frac{1}{2}W\left(1 - \frac{2x}{L}\right)$$

$M = \frac{1}{2}W\left(x - \frac{x^2}{L} - \frac{L}{6}\right)$

Max $+ M = \frac{1}{24}WL$ at $x = \frac{L}{2}$

Max $- M = -\frac{1}{12}WL$ at A and B

$y = -\frac{1}{24}\frac{Wx^2}{EIL}(2Lx - L^2 - x^2)$

Max $y = -\frac{1}{384}\frac{WL^3}{EI}$ at $x = \frac{L}{2}$

---

*From "Machine Design" by shigley pp. 492-494, Table A-2: Copy right 1956 by the McGraw-Hill Book Company, Inc., used with permission of McGraw-Hill Book Company, New York.

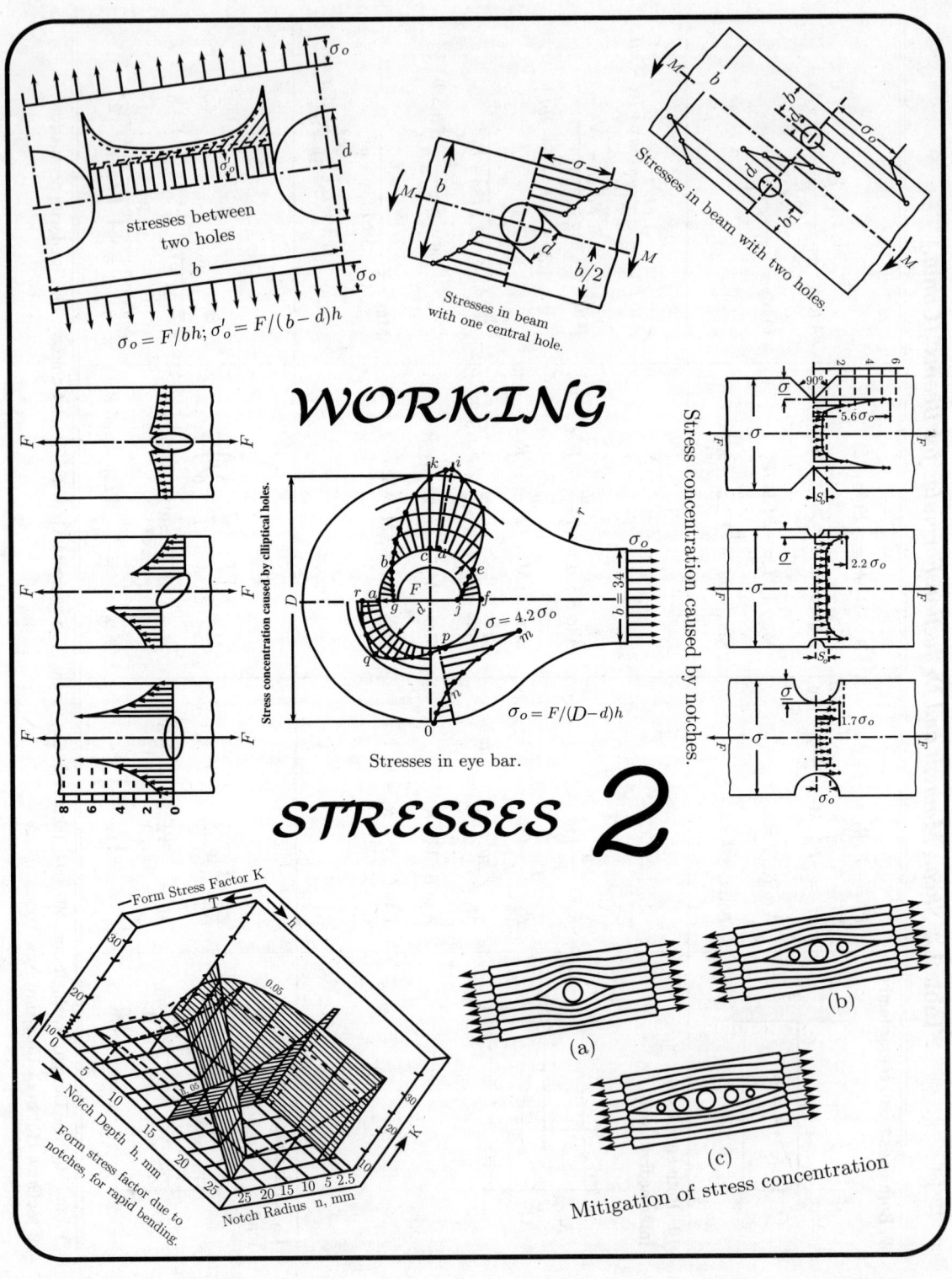

stresses between
two holes

$$\sigma_o = F/bh; \sigma'_o = F/(b-d)h$$

Stresses in beam
with one central hole.

Stresses in beam with two holes.

WORKING

Stress concentration caused by elliptical holes.

$\sigma = 4.2\sigma_o$

$b = 34$

$\sigma_o = F/(D-d)h$

Stresses in eye bar.

STRESSES 2

Stress concentration caused by notches.

$5.6\sigma_o$

$2.2\sigma_o$

$1.7\sigma_o$

Form Stress Factor K

0.05

Notch Depth h, mm

Form stress factor due to
notches, for rapid bending.

Notch Radius n, mm

(a)

(b)

(c)

Mitigation of stress concentration

Working Stresses

Symbols	Description and Units
A	correction factor for the type of loading
B	size factor
C	surface correction factor
F_m	average or mean load, N(kgf)
F_a	variable or alternating load, N(kgf)
K_t	theoretical stress concentration factor for normal stress (tension or bending)
K_s	theoretical stress concentration factor for shear stress
K'_t	theoretical combined stress concentration factor
K_{tf}	estimated fatigue stress concentration factor for normal stress
K'_{tf}	estimated combined fatigue factor for normal stres
K_{sf}	estimated fatigue stress concentration factor for shear stress
K_n	stress concentration factor in the tranverse direction
n	factor of safety
q	notch sensitivity factor for cyclic loading
R	reliability factor
U	internal elastic energy, mJ (mm-kgf)
δ	Static deformation under the action of the weight W, mm
δ'	Deformation under impact action, mm
σ	static stress, MN/m^2 (kgf/mm^2)
σ_b	bending stress, MN/m^2 (kgf/mm^2)
σ_d	design stress, MN/m^2 (kgf/mm^2)
σ_x, σ_y	direct stresses in x and y directions respectively, MN/m^2 (kgf/mm^2)
σ_1, σ_2	maximum and minimum principal stresses respectively, MN/m^2 (kgf/mm^2)
σ_{en}	endurance limit stress of the material in reversed bending, MN/m^2 (kgf/mm^2)
σ_{en-a}	endurance limit stress of the material in reversed axial loading, MN/m^2 (kgf/mm^2)
σ_{yp}	yield point stress, MN/m^2 (kgf/mm^2)

Symbols	Description and Units
σ_m	average or mean normal stress, MN/m^2 (kgf/mm^2)
σ_a	variable normal stress, MN/m^2 (kgf/mm^2)
σ_{dr}	design stress for completely reversed loads, MN/m^2 (kgf/mm^2)
σ_{da}	design stress for alternating loads, MN/m^2 (kgf/mm^2)
σ_u	ultimate stress, MN/m^2(kgf/mm^2)
σ'	impact stress, MN/m^2(kgf/mm^2)
τ	shear stress, MN/m^2(kgf/mm^2)
τ_{en}	endurance limit stress of the material in cyclic torsion, MN/m^2 (kgf/mm^2)
τ_m	average or mean shear stress, MN/m^2 (kgf/mm^2)
τ_a	variable shear stress, MN/m^2 (kgf/mm^2)
τ_{yp}	yield strength of the material in shear, MN/m^2 (kgf/mm^2)
τ'	the impact stress due to torsion, MN/m^2 (kgf/mm^2)
θ	static angular deflection, rad
θ'	angular deflection under impact loading, rad

Particular	Equation	Eqn. No.
Stress concentration in members:		
The maximum stresses at the discontinuity		
i) For a direct stress: (Fig. 2.1(a))	$\sigma_{max} = \sigma K_t = \dfrac{F}{A} K_t$	2.1(a)
ii) For bending: (Fig. 2.1(b))	$\sigma_{max} = \sigma_b K_t = \dfrac{Mc}{I} K_t = \dfrac{M}{Z} K_t$	2.1(b)
iii) For torsion: (Fig. 2.1(c))	$\tau_{max} = \tau K_s = \dfrac{Tr}{J} K_S = \dfrac{T}{Z_p} K_s$	2.1(c)

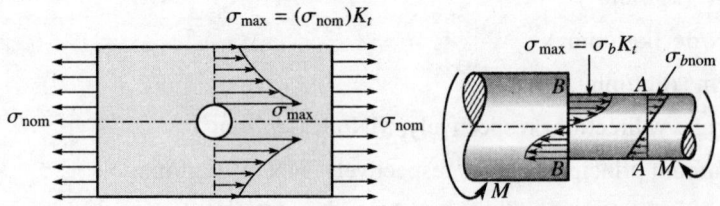 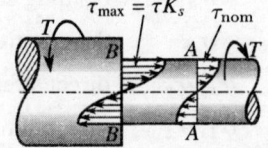

Fig. 2.1(a): *Tensile Stress*   **Fig. 2.1(b):** *Bending Stress*   **Fig. 2.1(c):** *Shear Stress*

Particular	Equation	Eqn. No.
Transverse stress induced around the hole in a plate of infinite width (Fig. 2.2)	$\sigma_{max} = \sigma K_n = \dfrac{F}{A} K_n$	2.2
When a plate with a hole is subjected to biaxial stresses σ_x and σ_y acting at right angles, then the combined maximum stress induced (super position)	$\sigma_{max} = K_t \sigma_x + K_n \sigma_y = K_t \sigma_1 + K_n \sigma_2$	2.3
The notch sensitivity index:	$q = \dfrac{K_{tf} - 1}{K_t - 1}$	2.4
Estimated fatigue stress concentration factor for normal stress	$K_{tf} = 1 + q(K_t - 1)$	2.5
Estimated combined fatigue factor for normal stress	$K'_{tf} = 1 + q(K'_t - 1)$	2.6
Estimated fatigue stress concentration factor for shear stress	$K_{sf} = 1 + q(K_s - 1)$	2.7

Theories of failure:

Particular	Equation	Eqn. No.
Stress according to the maximum normal stress theory or Rankine theory	$\sigma_e = \left(\dfrac{\sigma_x + \sigma_y}{2}\right) + \sqrt{\left(\dfrac{\sigma_x - \sigma_y}{2}\right)^2 + \tau_{xy}^2}$ $= \sigma_1$, maximum principle stress	2.8(a)

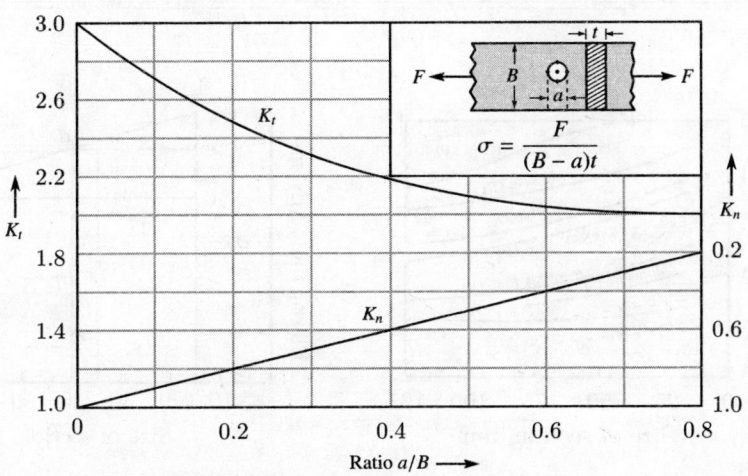

Fig. 2.2: *Form Stress Factor due to hole in a plate*

Particular	**Equation**	**Eqn. No.**

Stress according to the maximum strain theory or Saint-Vanant's theory

$$\sigma_e = (1 - \mu)\left(\frac{\sigma_x + \sigma_y}{2}\right) + (1 + \mu)\sqrt{\left(\frac{\sigma_x - \sigma_y}{2}\right)^2 + \tau_{xy}^2} = \sigma_1 - \mu\sigma_2 \qquad \text{2.8(b)}$$

Stress according to the maximum shear stress theory or Guest's theory

$$\sigma_e = 2\sqrt{\left(\frac{\sigma_x - \sigma_y}{2}\right)^2 + \tau_{xy}^2} = \sqrt{(\sigma_x - \sigma_y)^2 + 4\tau_{xy}^2} = (\sigma_1 - \sigma_2) \qquad \text{2.8(c)}$$

Stress according to shear energy theory or the Hencky-von Mises theory

$$\sigma_e = \sqrt{(\sigma_x^2 - \sigma_x\sigma_y + \sigma_y^2 + 3\tau_{xy}^2)} = \sqrt{\sigma_1^2 + \sigma_2^2 - \sigma_1\sigma_2} \qquad \text{2.8(d)}$$

Maximum total strain energy theory or Haigh's theory
$$\sigma_e = \sqrt{\sigma_1^2 + \sigma_2^2 - 2\mu\sigma_1\sigma_2} \qquad \text{2.8(e)}$$

Design for strength:

Influence of size:

The elastic limit σ_e' for any thickness h between 12.5 mm and 75 mm (Fig. 2.3 and 2.4)

$$\sigma_e' = \sigma_e - \frac{(\sigma_e - \sigma_{e_3})(h - 12.5)}{75 - 12.5} = \sigma_e B \qquad \text{2.9(a)}$$

where B is the size factor

$$1/B = \frac{250}{300 - 4h + (\sigma_{e_3}/\sigma_e)(4h - 50)} \qquad \text{2.9(b)}$$

value of the ratio (σ_{e_3}/σ_e) for a few materials are given in Table. 2.5

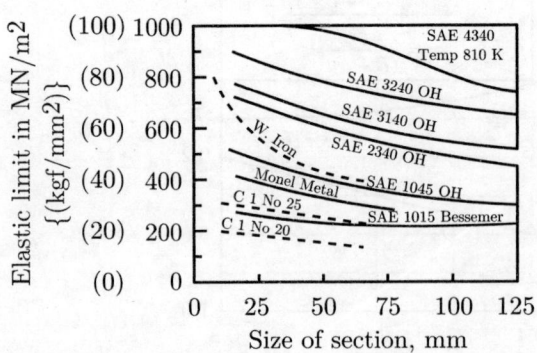

Fig. 2.3: *Influence of Size on Elastic Limit*

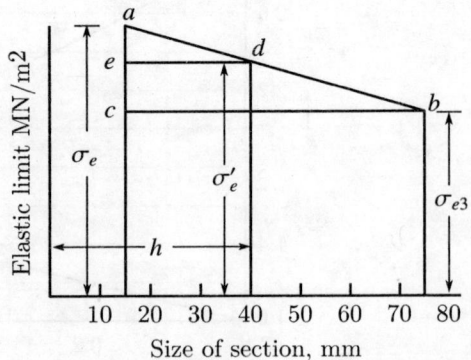

Fig. 2.4: *Change of Elastic Limit with Size of Section*

Particular	Equation	Eqn. No.
Static loads:		
The design stress for a static load	$\sigma_{ds} = \dfrac{\sigma_e B}{R K_t}$ where R is the reliability factor, Table. 2.7	2.10
The bearing stress	$\sigma_b = 1.81\sigma_e$	2.11
Design for fatigue:		
Endurance or fatigue stress concentration factor	$K_{tf} = \dfrac{\sigma_{en}}{\sigma_{enf}} = q(K_t - 1) + 1$	2.12(a)
	where σ_{en} is the Endurance limit without discontinuity σ_{enf} is the fatigue strength with discontinuity	
Design stress for completely reversed loads	$\sigma_{dr} = \dfrac{\sigma_{en} B}{R K_{tf}}$	2.12(b)
Relation between tensile strength and endurance limit:		
for steel	$\sigma_{en} = (1/2 \text{ to } 5/8)\,\sigma_u$	2.13(a)
for cast iron	$\sigma_{en} = 0.4\sigma_u$	2.13(b)
for nonferrous metals and alloys	$\sigma_{en} = (1/4 \text{ to } 1/3)\sigma_u$	2.13(c)
Direct stress endurance limit in terms of σ_{en} and σ_u		
For steel	$\sigma_{en\text{-}a} = (0.7 \text{ to } 1.0)\sigma_{en} = (0.35 \text{ to } 5/8)\sigma_u$	2.14(a)
For cast iron	$\sigma_{en\text{-}a} = (0.7 \text{ to } 1.0)\sigma_{en} = (0.28 \text{ to } 0.4)\sigma_u$	2.14(b)
For non-ferrous metals and alloys	$\sigma_{en\text{-}a} = (0.7 \text{ to } 1.0)\sigma_{en} = (0.175 \text{ to } 1/3)\sigma_u$	2.14(c)
Cyclic torsion endurance limit in terms of σ_{en} and σ_u		
For steel	$\tau_{en} = (0.5 \text{ to } 0.6)\sigma_{en} = (0.25 \text{ to } 0.3)\sigma_u$	2.15(a)
For cast iron	$\tau_{en} = 0.8\sigma_u$	2.15(b)
For non-ferrous metals and alloys	$\tau_{en} = 0.2\sigma_u$	2.15(c)
Static plus alternating simple loads:- **(Fig. 2.5)**		
The average or mean stress	$\sigma_m = \dfrac{\sigma_{max} + \sigma_{min}}{2}$	2.16(a)
The variable stress component	$\sigma_a = \dfrac{\sigma_{max} - \sigma_{min}}{2}$	2.16(b)

Particular	Equation	Eqn. No.
The design stress for alternating loads	$\sigma_{da} = \dfrac{\sigma_d(F_m + F_a)}{F_m + \left(\dfrac{\sigma_d}{\sigma_{dr}}\right)F_a}$	2.17(a)
	where $\quad F_m = \dfrac{F_{\max} + F_{\min}}{2}, \quad$ average or mean load $\quad\quad F_a = \dfrac{F_{\max} - F_{\min}}{2}, \quad$ alternating load	
The required cross-sectional area of the member for alternating loads	$A = \dfrac{F_{max}}{\sigma_{da}} = \dfrac{F_m + F_a}{\sigma_{da}}$	2.17(b)
The equivalent static load for a cyclic load $F_m \pm F_a$	$F'_m = F_m + (\sigma_d/\sigma_{dr})F_a$	2.18(a)
The equivalent static load for a bending load $M_m \pm M_a$	$M'_m = M_m + (\sigma_d/\sigma_{dr})M_a$	2.18(b)
The equivalent static load for a torsional load $T_m \pm T_a$	$T'_m = T_m + (\sigma_d/\sigma_{dr})T_a$	2.18(c)

Fatigue Failure Equations (Fig. 2.6)

Particular	Equation	Eqn. No.
Gerber's parabolic relationship for fluctuating stress	$\sigma_a = \sigma_{en}[1 - (\sigma_m/\sigma_u)^2]$ or $\dfrac{\sigma_a}{\sigma_{en}} + \left(\dfrac{\sigma_m}{\sigma_u}\right)^2 = 1$	2.19(a)
Goodman's relation for fluctuating stress	$\sigma_a = \sigma_{en}\left(\dfrac{1}{n} - \dfrac{\sigma_m}{\sigma_u}\right)$ or $\dfrac{\sigma_a}{\sigma_{en}} + \dfrac{\sigma_m}{\sigma_u} = \dfrac{1}{n}$	2.19(b)
Soderberg's relation for fluctuating stress	$\sigma_a = \sigma_{en}\left(\dfrac{1}{n} - \dfrac{\sigma_m}{\sigma_{yp}}\right)$ or $\dfrac{\sigma_a}{\sigma_{en}} + \dfrac{\sigma_m}{\sigma_{yp}} = \dfrac{1}{n}$	2.19(c)

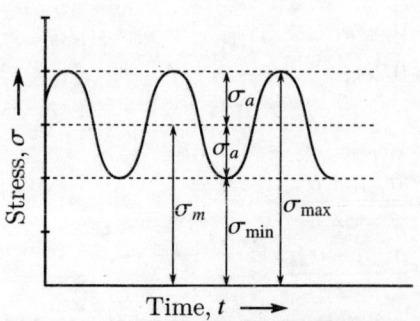

Fig. 2.5: *Fluctuating Stress*

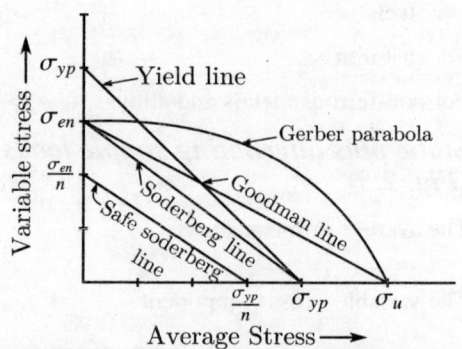

Fig. 2.6: *Fatigue Failure Equations*

Particular	Equation	Eqn. No.
Goodman's relation for fluctuating torsional stress	$\tau_a = \tau_{en}\left(\dfrac{1}{n} - \dfrac{\tau_m}{\tau_u}\right)$ or $\dfrac{\tau_a}{\tau_{en}} + \dfrac{\tau_m}{\tau_u} = \dfrac{1}{n}$	2.19(d)
Soderberg's relation for fluctuating tosional stress	$\tau_a = \tau_{en}\left(\dfrac{1}{n} - \dfrac{\tau_m}{\tau_{yp}}\right)$ or $\dfrac{\tau_a}{\tau_{en}} + \dfrac{\tau_m}{\tau_{yp}} = \dfrac{1}{n}$	2.19(e)

The maximum cyclic stress in terms of the endurance limit:

According to Goodman relation	$\sigma_{max} = \dfrac{\sigma_{en}}{n} + \sigma_m\left(1 - \dfrac{\sigma_{en}}{\sigma_u}\right)$	2.20(a)
According to Soderberg relation	$\sigma_{max} = \dfrac{\sigma_{en}}{n} + \sigma_m\left(1 - \dfrac{\sigma_{en}}{\sigma_{yp}}\right)$	2.20(b)
In the case of cyclic torsion the maximum stress according to Soderberg relation.	$\tau_{max} = \dfrac{\tau_{en}}{n} + \tau_m\left(1 - \dfrac{\tau_{en}}{\tau_{yp}}\right)$	2.20(c)

Taking the correction factors into account:

The Goodman's relationship

a) for ductile materials	$\dfrac{K_{tf}\sigma_a}{ABC\sigma_{en}} + \dfrac{\sigma_m}{\sigma_u} = \dfrac{1}{n}$	2.21(a)
b) for brittle materials	$\dfrac{K_{tf}\sigma_a}{ABC\sigma_{en}} + K_t\dfrac{\sigma_m}{\sigma_u} = \dfrac{1}{n}$	2.21(b)

The Soderberg relationship

a) for ductile materials	$\dfrac{K_{tf}\sigma_a}{ABC\sigma_{en}} + \dfrac{\sigma_m}{\sigma_{yp}} = \dfrac{1}{n}$	2.21(c)
b) for brittle materials	$\dfrac{K_{tf}\sigma_a}{ABC\sigma_{en}} + K_t\dfrac{\sigma_m}{\sigma_{yp}} = \dfrac{1}{n}$	2.21(d)
c) for ductile materials in shear	$\dfrac{K_{sf}\tau_a}{ABC\sigma_{en}} + \dfrac{\tau_m}{\tau_{yp}} = \dfrac{1}{n}$	2.21(e)

where $A = 1.0$ for reversed bending,

$= 0.7$ to 1.0 for reversed axial loading

$= 0.5$ to 0.6 for reversed torsional loading

B is the size correction factor (Eqn. 2.9(b))

C is the surface correction factor (Table 2.2)

n is the factor of safety (Table III-1)

Particular	Equation	Eqn. No.
The equivalent maximum shear and normal stresses:		
The equivalent normal stress	$\sigma_{eq-n} = \sigma_m + \left(\dfrac{\sigma_{yp}}{\sigma_{en}}\right)\dfrac{K_{tf}\sigma_a}{ABC}$	2.22(a)
The equivalent shear stress	$\tau_{eq} = \tau_m + \left(\dfrac{\tau_{yp}}{\sigma_{en}}\right)\dfrac{K_{sf}\tau_a}{ABC}$	2.22(b)
The equivalent maximum shear stress	$\tau_{eq}(\text{max}) = \sqrt{\left(\frac{1}{2}\sigma_{eq-n}\right)^2 + (\tau_{eq})^2} = \tau_{yp}/n$	2.23(a)

The equivalent maximum normal stress to be used when designing with brittle materials

$$\sigma_{eq-n}(\text{max}) = \frac{1}{2}\sigma_{eq-n} + \sqrt{\left(\frac{1}{2}\sigma_{eq-n}\right)^2 + (\tau_{eq})^2} = \frac{\sigma_{yp}}{n} \qquad 2.23(b)$$

Particular	Equation	Eqn. No.
Inertia stresses and Centrifugal loads:		
The general expression for the centrifugal force	$F_c = \dfrac{mv^2}{R} = \dfrac{W}{g}\dfrac{v^2}{R}$	2.24(a)

where, v = velocity, m/s

R = radius of curvature of the path of the motion of the mass, m.

W = weight, N(kgf)

g = acceleration due to gravity, m/s^2.

Particular	Equation	Eqn. No.
The centrifugal force per unit volume	$\overline{F}_c = \dfrac{w}{g}\dfrac{v^2}{R}$	2.24(b)

where w = the specific weight of the material, N/mm^3 (kgf/mm^3)

Particular	Equation	Eqn. No.
In the case of a coupling rod (Fig. 2.7), (i) The centrifugal force	$F_c = \dfrac{w}{g}\dfrac{v^2}{R}htL$	2.24(c)

where, h = height of coupling rod, mm

t = thickness of coupling rod, mm

and L = length of coupling rod, mm

Particular	Equation	Eqn. No.
(ii) Bending component of the centrifugal force	$F_{c_b} = \dfrac{w}{g}\dfrac{v^2}{R}htL\cos\alpha = \dfrac{W}{g}\dfrac{v^2}{R}\cos\alpha$	2.24(d)

where, α = crank angle, degrees

W = total weight of the coupling rod, N(kgf).

Particular	Equation	Eqn. No.
(iii) The maximum bending component of the centrifugal force (when $\alpha = 0°$, i.e. at b)	$F_{c_b}(\max) = \dfrac{w}{g}\dfrac{v^2}{R}htL = \dfrac{W}{g}\dfrac{v^2}{R}$	2.24(e)
(iv) The maximum bending moment (when $\alpha = 0°$, i.e. at b)	$M_{\max} = \dfrac{1}{8}F_{c_b}(\max)L = \dfrac{wv^2}{8gR}htL^2 = \dfrac{Wv^2L}{8gR}$	2.24(f)
(v) The axial component of the centrifugal force	$F_{ca} = \dfrac{w}{g}\dfrac{v^2}{R}htL\sin\alpha = \dfrac{W}{g}\dfrac{v^2}{R}\sin\alpha$	2.24(g)
(vi) The maximum axial component of the centrifugal force (when $\alpha = 90°$, i.e. at a')	$F_{ca} = \dfrac{W}{g}\dfrac{v^2}{R}$	2.24(h)
Impact Energy:		
Kinetic Energy	$E_k = \dfrac{Wv^2}{2g}$	2.25(a)
Impact energy of a body falling from a height, h	$E_k = Wh$	2.25(b)
The internal elastic energy	$U = W(h + \delta') = \dfrac{Wv^2}{2g} + W\delta'$	2.25(c)
If the velocity has a random direction, then the internal elastic energy	$U = \dfrac{Wv_1^2}{2g} + W\delta'\sin\alpha$	2.25(d)

where v_1 is the velocity of the moving body, mm/sec

g is the acceleration due to gravity, mm/s^2

Impact stress

The general equation for the impact stress

$$\sigma' = \sigma(1 + \sqrt{1 + 2h/\delta}) = \frac{W}{A}(1 + \sqrt{1 + 2hEA/WL}) \qquad \text{2.26(a)}$$

The general equation for the deformation under impact action	$\delta' = \delta(1 + \sqrt{1 + 2h/\delta})$	2.26(b)
The impact stress due to bending	$\sigma'_b = \sigma_b(1 + \sqrt{1 + 2h/y})$	2.26(c)

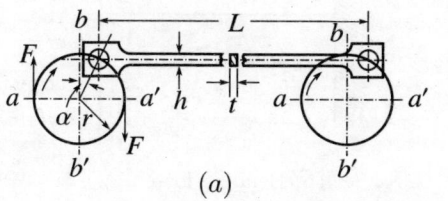   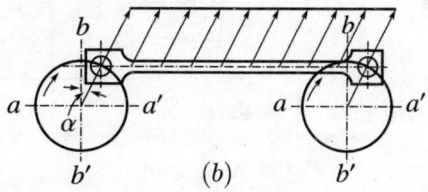

(a) (b)

Fig. 2.7: *Locomotive Coupling Rod*

Particular	Equation	Eqn. No.
Deflection under impact action due to bending	$y' = y(1 + \sqrt{1 + 2h/y})$	2.26(d)
The impact stress due to torsion	$\tau' = \tau(1 + \sqrt{1 + 2h/r\theta})$	2.26(e)
The angular deformation due to impact loading (torsion)	$\theta' = \theta(1 + \sqrt{1 + 2h/r\theta})$ where r is the moment arm of the load W	2.26(f)
Impact stress due to sudden load	$(\sigma' = 2\sigma)$, $(\sigma'_b = 2\sigma_b)$ and $(\tau' = 2\tau)$	2.26(g)
Deformation under impact action due to sudden load	$(\delta' = 2\delta)$, $(y' = 2y)$ and $(\theta' = 2\theta)$	2.26(h)
When a body having a wieght W strikes another body that has a wieght W' according to the laws of collision of two perfectly inelastic bodies, the impact energy Wh is reduced nWh. The value of n may be found by the formula	$n = \dfrac{1 + am}{(1 + bm)^2}$ where $m = W'/W$ a and b are coefficients (Table 2.8)	2.26(i)

Resilience:

The resilience of a body	$U = \dfrac{1}{2}F\delta$	2.27(a)

$$\text{where } F = \text{average applied force}$$

$$= W \text{ when load is applied without impact}$$

$$= \frac{W\delta'}{\delta} = \frac{W\sigma'}{\sigma}, \quad \text{when load is applied with impact}$$

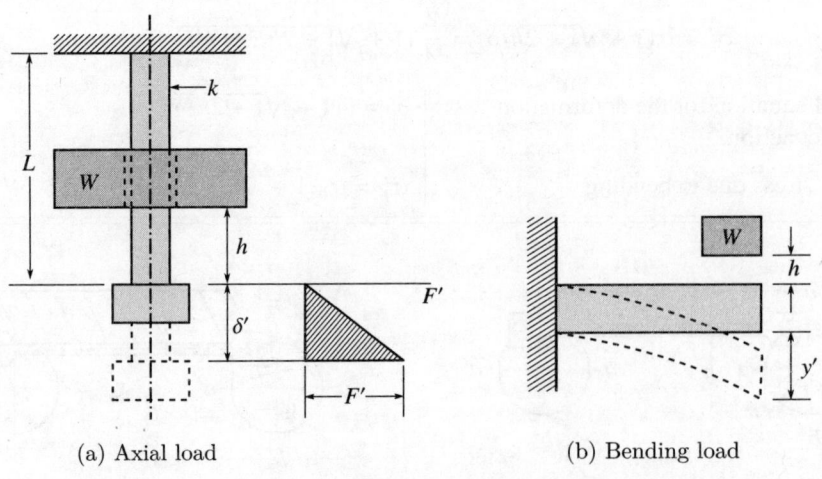

(a) Axial load   (b) Bending load

Fig. 2.8: *Impact Stresses*

Particular	Equation	Eqn. No.
Resilience in tension or compression	$U = \dfrac{\sigma^2 V}{2E}$ where $V = AL$, Volume of the body, mm^3	2.27(b)
Resilience in bending	$U = \left[\dfrac{K_2^2}{2K_1}\right]\left(\dfrac{k}{c}\right)^2 \dfrac{\sigma^2 AL}{E}$	2.27(c)

where $(k/c)^2 = (1/3)$, for rectangular sections

$\qquad\qquad = (1/4)$, for circular sections

$\quad K_1$ is the constant in the deflection equation $(y = FL^3/K_1 E)$ corresponding to the type of loading

$\quad K_2$ is the constant in the maximum moment equation $(M = FL/K_2)$ corresponding to the type of loading

$\quad k$ is the radius of gyration

Resilience in shear	$U_s = \dfrac{\tau^2 V}{2G}$	2.27(d)
Resilience in torsion	$U_s = \left(\dfrac{k_p}{c}\right)^2 \dfrac{\tau^2 AL}{2G}$ where k_p is the polar radius of gyration	2.27(e)

References

[1] *Siegel M.J., Maleev V. L., Hartman J. B., "Mechnaical Design of Machines"*, 4th edition, International Text Book Company, 1965.

[2] *Vallance A., Doughtie V. L., "Design of Machine Members"*, 3rd edition, McGraw-Hill Book Co., 1951.

[3] *Spotts M. E., "Design of Machine Elements"*, 3rd edition, Prentice Hall, Inc., Maruzen Co. Ltd.

[4] *Black P. H., "Machine Deisgn"*, 3rd edition, McGraaw Hill Book Company, Inc.

[5] *Faires V. M., "Design of Machine Elements"*, 2nd Edition, The Macmillan Company, 1941.

[6] *Shigley J. E., "Machine Design"*, McGraw Hill Book Company, Inc.

[7] *Hyland P. H., Kommers, J. B., "Machine Design"*, McGraw Hill Book Company, 1943.

[8] *Hall A. S., HoloWenko, A. R., Laughlin H. G., "Schaum's Outline of Theory and Problems of Machine Design"*, Schaum Publishing Co., 1961.

[9] *Slaymaker R. R., "Mechanical Design and Analysis"*, John Wiley and Son, Inc., 1958.

[10] *Roark R. J., "Formulas for stress and strain"*, McGraw Hill Book Company 1954.

Table 2.1 *Stress Concentration Factors*

Type of form irregularity or stress riser	Manner of loading	Equation for the stress concentration factor	Experimental value of the factor K_t or N or K_{tf}
1. A Round hole in a plate of infinite width (Fig. 2.9)	Tension	$K_t = \dfrac{1}{2}\left[2 + \left(\dfrac{a}{2x}\right)^2 + 3\left(\dfrac{a}{2x}\right)^4\right]$	$K_t = 3$
2. Round filled hole	Tension		$K_t = 2.5$
3. The pin in a hole transmits the load	Tension		$K_t = 2.5$ $K_n = 0.5$
4. For a small V-notch at the edge of the place Fig. 2.10	Tension	$K_t = 1 + 2\sqrt{h/r}$ where h = depth of the notch r = radius at the notch corner	
5. An Elliptical hole in a plate with major axis normal to the load (Fig. 2.11)	Tension	$K_t = 1 + 2\dfrac{b}{c}$	
6. An Elliptical hole in a plate, the major axis along the load	Tension	$K_t = 1 + \dfrac{2c}{b}$ b = semi major axis and c semi minor axis	

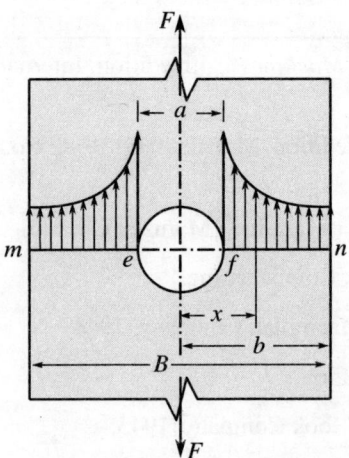

Fig. 2.9: *Stress concentration for a plate with hole in tension*

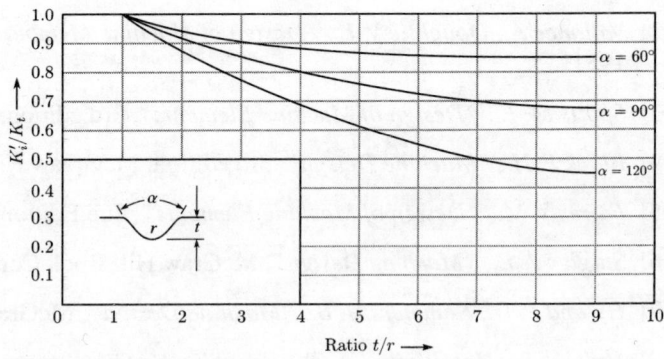

Fig. 2.10: *Form-Factor ratio due to notches of various shapes*

Table 2.1 *Stress Concentration Factors (Contd.)*

Type of form irregularity or stress riser	Manner of loading	Equation for the stress concentration factor	Experimental value of the factor K_t or N or K_{tf}
7. Key ways with $b = d/4$ and $h = b/2$			
(i) Profile key way	Shear		$K_s = 1.68$
(ii) Sled runner	Shear		$K_s = 1.44$
8. Screw thread			
(i) UNF threads	Tension		$K_{tf} = 2.5$ to 3.75
(ii) Whitworth	Tension		$K_{tf} = 1.5$ to 3.0
9. Press and shrink fit			
(i) Plain member			$K_t = 1.95$
(ii) Grooved member			$K_t = 1.34$
10. Rotating disc with hole			
(i) For $R_i/R_o \rightarrow 0$			$K_t = 2$
(ii) Thin Ring			$K_t = 1$
11. Helical spring	Shear	$K_s = \dfrac{4C - 1}{4C - 4} + \dfrac{0.615}{C}$ where C is the spring index	
12. Crane hook			$K_t = 1.56$
13. Gear teeth			
(i) At the root fillet of $14\frac{1}{2}°$ involute	Bending	$K_t = 0.22 + \left[\dfrac{t_g}{r}\right]^{0.20} \left[\dfrac{t_g}{l}\right]^{0.40}$	
(ii) At the root fillet of $20°$ involute	Bending	$K_t = 0.18 \left[\dfrac{t_g}{r}\right]^{0.15} \left[\dfrac{t_g}{l}\right]^{0.45}$	
14. Curved beam	Bending	$K_t = 1.0 + B \left[\dfrac{I}{bc^2}\right] \left[\dfrac{1}{r - c} + \dfrac{1}{r}\right]$	

where $B = 1.05$ for circular or elliptical sections

$= 0.5$ for other sections

c is distance of the extreme fiber from the centroidal axis

r is the radius of curvature

Table 2.2 *The average values of the surface correction factor C*

Ultimate stress $\sigma_u MN/m^2$ (Kgf/mm²)	C for Machine surface (Cold drawn)	C for hot rolled surface	Ultimate stress $\sigma_u MN/m^2$ (Kgf/mm²)	C for Machine surface (Cold drawn)	C for hot rolled surface
410 (42)	0.91	0.72	760 (77)	0.84	0.52
480 (49)	0.90	0.68	820 (84)	0.82	0.48
550 (56)	0.88	0.62	1030 (105)	0.78	0.38
620 (63)	0.86	0.58	1370 (140)	0.72	0.30
690 (70)	0.85	0.55	–	–	–

Table 2.3 *Chart for Guidance in Selecting Stress-Concentration Factors for Various Types of Loading and Materials*

Loading	Brittle material		Ductile material	
	Normal	Shear	Normal	Shear
Static	K_t	K_s	Neglect	Neglect
Cyclic	K_t	K_s	K'_{tf}	K_{sf}

Table 2.4 *Index of Sensitivity for Repeated Stresses*

Material	Average Index of Sensitivity, q		
	Annealed or soft	Heat treated and drawn at 920K (650°C)	Heat treated and drawn at 750K (480°C)
Armco iron, 0.02% C ..	0.15-0.20	..	..
Carbon steel :			
0.10%C ..	0.05-0.10	..	..
0.20%C (also cast steel) ..	0.10	..	..
0.30%C ..	0.18	0.35	0.45
0.50%C ..	0.26	0.40	0.50
0.85%C ..	..	0.45	0.57
Spring steel, 0.56%C, 2.3 Si, rolled ..	..	0.38	..
SAE 3140, 0.37% C; 0.6% Cr; 1.3% Ni ..	0.25	0.45	..
Cr – Ni steel, 0.8% Cr; 3.5% Ni	..	0.25	0.70
Stainless steel, 0.3% C; 8.3% Cr; 19.7% Ni ..	0.16	..	..
Cast iron ..	0-0.05	..	..
Copper, electrolitic ..	0.07	..	..
Duraluminium ..	0.05-0.13	..	..

Table 2.5 *Strength Ratios for Various Materials*

Material	Natural State	Annealed	Drawn at 923K (650°C)	Drawn at 813K (540°C)	Drawn at 703K (430°C)
Aluminiium, strong, wrought ..	0.93	..	..	..	..
Tobin bronze ..	0.90	..	..	..	..
Monel metal, forged ..	0.80	..	..	..	..
Ductile iron ..	0.80	0.98	..	..	..
Low-carbon steel, C< 0.20% ..	0.84	..	..	..	..
Medium-carbon steel, 0.30 to 0.50%C ..	0.85	0.72	0.59	0.53	
Nickel steel, SAE 2340 ..	..	0.86	0.80	0.74	..
Cr-Ni steel, SAE 3140 ..	..	0.80	0.75	0.70	0.65
Cast iron, Class No. 20 ..	0.55	..	..	..	..
Cast iron, Class No. 25 ..	0.73	..	..	..	..
Cast iron, Class No. 35 ..	0.60	..	..	..	..
Wrought iron ..	0.55	..	..	..	..

The table header spans: **Values of σ_{e3}/σ_e**

Table 2.6 *Comparision of Theories of Failure*

Type of load	Rankine Theory	Saint-Venant's Theory	Guest's Theory	Hencky von Mises theory
1. For pure tension i.e. $\sigma_x = \sigma, \sigma_y = 0, \tau = 0$	$\sigma = \sigma_e$	$\sigma = \sigma_e$	$\sigma = \sigma_e$	$\sigma = \sigma_e$
2. For pure shear i.e. $\sigma_x = 0, \sigma_y = 0$ and $\tau_{xy} = \tau$	$\tau = \sigma_e$	$\tau = 0.77\sigma_e$	$\tau = 0.5\sigma_e$	$\sigma = 0.58\sigma_e$

The table header spans: **Theories of failure**

Table 2.7 *Reliability Factor*

Sl. No.	Particular	Reliability factor, R
1.	When close dimensional control is exercised in production, and materials have been purchased to close tolerance specifications such as in the design of air craft and space vehicles.	1.0
2.	For reliable high grade materials, when loads and stresses can be determined very accurately and a low weight is desired.	1.1 to 1.5
3.	For the same above condition 2, when a low weight is not important or critical.	1.5 to 2.0
4.	For ordinary materials, where over load is possible and reliability is important.	2.0 to 3.0
5.	For cast iron and similar materials, where loading is uncertain in design applications and where the stresses cannot be determined accurately.	3 and over
6.	In mechanical design of steel and aluminium elements.	1.25 to 1.50
7.	If the material (steel or aluminium) is not of best quality, or if there is no definite information about its quality.	2.00

Table 2.8 *Coefficients in the Equation for Inertia, Equation* 2.26(*i*)

Type of impact	a	b
Longitudinal impact on bar	1/3	1/2
Centre impact on simple beam	17/35	5/8
Centre impact on beam with fixed ends	13/35	1/2
End impact on cantilever beam	4/17	3/8

Table 2.9 *Maximum Resilience Per Unit Volume*

Type of loading	Modulus of Resilience mJ* (mm-kgf) per cubic mm
Tension or compression	$\sigma_e^2/2E$
Shear, simple transverse	$\tau_e^2/2G$
Bending in beams with rectangular-sections: (For circular sections, multiply given values by 3/4):	
Cantilever, end load	$\sigma_e^2/18E$
Cantilever, uniform load	$\sigma_e^2/30E$
Simply supported, concentrated load	$\sigma_e^2/18E$
Simply supported, uniform load	$(4/45)\left(\sigma_e^2/E\right)$
Fixed at both ends, concentrated load	$\sigma_e^2/18E$
Fixed at both ends, uniform load	$\sigma_e^2/30E$
Uniform strength beam, concentrated load	$\sigma_e^2/6E$
Torsion	
Solid round bar	$\tau_e^2/4G$
Hollow round bar with D_1 greater then D_2	$\left[1 + (D_2/D_1)^2\right](\tau_e^2/4G)$
Springs	
Laminated with flat leaves of uniform strength ..	$\sigma_e^2/6E$
Flat spiral with rectangular section	$\sigma_e^2/24E$
Helical with round section and axial load	$\tau_e^2/4G$
Helical with round section and axial twist	$\sigma_e^2/8E$
Helical with rectangular section and axial twist ..	$\sigma_e^2/6E$

*mJ refers to milli Joules.

Table 2.10 *Resilience in Tension*

Material	Elastic Limit σ_e MN/m² (kgf/mm²)	Modulus of Elasticity $E \times 10^{-3}$ MN/m² (kgf/mm²)	Modulus of Resilience u mJ/mm³ (mm kgf/mm³)	Impact Strength (Izod number)
CAST IRON				
Class 20 (ordinary) ..	43.2* (4.40)	68.7 (7.00)	0.215 (0.022)	..
Class 25 ..	68.7* (7.00)	89.2 (9.10)	0.430 (0.044)	..
Nickel, Grade II ..	118.0* (12.00)	124.5 (12.70)	0.905 (0.092)	..
Malleable ..	138.3 (14.10)	172.6 (17.60)	0.905 (0.092)	7.9
Aluminium alloy, SAE 33 ..	48.1 (4.90)	66.7 (6.80)	0.280 (0.029)	..
Brass, SAE 40 or SAE 41 ..	68.7 (7.00)	82.4 (8.40)	0.452 (0.046)	2.7
Bronze, SAE 43 ..	193.2 (19.70)	110.8 (11.30)	2.770 (0.282)	..
MONEL METAL				
Hot-rolled ..	206.0 (21.10)	176.5 (18.00)	2.000 (0.203)	120
Cold-rolled, normalized ..	482.5 (49.20)	176.5 (18.00)	10.850 (1.106)	110
STEEL ––				
SAE 1010 ..	207.0 (21.10)	207.0 (21.10)	1.695 (0.173)	..
SAE 1030 ..	252.0 (25.70)	207.0 (21.10)	2.490 (0.254)	20
SAE 1050, annealed ..	334.4 (34.10)	206.0 (21.00)	4.290 (0.438)	..
SAE 1095, annealed ..	414.0 (42.20)	206.00 (21.00)	6.780 (0.691)	..
SAE 1095, tempered ..	516.8 (52.70)	216.0 (21.00)	10.620 (1.083)	..
SAE 2320, annealed ..	310.0 (31.60)	206.0 (21.00)	3.840 (0.392)	52
SAE 2320, tempered ..	690.0 (70.30)	206.0 (21.00)	18.870 (1.924)	40
SAE 3250, annealed ..	552.0 (56.25)	214.0 (21.80)	21.810 (2.224)	..
SAE 3250, tempered ..	1383.0 (141.00)	214.0 (21.80)	72.880 (7.431)	30
SAE 6150, annealed ..	427.6 (43.60)	214.0 (21.00)	7.005 (0.714)	..
SAE 6150, tempered ..	1100.0 (112.50)	214.0 (21.80)	52.650 (5.369)	..
Rubber ..	2.1 (0.21)	1.0×10^{-3} (0.11×10^{-3})	33.900 (3.456)	

*Cast iron has no well defined elastic limit, but, for all practical purposes, the values given may be safely used.

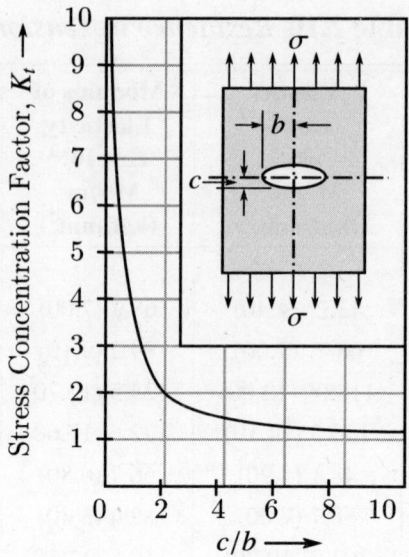

Fig. 2.11: *Stress Concentration at the Edge of an Elliptical Hole in a Plate*

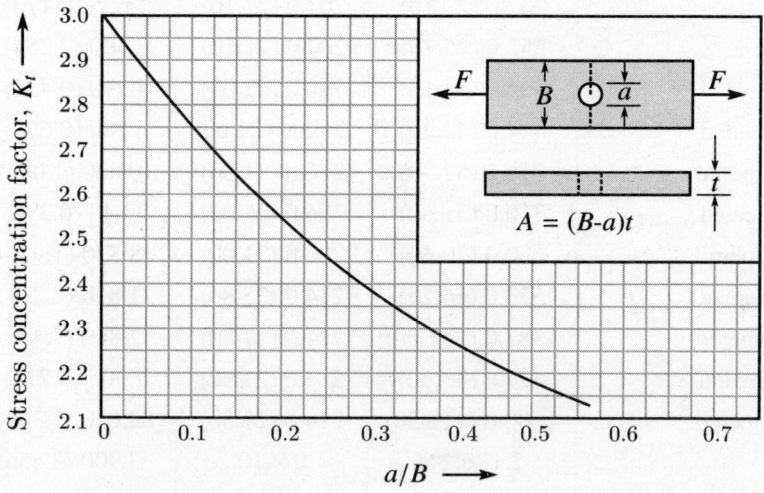

Fig. 2.12: *Stress Concentration Factor K_t for a plate with hole in tension*

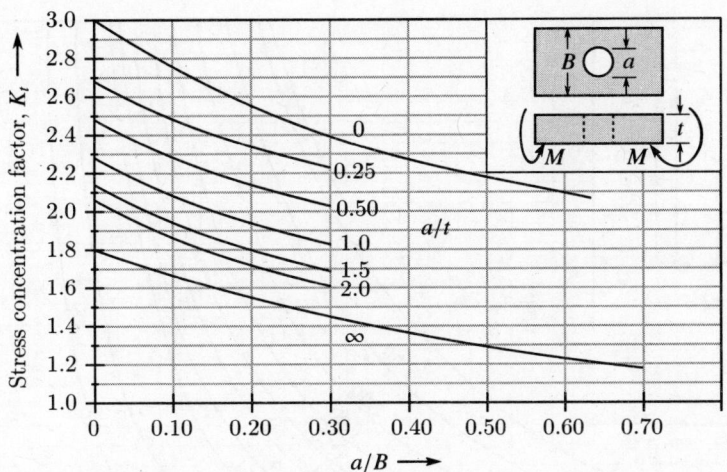

Fig. 2.13: *Stress concentration factor for a flat bar with a transverse hole in bending*

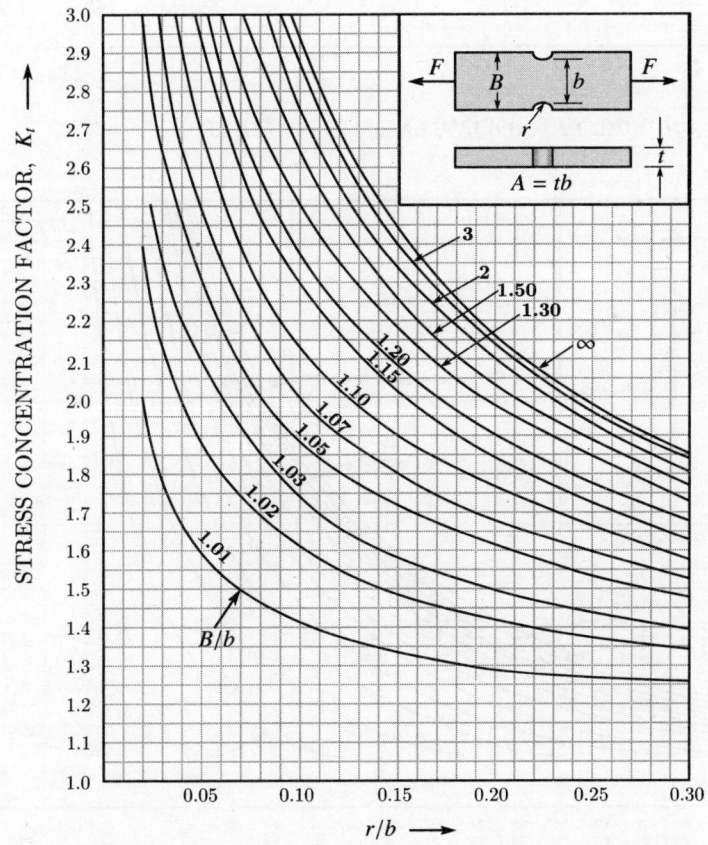

Fig. 2.14: *Stress concentration Factor K_t for a notched Flat bar in tension*

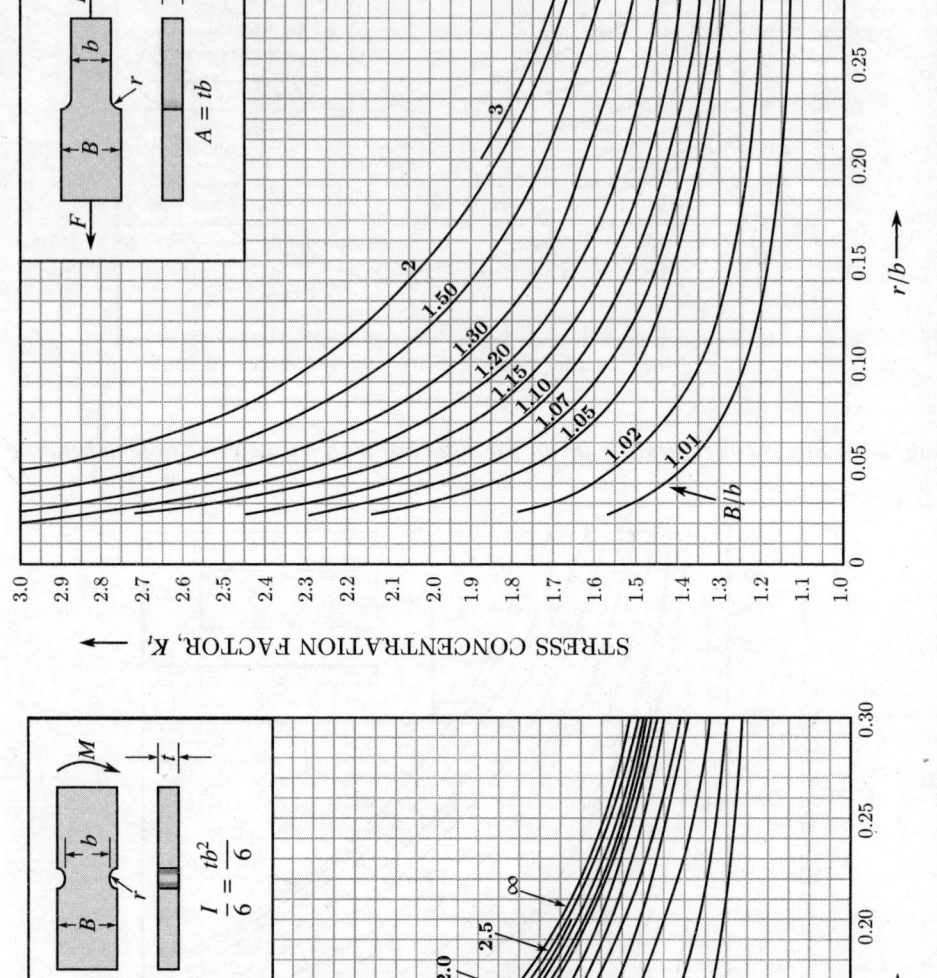

Fig. 2.16: *Stress Concentration Factor K$_t$ for Stepped flat bar in tension*

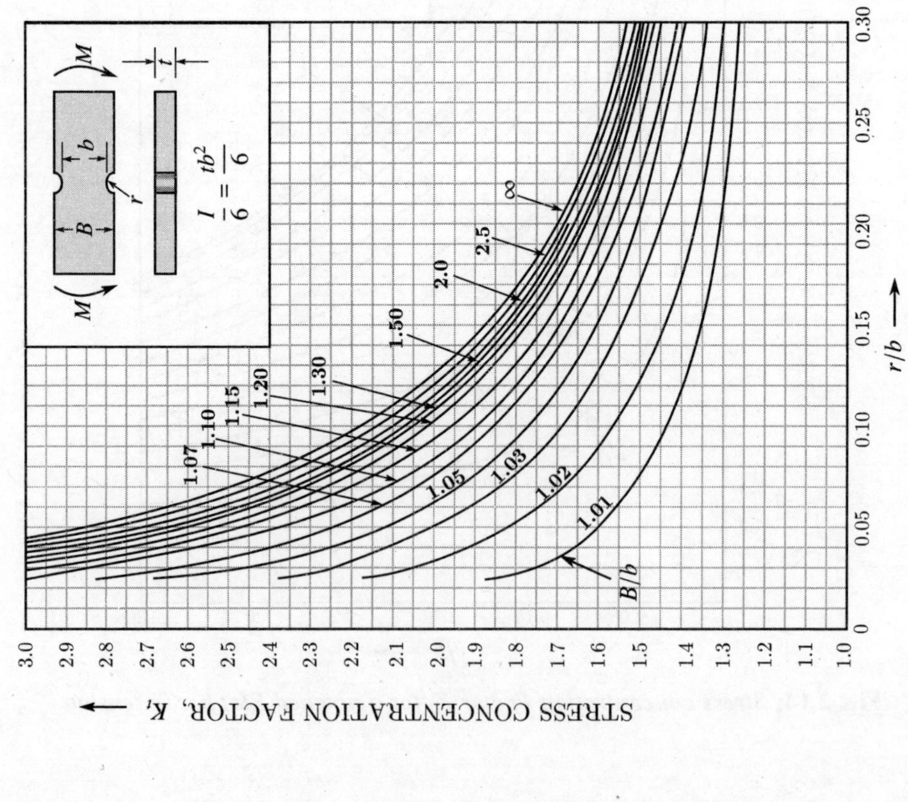

Fig. 2.15: *Stress concentration Factor K$_t$ for a notched Flat bar in bending*

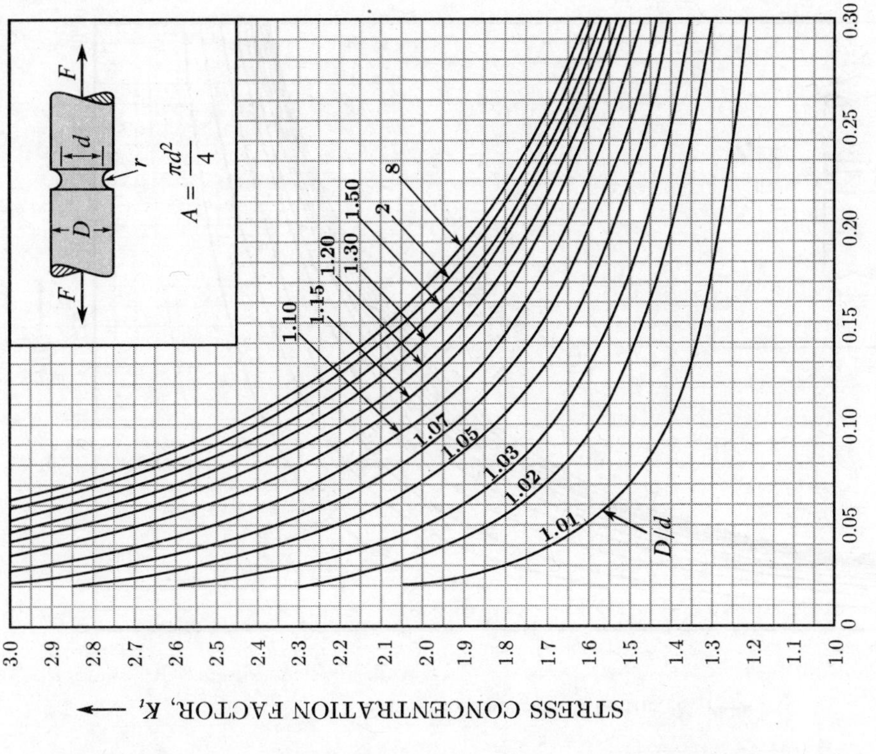

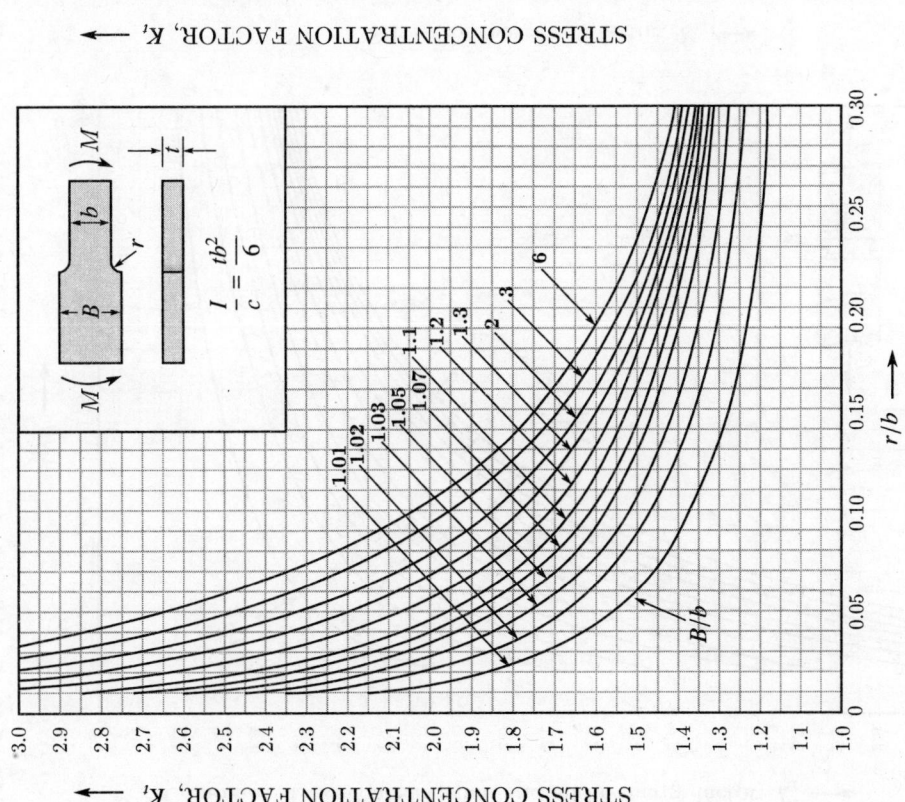

Fig. 2.18: *Stress Concentration Factor K_t for a grooved shaft in tension*

Fig. 2.17: *Stress Concentration Factor K_t for Stepped flat bar in Bending*

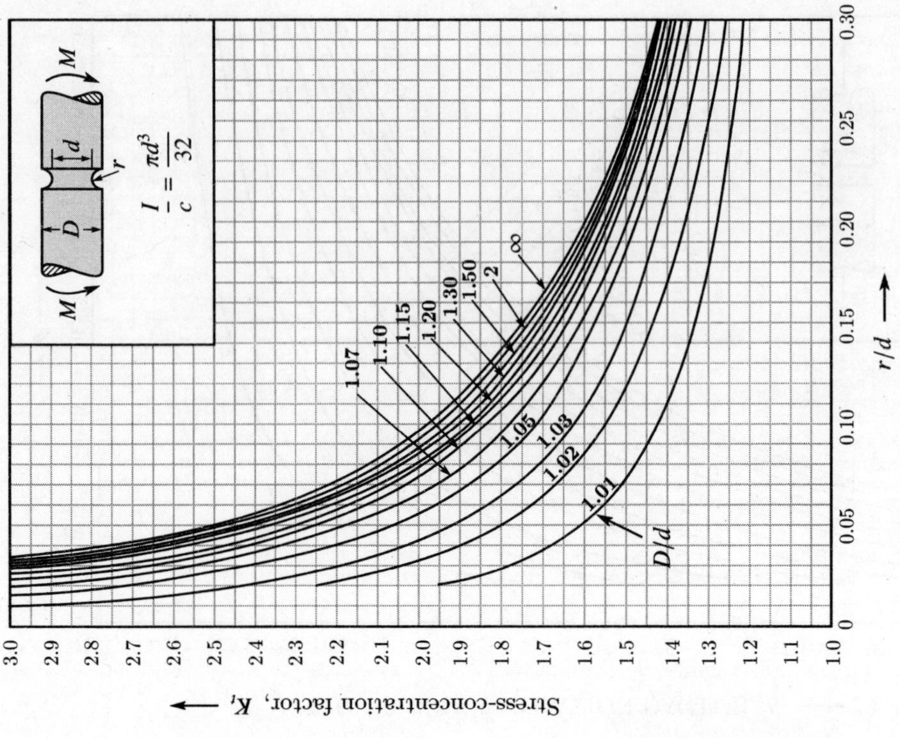

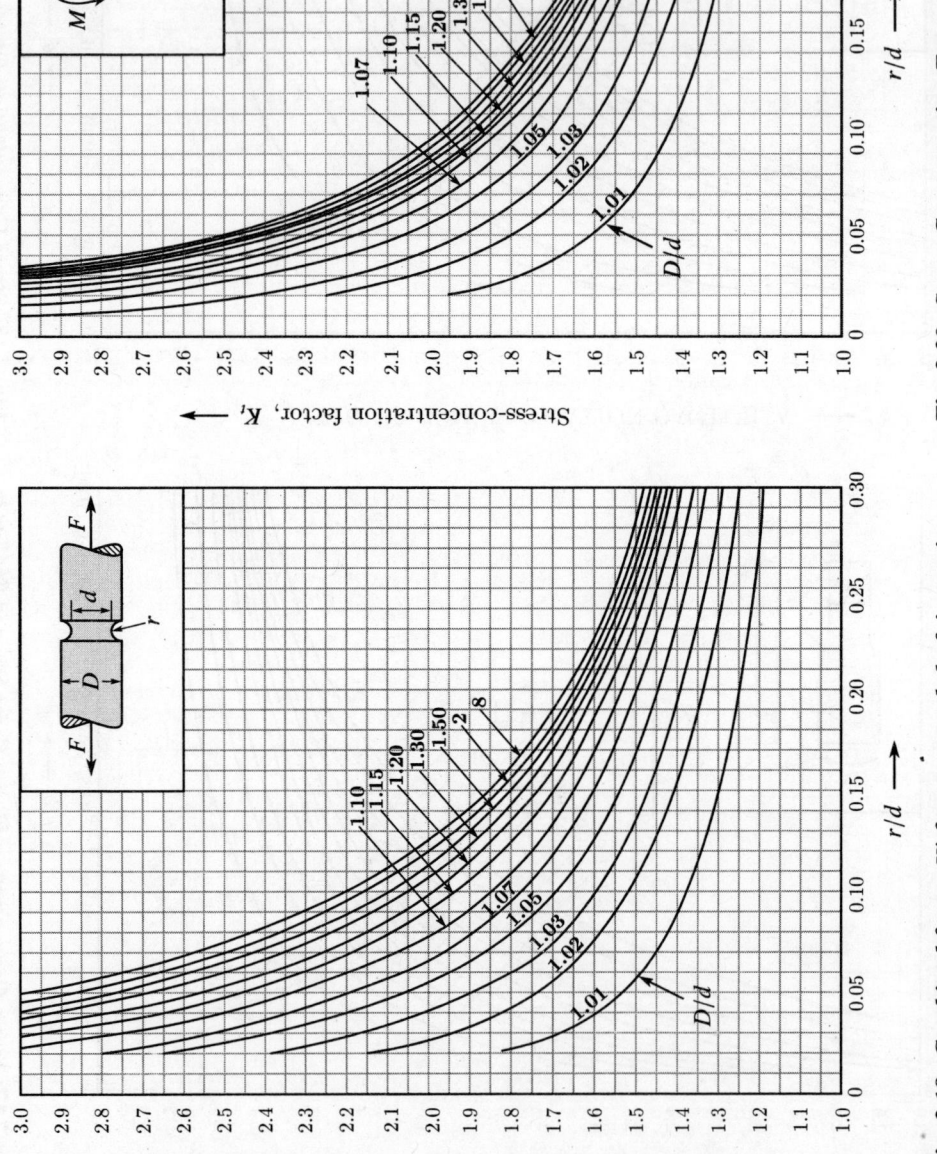

Fig. 2.20: *Stress Concentration Factor K_t for a grooved shaft in bending*

Fig. 2.19: *Combined factor K'_t for a grooved shaft in tension*

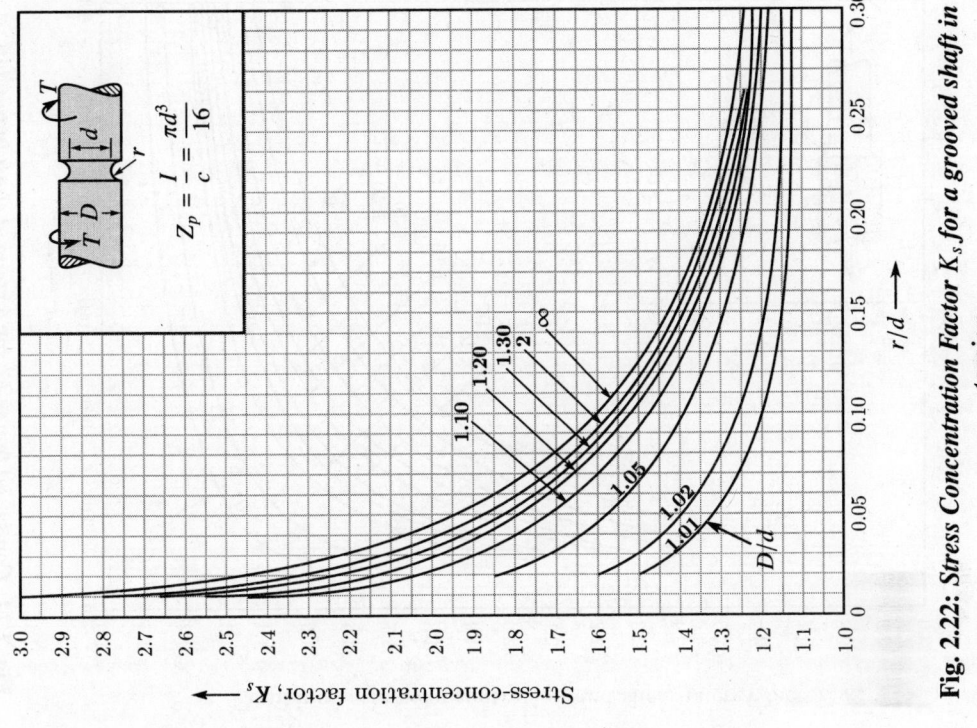

Fig. 2.22: *Stress Concentration Factor K_s for a grooved shaft in torsion*

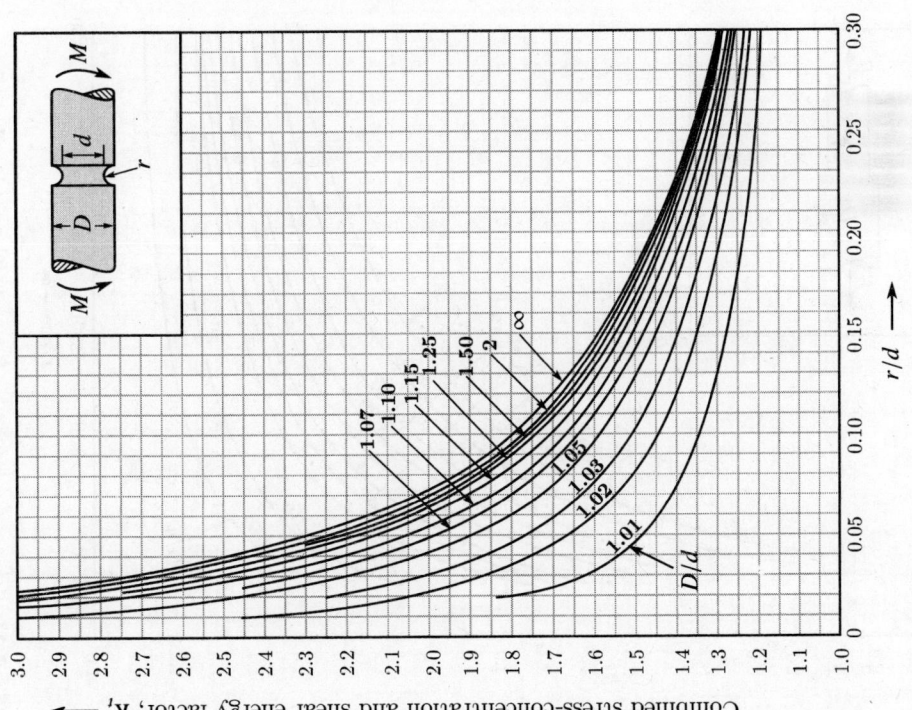

Fig. 2.21: *Combined factor K'_t for a grooved shaft in bending*

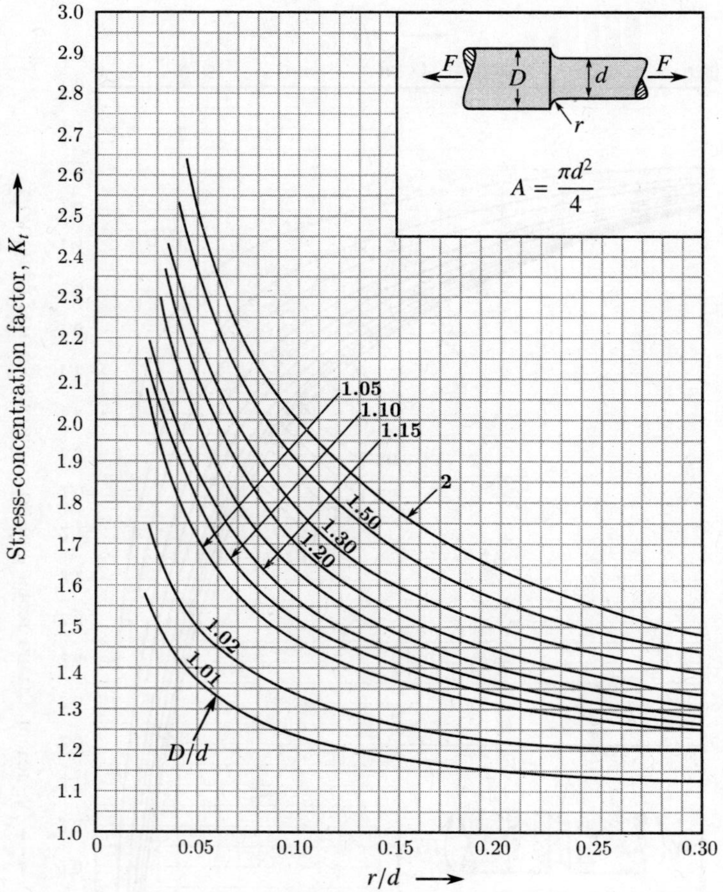

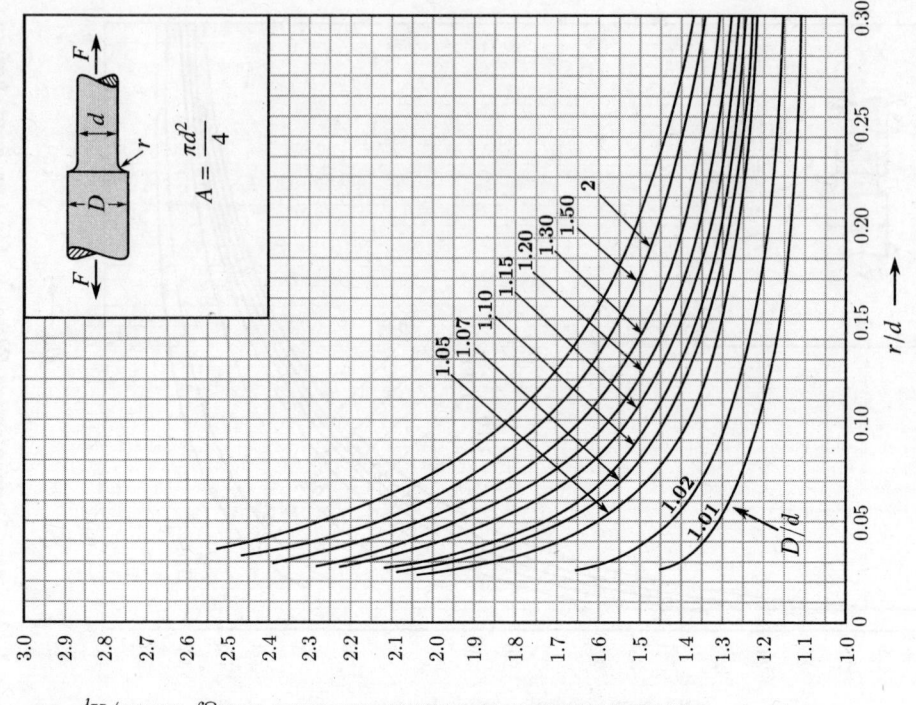

Fig. 2.24: *Combined factor K_t' for a stepped shaft in tension*

Combined stress-concentration and shear-energy factor, K_t'

Fig. 2.23: *Stress-concentration factor K_t for a stepped shaft in tension*

Stress-concentration factor, K_t

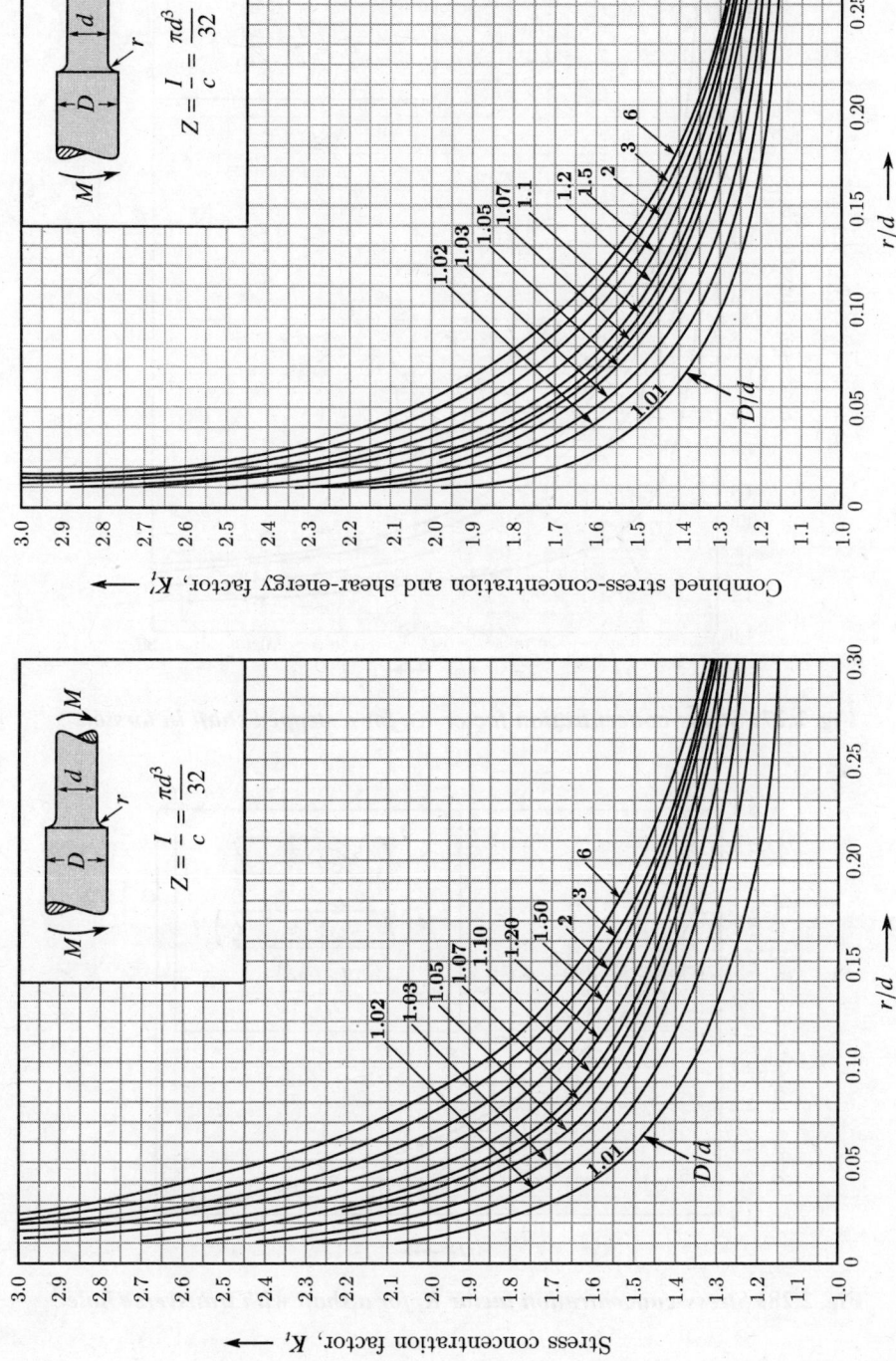

Fig. 2.26: *Combined factor K'_t for a stepped shaft in bending*

Fig. 2.25: *Stress-concentration factor K_t for a stepped shaft in bending*

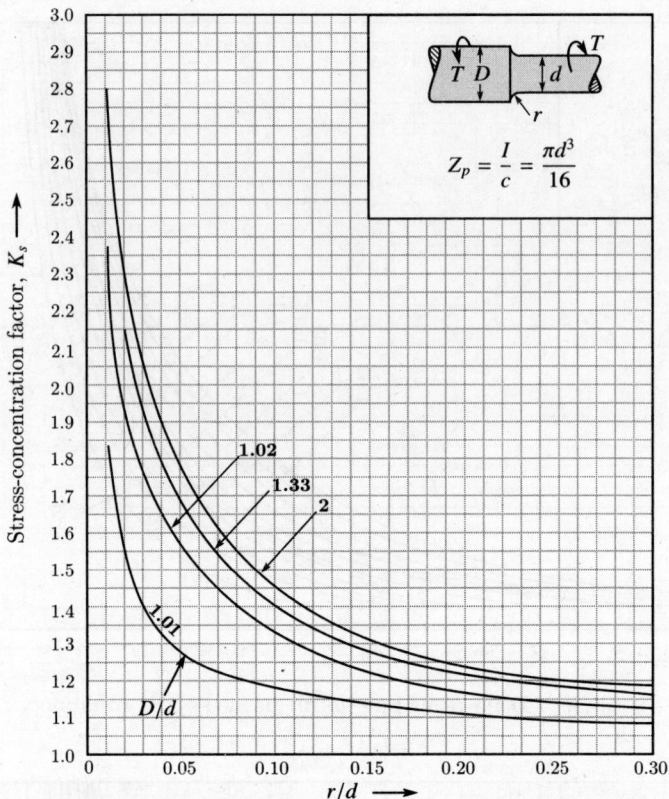

Fig. 2.27: *Stress-concentration factor K_{ts} for a stepped shaft in torsion*

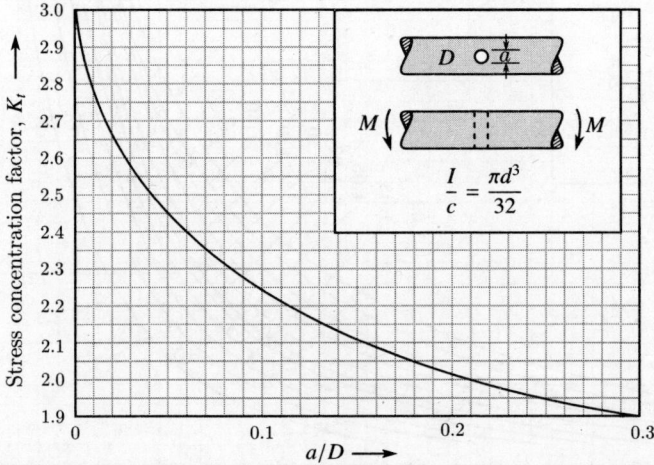

Fig. 2.28: *Stress-concentration factor K_t for a shaft with transverse hole*

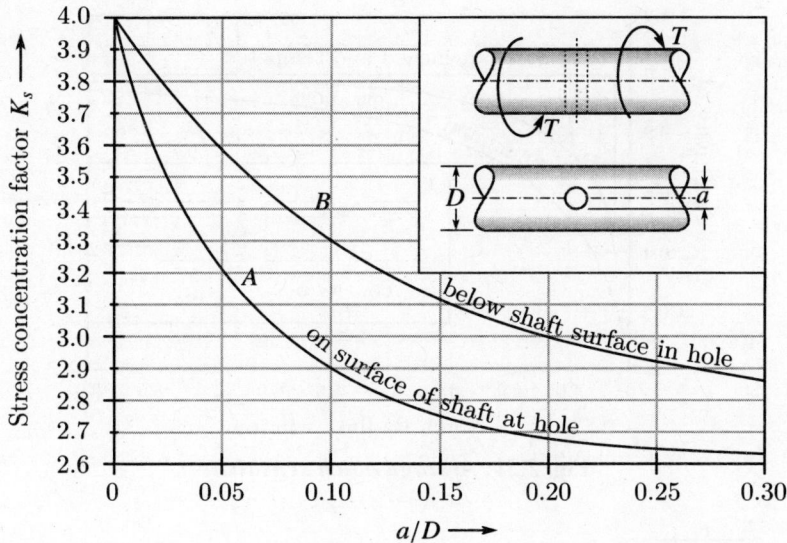

Fig. 2.29: *Stress concentration factor for a shaft with transverse hole in torsion*

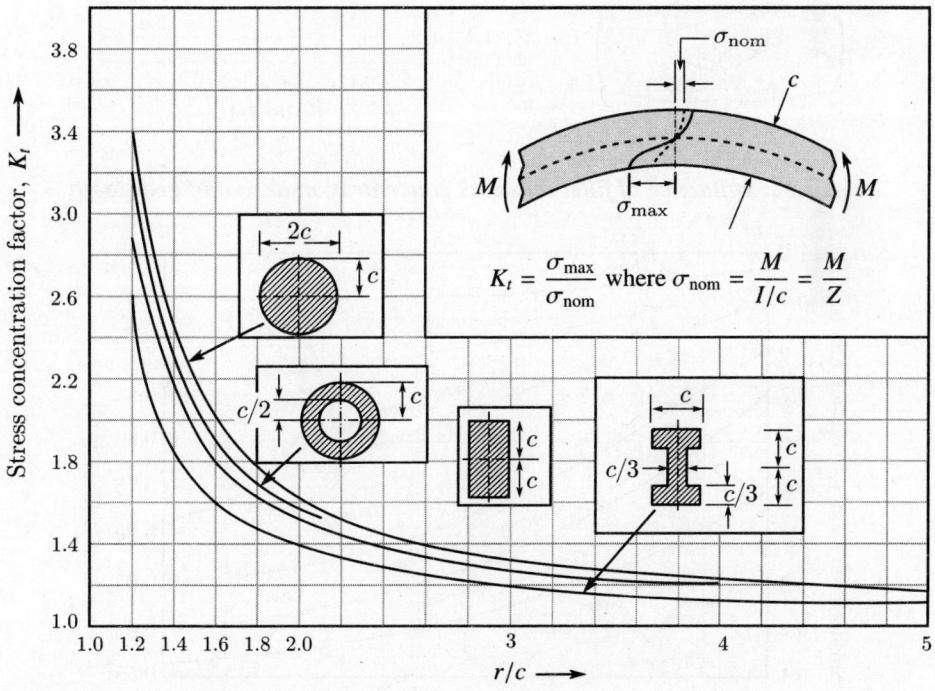

Fig. 2.30: *Theoretical stress-concentration factor K_t for a curved bar in bending*

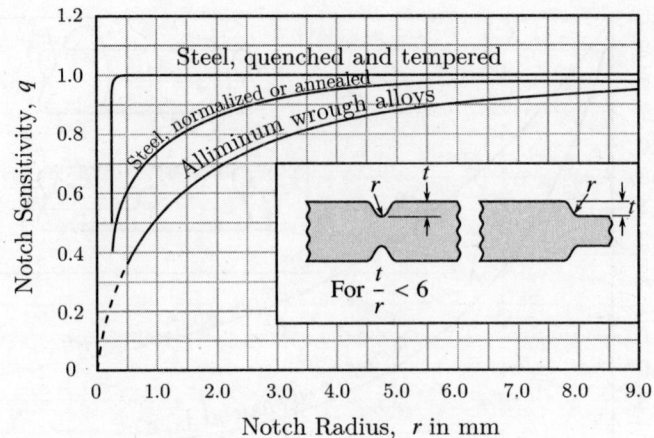

Fig. 2.31: *Average notch sensitivity*

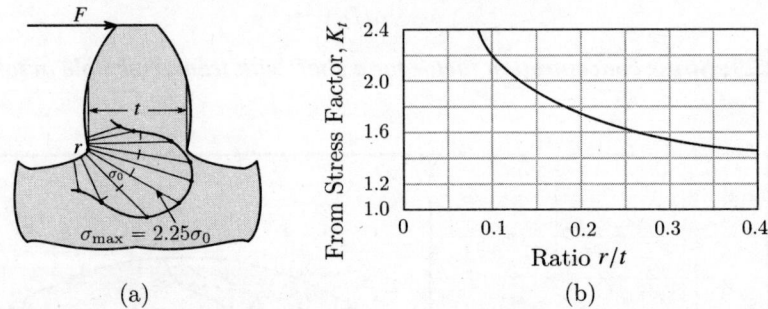

Fig. 2.32: *Influence of fillet on stress concentration at root of gear tooth*

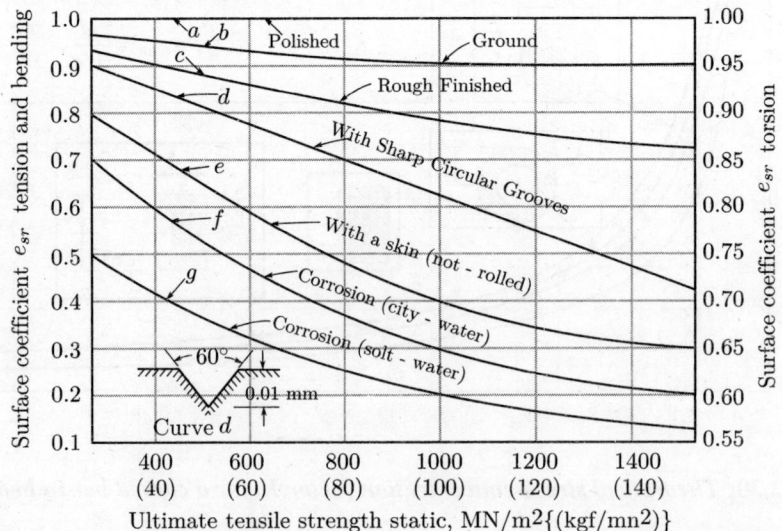

Fig. 2.33: *Reciprocals of Stress Concentration Factors Caused by Surface Conditions*

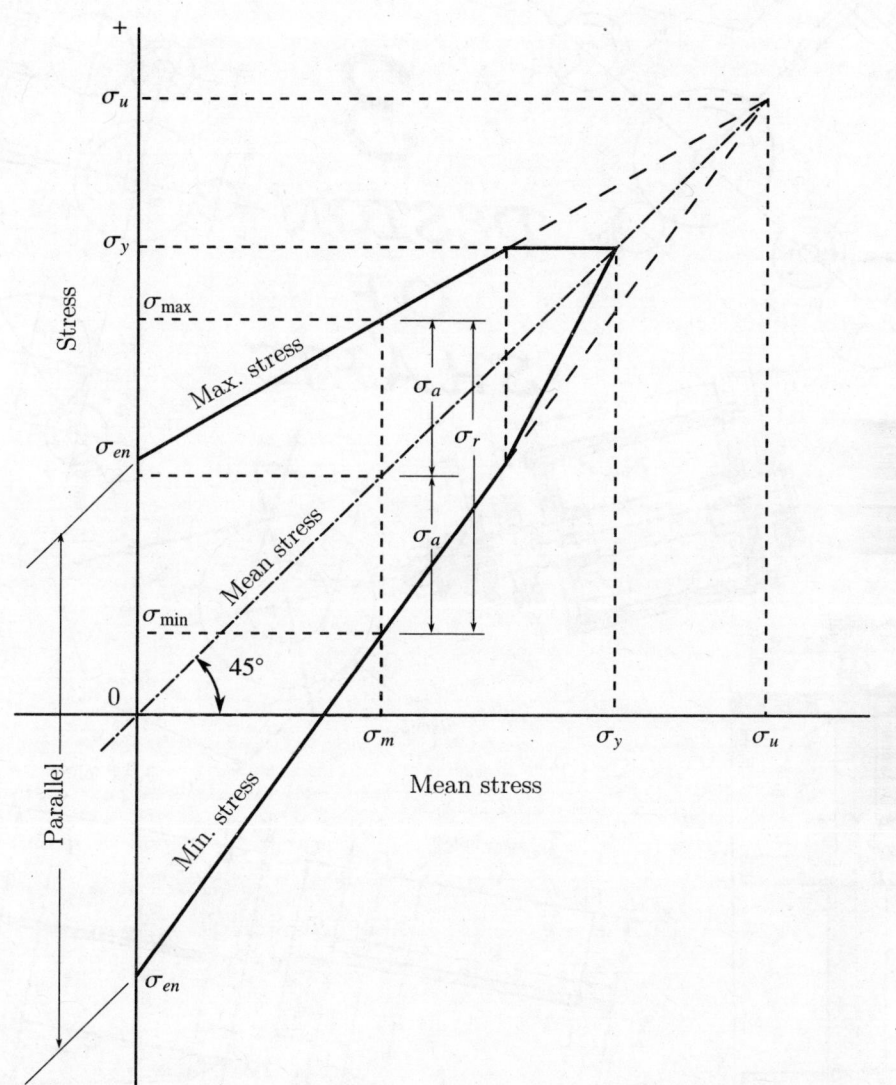

Modified Goodman Diagram

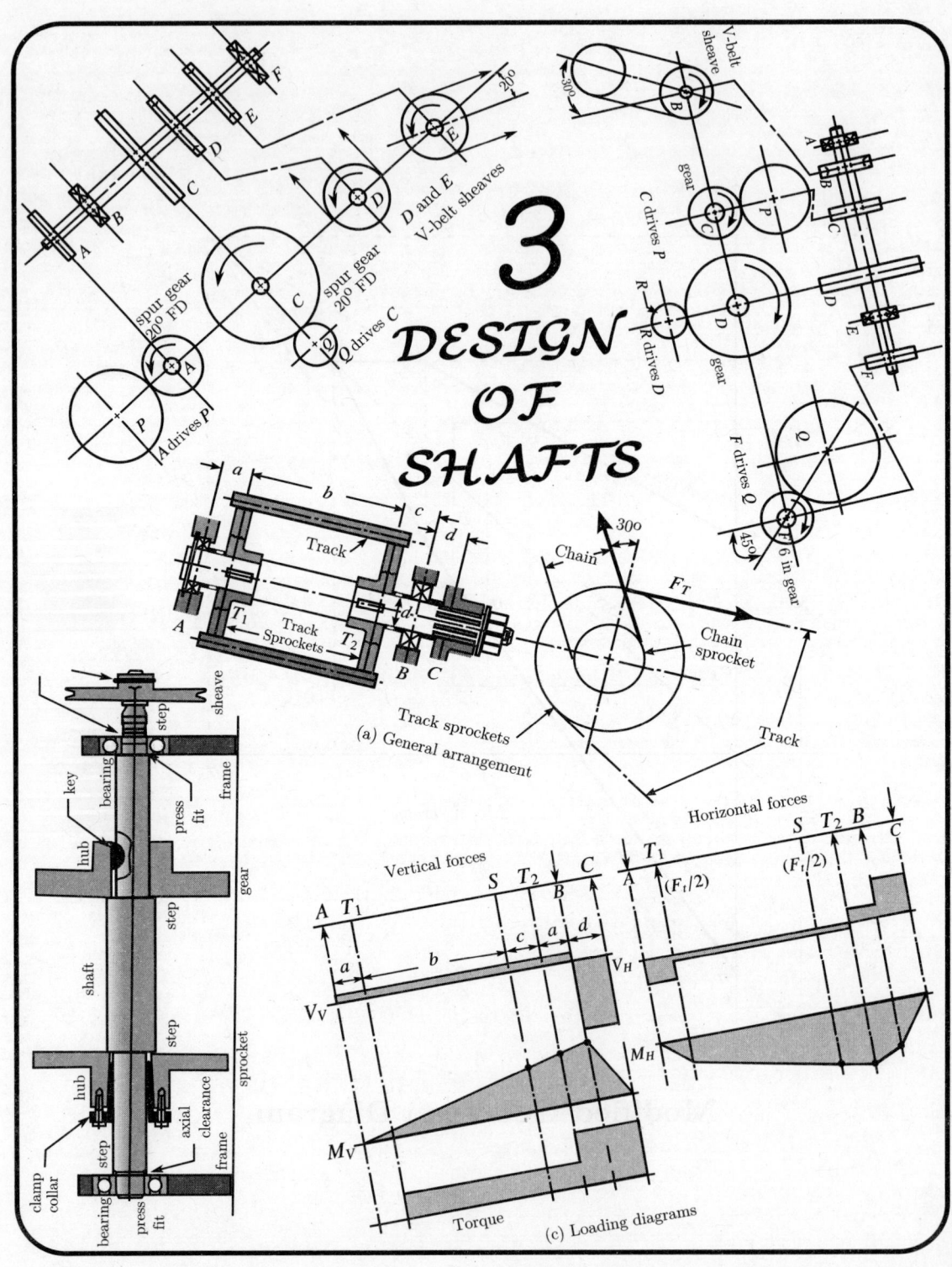

3

DESIGN

OF

SHAFTS

spur gear 20° FD

A drives P

spur gear 20° FD

Q drives C

D and E V-belt sheaves

V-belt sheave

C drives P

gear

R drives D

gear

F drives Q

6 in gear

a *b* *c* *d*

Track

Track Sprockets

T_1 T_2

d

A

B C

Chain

30°

F_T

Chain sprocket

Track sprockets

(a) General arrangement

Track

sheave

step

bearing

press fit

frame

key

hub

shaft

step

gear

step

hub

sprocket

clamp collar

bearing

step

press fit

frame

axial clearance

Vertical forces

A T_1

S T_2 C B

a *b* *c* *a* *d*

V_V

M_V

Horizontal forces

S T_2 B

A T_1 $(F_t/2)$ $(F_t/2)$ C

V_H

M_H

Torque

(c) Loading diagrams

$$3$$

Design of Shafts

Symbols	Description and Units
c	distance from neutral axis to outer most fiber, mm
C_m, C_t	the numerical combined shock and fatigue factors to be applied to the computed bending moment and torsional moment respectively (Table 3.1)
d	diameter of solid shaft, mm (Table 3.5)
d_i, d_0	inside and outside diameters of the hollow shaft respectively, mm
F_c	Force on the connecting rod, N (kgf)
F_p	Force on the piston, N (kgf)
F_r	radial force along the crank, N (kgf)
F_t	tangential force perpendicular to the crank, N (kgf)
J	polar moment of inertia of cross-sectional area about axis of rotation, mm^4
K	ratio of inside to outside diameter of hollow shaft
L	length of the shaft, mm
M	bending moment, N mm (kgf-mm)
n	speed of the shaft, rpm
P	power, kW
p_{bc}	allowable crank pin bearing pressure, MN/m^2 (kgf/mm^2) (Table 3.6)
p_{bs}	main bearing pressure, MN/m^2 (kgf/mm^2) (Table 3.6)
T	torsional moment, N mm (kgf-mm)
σ_b	stress due to bending, MN/m^2 (kgf/mm^2)
σ_d	design stress, MN/m^2 (kgf/mm^2) (Table 3.5(b))
σ_e	stress at the elastic limit, MN/m^2 (kgf/mm^2)
τ	torsional shear stress, MN/m^2 (kgf/mm^2)
τ_d	design shear stress, MN/m^2 (kgf/mm^2) (Table 3.5(b))
τ_e	shear stress at the elastic limit, MN/m^2 (kgf/mm^2)
ω	angular velocity, rad/s
θ	angle of twist, deg

Particular	Equation	Eqn. No.
Torsion of circular shafts:		
The maximum torsional shear stress due to torsional loading	$\tau = \dfrac{Tc}{J} = \dfrac{16T}{\pi d^3}$ for solid shafts	3.1
	$= \dfrac{16T}{\pi d_o^3}\left(\dfrac{1}{1-K^4}\right)$ for hollow shafts	
The angular deformation	$\theta = \dfrac{TL}{JG}$ rad $= \dfrac{584TL}{Gd^4}$ deg., for solid shaft	3.2
	$= \dfrac{584TL}{G(d_o^4 - d_i^4)}$ deg., for hollow shafts	
The torque to be transmitted by the shaft N-mm	$\left.\begin{aligned} T &= \dfrac{10^6 P}{\omega} \\ T &= \dfrac{9.55 \times 10^6 (P)}{n} \end{aligned}\right\}$ SI Units	3.3(a)
The torque transmitted by the shaft, kgf mm	$\left.\begin{aligned} T &= \dfrac{75 \times 10^3 (MHP)}{\omega} \\ &= \dfrac{7.16 \times 10^5 (MHP)}{n} \\ &= \dfrac{9.74 \times 10^5 (P)}{n} \end{aligned}\right\}$ Metric Units	3.3(b)
Hollow shaft:[*]		
The outside diameter of hollow shaft subjected to simple torsion	$d_o = \left[\dfrac{16T}{\pi \tau_d}\left(\dfrac{1}{1-K^4}\right)\right]^{\frac{1}{3}}$	3.4(a)
Out side diameter of hollow shaft subjected to simple bending	$d_o = \left[\dfrac{32M}{\pi \sigma_d}\left(\dfrac{1}{1-K^4}\right)\right]^{\frac{1}{3}}$	3.4(b)
	where $\tau_d = \dfrac{\tau_e B}{RK_s}$ and $\sigma_d = \dfrac{\sigma_e B}{RK_t}$	
The outside diameter of hollow shaft subjected to combined bending and torsion.	R is reliability factor Table 2.7 B is the size factor (Eqn. 2.9(b))	
a) According to maximum normal stress theory	$d_o = \left[\dfrac{16}{\pi \sigma_{\max}}\left(M + \sqrt{M^2 + T^2}\right) \times \left(\dfrac{1}{1-K^4}\right)\right]^{\frac{1}{3}}$	3.5(a)
b) According to maximum shear stress theory	$d_o = \left[\dfrac{16}{\pi \tau_{max}}\left(\sqrt{M^2 + T^2}\right) \times \left(\dfrac{1}{1-K^4}\right)\right]^{\frac{1}{3}}$	3.5(b)

[*]For solid shafts, substitute $K = 0$ and $d_0 = d$ in the above equaitons.

Particular	Equation	Eqn. No.

ASME Code for design of transmission shafting:

(a) According to maximum normal stress theory

$$d_o = \left[\frac{16}{\pi \sigma_{max}} \left(C_m M + \sqrt{(C_m M)^2 + (C_t T)^2} \right) \times \left(\frac{1}{1 - K^4} \right) \right]^{\frac{1}{3}}$$

3.6(a)

(b) According to maximum shear stress theory

$$d_o = \left[\frac{16}{\pi \tau_{max}} \left(\sqrt{(C_m M)^2 + (C_t T)^2} \right) \times \left(\frac{1}{1 - K^4} \right) \right]^{\frac{1}{3}}$$

3.6(b)

For fluctuating loads:

(a) According to maximum normal stress theory

$$d_o = \left[\frac{16}{\pi \sigma_{max}} \left(\left(M_m + \frac{K_t \sigma_{yp}}{\sigma_{en}} M_a \right) + \sqrt{\left(M_m + \frac{K_t \sigma_{yp}}{\sigma_{en}} M_a \right)^2 + \left(T_m + \frac{K_s \sigma_{yp}}{\sigma_{en}} T_a \right)^2} \right) \times \left(\frac{1}{1 - K^4} \right) \right]^{\frac{1}{3}}$$

3.7(a)

(b) According to maximum shear stress theory

$$d_o = \left[\frac{16}{\pi \tau_{max}} \left(\sqrt{\left(M_m + \frac{K_t \sigma_{yp}}{\sigma_{en}} M_a \right)^2 + \left(T_m + \frac{K_s \sigma_{yp}}{\sigma_{en}} T_a \right)^2} \right) \times \left(\frac{1}{1 - K^4} \right) \right]^{\frac{1}{3}}$$

3.7(b)

(c) According to Mises Hencky theory

$$d_o = \left[\frac{16}{\pi \sigma_{max}} \left(\sqrt{4M_m^2 + 3T_m^2} + \frac{K_t \sigma_{yp}}{\sigma_{en}} \sqrt{4M_a^2 + 3T_a^2} \right) \times \left(\frac{1}{1 - K^4} \right) \right]^{\frac{1}{3}}$$

3.7(c)

The out side diameter of hollow shaft subjected to an axial load F in addition to the torsional and bending loads.

(a) According to the maximum normal stress theory

$$d_o = \left[\frac{16}{\pi \sigma_{max}} \left\{ \left(C_m M + \frac{\alpha F d_o (1 + K^2)}{8} \right) + \sqrt{\left(C_m M + \frac{\alpha F d_o (1 + K^2)}{8} \right)^2 + (C_t T)^2} \right\} \times \left(\frac{1}{1 - K^4} \right) \right]^{\frac{1}{3}}$$

3.8(a)

(b) According to maximum shear stress theory

$$d_o = \left[\frac{16}{\pi \tau_{max}} \left\{ \sqrt{\left(C_m M + \frac{\alpha F d_o (1 + K^2)}{8} \right)^2 + (C_t T)^2} \right\} \times \left(\frac{1}{1 - K^4} \right) \right]^{\frac{1}{3}}$$

3.8(b)

Particular	Equation	Eqn. No.

where α = ratio of the maximum intensity of stress resulting from the axial load, to the average axial stress from Table 3.2

$$= \frac{1}{1 - 0.0044(L/k)} \text{ when } L/k < 115$$

$$= \frac{\sigma_{yp}}{n\pi^2 E}(L/k)^2 \text{ when } L/k > 115 \quad \text{(Euler's formula)}$$

where L is the length between supporting bearings, mm

k is the radius of gyration of the shaft, mm

σ_{yp} is the yield stress in compression, MN/m^2 (kgf/mm^2)

E is the modulus of elasticity, MN/m^2 (kgf/mm^2)

n = constant for the type of column end support,

= 1.0, for free end supports or hinged ends

= 2.25, for fixed ends

= 1.60, for both ends pinned, guided and partly restrained

Particular	Equation	Eqn. No.
The relation between the diameter of a solid shaft to a hollow shaft if their torsional strengths are equal	$d_o^3 = \dfrac{d^3}{1 - K^4}$	3.9

Effect of keyways:

Particular	Equation	Eqn. No.
H.F. Moore's formula for determining the shaft strength factor or the ratio of strength of shaft with keyway to the same shaft without keyway	$K_e = 1.0 - \dfrac{0.2b}{d} - \dfrac{1.1h}{d}$	3.10
Moore's formula for determining the ratio of the angular twist of the shaft with the key way to the same shaft without keyway	$K_e = 1.0 + 0.4\dfrac{b}{d} + 0.7\dfrac{h}{d}$	3.11

where b and h are width and depth of keyway, mm

Crank Shaft:

Forces on crank arm: (Fig. 3.1)

Particular	Equation	Eqn. No.
The force on the connecting rod	$F_c = \dfrac{F_p}{\cos\phi}$	3.12(a)
The tangential force or the rotative effort on the crank	$F_t = F_c \sin(\theta + \phi) = F_p \dfrac{\sin(\theta + \phi)}{\cos\phi}$	3.12(b)
The radial force along the crank	$F_r = F_c \cos(\theta + \phi) = F_p \dfrac{\cos(\theta + \phi)}{\cos\phi}$	3.12(c)
The diameter of the crank pin at the root (Fig. 3.2)	$d_{p1} = \sqrt[4]{\dfrac{16F_c^2}{\pi p_{bc}\sigma_b}}$	3.13(a)
The diameter of the crank pin or journal	$d_p = (d_{p1})$ to $(d_{p1} + 6.5\text{mm})$	3.13(b)

Particular	Equation	Eqn. No.
The length of the crank pin	$l_p = \dfrac{F_c}{d_{p1} p_{bc}}$	3.14
The diameter of the crank shaft at the root	$d_s = \sqrt[3]{\dfrac{16 F_c r}{\pi \tau_d}}$	3.15(a)
The diameter of the crank shaft or journal	$(d_{s1}) = d_s$ to $(d_s + 6.5\text{mm})$	3.15(b)
The length of the main bearing	$l_s = \dfrac{1.2 F_t}{d_s p_{bs}}$	3.15(c)
The diameter of the crank pin according to American Bureau of shipping method (Fig. 3.3)	$d_p = a\sqrt[3]{\dfrac{D^2 pc}{\sigma_d}}$	3.16

where a is the coefficient from Table 3.8

D is the diameter of cylinder bore, mm

p is the maximum gas pressure, MN/m^2 (kgf/mm^2)

c is the distance over the crank web plus 25 mm (Fig. 3.3)

σ_d is the allowable stress, MN/m^2 (kgf/mm^2)

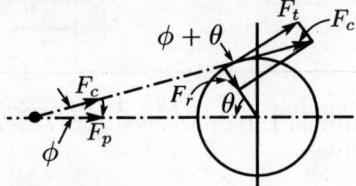

Fig. 3.1: *Forces on crank arm*

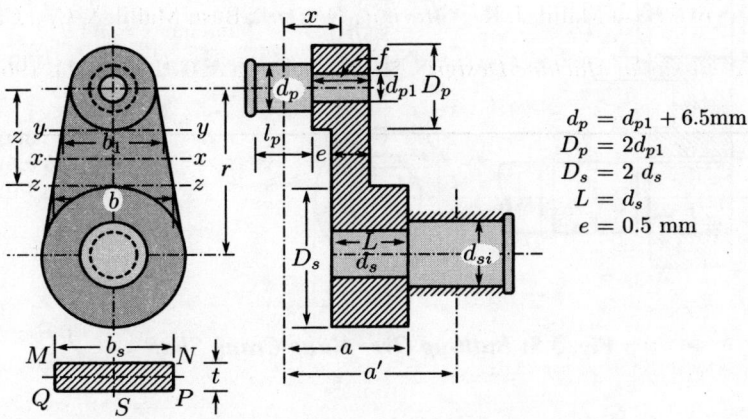

$d_p = d_{p1} + 6.5\text{mm}$
$D_p = 2 d_{p1}$
$D_s = 2\, d_s$
$L = d_s$
$e = 0.5$ mm

Fig. 3.2: *Typical Built-up Over Hung Crank Shaft*

Particular	Equation	Eqn. No.
Torsion of rectangular bars:		
Shear stress at the point A_1 (Fig. 3.4)	$T_1 = \dfrac{T}{\alpha_1 bc^2}$	3.17(a)
Shear stress at the point A_2 (Fig. 3.4)	$T_2 = \dfrac{T}{\alpha_2 bc^2}$	3.17(b)
The angle of twist, θ radians per mm of length where α_1, α_2 and β are constants, from Table 3.7	$\theta = \dfrac{T}{\beta Gbc^3}$	3.17(c)

Fig. 3.4

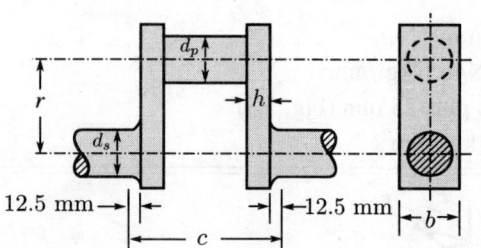

Fig. 3.3: *American Bureau of Shipping Method*

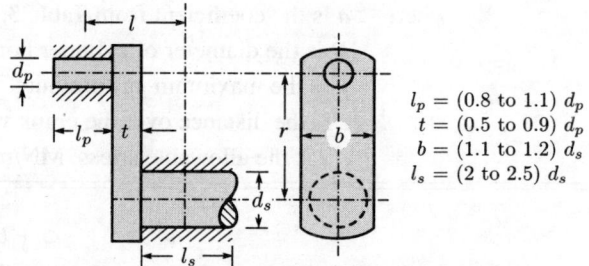

Fig. 3.4: *Forged Over Hung Crank Shaft*

$l_p = (0.8 \text{ to } 1.1)\, d_p$
$t = (0.5 \text{ to } 0.9)\, d_p$
$b = (1.1 \text{ to } 1.2)\, d_s$
$l_s = (2 \text{ to } 2.5)\, d_s$

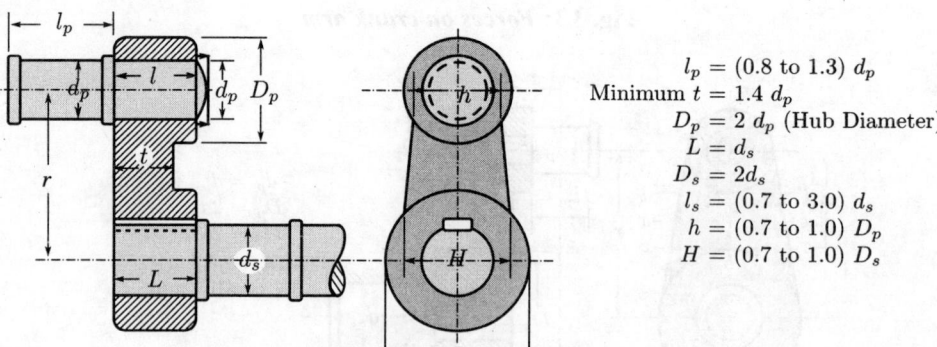

$l_p = (0.8 \text{ to } 1.3)\, d_p$
Minimum $t = 1.4\, d_p$
$D_p = 2\, d_p$ (Hub Diameter)
$L = d_s$
$D_s = 2d_s$
$l_s = (0.7 \text{ to } 3.0)\, d_s$
$h = (0.7 \text{ to } 1.0)\, D_p$
$H = (0.7 \text{ to } 1.0)\, D_s$

Fig. 3.5: *Built-up Over Hung Crank Shaft*

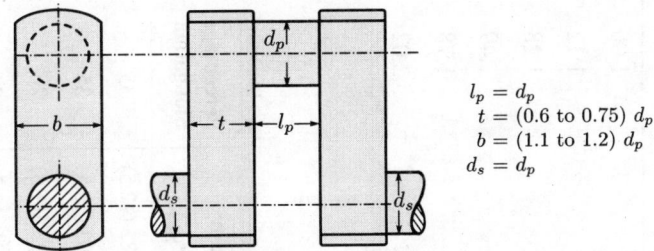

$l_p = d_p$
$t = (0.6 \text{ to } 0.75)\, d_p$
$b = (1.1 \text{ to } 1.2)\, d_p$
$d_s = d_p$

Fig. 3.6: *Forged Centre Crank*

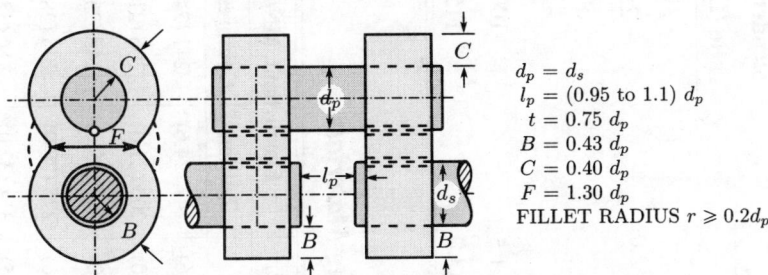

$d_p = d_s$
$l_p = (0.95 \text{ to } 1.1)\, d_p$
$t = 0.75\, d_p$
$B = 0.43\, d_p$
$C = 0.40\, d_p$
$F = 1.30\, d_p$
FILLET RADIUS $r \geqslant 0.2 d_p$

Fig. 3.7: *Buit-up Centre Crank Shaft*

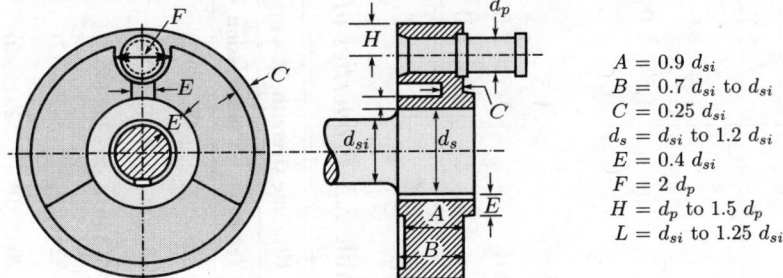

$A = 0.9\, d_{si}$
$B = 0.7\, d_{si} \text{ to } d_{si}$
$C = 0.25\, d_{si}$
$d_s = d_{si} \text{ to } 1.2\, d_{si}$
$E = 0.4\, d_{si}$
$F = 2\, d_p$
$H = d_p \text{ to } 1.5\, d_p$
$L = d_{si} \text{ to } 1.25\, d_{si}$

Fig. 3.8: *Cast Iron Crank Disc*

References

[1] Vallance A., Doughtie V. L., *"Design of Machine Members"*, 3rd edition, McGraw Hill Book Co. 1951.

[2] Spotts M. E., *"Design of Machine Elements"*, 3rd edition, Prentice Hall, Inc., Maruzen Co., Ltd.

[3] Bhattacharya S. C., Basu Mallik, J.R., *"Machine Design"*, basu Mallik & Co., Calcutta, 1966

[4] Low D. A., *"A Pocket Book for Mechanical Engineers"*, Longmans, Freen & Co., Ltd., London, 1955.

[5] Siegel M. J., Maleev V. L., Hartman J. B., *"Mechanical Design of Machines"*, 4th edition, International Text Book Company, 1965.

Table 3.1 *Constants for ASME Code (Shock and Endurance Factors)*

Nature of Loading	Value for	
	C_m	C_t
Stationary Shafts :		
Gradually applied load	1.0	1.0
Suddenly applied load	1.5 to 2.0	1.5 to 2.0
Rotating Shafts :		
Steady or gradually applied loads	1.5	1.0
Suddenly applied loads, minor shocks only	1.5 to 2.0	1.0 to 1.5
Suddenly applied loads, heavy shocks	2.0 to 3.0	1.5 to 3.0

Table 3.2 *Value of α to use in Equation 3.8(a) and 3.8(b)*

Slenderness ratio (L/k)	Factor, α
0	1.00
25	1.12
50	1.28
75	1.49
100	1.78
115	2.02

Table 3.3 *Properties of Shafting Materials*

Material	Percentage carbon	Ultimate strength, MN/m² (kgf/mm²)			Elastic limit, MN/m² (kgf/mm²)			Percentage Elongation
		Tension	Compression	Shear	Tension	Compression	Shear	
Commercial Cold rolled ...	0.10–0.25	482 (49.2)	482 (49.2)	241 (24.6)	241 (24.6)	241 (24.6)	122 (12.5)	35
Commercial turned ...	0.10–0.25	412 (42.0)	412 (42.0)	206 (21.0)	206 (21.0)	206 (21.0)	103 (10.5)	35
Hot rolled or forged ...	0.15–0.25	451 (46.0)	451 (46.0)	225 (23.0)	245 (25.0)	245 (25.0)	113 (11.5)	26
	0.25–0.35	482 (49.2)	482 (49.2)	241 (24.6)	275 (28.0)	275 (28.0)	121 (12.3)	24
	0.35–0.45	520 (53.0)	520 (53.0)	260 (26.5)	314 (32.0)	314 (32.0)	130 (13.2)	22
	0.45–0.55	553 (56.4)	553 (56.4)	276 (28.2)	345 (35.2)	345 (35.2)	138 (14.1)	20
$3\frac{1}{2}$% Nickel ...	0.15–0.25	588 (60.0)	588 (60.0)	294 (30.0)	392 (39.0)	382 (39.0)	147 (15.0)	26
Chrome Vandium ...	0.25–0.35	620 (63.2)	620 (63.2)	310 (31.6)	414 (42.2)	414 (42.2)	155 (15.8)	25

Table 3.4 *Fatigue Stress concentration Factors in bending for shafts with keyways based on section modulus of full area*

Steel	Tensile strength, MN/m^2 (kgf/ mm^2)	Yield strength (Plastic deformation 0.2%), MN/m^2 (kgf/mm^2)	For reversed bending stress	Chrome Nikel Heat treated		Medium Carbon normalised	
				σ_{en} MN/m^2 (kgf/mm^2)	K_{tf}	σ_{en} MN/m^2 (kgf/mm^2)	K_{tf}
Carbon Nickel (about SAE 3 140)	714.0 (72.8)	482.5 (49.2)	No Keyway ordinary tapered specimen	400.0 (40.0)	..	255.0 (26.0)	..
	–	–	Sledrunner keyway	248.0 (25.3)	1.61	193.0 (19.7)	1.32
	–	–	Profiled keyway	193.0 (19.7)	2.07	159.0 (16.2)	1.61
Medium Carbon (about SAE 1045)	552.0 (56.3)	310.0 (31.6)	Profiled Keyway 6.25mm transverse hole	–	–	83.0 (8.5)	3.06

Table 3.5 *(a) Standard shaft sizes in mm*

6	8	10	12	14	16	18	20	22	25	28	32
36	40	45	50	56	63	71	80	90	100	110	125
140	160	180	200	220	240	260	280	300	320	340	360
380	400	420	440	450	480	500	530	560	600	–	–

Table 3.5 *(b) Maximum Permissible Working Stresses for Shafts*

Grade of shafting	Simple bending MN/m^2 (kgf/mm^2)	Simple torsion MN/m^2 (kgf/mm^2)	Combined stress MN/m^2 (kgf/mm^2)
"Commercial Steel" shafting without allowance for keyways	110 (11.2)	55(5.6)	55(5.6)
"Commercial Steel" shafting with allowance for keyways	83 (8.5)	41 (4.2)	41(4.2)
Steel purchased under definite specification (without keyways)*	60% of the elastic limit but not over 36% of the ultimate in tension.	30% of the elastic limit but not over 18% of the ultimate in tension.	30% of the elastic limit but not over 18% of the ultimate in tension.

*The values are to be reduced by 25% if keyways are present.

Table 3.6 *Allowable bearing pressure*

Class of work	Main bearing pressure p_{bs}, MN/m² (kgf/mm²)	Crank pin pressure p_{bc}, MN/m² (kgf/mm²)
Automobile Engines	10.0—13.5 (1.0-1.40)	2.5—2.75 (0.25-0.28)
Diesel Engines	5.5—7.0 (0.56-0.70)	7.0—8.5 (0.70-0.85)
Marine Diesel Engines	2.75—3.5 (0.28-0.35)	7.0—10.0 (0.70-1.00)
Rail road, locomotive	1.2—1.4 (0.12-0.14)	10.0—12.0 (1.05-1.20)
Shear and punches, slow speed	20.5—27.5 (2.10-2.80)	34.0—54.0 (3.50-5.50)

Table 3.7 *Constant for torsion of rectangular bars*

b/c	1.00	1.20	1.50	1.75	2.00	2.50	3.00
α_1	0.208	0.210	0.231	0.239	0.246	0.258	0.267
α_2	0.208	0.235	0.269	0.291	0.309	0.336	0.355
β	0.141	0.116	0.196	0.214	0.229	0.249	0.263
b/c	4.00	5.00	6.00	8.00	10.00	∞	–
α_1	0.282	0.291	0.299	0.307	0.312	0.333	–
α_2	0.378	0.392	0.402	0.414	0.421	–	–
β	0.281	0.291	0.299	0.307	0.312	0.333	–

Table 3.8 *Coefficient 'a' in the American Bureau of Shipping Formula 3.16*

Type	Number of *cylinder*		Ratio of stroke to distance over crank webs = L/c							
	Four stroke	Two stroke	0.7	0.8	0.9	1.0	1.1	1.2	1.3	1.4
Explosion engines	1,2,4	1,2	1.17	1.17	1.17	1.17	1.17	1.17	1.17	1.17
	3,5,6	3	1.17	1.17	1.17	1.17	1.19	1.20	1.22	1.24
	8	4	1.17	1.19	1.21	1.23	1.25	1.28	1.30	1.32
	10,11,12	5,6	1.18	1.20	1.23	1.25	1.28	1.31	1.33	1.35
Air-injection diesel engines	1,2,4	1,2	1.17	1.19	1.22	1.25	1.28	1.31	1.34	1.36
	3,5,6,	3	1.19	1.22	1.25	1.28	1.32	1.35	1.38	1.41
	8	4	1.20	1.24	1.27	1.30	1.33	1.37	1.40	1.43
	12	5,6	1.22	1.25	1.29	1.32	1.36	1.39	1.42	1.45
	16	8	1.25	1.29	1.33	1.36	1.40	1.44	1.47	1.50

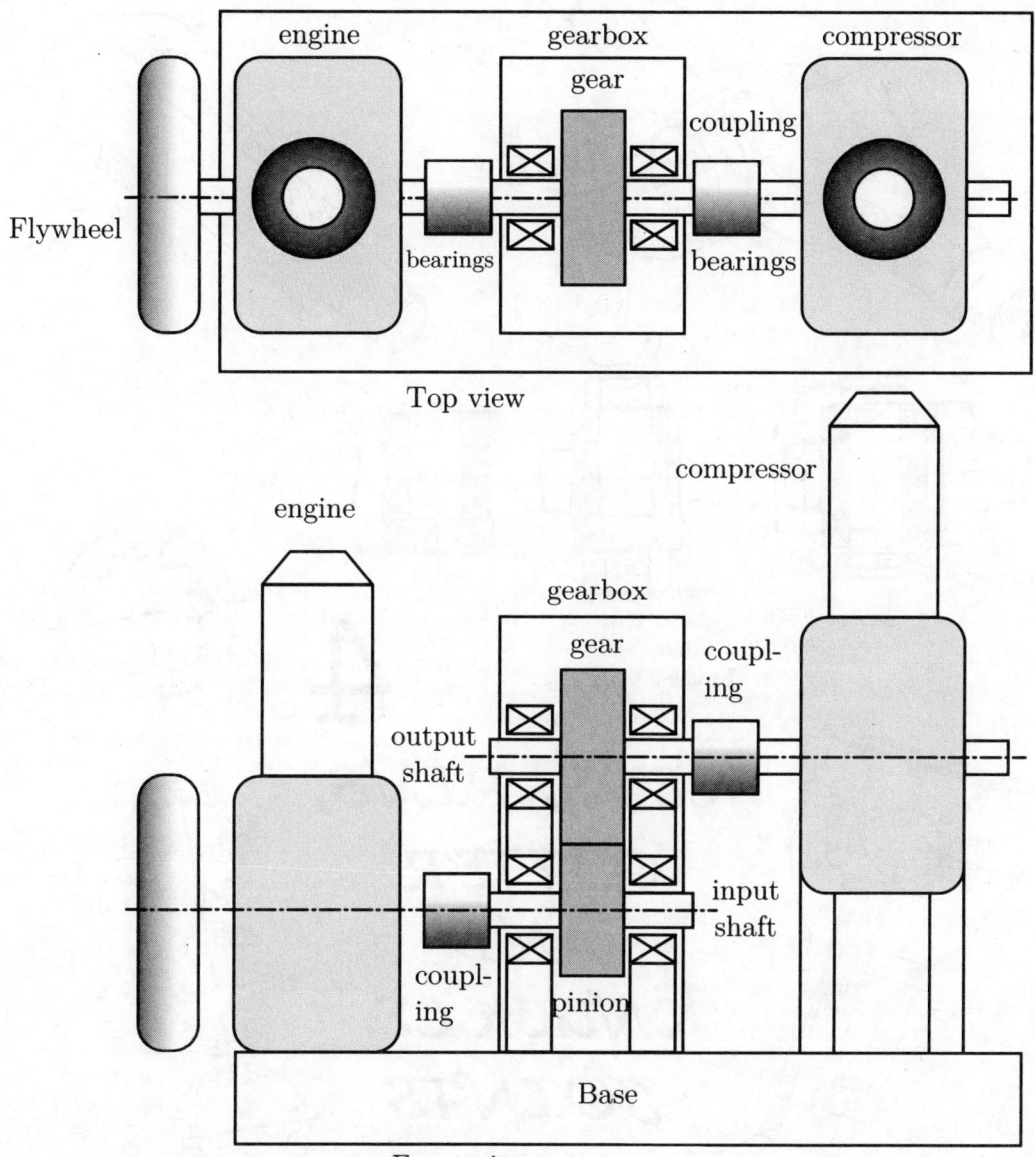

Schematic diagram of Gasoline-Engine-Powered Portable Air Compressor, Gearbox, Couplings, Shafts and Bearings.

Note: Excerpted from Norton, Machine Design Pearson Education (Singapore) Pvt. Ltd., Delhi.

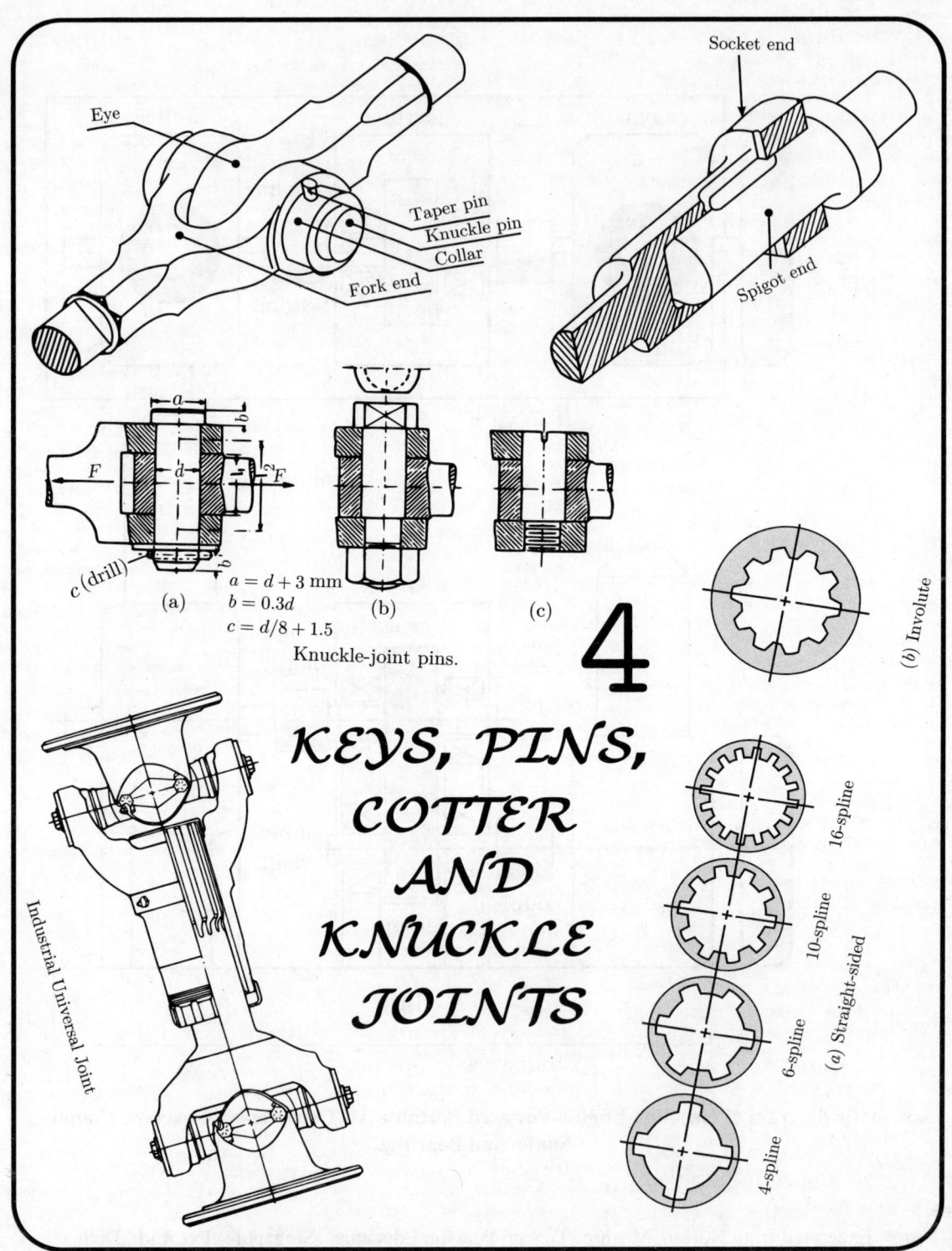

Eye

Taper pin
Knuckle pin
Collar

Fork end

Socket end

Spigot end

$a = d + 3$ mm
$b = 0.3d$
$c = d/8 + 1.5$

a

b

F

d

F

c (drill)

(a)

(b)

(c)

Knuckle-joint pins.

4

KEYS, PINS,
COTTER
AND
KNUCKLE
JOINTS

Industrial Universal Joint

(b) Involute

16-spline

10-spline

6-spline

4-spline

(a) Straight-sided

4

Keys, Pins, Cotter and Knuckle Joints

Symbols	Description and Units
b	width of key, mm
d	diameter of the shaft, mm
d_p	diameter of the pin, mm
F	pressure between the hub and the shaft, N (kgf)
F_t	circumferential force, N (kgf)
h	thickness of key, mm
l	length of key, mm
p	tangential pressure per unit length, MN/m^2 (kgf/mm^2)
p_1	maximum pressure where the shaft enters the hub, MN/m^2 (kgf/mm^2)
p_2	pressure at the end of key, MN/m^2 (kgf/mm^2)
T	Torque, N mm (kgf-mm)
σ_{b1}	nominal bearing stress at the dangerous point, MN/m^2 (kgf/mm^2)
τ_1	nominal shear stress at the dangerous point, MN/m^2 (kgf/mm^2)
μ_1	coefficient of friction between the shaft and the hub
μ_2	coefficient of friction on both the top and bottom surfaces of the key

Particular	Equation	Eqn. No.
Square and Rectangular keys: (Fig. 4.1(a)) (Table 4.1)		
The width of the square key	$b = \frac{1}{4}d$	4.1
The width of the rectangular key	$b = \frac{1}{4}d$	4.2(a)
The height of the rectangular key	$h = \frac{1}{6}d$	4.2(b)
a) *Crushing strength:*		
The tangential pressure per unit length of the key at any intermediate distance l_x from the hub edge (Fig. 4.1(b))	$p = p_1 - l_x \tan \alpha$	4.3

Particular	Equation	Eqn. No.
	where $\tan \alpha = \dfrac{p_1 - p}{l_x} = \dfrac{p_1 - p_2}{l_z} = \dfrac{p_1 - p_2}{l} = \dfrac{p_1}{l_o}$	
Torque transmitted by the key can be expressed by the equation	$T = \frac{1}{2} p_1 dl - \dfrac{dl^2}{r} \tan \alpha$	4.4(a)
The general equation for torgue transmitted	$T = \frac{1}{4} \sigma_{b1} hdl - \frac{1}{18} \sigma_{b1} hl^2$	4.4(b)
	when $p_2 = 0$ and $l = l_o = 2.25d$	
	$\tan \alpha = p_1/l_o = \dfrac{\sigma_{b1} h}{4.5d}$	4.4(c)
b) *Strength in shear:*		
The general expression for torque transmitted	$T = \frac{1}{2} \tau_1 bdl - \frac{1}{9} \tau_1 bl^2$	4.5(a)
	when $\tan \alpha = \dfrac{p_1}{l_o} = \dfrac{\tau_1 b}{2.25d}$	4.5(b)
	where $\tau_1 = \dfrac{T}{lb(0.5d - 0.11l)}$	4.5(c)
2) *Taper keys: (Table 4.2)*		
The relation involving the circumferential force F_t and the pressure F between the shaft and hub (Fig. 4.2)	$F_t = \mu_1 F$	4.6
	where $\mu_1 = 0.25$, coefficient of friction between the shaft and hub	
The pressure F between the shaft and hub	$F = blp$	4.7

where p is the pressure, or compressive stress in the key, MN/m^2 (kgf/mm^2)

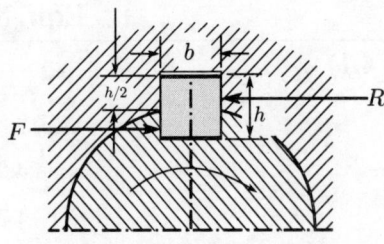

Fig. 4.1(a): *Rectangular Key*

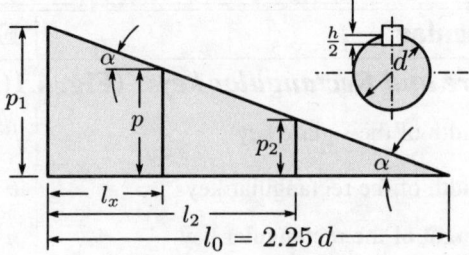

Fig. 4.1(b): *Pressures between key and key seat*

Particular	Equation	Eqn. No.
The relation between the torque T and the force F_t	$T = \frac{1}{2}F_t d = \frac{1}{2}\mu_1 blpd$	4.8
The necessary key length	$l = \dfrac{2T}{\mu_1 bpd}$	4.9
The axial effort F_a necessary to drive the key home (Fig. 4.2)	$F_a = H + R = 2F\mu_2 + F\tan\beta = 0.21\ pbl$	4.10

where $\mu_2 = 0.10 \tan\beta = 0.0104$, if the taper is 10.5 mm/metre

3) Friction of Feather keys: (Fig. 4.3)

a) *One feather key:*

If one feather key is used, the torque	$T = F_{t_1} a$	4.11(a)
Circumferential force due to the torque T	$F_{t_1} = T/a$	4.11(b)
The two opposite forces F_1' and F_1'', applied in the centre plane	$F_1' = F_1'' = F_{t_1}$	4.11(c)
When the hub is shifted lengthwise, the resistance on the key and on the shaft	$R_1 = \mu F_{t1} + \mu_2 F_1' = 2\mu F_1' = 2\mu F_{t_1} = 2\mu\dfrac{T}{a}$ where $\mu \approx \mu_2$	4.11(d)

b) *Two feather keys:*

If two feather keys are used, the torque	$T = F_{t_2} a + F_{t2} a = 2F_{t2} a$	4.12(a)
	From which $F_{t2} = \dfrac{1}{2}F_{t1}$	4.12(b)
The opposite forces applied in the centre plane	$F_2' = F_2'' = F_{t_2}$	4.12(c)
Circumferential force due to torque	$F_{t_2} = \dfrac{T}{2a}$	4.12(d)
When the hub is shifted lengthwise, the resistance on the key and shaft	$R_2 = 2\mu\, F_{t_2} = 2\mu\left(\dfrac{T}{2a}\right) = \dfrac{1}{2}R_1$	4.12(e)

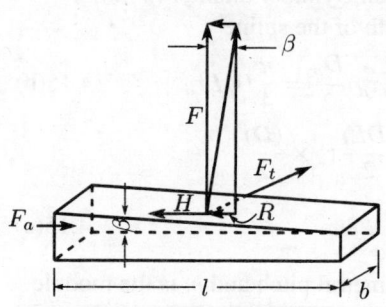

Fig. 4.2: *Diagram of forces acting on a taper key*

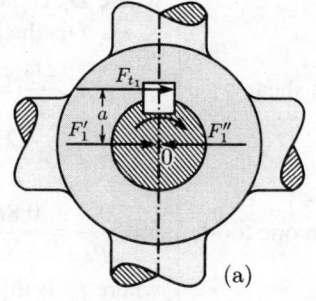
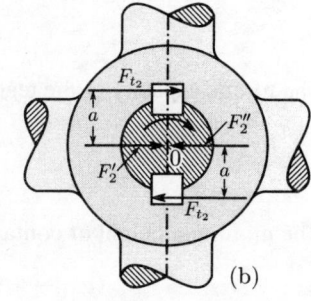

Fig. 4.3: *Feather keys*

Particular	Equation	Eqn. No.
Round Taper Pin Keys: (Table 4.3(a) and (b))		
Large diameter of the pin key	$d_p = 1.9\sqrt{d}$ to $2.2\sqrt{d}$	4.13(a)
The diameter d_s at the small end can be found by the relation	$d_s = d_p - 0.028l$ where d_p is the diameter at large end	4.13(b)
The mean diameter of the pin	$d_m = 0.20d$ to $0.25d$	4.13(c)

Parallel Side Splines/Straight sided splines (Table 4.4)

In case of Integral multiple Shaft, the torque Transmitted between the sides of spline	$T = \frac{1}{2}p_b h l N(D - h)$	4.14

where D is the diameter of the shaft, mm

h is the height of the spline, mm

$h = h_{min}h_1$, for press fit or permanent fit

$h = 1.5h_1$, for close fit (hub to slide when not under load)

$h = 2h_1$, for close fit (hub to slide when under load)

p_b is the allowable bearing pressure, MN/m^2 (kgf/mm^2)

$p_b = 7$ MN/m^2 (kgf/mm^2), for sliding fit

$\quad = 14$ MN/m^2 (kgf/mm^2), for close fit

$\quad = 21$ MN/m^2 (kgf/mm^2), for press fit

N is the number of splines

L is the engaged length of each spline, mm

Involute Splines (Table 4.5)

The area of resisting shear	$A_s = \dfrac{\pi D_p L}{2}$ where D_p is the pitch Cylinder diamter in mm $\qquad L$ is the length of the spline	4.15(a)
The torque capacity of the teeth in shear	$T = F_s\dfrac{D_p}{2} = (A_s\tau_d)\dfrac{D_p}{2} = \dfrac{\pi}{4}D_p^2 L\tau_d$ $T = F_s \times \dfrac{D}{2} = \dfrac{(DL)}{2}\tau_d \times \dfrac{(D)}{2}$	4.15(b)
The minimum height of contact on one tooth	$h = \dfrac{0.8}{p_d} = \dfrac{0.8D}{N} = 0.8m$ where p_d is the diametral pitch and m is the module	4.15(c)

Particular	Equation	Eqn. No.
Area of contact of all 'N' teeth	$A_c = \dfrac{(0.8D_p)}{N}(LN) = 0.8DL$	4.16(d)
The torque capacity of spline in bearing stress	$T_b = (0.8D_pL)\left(\dfrac{D_p}{2}\right)\sigma_b$ $= (0.8D_pL)\left(\dfrac{D_p}{2}\right)2\sigma_{dc}$ $= 0.8D_p^2L\sigma_{dc}$ where $\sigma_b = 2\sigma_{dc}$, bearing stress σ_{dc} is the allowable stress in compression	4.15(e)
Torque capacity	$T = \dfrac{\pi}{16}D^3T_d$	4.15(f)
Assuming only about 25 percent of the teeth are in actual contact, the length of the spline (Equating torque from equations 4.16(b) and 4.16(f))	$L = D_p$	4.15(g)

Cotter Joint: (Fig. 4.4)

a) *Design of the rod:*

Particular	Equation	Eqn. No.
The tearing resistance of the solid rod	$P = \dfrac{\pi}{4}d^2\sigma_t$	4.16(a)
The resistance of cotter and rod end to crushing	$P = d_1t\sigma_c$	4.16(b)
The tearing resistance of the rod end through the cotter hole	$P = \left(\dfrac{\pi}{4}d_1^2 - d_1t\right)\sigma_t$	4.16(c)
When the joint is in compression the resistance of collar in compression	$P = \dfrac{\pi}{4}(d_2^2 - d_1^2)\sigma_c$	4.16(d)
The resistance of thrust collar to shearing	$P = \pi d_1t_1\tau$	4.16(e)
Equating the bending moment on the collar to the resistance moment, the thickness of the collar	$t_1 = \left[\dfrac{3}{2}\dfrac{P(d_2 - d_1)}{\pi d_1\sigma_b}\right]^{\frac{1}{2}}$	4.16(f)
The shearing resistance of the rod end	$P = 2d_1l_1\tau'$	4.16(g)

	Symbol	Proportions used in practice
Diameter of rod end	d_1	$1.25d$
Thickness of cotter	t	$0.25d_1$
Width of cotter	$B = b$	$1.25d_1$ or $5t$
Diameter of the socket	D	$2.00d_1$
Diameter of socket across cotter note	D_1	$1.75d$ to $2.00d$
Diameter of the collar	d_2	$1.5d$
Length	l_1 and l	$0.75d$ to $1.25d$
Thickness of the collar	t_1	$0.50d$
Thickness of socket end	t_2	$0.50d$
Clearance	C	2mm to 3mm
Diameter of solid rod	d	–

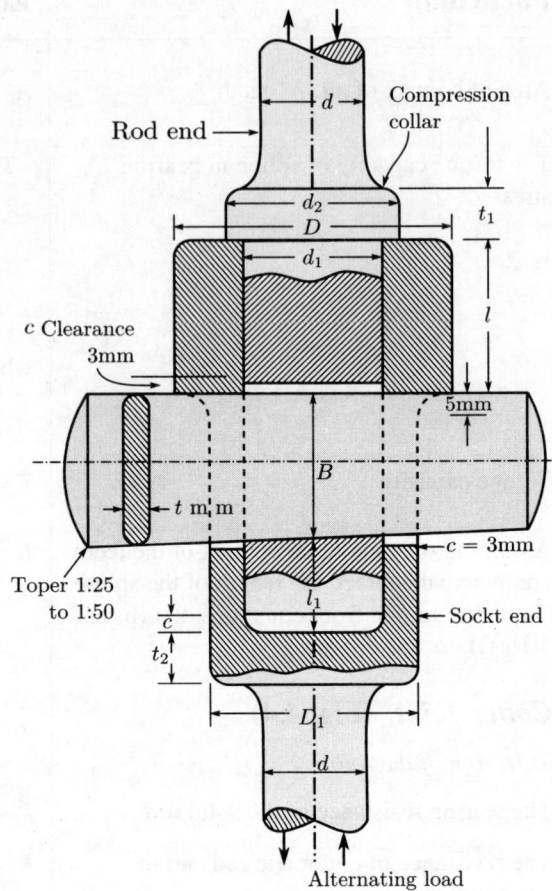

Fig. 4.4: *Cotter Joint*

σ_c allowable crushing stress, MN/m^2 (kgf/mm^2)

σ_b allowable bending stress, MN/m^2 (kgf/mm^2)

σ_t allowable tensile stress, MN/m^2 (kgf/mm^2)

τ allowable shear stress, MN/m^2 (kgf/mm^2)

τ' allowable shear stress parallel with fibre, MN/m^2 (kgf/mm^2)

Particular	Equation	Eqn. No.
b) *Design of the socket:*		
The tearing resistance of the socket end through the cotter hole	$P = \left[\dfrac{\pi}{4}(D_1^2 - d_1^2) - (D_1 - d_1)t\right]\sigma_t$	4.17(a)
The resistance of cotter and socket end to crushing	$P = (D - d_1)t\sigma_c$	4.17(b)
The shearing resistance of socket end in front of cotter	$P = 2(D - d_1)l\tau'$	4.17(c)
The diameter of the socket end	$D \geq 2d_1$	4.17(d)
The shearing resistance of the solid rod from the socket end	$P = \pi d t_2 \tau'$	4.17(e)
c) *Design of cotter:*		
The shearing resistance of the cotter	$P = 2bt\tau$	4.18(a)
Equating the maximum bending moment to resisting moment	$P = \dfrac{4}{3}\dfrac{tb^2\sigma_b}{D}$	4.18(b)

Design of Knuckle Joint: (Fig. 4.5)

Particular	Equation	Eqn. No.
Tearing resistance of the tod	$P = \dfrac{\pi}{4}d^2\sigma_t$	4.19(a)
The tearing resistance of the two sections across the fork	$P = 2Ad_2\sigma_t$	4.19(b)
	where $d_2 = S$ = width of the square section, mm	
The resistance to shearing of the pin	$P = \dfrac{\pi}{4}d_1^2\tau \times 2 = \dfrac{\pi}{2}d_1^2\tau$	4.20(a)
The tearing resistance of the square section	$P = d_2^2\sigma_t$	4.20(b)
Equating the shearing resistance of the pin to the tearing resistance of the square section the diameter of the pin	$d_1 = \left[\dfrac{(1.44d^2 \times 2 \times \sigma_t)}{\pi\tau}\right]^{\frac{1}{2}}$	4.20(c)
The tearing resistance of the two sections across the forked and along the plane through the pin axis	$P = 2(D - d_1)B\sigma_t$	4.21(a)
The tearing resistance of the section across the eye and along a plane through the pin axis	$P = F(D - d_1)\sigma_t$	4.21(b)
The resistance of the rod end to crushing	$P = Fd_1\sigma_c$	4.21(c)
The resistance of fork end to crushing	$P = 2Bd_1\sigma_c$	4.21(d)

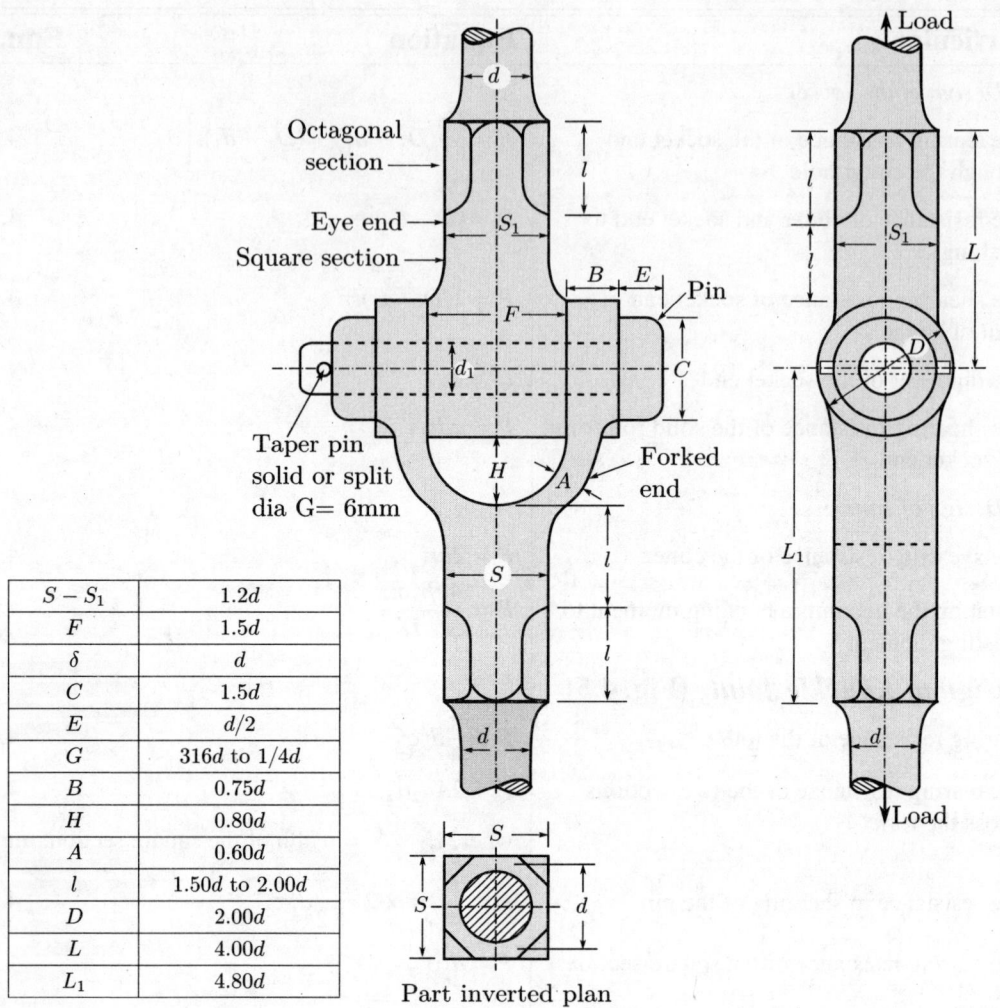

$S - S_1$	$1.2d$
F	$1.5d$
δ	d
C	$1.5d$
E	$d/2$
G	$316d$ to $1/4d$
B	$0.75d$
H	$0.80d$
A	$0.60d$
l	$1.50d$ to $2.00d$
D	$2.00d$
L	$4.00d$
L_1	$4.80d$

Part inverted plan

Fig. 4.5: *Knuckle Joint*

References

[1] Siegel M. J., Maleev V. L., Hartman, J. B., *"Mechanical Design of Machines"*, 4th edition, International Text Book Company, 1965.

[2] Vallance A., Doughtie V. L., *"Design of Machine Members"*, 3rd edition, McGraw Hill Book Company, 1951.

[3] Ghosh A. K., *"Practical Machine Design"*, S. Bhattacharya & Co., Calcutta. 1969.

[4] Bhattacharya S. C., Basu Mallik J. R., *"Machine Design"*, Basu Mallik & Co., Calcutta, 1966.

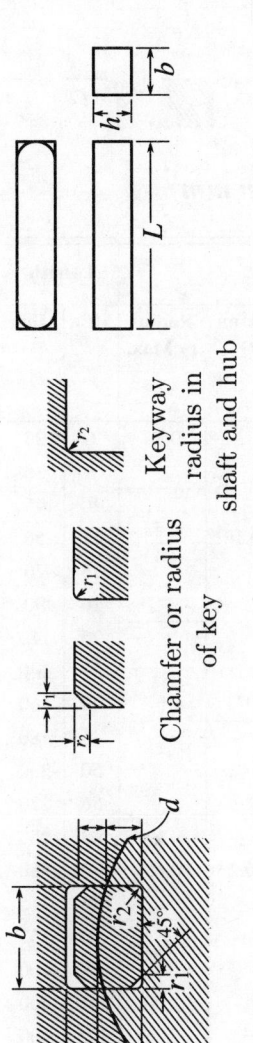

Chamfer or radius of key

Keyway radius in shaft and hub

Table 4.1 Dimensions of Parallel keys and keyways (All Dimensions in mm)

	6	8	10	12	17	22	30	38	44	50	58	65	75	85	95	110	130	150	170	200	230	260	290	330	380	400
For shaft diameters — Up to	8	10	12	17	22	30	38	44	50	58	65	75	85	95	110	130	150	170	200	230	260	290	330	380	400	500
Key cross section — Width b	2	3	4	5	6	8	10	12	14	16	18	20	22	25	28	32	36	40	45	50	56	63	70	80	90	100
Key cross section — Height h	2	3	4	5	6	7	8	8	9	10	11	12	14	14	16	18	20	22	25	28	32	32	36	40	45	50
Keyway depth (nominal) — in shaft t_1	1.2	1.8	2.5	3.0	3.5	4.0	5.0	5.0	5.5	6.0	7.0	7.5	8.5	9.0	10	11	12	13	15	17	19	20	22	25	28	31
Keyway depth (nominal) — in hub t_2	1.0	1.4	1.8	2.3	2.8	3.3	3.3	3.3	3.8	4.3	4.4	4.9	4.9	5.4	6.4	7.4	8.4	9.4	10.4	11.4	12.4	13.4	14.4	15.4	17.4	19.5
Tolerance on t_1				+ 0.1									+ 0.2									+ 0.3				
Keyway depth t_2				+ 0.1									+ 0.2									+ 0.3				
Chamfer or radius r_1 of key — Max		0.25		0.25			0.35				0.55				0.80			1.30			2.00			2.95		
Chamfer or radius r_1 of key — Min		0.16		0.16			0.25				0.40				0.60			1.00			1.60			2.50		
keyway radius r_2 — Max		0.16		0.16			0.25				0.40				0.60			1.00			1.60			2.50		
Length of key L — Min	6	6	8	10	14	18	22	28	36	45	50	56	63	70	80	90	100	110	125	140	160	180	200	220	250	280
Length of key L — Max	20	36	45	56	70	90	110	140	160	180	200	220	250	280	320	360	400	400	400	400	400	400	400	400	400	400

Designation: A Parallel Key of width 10 mm, height 8 mm, and length 50 mm shall be designated as: Parallel Key $10 \times 8 \times 50 \times$ LS:2048

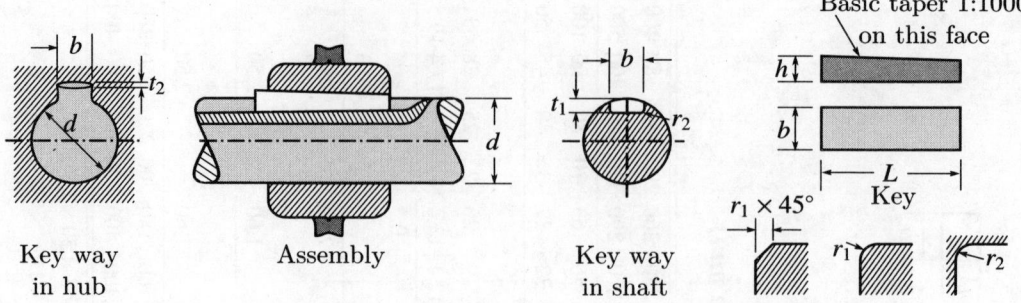

Key way in hub   Assembly   Key way in shaft   Key

Table 4.2 *Taper keys and keyways (All dimensions in mm)*

Shaft Diametre, d		Key			Keyway in Shaft and Hub						Length	
Above	Upto & Includ-ing	Cross Section		Chamfer or Radius r_1 (Min)	Keyway width b (D 10)	Depth in Shaft t_1	Tol. on t_1	Depth in hub t_2	Tol. on t_2	Radius r_2 Max.	Min.	Max.
		Width, b ($h9$)	Height h									
6	8	2	2	0.16	2	1.2	+0.05	0.5		0.16	6	20
8	10	3	3		3	1.8		0.9			8	36
10	12	4	4		4	2.5		1.2			10	45
12	17	5	5	0.25	5	3.0		1.7	+0.10	0.25	12	56
17	22	6	6		6	3.5		2.1			16	70
22	30	8	7		8	4.0	+ 0.1	2.5			20	90
30	38	10	8		10	5.0		2.5			25	110
38	44	12	8		12	5.0		2.5			32	140
44	50	14	9	0.40	14	5.5		2.9			40	160
50	58	16	10		16	6.0		3.4			45	180
58	65	18	11		18	7.0		3.4			50	200
65	75	20	12		20	7.5		3.8			56	220
75	85	22	14		22	8.5		3.8			63	250
85	95	25	14	0.60	25	9.0		4.3	+0.2	0.60	70	280
95	110	28	16		28	10.0		5.3			80	315
110	130	32	18		32	11.0		6.2			90	355
130	150	36	20		36	12.0		7.2			100	400
150	170	40	22	1.00	40	13.0	+0.15	8.2		1.00	110	400
170	200	45	25		45	15.0		9.2			125	400
200	230	50	28		50	17.0		10.1			140	400
230	260	56	32		56	19.0		12.1				
260	290	63	33	1.6	63	20.0		12.1		1.60		
290	330	70	36		70	22.0		13.1	+0.3			
330	380	80	40		80	25.0		14.1				
380	440	90	45	2.5	90	28.0		16.1		2.50		
440	500	100	50		100	31.0		18.1				

IS: 2292-1963

Table 4.3 *(a) Standard right duty Taper Pins*

Small Diameter d_s, mm	Lengths Available mm	Small Diameter d_s, mm	Lengths Available mm	Small Diameter d_s, mm	Lengths Available mm
1.5	8-25	5	20-60	16	40-180
2.0	10-35	6	25-90	20	45-200
2.5	10-35	8	25-130	25	50-200
3.0	12-45	10	30-160	30	55-200
4.0	14-55	12	35-180	40	60-200

Table 4.3 *(b) Standard heavy duty Taper Pins*

Nominal diameter mm	Preferred length mm	Nominal diameter mm	Prefered length mm
1.6	8-25	10	35-150
2.0	10-30	12	35-180
2.5	12-35	16	40-200
3.0	14-45	20	45-200
4.0	16-60	25	60-200
5.0	20-70	32	70-200
6.0	25-90	40	70-200
8.0	30-100	50	80-200

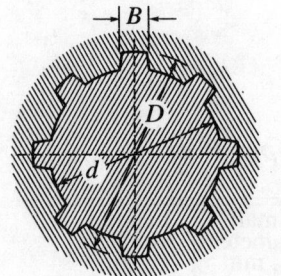

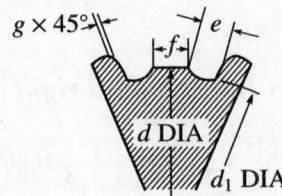

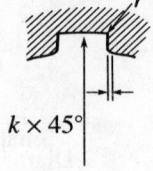

All dimensions in milimetres.

Splined shuft and hub profile   Splined shaft   Splined hub

Table 4.4 *Straight sided splines*

Nominal size $N \times d \times D$	No. of Splines N	Minor Dia d	Major Dia D	Width B	d_1^* Min	e^* Max	f^*	g Max	k Max	r Max	Centering on
Light Duty Series											
$6 \times 23 \times 26$	6	23	26	6	22.1	1.25	3.54	0.3	0.3	0.2	Inside* diameter
$6 \times 26 \times 30$	6	26	30	6	24.6	1.84	3.85	0.3	0.3	0.2	
$6 \times 28 \times 32$	6	28	32	7	26.7	1.77	4.03	0.3	0.3	0.2	
$8 \times 32 \times 36$	8	32	36	6	30.4	1.80	2.71	0.4	0.4	0.3	
$8 \times 36 \times 40$	8	36	40	7	34.5	1.78	3.46	0.4	0.4	0.3	
$8 \times 42 \times 46$	8	42	46	8	40.4	1.68	5.03	0.4	0.4	0.3	
$8 \times 46 \times 50$	8	46	50	9	44.6	1.61	5.75	0.4	0.4	0.3	
$8 \times 52 \times 58$	8	52	58	10	49.7	2.72	4.89	0.5	0.5	0.5	Inside** diameter or flanks
$8 \times 56 \times 68$	8	56	62	10	53.6	2.76	6.38	0.5	0.5	0.5	
$8 \times 62 \times 68$	8	62	68	12	59.8	2.48	7.31	0.5	0.5	0.5	
$10 \times 72 \times 78$	10	72	78	12	69.6	2.54	5.45	0.5	0.5	0.5	
$10 \times 82 \times 88$	10	82	88	12	79.3	2.67	8.62	0.5	0.5	0.5	
$10 \times 92 \times 98$	10	92	98	14	89.4	2.36	10.08	0.5	0.5	0.5	
$10 \times 102 \times 108$	10	102	108	16	99.9	2.23	11.40	0.5	0.5	0.5	
$10 \times 112 \times 120$	10	112	120	18	108.8	3.23	10.72	0.5	0.5	0.5	
Medium Duty Series											
$6 \times 11 \times 14$	6	11	14	3	9.9	1.55	-	0.3	0.3	0.2	Inside* diameter
$6 \times 13 \times 16$	6	13	16	3.5	12.0	1.50	0.32	0.3	0.3	0.2	
$6 \times 16 \times 20$	6	16	20	4	14.5	2.10	0.16	0.3	0.3	0.2	
$6 \times 18 \times 22$	6	18	22	5	16.7	1.93	0.45	0.3	0.3	0.2	
$6 \times 21 \times 25$	6	21	25	5	19.5	1.95	1.95	0.3	0.3	0.2	
$6 \times 23 \times 28$	6	23	28	6	21.3	2.30	1.34	0.3	0.3	0.2	
$6 \times 26 \times 32$	6	26	32	6	23.4	2.94	1.65	0.4	0.4	0.3	
$6 \times 28 \times 34$	6	28	34	7	25.9	2.94	1.70	0.4	0.4	0.3	
$8 \times 32 \times 38$	8	32	38	6	29.4	3.30	0.15	0.4	0.4	0.3	
$8 \times 36 \times 42$	8	36	42	7	33.5	3.01	1.02	0.4	0.4	0.3	
$8 \times 42 \times 48$	8	42	48	8	39.5	2.91	2.57	0.4	0.4	0.3	
$8 \times 46 \times 54$	8	46	54	9	42.7	4.10	0.86	0.5	0.5	0.5	
$8 \times 52 \times 60$	8	52	60	10	48.7	4.00	2.44	0.5	0.5	0.5	Inside** diameter or flanks
$8 \times 56 \times 65$	8	56	65	10	52.2	4.74	2.50	0.5	0.5	0.5	
$8 \times 62 \times 72$	8	62	72	12	57.8	5.00	2.40	0.5	0.5	0.5	
$10 \times 72 \times 82$	10	72	82	12	67.4	5.43	-	0.5	0.5	0.5	
$10 \times 82 \times 92$	10	82	92	12	77.1	5.40	3.00	0.5	0.5	0.5	
$10 \times 92 \times 102$	10	92	102	14	87.3	5.20	4.50	0.5	0.5	0.5	
$10 \times 102 \times 112$	10	102	112	16	97.7	4.00	6.30	0.5	0.5	0.5	
$10 \times 112 \times 125$	10	112	125	18	106.3	6.40	4.40	0.5	0.5	0.5	

*These values are based on the generating process.   IS: 2327-1963
**Inside centering is not always possible with generating processes.

Table 4.5 Dimensions for involute splines for different modules

	D × d	m = 2mm		D × d	m = 3mm		D × d	m = 4mm		D × d	m = 5mm	
		n	t		n	t		n	t		n	t
1)	15 × 11	6	3.603	25 × 19	7	5.117	35 × 27	7	7.784	40 × 30	6	10.452
2)	18 × 14	7	4.181	30 × 24	8	6.271	40 × 32	8	8.362	50 × 40	8	10.452
3)	20 × 16	8	4.181	35 × 29	10	5.694	50 × 42	11	7.207	60 × 50	10	10.452
4)	25 × 21	11	3.603	40 × 34	12	5.117	60 × 52	14	6.052	75 × 65	14	7.565
5)	30 × 26	14	3.026	50 × 44	15	5.694	70 × 62	16	7.207	90 × 80	16	10.452
6)	35 × 31	16	3.603	60 × 54	18	6.271	80 × 72	18	8.362	100 × 90	18	10.452
7)	40 × 36	18	4.181	70 × 64	22	5.117	90 × 82	21	7.207	120 × 110	22	10.452
8)	45 × 41	21	3.603	80 × 74	25	5.694	100 × 92	24	6.052	150 × 140	28	10.452
9)	50 × 46	24	3.026	90 × 84	28	6.271	110 × 102	26	7.207	200 × 190	38	10.452
10)	55 × 51	26	3.603	100 × 94	32	5.117	120 × 112	28	8.362	210 × 200	40	10.452
11)	60 × 56	28	4.181	110 × 104	35	5.694	130 × 122	31	7.207	220 × 210	42	10.452
12)	65 × 61	31	3.603	120 × 114	38	6.271	140 × 132	34	6.052	240 × 230	46	10.452
13)	70 × 66	34	3.026	130 × 124	42	5.117	150 × 142	36	7.207	250 × 240	48	10.452
14)	75 × 71	36	3.603	140 × 134	45	5.694	160 × 152	38	8.362	260 × 250	50	10.452
15)	80 × 76	38	4.181	150 × 144	48	6.271	170 × 162	41	7.207	280 × 270	54	10.452

IS: 3665–1966

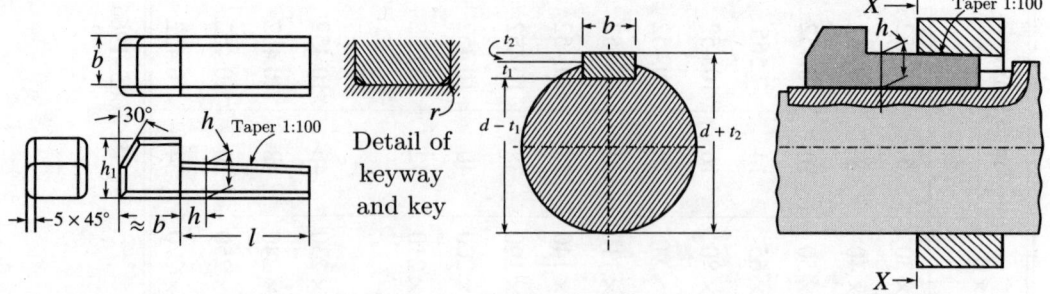

Table 4.6 *Gib-Head keys and keyways All dimensions in millimeters.*

Range of Shaft Dia.d		Key				Keyway									Range of Key Lenght:	
													r			
Above	Upto	$b \times h$	h_1	b	Tol on b D 10	t_1	Tol on t_1	t_2	Tol on t_2	min	max				min	max
10	12	4×4	7	4		2.5		1.2		0.08	0.16				14	45
12	17	5×5	8	5	+ 0.078	3.0	+0.1	1.7	+0.1	0.16	0.25				14	56
17	22	6×6	10	6	+ 0.030	3.5	0	2.2	0	0.16	0.25				16	70
22	30	8×7	11	8	+0.098	4.0		2.4		0.16	0.25				20	90
30	38	10×8	12	10	+ 0.040	5.0		2.4		0.25	0.40				25	110
38	44	12×8	12	12		5.0		2.4		0.25	0.40				32	140
44	50	14×9	14	14	+0.120	5.5		2.9		0.25	0.40				40	160
50	58	16×10	16	16	+ 0.050	6.0	+0.2	3.4	+ 0.2	0.25	0.40				45	180
58	65	18×11	18	18		7.0	0	3.4	0	0.25	0.40				50	200
65	75	20×12	20	20		7.5		3.9		0.40	0.60				56	220
75	85	22×14	22	22	+ 0.149	9.0		4.4		0.40	0.60				63	250
85	95	25×14	22	25	+ 0.065	9.0		4.4		0.40	0.60				70	280
95	110	28×16	25	28		10.0		5.4		0.40	0.60				80	320
110	130	32×18	28	32		11.0		6.4		0.40	0.60				90	360
130	150	36×20	32	36	+ 0.180	12.0		7.1		0.70	1.00				100	400
150	170	40×22	36	40	+ 0.080	13.0		8.1		0.70	1.00				110	400
170	200	45×25	40	45		15.0		9.1		0.70	1.00				125	400
200	230	50×28	45	50		17.0		10.1		0.70	1.00				140	400
230	260	56×32	50	56		20.0		11.1		1.20	1.60				-	-
260	290	63×32	50	63	+0.220	20.0	+0.3	11.1	+0.3	1.20	1.60				-	-
290	330	70×36	56	70	+ 0.100	22.0	0	13.1	0	1.20	1.60				-	-
330	380	80×40	63	80		25.0		14.1		2.00	2.50				-	-
380	440	90×45	70	90	+ 0.260	28.0		16.1		2.00	2.50				-	-
440	500	100×50	80	100	+0.120	31.0		18.1		2.00	2.50				-	-

IS: 2293-1974

Designation: A Gib-Head Key of b = 12mm, h = 8mm and l = 50mm shall be designated as $12 \times 18 \times 50$

Table 4.7 *Relationship of shaft diameter to key size (woodruff)*
All dimensions in millimetres.

Shaft Diameter d				Key Size $b \times h_1 \times D$
Series 1*		Series 2**		
over	Including	Over	Including	
3	4	3	4	$1.0 \times 1.4 \times 4.0$
4	5	4	6	$1.5 \times 2.6 \times 7.0$
5	6	6	8	$2.0 \times 2.6 \times 7.0$
6	7	8	10	$2.0 \times 3.7 \times 10.0$
7	8	10	12	$2.5 \times 3.7 \times 10.0$
8	10	12	15	$3.0 \times 5.0 \times 13.0$
10	12	15	18	$3.0 \times 6.5 \times 16.0$
12	14	18	20	$4.0 \times 6.5 \times 16.0$
14	16	20	22	$4.0 \times 7.5 \times 19.0$
16	18	22	25	$5.0 \times 6.5 \times 16.0$
18	20	25	28	$5.0 \times 7.5 \times 19.0$
20	22	28	32	$5.0 \times 9.0 \times 22.0$
22	25	32	36	$6.0 \times 9.0 \times 22.0$
25	28	36	40	$6.0 \times 10.0 \times 25.0$
25	32	40	-	$8.0 \times 11.0 \times 28.0$
32	38	-	-	$10.0 \times 13.0 \times 32.0$
*Series 1 - For Torque Applications				IS : 2294–1980
**Series 2 - For Positional Applications				

Designation: A woodruff key of width 4mm and height 6.5mm shall be designated as
"woodrull key 4×6.5

Table 4.8 *Dimensions and Tolerances of keys (Woodruff)*

All dimensions in millimetres.

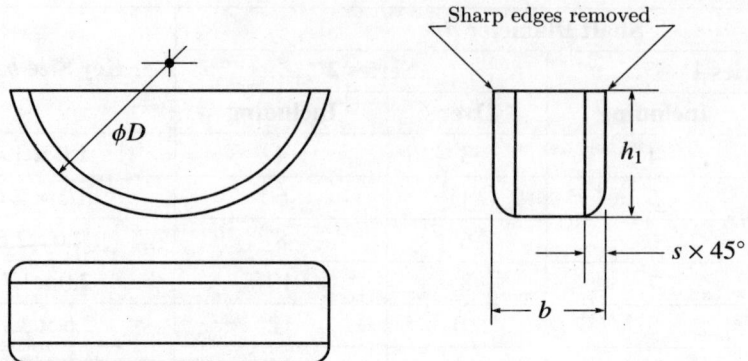

b	Tol on b hg*	h₁	Tol on h₁ h11	D	Tol on D h12	s	
						Min	Max
1.0		1.4		4.0	0 −0.120	0.16	0.25
1.5		2.6	0 −0.060	7.0		0.16	0.25
2.0		2.6		7.0	0 −0.150	0.16	0.25
2.0	0 −0.025	3.7		10.0		0.16	0.25
2.5		3.7	0 −0.075	10.0		0.16	0.25
3.0		5.0		13.0		0.16	0.25
3.0		6.5		16.0	0 −0.180	0.16	0.25
4.0		6.5		16.0		0.25	0.40
4.0		7.5		19.0	0 −0.210	0.25	0.40
5.0		6.5		16.0	0 −0.180	0.25	0.40
5.0	0 −0.030	7.5	0 −0.090	19.0		0.25	0.40
5.0		9.0		22.0		0.25	0.40
6.0		9.0		22.0	0 −0.210	0.25	0.40
6.0		10.0		25.0		0.25	0.40
8.0	0 −0.036	11.0	0 −0.110	28.0		0.40	0.60
10.0		13.0		32.0	0 −0.250	0.40	0.60

*A closer tolerance may be adopted subject to agreement between the suppller and the purchaser.

Table 4.9 *Dimensions and Tolerances of keyways (Woodruff)*

All dimensions in millimeters.

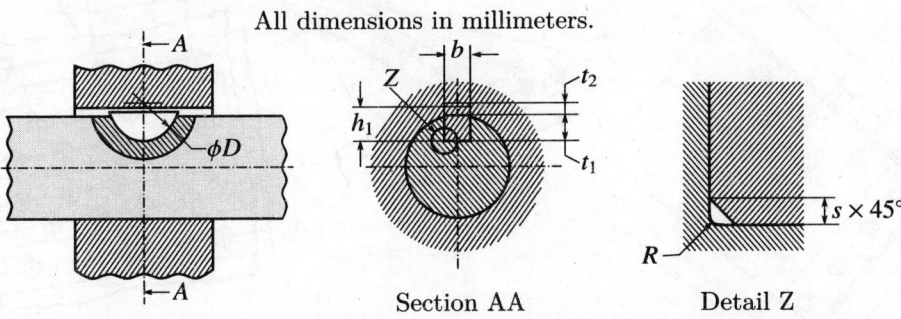

Section AA   Detail Z

Key $b \times h_1 \times D$	b Nom	Tolerance on b — Normal Shaft N9	Tolerance on b — Fit Hub Js9	Tolerance on b — Close Fit Shaft & Hub P9	t_1	Tol on t_1	t_2	Tol on t_2	R Max	R Min
$1.0 \times 1.4 \times 4.0$	1.0				1.0		0.6		0.16	0.08
$1.5 \times 2.6 \times 7.0$	1.5				2.0		0.8		0.16	0.08
$2.0 \times 2.6 \times 7.0$	2.0				1.8	+0.1 / 0	1.0		0.16	0.08
$2.0 \times 3.7 \times 10.0$	2.0	-0.004 / -0.029	+0.012 / -0.012	-0.006 / -0.031	2.9		1.0		0.16	0.08
$2.5 \times 3.7 \times 10.0$	2.5				2.7		1.2		0.16	0.08
$3.0 \times 5.0 \times 13.0$	3.0				3.8		1.4		0.16	0.08
$3.0 \times 6.5 \times 16.0$	3.0				5.3		1.4	+0.1 / 0	0.16	0.08
$4.0 \times 6.5 \times 16.0$	4.0				5.0	+0.2 / 0	1.8		0.25	0.16
$4.0 \times 7.5 \times 19.0$	4.0				6.0		1.8		0.25	0.16
$5.0 \times 6.5 \times 16.0$	5.0				4.5		2.3		0.25	0.16
$5.0 \times 7.5 \times 19.0$	5.0	0 / -0.030	+0.015 / -0.015	-0.012 / -0.042	5.5		2.3		0.25	0.16
$5.0 \times 9.0 \times 22.0$	5.0				7.0		2.3		0.25	0.16
$6.0 \times 9.0 \times 22.0$	6.0				6.5		2.8		0.25	0.16
$6.0 \times 10.0 \times 25.0$	6.0				7.5	+0.3 / 0	2.8		0.25	0.16
$8.0 \times 11.0 \times 28.0$	8.0	0 / -0.036	+0.018 / -0.018	-0.015 / -0.051	8.0		3.3	+0.2 / 0	0.40	0.25
$10.0 \times 13.0 \times 32.0$	10.0				10.0		3.3		0.40	0.25

Note- The diameter of the keyways in the shaft shall be equal to nominal diameter 'D' of the key with a tolerance of +0.5 mm.

IS: 2294-1980

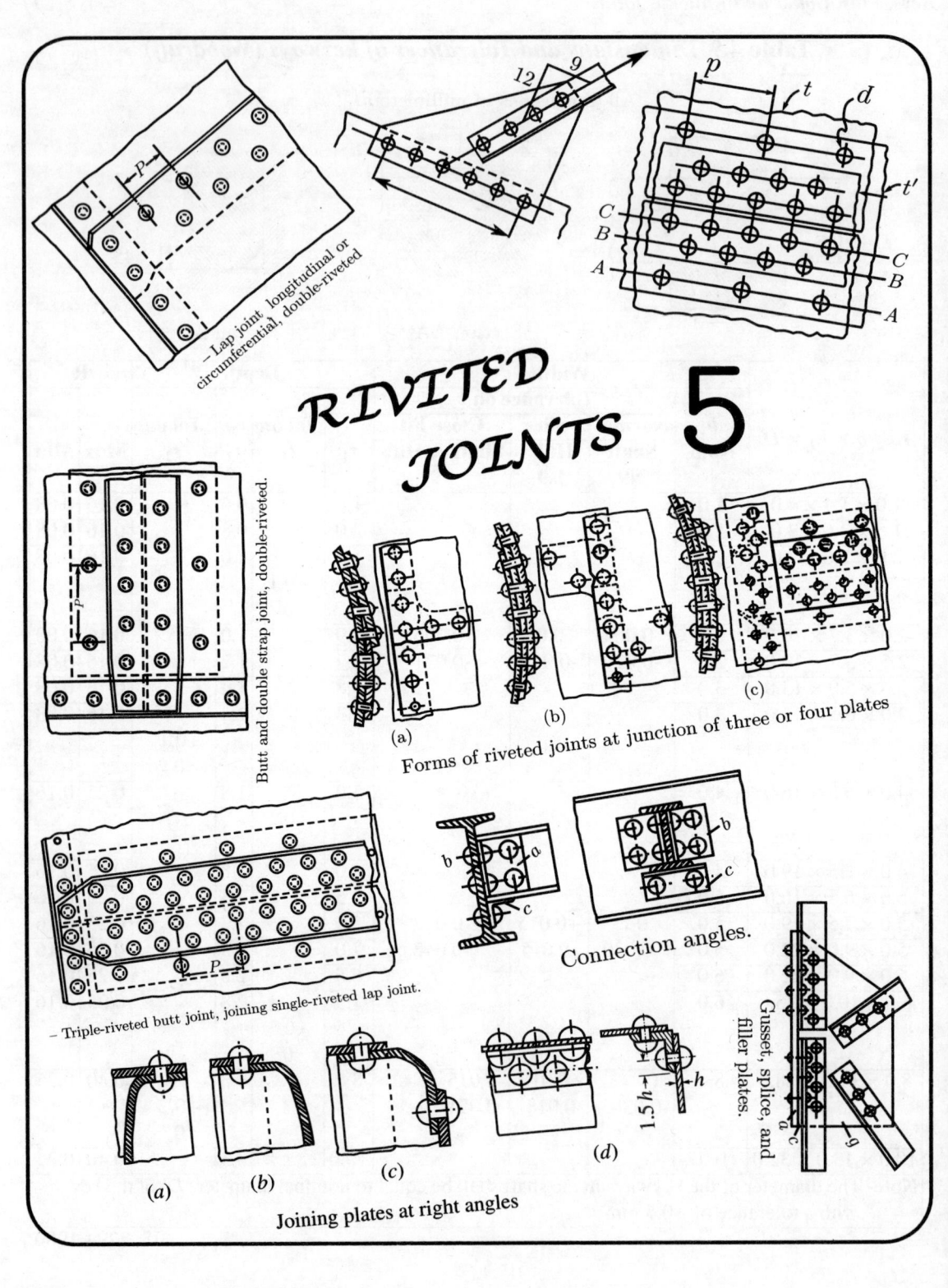

RIVITED JOINTS **5**

– Lap joint, longitudinal or circumferential, double-riveted

Butt and double strap joint, double-riveted.

(a) (b) (c)

Forms of riveted joints at junction of three or four plates

– Triple-riveted butt joint, joining single-riveted lap joint.

Connection angles.

Gusset, splice, and filler plates.

(a) (b) (c) (d)

Joining plates at right angles

5

Riveted Joints

Symbols	Description and Units
d	diameter of the rivet hole, mm (Table 5.3(b))
D	internal diameter of the pressure vessel, mm
n_1	number of rivets in single shear
n_2	number of rivets in double shear
p	pitch on the gage line or longitudinal pitch, mm (Table 5.4(b))
p_d	diagonal pitch, mm
p_i	pressure acting inside the boiler, MN/m^2 (kgf/mm^2)
p_t	transverse pitch, mm
t	thickness of the shell or main plate, mm (Table 5.3(a))
t_i	thickness of inner cover plate, mm
t_o	thickness of outer cover plate, mm
η	efficiency of longitudinal joint (Table 5.1)
σ_c	allowable crushing stress for rivets or plate, MN/m^2 (kgf/mm^2) (Table 5.5)
σ_t	allowable tensile stress of shell plate, MN/m^2 (kgf/mm^2) (Table 5.5)
τ	allowable shearing stress of rivets, MN/m^2 (kgf/mm^2)

Particular	Equation	Eqn. No.
The thickness of shell	$t = \dfrac{p_i D}{2\sigma_t \eta}$	5.1
The diagonal pitch of lap joint (staggered)	$p_d = \dfrac{2p + d}{3}$	5.2
In staggered riveting the transverse pitch of lap joint	$p_t = \left[\left(\dfrac{2p + d}{3} \right)^2 - \left(\dfrac{p}{2} \right)^2 \right]^{\frac{1}{2}}$	5.3
Thickness of the cover plates according to Indian Boiler Code:		
Thickness of single butt strap having ordinary riveting	$t_i = 1.125t$	5.4(a)

Particular	Equation	Eqn. No.
Thickness of single butt strap having alternate rivet in the outer rows omitted	$t_i = 1.125t\dfrac{(p-d)}{(p-2d)}$	5.4(b)
Thickness of double butt strap of equal width having ordinary riveting	$t_i = t_o = 0.625t$	5.4(c)
Thickness of double butt straps of equal width having every alternate rivet in the outer rows omitted	$t_i = t_o = 0.625\left\{\dfrac{(p-d)}{(p-2d)}\right\}t$	5.4(d)
Thickness of the double butt straps of unequal width either having ordinary riveting or having every alternate rivet in the outer rows omitted	$t_0 = 0.625t$ $t_i = 0.750t$	5.4(e) 5.4(f)
Length of the shank of the rivet	$L = \sum t + (1.5\text{to}1.7)d$	5.5

Strength of riveted joints:

The tearing resistance or tensile strength of solid plate of a unit strip	$P = pt\sigma_t$	5.6(a)
The tearing resistance or tensile strength of a unit strip of plate along its weakest section	$P_t = (p-d)t\sigma_t$	5.6(b)
According to Indian Boiler Regulations, the strength of a rivet in double shear	$P_s = 1\frac{7}{8}$ times the strength in single shear $= 1.875\left(\dfrac{\pi d^2}{4}\right)\tau$	5.6(c)
The general expression for the resistance to shear of all the rivets in a unit strip	$P_s = (1 + 1.875n_2)\left(\dfrac{\pi d^2}{4}\right)\tau$	5.6(d)
The general expression for the resistance to crushing of the rivets	$P_c = (n_1t_i + n_2t)d\sigma_c$	5.6(e)
The theoretical efficiency of the riveted joint*	$\eta = \dfrac{(n_1 + 1.875n_2)\pi d^2\tau}{4pt\sigma_t} = \dfrac{(n_1t_i/t + n_2)\sigma_c}{(n_1t_i/t + n_2)\sigma_c + \sigma_t}$	5.7

In multirow riveted joint failure of the rivets through combined action:

The total resistance against failure of a unit strip of plate due to tearing of the plate at the inner row and shearing of the rivets in the outer row	$P_{ts} = (p-2d)t\sigma_t + k\dfrac{\pi}{4}d^2\tau$	5.8(a)
	$\eta_{ts} = \dfrac{(p-2d)t\sigma_t + k\frac{\pi}{4}d^2\tau}{pt\sigma_t}$	5.8(b)
	where $k = 1$ for rivets in single shear	
	$= 1.875$ for rivets in double shear	

---

*to find the efficiency of lap joint put $t_i/t = 1$ and $n_2 = 0$

Particular	Equation	Eqn. No.
The total resistance against failure of a unit strip of plate due to combined action of tearing of the plate at the inner row and crushing of rivets in the outer row	$P_{tc} = (p - 2d)t\sigma_t + dt\sigma_c$ $\eta_{tc} = \dfrac{(p - 2d)t\sigma_t + dt\sigma_c}{pt\sigma_t}$	5.9(a) 5.9(b)
The total resistance against failure of a unit strip of plate due to the combined action of shearing of the rivets in the outer row and crushing of the rivets in the inner rows	$P_{sc} = \frac{\pi}{4}d^2\tau + ndt\sigma_c$ $\eta_{sc} = \dfrac{\frac{\pi}{4}d^2\tau + ndt\sigma_c}{pt\sigma_t}$	5.9(c) 5.9(d)
Plate efficiency	$\eta_t = \dfrac{p - d}{p}$	5.9(e)
Rivet efficiency	$\eta_s = \dfrac{\frac{\pi}{4}d^2(n_1 + 1.875n_2)\tau}{pt\sigma_t}$	5.9(f)
Rivet size:		
General expression for the diameter of rivet hole[†]	$d = \dfrac{4(n_1t_i + n_2t)}{\pi(n_1 + 1.875n_2)} \times \dfrac{\sigma_c}{\tau}$	5.10(a)
For lap joint ($t_i = t$ and $n_2 = 0$)	$d = \dfrac{4t\sigma_c}{\pi\tau}$	5.10(b)
For equal cover butt joint ($n_1 = 0$)	$d = \dfrac{4t\sigma_c}{1.875\pi\tau}$	5.10(c)
The empirical formula to determine the diameter of steel rivet hole		
a) for lap joint ($t \leq 10$mm)	$d = 2t$	5.11(a)
b) for lap joint ($t > 10$mm)	$d \geq t + 2$ mm	5.11(b)
c) for butt joint	$d = t + 6$ mm	5.11(c)
d) Prof. Unwin's formula for lap and butt joints	$d = (6.07\sqrt{t})$ to $(6.325\sqrt{t})$	5.11(d)

Pitch:

The general expression to determine the optimum pitch of the riveted joint[‡]

$$p = \frac{(n_1 + 1.875n_2)\pi d^2\tau}{4t\sigma_t} + d = \left[(n_1t_i/t + n_2)\frac{\sigma_c}{\sigma_t} + 1\right]\left[\frac{4(n_1t_i/t + n_2)\sigma_c}{\pi(n_1 + 1.875n_2)\tau}\right]t \qquad \text{5.12(a)}$$

According to IBR, the maximum shorter pitch of the rivet in the longitudinal joint	$p = k_1t + 41$ mm where, k_1 is a constant (Table 5.4(a))	5.12(b)
Minimum pitch	$p = (2.25d)$ to $(2.5d)$	5.12(c)

[†]For lap joint put $t_i = t$ and $n_2 = 0$.
[‡]For equal double cover butt joint put $n_1 = 0$

Particular	Equation	Eqn. No.
For staunchness of the joint, i.e. to make the joint leakproof, the pitch	$p \leq 6d$	5.12(d)
For low pressure vessels, the pitch along the caulking edge.	$p \leq 8t_o$	5.12(e)
For high pressure vessels the permissible pitch along the caulking edge to outside cover plate (Haven and Swett)	$p = d + 3.45 \sqrt[4]{t_o^3 / p_i}$	5.12(f)
Transverse pitch:		
In chain riveting the transverse pitch for butt joints	$p_t = (2d)$ to $(2.5d)$	5.13(a)
In staggered riveting the transverse pitch for butt joints	$p_t \geq \sqrt{0.5pd + 0.25d^2}$	5.13(b)
For longitudinal joint the minimum value of transverse pitch (ASME Boiler code)	$p_t = 1\frac{3}{4}d$ if $\frac{p}{d} = 4$ or less	5.13(c)
	$p_t = 1\frac{3}{4}d + 0.1(p - d)$ if $\frac{p}{d} > 4$	5.13(d)

where p is the pitch in the outer row, when a rivet in the inner row comes midway between two rivets in the outer row; or p is the pitch in the outer row less the pitch in the inner row when two rivets in the inner row come between two rivets in the outer row.

According to Indian Boiler Code:		
(a) The transverse pitch for equal number of rivets in the rows:		
(i) For chain riveting	$p_t \geq 2d$	5.14(a)
(ii) For staggered riveting	$p_t \geq 0.33p + 0.67d$	5.14(b)
(b) In joints where the longer pitch is double the shorter one and the inner rows are chain riveted:		
(i) the transverse pitch between the outer row and the inner row	$p_t \geq 2d$ or	5.14(c)
	$p_t \geq 0.33p + 0.67d$	
(ii) the transverse pitch between the successive inner rows	$p_t \geq 2d$	5.14(d)
(c) In joints where the longer pitch is double the shorter one and the inner rows are zig-zag riveted:		
(i) the transverse pitch between the outer row and the inner row	$p_t \geq 0.2p + 1.15d$	5.15(a)

Particular	Equation	Eqn. No.
(ii) the transverse pitch between the successsive inner rows	$p_t \geq 0.165p + 0.67d$	5.15(b)
According to Indian Boiler code, the margin	$m = 1.5d$	5.16
In staggered joint the diagonal pitch	$p_d \geq \dfrac{(p + d)}{2}$	5.17(a)
	$p_d = (2.25d)$ to $(2.5d)$	5.17(b)

Eccentric Loads on structural connections: (Fig. 5.1)

The direct or primary shear stress	$\tau' = \dfrac{F}{nA} = \dfrac{F'}{A}$ where $F' = F/n$, the primary force, $N(kgf)$	5.18
The secondary shear stress	$\tau'' = \dfrac{Tc}{\sum Ac^2} = \dfrac{Tc}{J}$	5.19

where $\sum Ac^2 = J$, polar moment of inertia of the rivet areas about the center of gravity, mm^4

$\qquad T = Fe$, Torsional moment, N-mm

$\qquad c =$ the distance from the centre of gravity to the centre of the rivet, mm

The secondary force	$F'' = \tau'' A' = \dfrac{Tc}{J}A'$ where $A' =$ area of rivet under consideration mm^2	5.20
The resultant shear force on the rivet	$F_R = \sqrt{F'^2 + F''^2 + 2F'F'' \cos\theta}$ where $\theta =$ the angle between the primary and secondary shear forces	5.21

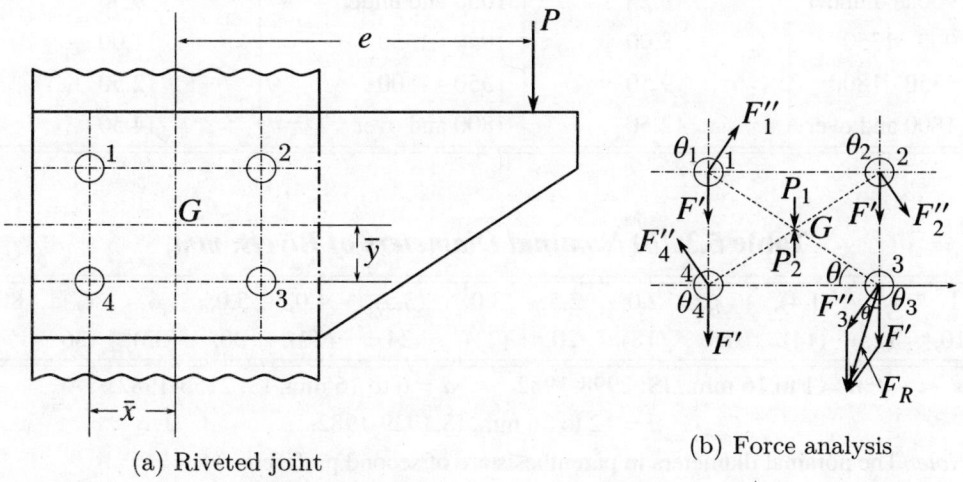

(a) Riveted joint (b) Force analysis

Fig. 5.1: *Rivet Joint with eccentric load*

Table 5.1 *Efficiency of Commercial Boiler Joints*

Type of joint	No. of rivets per pitch	% Efficiency
Single riveted lap joint	1	40 – 60
Double row lap joint	2	60 – 72
Triple row lap joint	3	72 – 82
Single row butt joint with two cover plates	1	60 – 72
Double row butt joint with two cover plates	2	72 – 82
Triple row butt joint with two cover plates	3	80 – 90
Quadruple row butt joint with two cover plates	4	85 – 94

Table 5.2 *Recommended Types of Joints*

Diameter of shell, mm	Thickness of shell, mm	Type of joint Butt
600 - 1800	6.25 - 12.50	Double riveted
900 - 2100	8.00 - 25.00	Triple riveted
1500 - 2700	9.50 - 45.00	Quadruple riveted

Table 5.3 *(a) Minimum Thickness of Boiler Plates*

Shell plates		Tube sheets of fire tube boiler	
Diameter of shell, mm	Minimum thickness after flanging, mm	Diameter of tube sheet, mm	Minimum thickness, mm
900 and under	6.25	1050 and under	9.50
900 - 1350	8.00	1050 - 1350	11.00
1350 - 1800	9.50	1350 - 1800	12.50
1800 and over	12.50	1800 and over	14.50

Table 5.3 *(b) Nominal Diameters of Rivets, mm,*

1.	1.2,	(1.4),	1.6,	2.0,	2.5,	3.0,	(3.5),	4.0,	5.0,	6,	(7),	8,	
10,	12,	(14),	16,	(18),	20,	(22),	24,	(27),	30,	(33),	36		

d = 1 to 16 mm., IS: 2998-1982. d = 6 to 16 mm, IS: 2155-1982.

d = 12 to 36 mm, IS:1929-1982.

Note: The nominal diameters in parenthesis are of second preference.

Designation: Snap Head Rivet 16 × 70 IS: 1929.

Table 5.3 *(c) Thickness of Steel Plates for Structural Works, Pressure Vessels and Boilers, mm.*

0.5, 0.8, 1.0, 1.25, 1.40, 1.6, 1.8, 2.0, 2.24, 2.50, 2.80, 3.15, 3.55, 4.0,
IS 1730-1961.
5, 6, 7, 8, 10, 12, 14, 16, 18, 20, 22, 25, 28, 32, 36, 40, 45, 50, 56, 63.
IS: 2002-1982,   IS: 1730-1974

Table 5.4 *(a) Coefficient k_1 in equation 5.12(b)*

No. of rivets per pitch	Coefficients for Lap joints	Coefficients for single butt-strapped joints	Coefficients for double butt-strapped joints
1	1.31	1.53	1.75
2	2.62	3.06	3.50
3	3.47	4.05	4.63
4	4.14	–	5.52
5	–	–	6.00

Table 5.4 *(b) Recommended values for Rivet hole diameter, pitch and efficiency*

Type of seam	$\dfrac{DP_i}{2}$ N/mm (kgf/mm)	Diameter of rivet hole, mm	Max. allowable pitch p, mm	efficiency $\eta_t = \left(\dfrac{p-d}{p}\right)100$
Single riveted lap joint	Upto 500 (50)	$t + 8$ mm	$2t + 40$ mm	56% to 60 %
Double riveted lap joint	350-950 (35-95)	$t + 8$ mm	$2.62t + 40$ mm	70 %
Triple riveted lap joint	450-1350 (45-135)	$t + (6$ to $8)$ mm	$3\,t + 40$ mm	75 %
Double riveted two strap butt joint	450-1350 (45-135)	$t + (5$ to $6)$ mm	$3.5t + 40$ mm	75 %
Triple riveted two strap butt joint (Diamond Riveting)	450-2300 (45-230)	$t + 5$ mm	$6t + 40$ mm	85%

Table 5.5 *Recommended Values of Allowable Stress for Structural Joints, MN/m^2 (kgf/mm^2)*

	Shop assembly	Field assembly
Tensile stress of the plate	115 (11.7)	115 (11.7)
Shear stress of the rivet	86 (8.8)	70 (7.1)
Crushing stress of the rivet	210 (21.4)	140 (14.2)

Table 5.6 *Values of working stress at elevated temperatures*

Maximum temperature t, °C	Minimum of the specified range of tensile strength of the material, MN/m² (kgf/mm²)				
	315 (32)	340(35)	380 (39)	410 (42)	520 (53)
0-370	63 (6.40)	68 (7.00)	76 (7.80)	82 (8.40)	104 (10.60)
400	57 (5.80)	63 (6.40)	69 (7.00)	76 (7.75)	90 (9.15)
425	45 (4.60)	51 (5.15)	55 (5.60)	62 (6.30)	71 (7.20)
455	37 (3.80)	42 (4.24)	47 (4.75)	51 (5.20)	57 (5.80)
480	29 (3.00)	33 (3.40)	38 (3.85)	38 (3.90)	41 (4.20)
510	22 (2.25)	25 (2.50)	28 (2.80)	28 (2.80)	28 (2.80)

Note: Design stresses for pressure vessels are based on a factor of safety of 5

References

[1] Siegel M. J., Maleev V. L., Hartman J. B., *"Mechanical Design of Machines"*, 4th edition, International Text Book Company, 1965.

[2] Vallance A., Doughtie V. L., *"Design of Machine Members"*, 3rd edition, McGraw Hill Book Co., 1951.

[3] Bhattacharya S. C., Basu Mallik J. R., *"Machine Design"*, Basu Mallik & Co., Calcutta, 1966.

[4] Ghosh A. K., *"Practical Machine Design"*, S. Bhattacharya & Co., Calcutta, 1969.

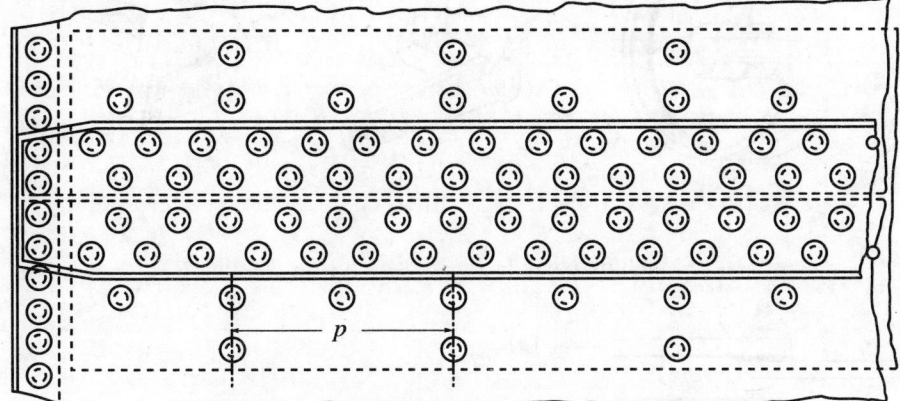

Quadruple-riveted butt and double strap joint.

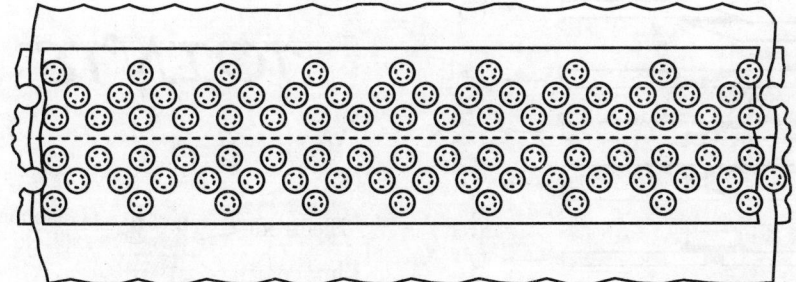

Triple-riveted butt and double strap joint with straps of equal width.

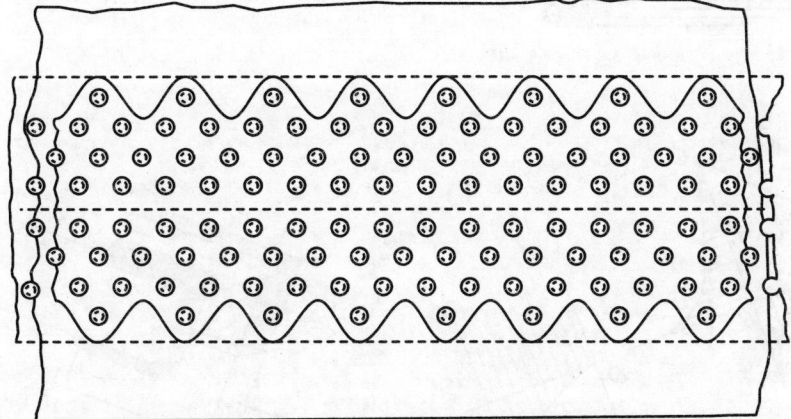

Quadruple-riveted butt and double strap joint of the saw-tooth type.

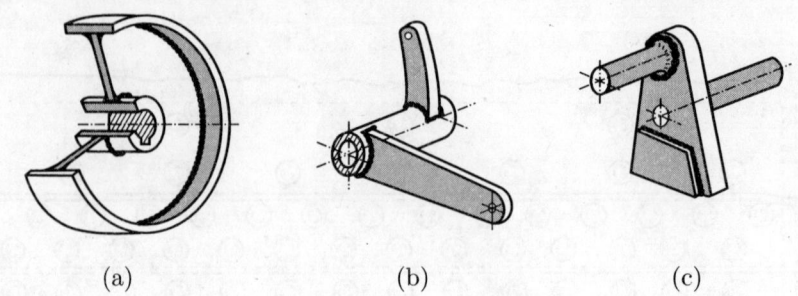

(a)   (b)   (c)

Machine parts fabricated by fusion welding

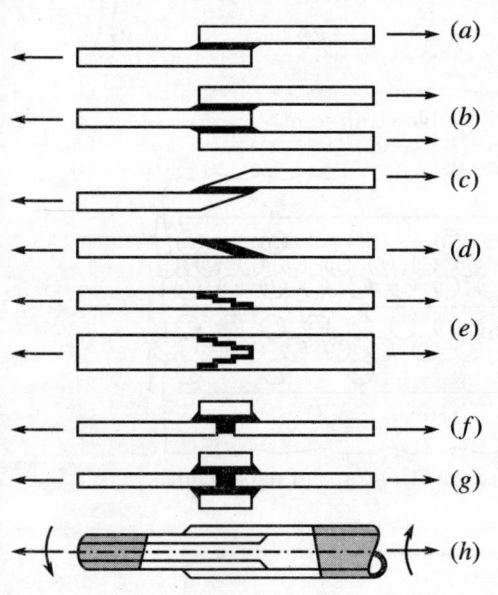

WELDED JOINTS

6

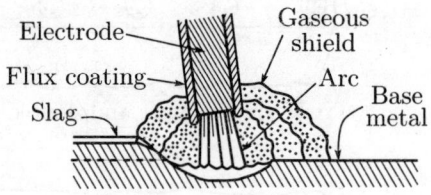

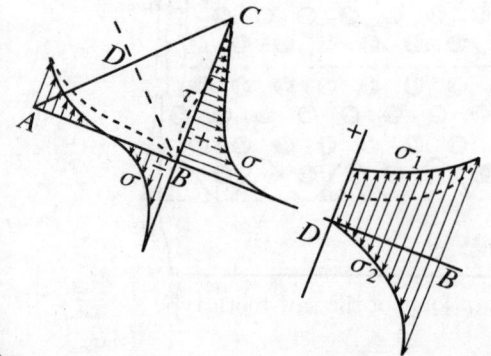

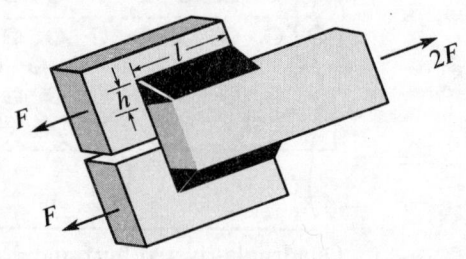

6

Welded Joints

Symbols	Description and Units
h	thickness of plate or size of weld leg, mm
h_t	weld depth of throat, mm
F	force or external load, N (kgf)
L	length of the weld, mm
M	bending moment, N mm (kgf-mm)
σ	normal stress, MN/m^2 (kgf/mm^2)
τ	shear stress, MN/m^2 (kgf/mm^2)
τ'	primary shear stress, MN/m^2 (kgf-mm^2)
τ''	secondary shear stress, MN/m^2 (kgf/mm^2)

Particular	Equation	Eqn. No.
The average normal stress for single V-Groove butt weld in tension (Fig. 6.1(a))	$\sigma = \dfrac{P}{A_t} = \dfrac{P}{h_t L} = \dfrac{P}{hL}$	6.1(a)
	where $A_t = h_t L = hL$, throat area of weld, mm^2	
	$h_t = h$, throat length or weld depth of throat, mm	
The average shear stress for single V-Groove Butt weld in shear (Fig. 6.1(b))	$\tau = \dfrac{P}{A_t} = \dfrac{P}{h_t L} = \dfrac{P}{hL}$	6.1(b)
The average normal stress for single V-Groove butt weld in bending (Fig. 6.1(c))	$\sigma = \dfrac{M}{Z} = \dfrac{6M}{Lh_t^2} = \dfrac{6M}{Lh^2}$	6.1(c)

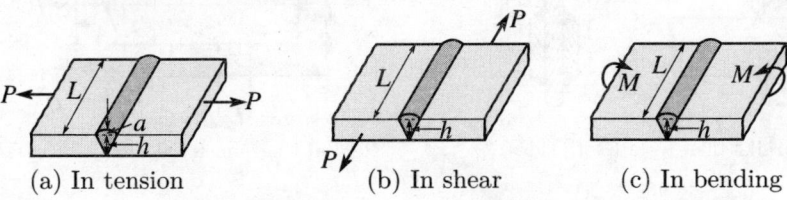

(a) In tension   (b) In shear   (c) In bending

Fig. 6.1: *Single V-Groove Butt Weld Joint*

Particular	Equation	Eqn. No.
The average normal stress for single fillet transverse lap weld in tension (Fig. 6.2(a))	$\sigma = \dfrac{P}{A_t} = \dfrac{P}{h_t L} = \dfrac{P}{h \cos 45° \times L}$ $= \dfrac{P}{0.707 hL} = \dfrac{1.414 P}{hL}$	6.2(a)
The average normal stress for double fillet transverse lap weld in tension (Fig. 6.2(b))	$\sigma = \dfrac{P}{2A_t} = \dfrac{P}{2h_t L} = \dfrac{0.707 P}{hL}$	6.2(b)
The average normal stress for double fillet parallel lap weld in tension (Fig. 6.2(c))	$\sigma = \dfrac{P}{2A_t} = \dfrac{P}{2h_t L} = \dfrac{0.707 P}{hL}$	6.2(c)
The normal stress for double fillet lap weld (both sides) in tension (Fig. 6.2(d))	$\sigma = \dfrac{P}{4A_t} = \dfrac{P}{4h_t L} = \dfrac{0.354 P}{hL}$	6.2(d)

Unsymmetrical Sections:

Average normal stress on unsymmetrical sections of fillet weld in tension (Fig. 6.2(e))	$\sigma = \dfrac{1.414 P}{h(L_1 + L_2)}$	6.2(e)
The lengths of the weld so that the sum of the resisting moments of the welds about the gravity axis is zero (Fig. 6.2(e))	$L_1 = \dfrac{L e_2}{e_1 + e_2} = \dfrac{1.414 P e_2}{\sigma h b}$	6.2(f)
	$L_2 = \dfrac{L e_1}{e_1 + e_2} = \dfrac{1.414 P e_1}{\sigma h b}$	6.2(g)

where $L = L_1 + L_2$, total length of the weld, mm

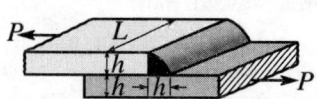

(a) Single transverse fillet weld

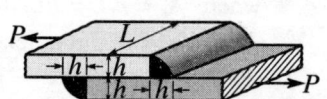

(b) Double transverse fillet weld

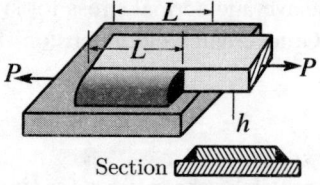

(c) Double parallel fillet weld

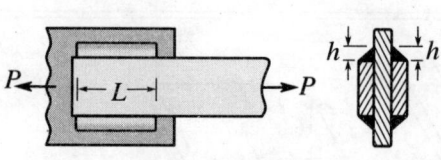

(d) Double parallel fillet weld (Both sides)

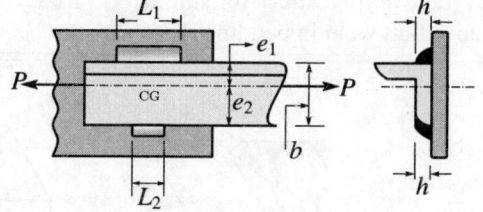

(e) Unsymmetrical weld joint in tension

Fig. 6.2: *Lap Weld Joints*

Particular	Equation	Eqn. No.
Eccentric Loads:		
Primary shear stress	$\tau' = \dfrac{P}{h_t L} = \dfrac{P}{(h\cos 45°)L}$	6.3(a)
Maximum secondary shear stress (Fig. 6.3)	$\tau'' = \dfrac{Pe\sqrt{m^2 + n^2}}{2J}$	6.3(b)
	where J is the polar moment of inertia of the weld (Table 6.7)	
The maximum resultant shear stress where θ is the angle between the primary and secondary shear stresses	$\tau_{max} = \sqrt{\tau'^2 + \tau''^2 + 2\tau'\tau''\cos\theta}$	6.3(c)
	$\cos\theta = \dfrac{n}{\sqrt{m^2 + n^2}}$	6.3(d)

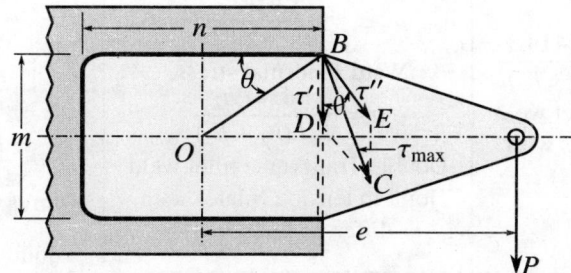

Fig. 6.3: *Eccentrically loaded welded joint*

References

[1] Vallance, A., Doughtie, V. L., *"Design of Machine Members"*, 3rd edition, McGraw Hill Book Co., 1951.

[2] Faires, V. M., *"Design of Machine Elements"*, 2nd edition, The macmillan Company, 1941.

[3] Shigley, J. E., *"Machine Design"*, McGraw Hill Book Company, Inc.

Table 6.1 *Stresses in Welds*

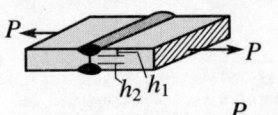

Normal stress, $\sigma = \dfrac{P}{(h_1 + h_2)L}$

Double V-grooved Butt weld joint in tension

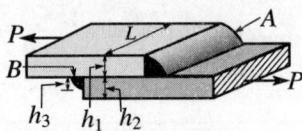

Normal stress, $\sigma = \dfrac{0.707P}{hL}$

Transverse fillet weld in tension

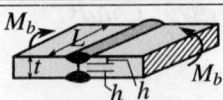

Normal stress,

$\sigma = \dfrac{3tM}{Lh(3t^2 - 6th + 4h^2)}$

Double V-grooved Butt-joint in bending

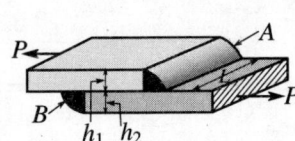

Normal stress, $\sigma = \dfrac{1.414P}{(h_1 + h_2)L}$

Double Transverse fillet weld joint in tension (plates with different thickness)

Weld A normal stress,

$\sigma = \dfrac{1.414P}{(h_1 + h_2)L}$

Weld B normal stress,

$\sigma = \dfrac{1.414Ph_2}{h_3L(h_1 + h_2)}$

Double Transverse fillet weld joint in tension (plates with different thickness)

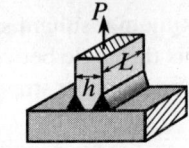

Normal stress, $\sigma = \dfrac{P}{hL}$

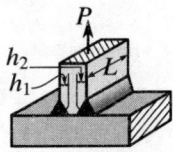

Normal stress, $\sigma = \dfrac{P}{(h_1 + h_2)L}$

T-joint Transverse fillet weld

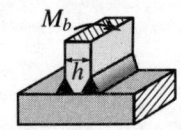

Normal stress, $\sigma = \dfrac{6M}{Lh^2}$

T-joint fillet weld in bending

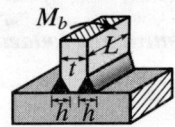

Normal stress,

$\sigma = \dfrac{3tM}{Lh(3t^2 - 6th + 4h^2)}$

T-joint fillet weld in bending

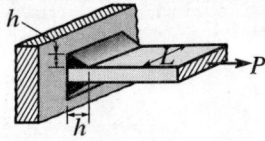

Normal stress, $\sigma = \dfrac{0.707P}{hL}$

Transverse fillet weld in tension

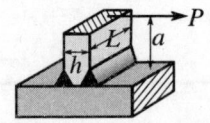

Normal stress, $\sigma = \dfrac{6Pa}{Lh^2}$

Shear stress, $\tau = \dfrac{P}{Lh}$

T-Joint fillet weld in bending

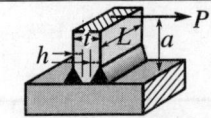

Normal stress,

$\sigma = \dfrac{3tPa}{Lh(3t^2 - 6th + 4h^2)}$

Shear stress, $\tau = \dfrac{P}{2Lh}$

T-Joint fillet weld in bending

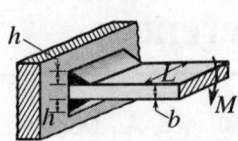

Normal stress, $\sigma = \dfrac{1.414M}{hL(b + h)}$

T-Joint Transverse fillet weld

Table 6.1 *Stresses in Welds – (Contd..)*

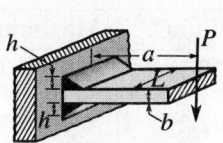

Average shear stress,

$$\tau_m = \frac{0.707P}{hL}$$

Maximum normal stress,

$$\sigma_{max} = \frac{P}{hL(b+h)} \sqrt{2a^2 + \frac{(b+h)^2}{2}}$$

T-Joint Transverse fillet weld

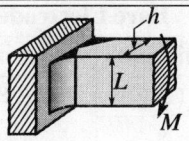

Normal stress, $\sigma = \dfrac{6M}{hL^2}$

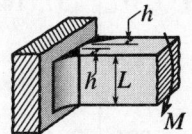

Normal stress, $\sigma = \dfrac{3M}{hL^2}$

T-Joint parallel fillet weld

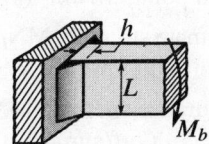

Normal stress, $\sigma = \dfrac{4.24M}{hL^2}$

T-Joint parallel fillet weld

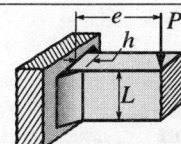

Average shear stress,

$$\tau_m = \frac{0.707P}{hL}$$

Maximum normal stress,

$$\sigma_{max} = \frac{4.24Pe}{hL^2}$$

T-Joint parallel fillet weld

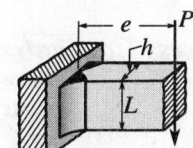

Normal stress, $\sigma = \dfrac{6Pe}{hL^2}$

Shear stress, $\tau = \dfrac{P}{hL}$

T-Joint parallel fillet weld

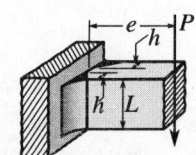

Normal stress, $\sigma = \dfrac{3Pe}{hL^2}$

Shear stress, $\tau = \dfrac{P}{2hL}$

T-Joint parallel fillet weld

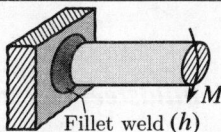

Fillet weld (h)

Normal stress, $\sigma = \dfrac{5.66M}{\pi hD^2}$

Annular fillet weld in bending

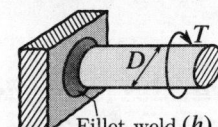

Fillet weld (h)

Shear stress, $\tau = \dfrac{2.83T}{\pi hD^2}$

Annular fillet weld in Torsion

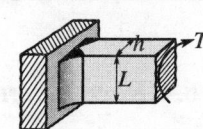

Shear stress, $\tau = \dfrac{T(3L + 1.8h)}{h^2L^2}$

T-Joint fillet weld in Torsion

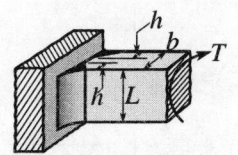

Shear stress, $\tau = \dfrac{T}{(b-h)(L-h)h}$

T-Joint fillet weld in Torsion

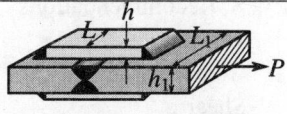

Fillet weld (h)

Normal stress,

$$\sigma = \frac{4.24M}{h[h^2 + 3L(b+h)]}$$

T-Joint fillet weld

Normal stress, (Fillet weld)

$$\sigma = \frac{1.414P}{2hL + h_1L_1}$$

Normal stress, (Butt weld)

$$\sigma = \frac{P}{2hL + h_1L_1}$$

Combined fillet and butt weld

Table 6.2 *Properties of Deposited weld metal*

Property	Bare Electrode		Coated Electrode	
	Minimum	Maximum	Minimum	Maximum
Yield point, MN/m^2 (kgf/mm^2)	235 (24.0)	275 (28.0)	290 (29.5)	380 (38.7)
Ultimate strength, MN/m^2 (kgf/mm^2)	310 (31.6)	380 (38.7)	415 (42.2)	482 (49.2)
Endurance strength, MN/m^2 (kgf/mm^2)	110 (11.3)	137 (14.0)	180 (18.3)	210 (21.1)
% Elongation, 50 mm	8	15	25	35
% Reduction of area	15	20	45	65
Impact strength, Izod, N mm (kgf-mm)	6870 (700)	20600 (2100)	53940 (5500)	67700 (6900)
Density, kg/mm^3	7.5 ×10^{-6}	7.6 ×10^{-6}	7.81 ×10^{-6}	7.85 ×10^{-6}

Table 6.3 *Stress Concentrstion Factors*

Type of weld	Stress concentration factor
Reinforced butt weld	1.2
Toe of transverse fillet weld	1.5
T-Butt joint with short corners	2.0
End of longitudinal fillet weld	2.7

Table 6.4 *Recommended design stresses for welds made with mildsteel electrodes, MN/m^2 (kgf/mm^2)*

Type of load	Bare Electrode		Coated Electrode	
	Steady loads	Reversed loads	Steady loads	Reversed loads
A.W.S. Recommendations				
Tension	90 (9.10)	35 (3.60)		
Compression	124 (12.65)	48 (4.90)		
Shear	78 (7.95)	24 (2.40)		
C.W. Jennings				
Recommendations Butt welds				
Tension	90 (9.10)	34 (3.50)	110 (11.20)	55 (5.60)
Compression	103 (10.50)	34 (3.50)	124 (12.65)	55 (5.60)
Shear	55 (5.60)	21 (2.10)	69 (7.00)	34 (3.50)
Fillet welds (all)	78 (7.95)	21 (2.10)	96 (9.80)	34 (3.50)

Table 6.5 *Strength of Shield arc steel welds subjected to repeated loads*

Type of joint	Kind of stress	Recommended stress, MN/m² (kgf/mm²)	
		Load varies from O to F	Load varies from $+F$ to $-F$
Butt-welded from both sides	Tension or compression	93 (9.5)	62 (6.3)
Butt-welded from both sides	Shear	62 (6.3)	41 (4.2)
Fillet welded	Tension, Compression or shear	49 (5.0)	33 (3.4)

Table 6.6 *(a) Plate Thickness and the Minimum Size of Fillet Weld.*

Plate thickness (mm)	Minimum weld size (mm)	Plate thickness (mm)	Minimum weld size (mm)
3 to 5	3	18 to 24	10
6 to 8	5	26 to 35	15
10 to 16	6	Over 38	20

Table 6.6 *(b) Allowable loads on Mild Steel Fillet Welds*

Size of weld, mm.	Allowable static load per linear mm of weld, N (kgf)			
	Bare welding rod		Shield arc	
	Normal weld	Parallel weld	Normal weld	Parallel weld
3 by 3	165 (16.8)	132 (13.5)	206 (21.0)	165 (16.8)
5 by 5	275 (28.0)	220 (22.5)	342 (35.0)	275 (28.0)
8 by 8	440 (44.8)	350 (36.0)	550 (56.0)	440 (44.8)
10 by 10	550 (56.0)	440 (45.0)	686 (70.0)	550 (56.0)
12 by 12	660 (67.2)	530 (54.0)	825 (84.0)	660 (67.2)
15 by 15	825 (84.0)	662 (67.5)	1030 (105.0)	825 (84.0)
20 by 20	1100 (112.0)	880 (90.0)	1370 (140.0)	1100 (112.0)

Table 6.6 *(c) Allowable Loads on Mild Steel Butt Welds*

Plate thickness mm	Allowable static load per linear mm of weld, N (kgf).			
	Bare welding rod		Shield arc	
	Normal weld (Tension & compression)	Parallel weld (shear)	Normal weld (Tension & compression)	Parallel weld (shear)
3	300 (31.0)	190 (19.5)	380 (38.7)	240 (24.5)
5	450 (46.0)	285 (29.0)	570 (58.0)	360 (36.7)
10	900 (91.7)	570 (58.0)	1140 (116.0)	720 (73.4)
12	1240 (126.4)	775 (79.0)	1550 (158.0)	970 (99.0)
16	1545 (157.0)	960 (98.0)	1930 (197.0)	1200 (122.0)
20	1800 (183.5)	1140 (116.0)	2280 (232.0)	1440 (147.0)
25	2472 (252.0)	1544 (157.0)	3090 (315.0)	1930 (197.0)

Table 6.7 *Section modulus in bending (Z) and polar moment of inertia in torsion (J) for typical fillet welded connections.*

Type of weld	Section modulus in Bending (Z), mm³ (about horizontal axis-x-x)	Polar moment of inertia in torsion (J), mm⁴
1	2	3
	$Z = \dfrac{nh_t^2}{6}$	$j = \dfrac{h_t n^3}{12}$
	$Z = \dfrac{h_t m^2}{6}$	$J = \dfrac{h_t m^3}{12}$
	$Z = h_t nm$	$J = \dfrac{h_t n(3m^2 + n^2)}{6}$
	$Z = \dfrac{h_t m^2}{3}$	$J = \dfrac{h_t m(m^2 + 3n^2)}{6}$
$m_x = \dfrac{m^2}{2(n+m)}$ $n_y = \dfrac{n^2}{2(n+m)}$	$Z = h_t\left(\dfrac{4nm + m^2}{6}\right)$ top $Z = h_t\left\{\dfrac{m^2(4nm + m)}{6(2n+m)}\right\}$ bottom	$J = h_t\dfrac{(n+m)^4 - 6n^2m^2}{12(n+m)}$
$n_y = \dfrac{n^2}{2(n+m)}$	$Z = h_t\left(nm + \dfrac{m^2}{6}\right)$	$J = h_t\left\{\dfrac{(2n+m)^3}{12} - \dfrac{n^2(n+m)^2}{(2n+m)}\right\}$

Table 6.7 *Section modulus in bending (Z) and polar moment of inertia in torsion (J) for typical fillet welded connections. – (Contd..)*

1	2	3
$m_x = \dfrac{m^2}{n+2m}$	$Z = h_t\left(\dfrac{2nm + m^3}{3}\right)$ top $Z = h_t\left\{\dfrac{m^2(2n+m)}{3(n+m)}\right\}$ bottom	$J = h_t\left\{\dfrac{(n+2m)^3}{12} - \dfrac{m^2(n+m)^2}{(n+2m)}\right\}$
	$Z = h_t\left(nm + \dfrac{m^2}{3}\right)$	$J = \dfrac{h_t(n+m)^3}{6}$
$m_x = \dfrac{m^2}{n+2m}$	$Z = \dfrac{h_t(2nm + m^2)}{3}$ top $Z = h_t\left\{\dfrac{m^2(2n+m)}{3(n+m)}\right\}$ bottom	$J = h_t\left\{\dfrac{(n+2m)^3}{12} - \dfrac{m^2(n+m)^2}{(n+2m)}\right\}$
$m_x = \dfrac{m^2}{2(n+m)}$	$Z = \dfrac{h_t(4nm + m^2)}{3}$ top $Z = h_t\left(\dfrac{4nm^2 + m^3}{6n + 3m}\right)$ bottom	$J = h_t\left\{\dfrac{m^3(4n+m)}{6(n+m)} + \dfrac{n^3}{6}\right\}$
	$Z = h_t\left(nm + \dfrac{m^2}{3}\right)$	$J = h_t\left(\dfrac{n^3 + 3nm^2 + m^3}{6}\right)$
	$Z = h_t\left(2nm + \dfrac{m^2}{3}\right)$	$J = h_t\left(\dfrac{2n^3 + 6nm^2 + m^3}{6}\right)$
	$Z = \dfrac{\pi m^2 h_t}{4}$	$J = \dfrac{\pi m^3 h_t}{4}$

CYLINDERS, PIPES AND TUBES 7

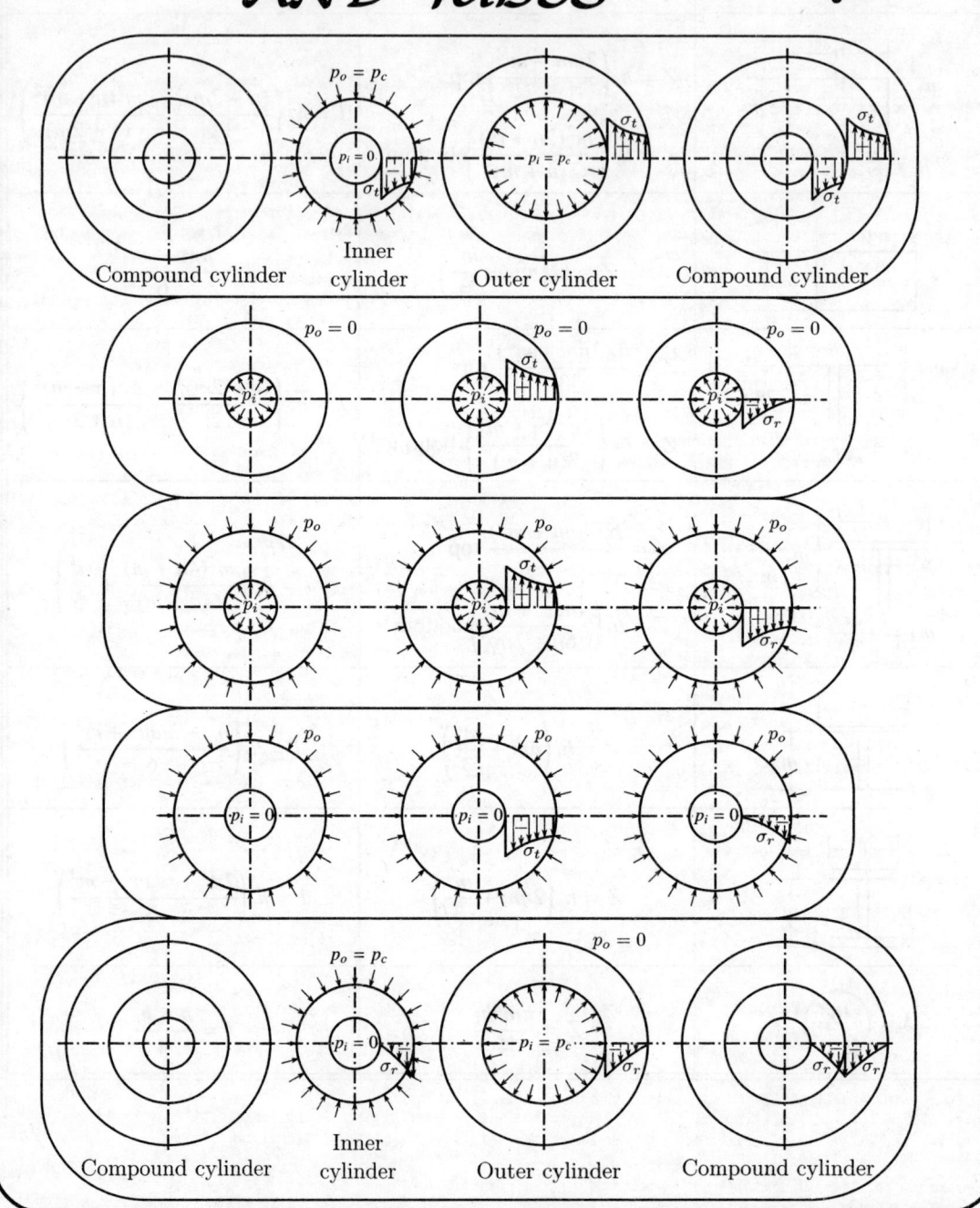

Compound cylinder Inner cylinder Outer cylinder Compound cylinder

Compound cylinder Inner cylinder Outer cylinder Compound cylinder

7

Cylinders, Pipes and Tubes

Symbols	Description and Units
B	Total shrinkage allowance, mm
d_c	diameter of the contact surface in compound cylinders, mm
d_i	inside diameter of pipe or cylinder, mm
d_o	outside diameter of pipe or cylinder, mm
f	cofficient of friction (ranges from 0.04 to 0.25, average value of $f = 0.08$)
p	working pressure, MN/m^2 (kgf/mm^2)
p_c	pressure at the contact surface of compound cylinders, MN/m^2 (kgf/mm^2)
p_{cr}	critical or collapsing pressure, MN/m^2 (kgf/mm^2)
p_i	internal pressure, MN/m^2 (kgf/mm^2)
p_o	external pressure, MN/m^2 (kgf/mm^2)
r	radius at any point in the cylinder wall, mm
t	wall thickness, mm
α	coefficient of expansion
σ	Permissible working stress, MN/m^2 (kgf/mm^2) (Table 7.1)
σ_r	radial stress, MN/m^2 (kgf/mm^2)
σ_t	tangential stress, MN/m^2 (kgf/mm^2)
μ	Poisson's ratio of laternal contraction

Particular	Equation	Eqn. No.
Thin Cylinders:		
For thin cylinders	$t/d < 0.07$	7.1(a)
Circumferential tensile stress or the tangentail stress (hoop stress)	$\sigma_t = \dfrac{pd_i}{2t}$	7.1(b)
When there is a seam or joint in the clyinder,	$\sigma_t = \dfrac{pd_i}{2\eta t}$	7.1(c)

Particular	Equation	Eqn. No.
Longitudinal tensile stress or the stress in the cylinder wall parallel to it axis	$\sigma_t = \dfrac{pd_i}{4t}$	7.1(d)
when there is a seam of joint in the cylinder the longitudinal tensile stress	$\sigma_t = \dfrac{pdi}{4\eta t}$ where η is the efficiency of the joint	7.1(e)

Long thin tubes with internal pressure:

The permissible steam pressure on steel and iron pipes (according to **ASME** Boiler code)

a) for nominal diameters between 6 mm to 125 mm.	$p = \dfrac{2\sigma}{d_o}(t - 1.65) - 0.862 \quad (SI\ units)$ $= \dfrac{2\sigma}{d_o}(t - 1.65) - 0.0879 \ (Metric\ units)$	7.2(a)
b) for nominal diameters over 125 mm	$p = \dfrac{2\sigma}{d_o}(t - 2.5)$	7.2(b)

The permissible pressure in wrought iron and steel tubes
for water tube boilers (according to **ASME** Boiler code).

seamless tubes at all pressures, welded steel tubes at pressures below 6.03 MN/m² (0.615 kgf/mm²) and lap welded wrought iron tubes at pressure below 2.45 MN/m² (0.25 kgf/mm²)	$p = \left[\dfrac{t - 0.99}{d_o}\right]124 - 1.726 \quad (SI\ units)$ $= \left[\dfrac{t - 0.99}{d_o}\right]12.65 - 0.176 \ (metric\ units)$	7.2(c)
welded steel tubes at pressure of 6.03 MN/m² (0.615 kgf/mm²) and above	$p = \left[\dfrac{t - 0.99}{d_o}\right]96.5 \ (SI\ units)$ $= \left[\dfrac{t - 0.99}{d_o}\right]9.84 \quad (Metric\ units)$	7.2(d)
lap welded wrought iron tubes at pressure of 2.45 MN/m² (0.25 kgf/mm²) and above	$p = \left[\dfrac{t - 0.99}{d_o}\right]72.8 \quad (SI\ units)$ $= \left[\dfrac{t - 0.99}{d_o}\right]7.45 \quad (Metric\ units)$	7.2(e)

Engine and press cylinders:

The wall thickness of engine and press cylinders.	$t = \dfrac{pd_i}{2\sigma_t} + 8.0mm$ where $\sigma_t = 8.825$ MN/-m² (0.90 kgf/mm²) for ordinary grade of cast iron	7.3

Particular	**Equation**	**Eqn. No.**

Openings in cylindrical drums:

According to D. S. Jacobus the largest permissible diameter or opening, mm.

$$d' = 8.3161 \sqrt[3]{d_o t (1.0 - K)}$$ 7.4(a)

where K is the ratio of the stress in the solid plate to one fifth the minimum tensile strength of the steel used in the shell, or

$$K = \left[\frac{p d_o}{2t} \right] (5/\sigma_u)$$ 7.4(b)

where d_o is the outside diameter of drum, mm

The minimum diameter of the unreinforced holes should be limited to 200 mm and should not exceed 0.60 d

Thin tubes with external pressure:

The collapsing pressure for seamless steel tubes (Professor A.P. Carman's formula)

a) when $(t/d_o) < 0.025$

$$p_{cr} = 346122(t/d_o)^3 \; (SI \; units)$$

$$= 35295(t/d_o)^3 \; (Metric \; units)$$ 7.5(a)

b) when $\dfrac{t}{d_o} > 0.03$

$$p_{cr} = 658.6 \frac{t}{d_o} - 14.5 \; (SI \; units)$$

$$= 67.16 \frac{t}{d_o} - 1.47 \; (Metric \; units)$$ 7.5(b)

Prof. A. P. Carman's formula for the collapsing pressure for lap-welded:

a) Steel tubes

$$p_{cr} = 574.28 \frac{t}{d_o} - 7.06 \; (SI \; units)$$

$$= 58.56 \frac{t}{d_o} - 0.72 \; (Metric \; units) \quad when \; t/d_o > 0.03$$ 7.6(a)

b) brass tubes

$$p_{cr} = 173406(t/d_o)^3 \; (SI \; units)$$

$$= 17682.5 \left(\frac{t}{d_o} \right)^3 \; (Metric \; units) \quad when \; t/d_o < 0.025$$ 7.6(b)

$$p_{cr} = 643.7 t/d_o - 17.06 \; (SI \; units)$$

$$65.64 \frac{t}{d_o} - 1.74 \; (Metric \; units) \quad when \; t/d_o > 0.03$$ 7.6(c)

Particular	Equation	Eqn. No.
Short tubes with external pressure:		
The collapsing pressure for short tubes, i.e. when $L < 6d_o$, (Sir William Fairbairn formula)	$p_{cr} = 35980 \dfrac{t^{2.19}}{Ld_o}$ *(SI units)* $= 3669 \dfrac{t^{2.19}}{Ld_o}$ *(Metric units)*	7.7(a)
The crushing stress for short tubes.	$\sigma_c = \dfrac{p_o d_o}{2t}$	7.7(b)
Unfired pressure vessels with external pressure:		
Critical pressure or collapsing pressure of large cylinder	$p_{cr} = \dfrac{2.6E(t/d_o)^{2.5}}{(L/d_o) - 0.45(t/d_o)^{0.5}}$	7.8

where L = maximum distance between supports or stiffening rings, mm

p_{cr} = the critical pressure, MN/m^2 (kgf/mm^2)

= 5 times the working pressure and in no case should the vessel be designed for less than 0.1 MN/m^2 (0.01 kgf/mm^2) working pressure

E = modulus of Elasticity, MN/m^2, (kgf/mm^2)

The moment of inertia of the stiffening ring, mm^4 $\qquad I = \dfrac{p_{cr}d^3L}{24E}$ $\qquad$ 7.9

where p_{cr} for the rings is about 10 percent larger than that of the shell proper

Thick Cylinders :   *Lame's Equations*

The tangential stress in the cylinder wall at radius r

$$\sigma_t = \frac{p_i d_i^2 - p_o d_o^2}{d_o^2 - d_i^2} + \frac{d_i^2 d_o^2 (p_i - p_o)}{4r^2(d_o^2 - d_i^2)} = a + \frac{b}{r^2} \qquad 7.10(a)$$

The radial stress in the cylinder wall at radius r

$$\sigma_r = \frac{p_i d_i^2 - p_o d_o^2}{d_o^2 - d_i^2} - \frac{d_i^2 d_o^2 (p_i - p_o)}{4r^2(d_o^2 - d_i^2)} = a - b/r^2 \qquad 7.10(b)$$

where a and b are constants for any given values of pressures and diameters

$$a = \frac{p_i d_i^2 - p_o d_o^2}{d_o^2 - d_i^2}, \qquad b = \frac{d_i^2 d_o^2 (p_i - p_o)}{4(d_o^2 - d_i^2)} \qquad 7.10(c)$$

Particular	Equation	Eqn. No.
Lame's equation for internal pressure:		
The tangential stress at radius r	$\sigma_t = \dfrac{p_i d_i^2}{4r^2}\left(\dfrac{4r^2 + d_o^2}{d_o^2 - d_i^2}\right)$	7.11(a)
The radial stress at radius r	$\sigma_r = \dfrac{p_i d_i^2}{4r^2}\left(\dfrac{4r^2 - d_o^2}{d_o^2 - d_i^2}\right)$	7.11(b)
The maximum tangential stress at the inner surface	$\sigma_{t\,max} = \dfrac{p_i(d_o^2 + d_i^2)}{d_o^2 - d_i^2}$	7.11(c)
The maximum radial stress at the inner surface	$\sigma_{r\,max} = -p_i$	7.11(d)
The maximum shear stress at the inner surface	$\tau_{max} = \dfrac{p_i d_o^2}{d_o^2 - d_i^2}$	7.11(e)
The equivalent maximum tension in the cylinder wall according to maximum shear theory	$\sigma_{t\,max} = \dfrac{2p_i d_o^2}{d_o^2 - d_i^2}$	7.11(f)
The cylinder wall thickness for birttle materials based on the maximum normal stress theory	$t = \dfrac{d_i}{2}\left[\left(\dfrac{\sigma_t + p_i}{\sigma_t - p_i}\right)^{\frac{1}{2}} - 1\right]$	7.11(g)
The cylinder wall thickness for ductile materials based on the maximum shear theory	$t = \dfrac{d_i}{2}\left[\left(\dfrac{\sigma_t}{\sigma_t - 2p_i}\right)^{\frac{1}{2}} - 1\right]$	7.11(h)
Clavarino's Equations for closed cylinders:	(Based on the maximum strain theory)	
The general equation for the tangential stress at radius r	$\sigma_t' = (1 - 2\mu)a + \dfrac{(1 + \mu)b}{r^2}$	7.12(a)
The radial stress at radius r	$\sigma_r'' = (1 - 2\mu)a - \dfrac{(1 + \mu)b}{r^2}$	7.12(b)
The cylinder wall thickness	$t = \dfrac{d_i}{2}\left[\left(\dfrac{\sigma_t' + (1 - 2\mu)p_i}{\sigma_t' - (1 + \mu)p_i}\right)^{\frac{1}{2}} - 1\right]$	7.12(c)
Birnie's Equations for open cylinders:		
The tangential stress at radius r, according to Birnie's equation for open cylinders	$\sigma_t' = (1 - \mu)a + (1 + \mu)\dfrac{b}{r^2}$	7.13(a)

Particular	Equation	Eqn. No.
The radial stress at radius r, for open cylinders	$\sigma'_r = (1 - \mu)a - (1 + \mu)\dfrac{b}{r^2}$	7.13(b)
The cylinder wall thickness, for open cylinders	$t = \dfrac{d_i}{2}\left[\left(\dfrac{\sigma'_t + (1 - \mu)p_i}{\sigma'_t - (1 + \mu)p_i}\right)^{\frac{1}{2}} - 1\right]$	7.13(c)

where a and b have the same meaning as in equation 7.10(c)

Barlow's equations:

| The tangential stress according to Barlow's equation (High pressure oil and gas pipes) | $\sigma_t = \dfrac{p_i d_o}{2t}$ | 7.13(d) |

values of σ_t can be taken from table 7.2.

Changes in cylinder diameter due to pressure:

| The increase in internal diameter of the cylinder due to internal pressure only | $\Delta d_i = \dfrac{p_i d_i}{E}\left[\dfrac{d_o^2 + d_i^2}{d_o^2 - d_i^2} + \mu\right]$ | 7.14(a) |
| The decrease in external diameter of a cylinder subjected to external pressure only | $\Delta d_o = \dfrac{p_o d_o}{E}\left[\dfrac{d_o^2 + d_i^2}{d_o^2 - d_i^2} - \mu\right]$ | 7.14(b) |

Compound cylinders:

| The tangential stress at any radius r for a cylinder open at both ends and subjected to internal pressure (Birnie's equation) | $\sigma_t = (1 - \mu)\dfrac{p_i d_i^2}{d_o^2 - d_i^2} + (1 + \mu)\dfrac{p_i d_i^2 d_o^2}{4r^2(d_o^2 - d_i^2)}$ | 7.15(a) |
| The radial stress at any radius r for a cylinder open at both ends and subjected to internal pressure (Birnie's equation) | $\sigma_r = (1 - \mu)\dfrac{p_i d_i^2}{d_o^2 - d_i^2} - (1 + \mu)\dfrac{p_i d_i^2 d_o^2}{4r^2(d_o^2 - d_i^2)}$ | 7.15(b) |

Press and Shrink fits

| The tangential stress at the inner surface of the inner cylinder (Fig. 7.1) | $\sigma_{t\text{-}i} = \dfrac{-2p_c d_c^2}{d_c^2 - d_i^2}$ | 7.16(a) |

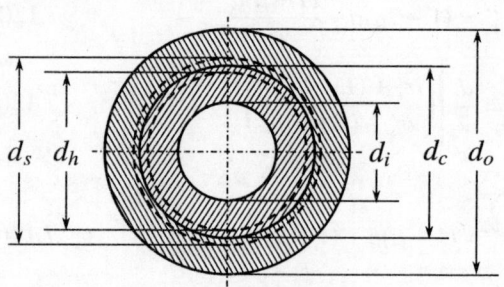

Fig. 7.1 *Shrink fit.*

d_i is the inside diameter of the inner cylinder
d_s is the outside diameter of the inner cylinder
d_n is the inside diameter of the outer cylinder
d_o is the outside diameter of the outer cylinder

Particular	Equation	Eqn. No.
The tangential stress at the outer surface of the inner cylinder	$$\sigma_{t\text{-}c} = -p_c\left(\frac{d_c^2 + d_i^2}{d_c^2 - d_i^2} - \mu\right)$$	7.16(b)
The tangential stress at the inner surface of the outer cylinder	$$\sigma_{t\text{-}c} = p_c\left(\frac{d_o^2 + d_c^2}{d_o^2 - d_c^2} + \mu\right)$$	7.16(c)
The tangential stress at the outer surface of the outer cylinder	$$\sigma_{t\text{-}o} = \frac{2p_c d_c^2}{d_o^2 - d_c^2}$$	7.16(d)

Radial pressure between the cylinders:

The total shrinkage allowance:

$$B = \frac{p_c d_s}{E_s}\left(\frac{d_s^2 + d_i^2}{d_s^2 - d_i^2} - \mu_s\right) + \frac{p_c d_h}{E_h}\left(\frac{d_o^2 + d_h^2}{d_o^2 - d_h^2} + \mu_h\right)$$

$$\approx p_c d_c\left[\frac{d_c^2 + d_i^2}{E_s(d_c^2 - d_i^2)} + \frac{d_o^2 + d_c^2}{E_h(d_o^2 - d_c^2)} - \frac{\mu_s}{E_s} + \frac{\mu_h}{E_h}\right] \qquad 7.17(a)$$

when both the cylinders are made of same material the pressure between the cylinders is given by the equation	$$p_c = \frac{BE(d_c^2 - d_i^2)(d_o^2 - d_c^2)}{2d_c^3(d_o^2 - d_i^2)}$$	7.17(b)

Forces resulting in interference fits:

The total axial force required to assemble a force fit (approximately)	$$F_a = \pi d L f p_c$$	7.18(a)
The torque transmitted	$$T = \frac{F_a d}{2} = \frac{\pi d^2 L f p_c}{2}$$	7.18(b)

where L = length of the external memeber or hub, mm

d = outer diameter of the internal member, mm

f = coefficient of friction

Stress due to Force and Shrink fits:

When relatively thin bands are shrunk on heavy internal members, the shrinkage stress in the band (approximately)	$$\sigma_t = E\delta = \frac{EB}{d_c}$$	7.19(a)

Particular	Equation	Eqn. No.
The temperature to which a piece to be shrunk must be heated for assembling	$$t_2 \geq \left(\frac{B}{a d_c} + t_1 \right)$$ where t_1 = original temperature of the parts (i.e. shaft) in shrink fit assembly	7.19(b)

References

[1] Vallance A., Doughtie V. L., *"Design of Machine Members"*, 3rd Ed. McGraw Hill, Book Co., 1951.

[2] Spotts M. E., *"Design of Machine Elements"*, 3rd edition, Prentice Hall, Inc., Maruzen Co. Ltd.

[3] Hall A. S., Holowenko A. R., Laughlin, H. G., Schaum's Outline of: *"Theory and Problems of Machine Design"*, Schaum Publishing Co., 1961.

Table 7.1 Values of σ to be used in equations 7.2(a) and 7.2(b)

Material	Spec. no.	243 (-30) to 613 (340)	For temperature in $K(°C)$ not to exceed						
			643 (370)	673 (400)	698 (425)	728 (455)	753 (480)	783 (510)	813 (540)
Seamless medium carbon steel	S – 18	82.4 (8.4)	82.4 (8.4)	71.6 (7.3)	57.5 (5.9)	43.5 (4.5)	30.5 (3.1)	18.0 (1.85)	—
Seamless low carbon steel	S – 18	65.0 (6.6)	62.0 (6.3)	59.0 (6.1)	49.0 (5.0)	40.0 (4.1)	30.5 (3.1)	18.0 (1.85)	—
Fusion welded steel	S – 1	75.5 (7.7)	71.0 (7.3)	66.0 (6.7)	55.0 (5.6)	43.5 (4.5)	30.5 (3.1)	18.0 (1.85)	—
Fusion welded steel:									
Grade *B*	S – 2	68.6 (7.0)	66.2 (6.8)	62.0 (6.3)	51.5 (5.3)	41.0 (4.2)	30.5 (3.1)	18.0 (1.85)	—
Grade *A*	S – 2	62.0 (6.3)	61.0 (6.2)	58.0 (5.9)	47.5 (4.9)	39.0 (4.0)	30.5 (3.1)	18.0 (1.85)	—
Lap-welded steel	S – 18	62.0 (6.3)	61.0 (6.2)	58.0 (5.9)	47.5 (4.9)	39.0 (4.0)	30.5 (3.1)	18.0 (1.85)	—
Butt-welded steel	S – 18	62.0 (6.3)	61.0 (6.2)	58.0 (5.9)	—	—	—	—	—
Lap-welded wrought iron	S – 19	55.0 (5.6)	53.0 (5.4)	47.5 (4.9)	—	—	—	—	—
Butt-welded wrought iron	S – 19	55.0 (5.6)	53.0 (5.4)	47.5 (4.9)	—	—	—	—	—
Seamless alloy steel, Grade P1	S – 45	75.5 (7.7)	75.5 (7.7)	75.5 (7.7)	74.0 (7.6)	72.5 (7.4)	68.6 (7.0)	55.0 (5.6)	34.0 (3.5)

The thickness subtraction factor in equations 7.2(a) and 7.2(b) limits the actual working stress to a value less than σ in order to allow for cross strains and mechanical or thermal stresses that cannot be determined accurately.

Table 7.2 Values of σ_t to be used in equation 7.13(d) for non-ferrous seamless tubes and pipes

Material	Spec. no.	For temperature in $K(°C)$ not to exceed						
		253 (–20) to 338 (65)	393 (120)	448 (175)	473 (200)	503 (230)	533 (260)	563 (290)
Muntz metal tubing and high brass tubing	S – 24	34.0 (3.5)	27.5 (2.8)	17.2 (1.75)	—	—	—	—
Muntz metal condenser tubes	S – 47	34.0 (3.5)	27.5 (2.8)	17.2 (1.75)	—	—	—	—
Red brass tubes	S – 24	41.2 (4.2)	37.8 (3.9)	34.0 (3.50)	30.9 (3.15)	—	—	—
Copper tubes	S – 22	41.2 (4.2)	34.0 (3.5)	30.9 (3.15)	27.5 (2.80)	—	—	—
Copper pipes	S – 23	41.2 (4.2)	34.0 (3.5)	30.9 (3.15)	27.5 (2.80)	—	—	—
Admiralty tubing	S – 24	48.0 (4.9)	45.0 (4.6)	41.2 (4.20)	37.8 (3.85)	30.9 (3.15)	—	—
Admiralty condenser tubes	S – 47	48.0 (4.9)	45.0 (4.6)	41.2 (4.20)	37.8 (3.85)	30.9 (3.15)	—	—
Steam bronz	S – 41	47.1 (4.8)	43.2 (4.4)	40.2 (4.10)	37.3 (3.80)	34.0 (3.50)	28.9 (2.95)	22.6 (2.30)

Stress in this table when used with equation 7.13(d) are applicable only to diameters 12.5 mm to 150 mm outside diameter inclusive, and for wall thickness not less than No. 18 *BWG* (0.049 in or 1.25 mm.)

Additional wall thickness should be provided where corrosion, or wear due to cleaning operations, is expected.

Where tube ends are threaded wall thickness of $\dfrac{8}{\text{no. of threads}}$ is to be provided.

Requirements for rolling or otherwise setting tubes in tube plates, may require additional thickness.

8

Shells, Flat Plates and Cylinder Heads

Symbols	Description and Units
a	short span of non-circular heads, mm
b	long span of non-circular heads or covers measured perpendicular to short span, mm
C	a factor depending upon the method of attachment to shell (Table 8.1)
D	diameter or short span measured as in Table 8.1, mm
D_i	inside diameter of the shell, mm
D_o	outside diameter of the shell, mm
E	modulus of elasticity at the operating temperature, MN/m^2 (kgf//mm^2) (Table 8.4)
F_B	total bolt load, N (kgf)
h_g	gasket moment arm equal to the radial distance from the centre line of the bolts to the line of gasket reaction, mm
J	Joint factor (Table 8.2)
K	the ratio of the elastic modulus E of the material at the design metal temperature to the room temperature elastic modulus (refer Table 8.4(a) to 8.4(d))
l	length of the flange of flanged heads, mm
L	effective length of the shell, mm
M	longitudinal bending moment, N mm (kgf-mm)
p	internal (design or test as appropriate) pressure, MN/m^2 (kgf/mm^2)
t	minimum thickness of shell plate exclusive of corrosion allowance, mm
t_r, t_s	required and actual thickness of the shell under design conditions, exclusive of corrosion allowance, mm
T	torque about vessel axis, N mm (kgf-mm)
W	weight (vertical vessel only), N (kgf)
	(for points above plane of support–weight of vessel, fittings, attachments and fluid supported above the point considered, the sum to be given a negative sign in equation 8.3(a); for points below plane of support-weight of vessel, fittings, attachment below the point considered, plus weight of fluid contents, the sum to be given a positive sign in equation 8.3(a))

Symbols	Description and Units
σ	allowable stress value, MN/m² (kgf/mm²) (Table 8.3)
σ_e	elastic limit stress (shear strain energy basis), MN/m² (kgf/mm²)
σ_z	longitudinal stress, MN/m² (kgf/mm²)
σ_θ	hoop stress, MN/m² (kgf/mm²)
τ	shearing stress, MN/m² (kgf/mm²)

Particular	Equation	Eqn. No.
Shells Subjected to Internal Pressure *(Unfired pressure vessels)**		
The minimum thickness of shell plates exclusive of corrosion allowance in mm		
a) For cylindrical shells:	$t = \dfrac{pD_i}{2\sigma J - p} = \dfrac{pD_o}{2\sigma J + p}$	8.1
b) For spherical shells:	$t = \dfrac{pD_i}{4\sigma J - p} = \dfrac{pD_o}{4\sigma J + p}$	8.2
The stress equivalent to the membrane stress on the shear strain energy criterion is given by the Huber-Hencky equation	$\sigma_e = \left[\sigma_\theta^2 - \sigma_\theta\sigma_z + \sigma_z^2 + 3\tau^2\right]^{\frac{1}{2}}$	8.3

where σ_z = longitudinal stress (tensile) MN/m² (kgf/mm²)

$$= \frac{\frac{\pi}{4}pD_i^2 + W \pm 4\dfrac{M}{D_i}}{\pi t(D_i + t)} \le \sigma \qquad \text{8.3(a)}$$

σ_z = longitudinal stress (compressive) $\le 0.125E\left(\dfrac{t}{D_o}\right)$

	$\sigma_\theta = \dfrac{p(D_i + t)}{2t}$	8.3(b)
	$\tau = \dfrac{2T}{\pi t D_i(D_i + t)}$	8.3(c)
Shells Subjected to External Pressure:		
The thickness of the cylindrical shells under external pressure is given by equations	$t = \dfrac{D_o}{100}\left[\dfrac{115p}{\sigma} + 0.053\left(\dfrac{K\sigma L}{D_o}\right)^{\frac{2}{3}}\right]$	8.4(a)

$$\text{when} \quad \frac{L}{D_o} < \frac{0.58(1000p/\sigma)^{\frac{5}{2}}}{100pK} \quad \text{or} \quad < \frac{38(100t/D_o)^{\frac{3}{2}}}{K\sigma}$$

*Indian Standard Code for unfired pressure vessels.

Particular	Equation	Eqn. No.
	$t = 1.03 \dfrac{D_o}{100}(100pK)^{\frac{1}{3}}$ but not less than $\dfrac{3.5pD_o}{2\sigma}$	8.4(b)

$$\text{when} \quad \frac{L}{D_o} > \frac{14.4}{(100pK)^{\frac{1}{6}}} \text{ or } > \frac{14.9}{(100t/D_o)^{\frac{1}{2}}} \text{ or } \frac{0.58(1000p/\sigma)^{\frac{5}{2}}}{100pK} > 14.4/(100pK)^{\frac{1}{6}}$$

$$\text{or } 38\frac{(100t/D_0)^{\frac{3}{2}}}{K\sigma} > \frac{14.6}{(100t/D_o)^{\frac{1}{2}}}$$

In all other cases the thickness	$t = \dfrac{D_o}{100}\left[7.5p\dfrac{L}{D_o}K\right]^{\frac{2}{5}}$	8.4(c)
Thickness of spherical shells under external pressure	$t = \dfrac{pD_o}{0.80\sigma}$	8.5

where $\sigma = 0.2$ percent proof stress in MN/m^2 (kgf/mm^2)

Unstayed Flat Heads and Covers
Thickness of Flat heads and covers:

The thickness of flat unstayed circular heads and covoers shall be calculated by the formula when the head or cover is attached by bolt's causing an edge movement

$$t = CD\sqrt{p/\sigma} \quad \text{For 'C' and 'D' refer Table 8.1} \qquad 8.6$$

The thickness of flat unstayed non-circular heads and covers shall be calculated by the formula

$$t = CZa\sqrt{p/\sigma} \qquad 8.7$$

where Z = the factor for non-circular heads depending
upon the ratio of short span to long span a/b (Fig. 8.1)

Spherically dished covers:

The thickness of spherically dished ends secured to the shell to a flange connection by means of bolts shall be calculated by the formula (provided that the inside crown radius R of the dished cover does not exceed 1.3 times the shell inside diameter D_i and the value of $100t/R$ is not greater than 10)

$$t = \frac{3}{2}\frac{pD_i}{\sigma J} \quad \text{where } J = \text{joint factor (Table 8.2)} \qquad 8.8$$

Stayed and Braced Plates:

The thickness of the stayed and braced plates shall be calculated by the formula	$t = C_1 D_1 \sqrt{p/\sigma}$ 8.9

where D_1 = diameter of the largest circle in mm which may be inscribed between the supporting points of the plates (Fig. 8.2)

C_1 = A factor depending on the mode of support and is given by Fig. 8.3(A) to 8.3(F). When the plate is supported in different ways on the circumference of the inscribed circle of diameter D_1, a mean value is to be adopted for C_1

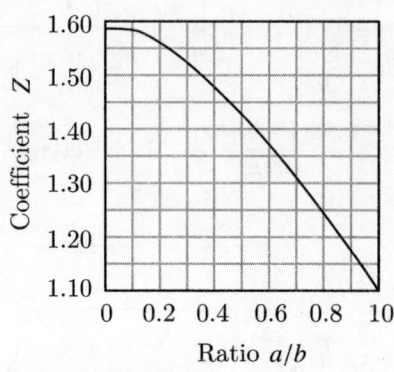

Fig. 8.1: *Value of Coefficient z for Non-Circular Flat Heads*

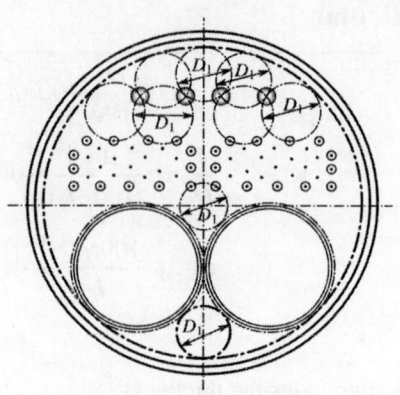

Fig. 8.2: *Stayed Flat Plate*

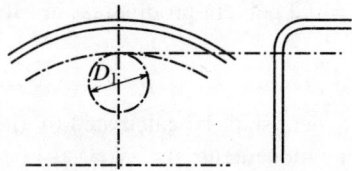

(A) Flange of a flanged head $C_1 = 0.45$

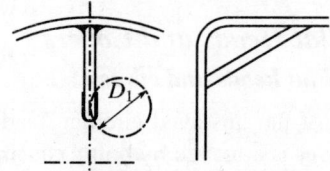

(B) Welded brace $C_1 = 0.45$

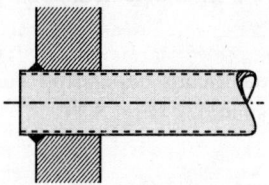

(C) Welded tube stay $C_1 - 0.55$

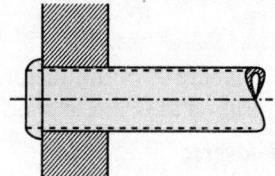

(D) Expanded and beaded tubular stay $C_1 - 0.55$

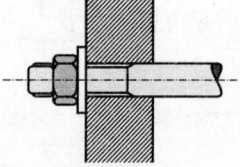

(E) Bar stay with washer of dia not less than times the stay dia $C_1 - 0.45$

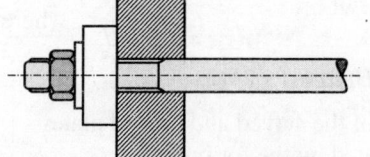

(F) Bar stay with washer and reinforcing plate of dia not less than 0.3 D $C_1 - 0.40$

Fig. 8.3: *Values of Co-Efficient C_1 Depending on the Type of Stay*

Particular	Equation	Eqn. No.
Circular plate uniformly loaded:		
The thickness of the plate with a diameter D supported at the circumference and subjected to a uniformly distributed pressure p over the total area.	$t = c_1 D \sqrt{p/\sigma}$	8.10
The maximum deflection	$y = \dfrac{c_2 D^4 p}{Et^3}$ where c_1 and c_2 are coefficients from Table 8.5	8.11
Circular plate loaded centrally:		
The thickness of a flat cast iron plate supported freely at the circumference with a diameter D and subjected to a load F distributed uniformly over an area $\dfrac{\pi D_o^2}{4}$	$t = 1.2 \sqrt{(1 - 0.670 D_o/D)\dfrac{F}{\sigma}}$	8.12
The deflection in mm	$y = \dfrac{0.12 D^2 F}{Et^3}$	8.13
Grashof's formula for the thickness of a plate rigidly fixed around the circumference with the above given type of loading	$t = 0.65 \left[\dfrac{F}{\sigma} \log_e (D/D_o)\right]^{\frac{1}{2}}$	8.14
The deflection in mm	$y = \dfrac{0.055 D^2 F}{Et^3}$	8.15
Rectangular plates:		
The thickness of a rectangular plalte subjected to uniform load (Grashoof and Bach)	$t = abc_3 \left[\dfrac{p}{\sigma(a^2 + b^2)}\right]^{\frac{1}{2}}$	8.15
The thickness of a rectangular plate on which a concentrated load F acts at the intersection of diagonals	$t = c_4 \left[\dfrac{abF}{\sigma(a^2 + b^2)}\right]^{\frac{1}{2}}$ where a = length of plate, mm b = breadth of plate, mm c_3, c_4 = coefficients from Table 8.5	8.16
Elliptical plate:		
The thickness of uniformly loaded elliptical plate	$t = abc_5 \left[\dfrac{p}{\sigma(a^2 + b^2)}\right]$ where a = minor axis, mm b = major axis, mm c_5 = coefficient, from Table 8.5	8.17

References

[1] Vallance A., Doughtie V. L., *"Design of Machine Members"*, 3rd edition, McGraw Hill Book Company, 1951.

[2] Indian Standard Code for Unfired pressure vessels.

Table 8.1 *Values of 'D' and 'C' for Typical Unstayed Flat Heads*

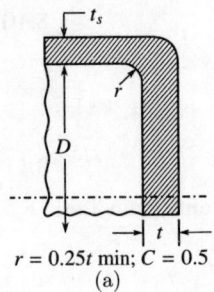
$r = 0.25t$ min; $C = 0.5$
(a)

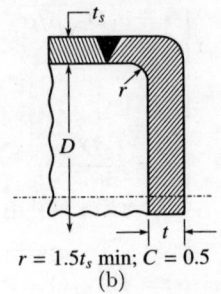
$r = 1.5t_s$ min; $C = 0.5$
(b)

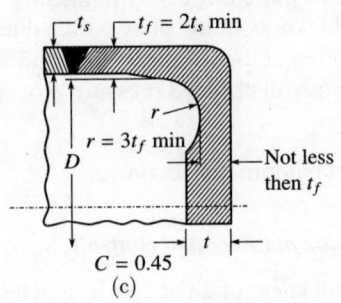
$C = 0.45$
(c)

Forged heads

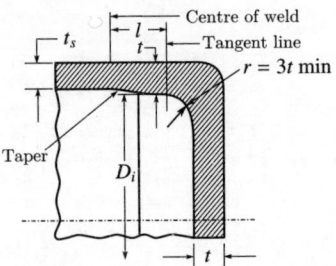

$C = 0.35$ when

$t \geq \left(1.1 - 0.8\dfrac{t_s^2}{t^2}\right) \sqrt{D_i t}$

$r \geq 2t$

$D = D_i - r$ and

taper is 1 : 4

$C = 0.45$ when

$r \geq 2t$

$D = D_i - r$ and

taper is 1 : 4

$C = 0.5$ when

$D = D_i$ and

$0.25t \leq r < 2t$

Flanged flat heads butt welded to the vessel

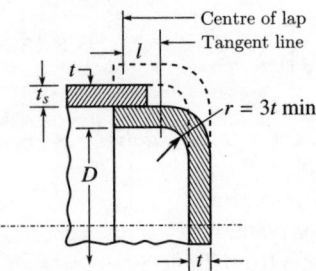

$C = 0.45$ when $t \geq \left(1.1 - 0.8\dfrac{t_s^2}{t^2}\right) \sqrt{Dt}$ and

$C = 0.55$ in other cases

Heads lap welded or brazed to the shell

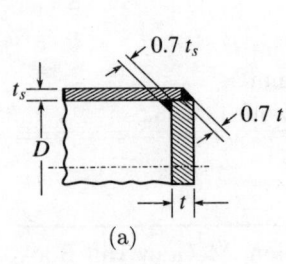
(a)

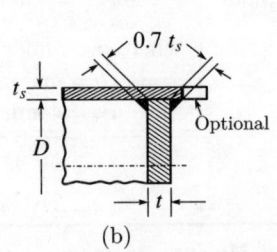
(b)

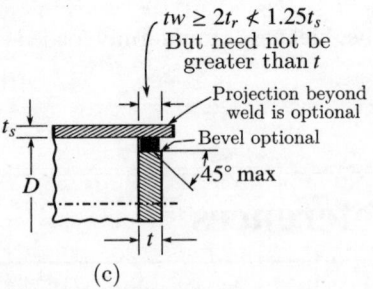
(c)

$$C = 0.7 \sqrt{\frac{t_r}{t_s}} \text{ but not less than } 0.55$$

Plates welded to the inside of the vessel

Reference: P 35-28: Indian Standard Code for unfired pressure vessels.

Table 8.1 *Values of 'D' and 'C' for Typical Unstayed Flat Heads – (Contd...)*

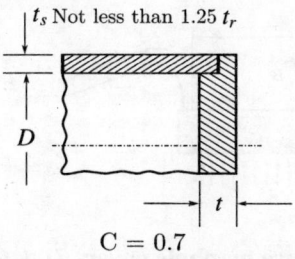

$C = 0.7$

Plates welded to the end of the shell

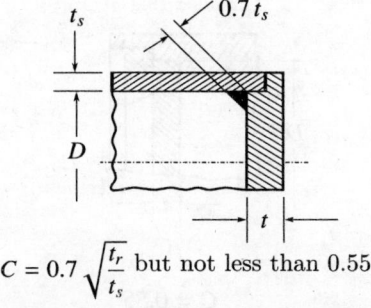

$C = 0.7 \sqrt{\dfrac{t_r}{t_s}}$ but not less than 0.55

Plates welded to the end of the shell with an additional fillet weld on the inside.

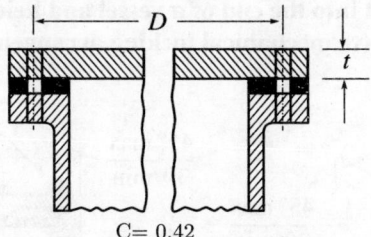

$C = 0.42$

Covers riveted or bolted with a full face gaskets to shells, flanges or side plates

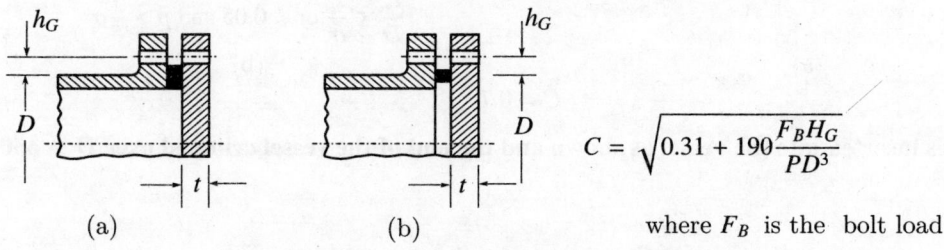

$$C = \sqrt{0.31 + 190\dfrac{F_B H_G}{PD^3}}$$

(a)   (b)   where F_B is the bolt load

Covers with a narrow face bolted flange joint

Table 8.1 *Values of 'D' and 'C' for Typical Unstayed Flat Heads – (Contd...)*

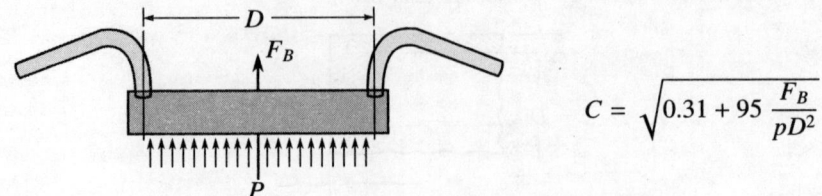

$$C = \sqrt{0.31 + 95\,\frac{F_B}{pD^2}}$$

Autoclave manhole covers $D \not> 610$ mm

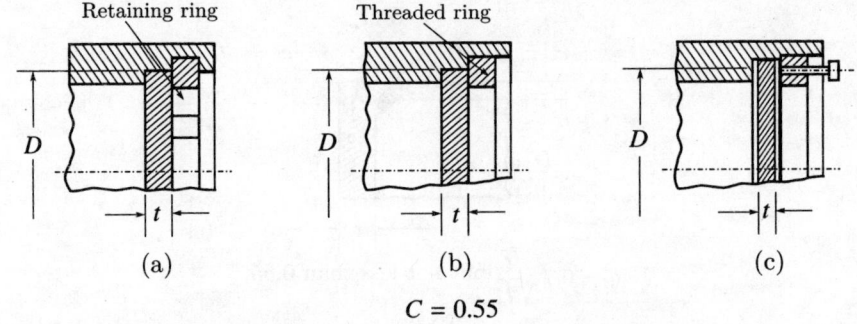

$$C = 0.55$$

All means of failures shall be resisted with a factor
of safety of at least 4 seal welds may be used if desired

**Plates inserted into the end of a vessel and held in place by a
positive mechanical locking arrangement.**

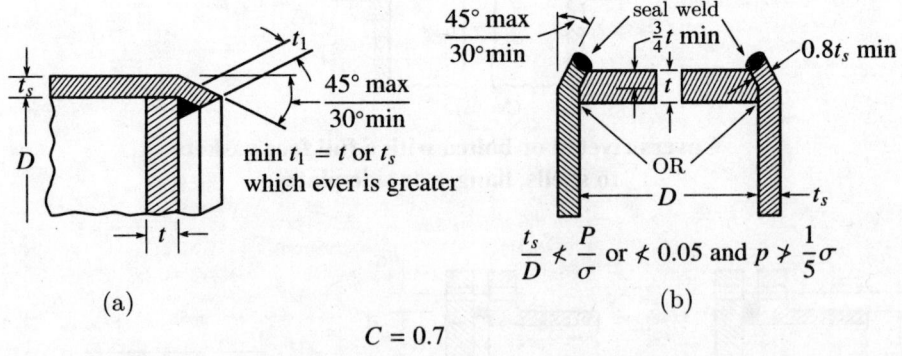

$$C = 0.7$$

Plates inserted into the vessel as shown and the end of the vessel crimped over $D \not> 450$ mm

Table 8.2 *Classification of pressure vessels and weld joint efficiency factor (J)*

Sl. No. (1)	Requirement (2)	Class I (3)	Class II (4)	Class III (5)	(6)	(7)
1.	Weld joint efficiency factor (J)	1.00	0.85	0.70	0.60	0.50
2.	Shell or end plate thickness	No limitation on thickness	Maximum thickness 38 mm after adding corrosion allowance	Maximum thickness 16 mm. before corrosion allowance is added	Maximum thickness 16 mm. before corrosion allowance is added	Maximum thickness 16 mm. before corrosion allowance is added
3.	Type of joints	i) Double welded butt joint with full penetration excluding butt joints with metal backing strips which remain in plate ii) Single welded butt joints with backing strip $J = 0.9$	i) Double welded butt joint with full penetration excluding butt joints with metal backing strips which remain in place ii) Single welded butt joints with backing strip $J = 0.80$	i) Double welded butt joints with full penetration excluding butt joints with metal backing strip which remain in place ii) Single welded butt joints with backing strip $J = 0.65$	i) Single welded butt joints with backing strip not over 16 mm. thickness or over 600 mm outside dia ii) Single welded butt joints with out backing strip $J = 0.55$	i) Single full fillet lap joints for circomferential seams only — —

Note: Columns (5), (6) and (7) are grouped under the heading **Class III**.

Table 8.3 Allowable stress values* for carbon and low alloy steel in tension

Material Specification	Grade or Designation	Mechanical Properties			Allowable stress values in MN/m² at Design Temperature °C										
		Tensile strength Min. MN/m² R_{20}	Yield stress Min. MN/m² E_{20}	Percentage Elongation Min. on gauge length $= 5.65\sqrt{S_o}$	Up to 250	Up to 300	Up to 350	Up to 375	Up to 400	Up to 425	Up to 450	Up to 475	Up to 500	Up to 525	Up to 550
					(a) Plates										
IS:2002-1962	I	363	$0.55R_{20}$	26	93.2	85.3	76.5	73.6	70.6	57.9	42.2	35.3	—	—	—
IS:2002-1962	SA	412	$0.50R_{20}$	25	96.1	88.3	79.4	75.5	72.6	57.9	42.2	35.3	—	—	—
IS:2002-1962	2B	501	$0.50R_{20}$	20	118.7	108.8	98.1	93.2	81.4	57.9	42.2	35.3	—	—	—
IS:2041-1962	$20M_o55$	471	275	20	140.2	129.5	120.6	116.7	112.8	109.8	105.9	75.5	54.9	36.3	—
IS:2041-1962	20Mn2	501	294	20	137.3	125.5	113.8	107.9	81.4	57.9	42.2	35.3	—	—	—
IS:1570-1961	$15Cr90\,M_o55$	490	294	20	157.0	149.1	141.2	135.3	131.4	127.5	123.0	114.7	84.3	56.9	34.3
IS:1570-1961	C15Mn75	412	226	25	105.0	96.1	87.3	82.4	79.4	57.9	42.2	35.3	—	—	—
					(b) Tubes and Pipes										
IS:3609-1966	$1\%Cr\tfrac{1}{2}M_o$ tube Normalized and tempered.	432	235	$950/R_{20}$	125.5	118.7	112.8	108.8	104.9	102	98.1	95.1	84.3	56.9	34.3
IS:3609-1966	$2.25\%Cr$ $1\%\,M_o$	481	245	$950/R_{20}$	137.3	132.4	125.5	123.6	120.6	117.7	113.8	110.8	94.1	68.7	48.1
IS:1570-1961	$20M_o55$	451	245	$950/R_{20}$	125.5	115.7	107.9	140.0	101.0	98.1	94.1	75.5	54.9	36.3	—
IS:1914-1961	314MN/m² min. Tensile strength.	314	$0.50R_{20}$	$950/R_{20}$	72.6	66.7	60.8	56.9	54.9	49.0	42.2	35.3	—	—	—
IS:1914-1961	422MN/m²	422	$0.50R_{20}$	$950/R_{20}$	98.1	90.2	81.4	77.5	74.5	57.9	42.2	35.3	—	—	—
IS:1978-1961	St 18	310	173	—	80.4	73.6	65.7	62.8	60.8	57.9	42.2	35.3	—	—	—
	St 20	331	193	—	90.2	82.4	74.5	70.6	67.7	57.9	42.2	35.3	—	—	—
	St 21	331	207	—	96.1	88.3	79.4	75.5	72.6	57.9	42.2	35.3	—	—	—
	St 25	414	241	—	112.8	103.0	93.2	88.3	81.4	57.9	42.2	35.3	—	—	—
IS:1979-1961	St 30	414	289	—	135.3	123.6	112.8	106.0	81.4	57.9	42.2	35.3	—	—	—
	St 32	434	317	—	147.1	135.3	122.6	115.7	81.4	57.9	42.2	35.3	—	—	—
	St 37	455	359	—	167.7	153.0	138.3	131.4	81.4	57.9	42.2	35.3	—	—	—

Note. Allowable stress values in Kgf/mm² can be obtained by dividing the above values with 9.807.

Table 8.4 (a) Values of E* for ferrous Materials, MN/m²

Material	Design Temperature °C						
	0	20	100	200	300	400	500
Carbon Steels } ≤ C 0.30%	192.2×10^3	192.2×10^3	191.2×10^3	186.3×10^3	178.5×10^3	166.7×10^3	—
> C 0.30%	206.9×10^3	206.9×10^3	203.0×10^3	195.2×10^3	186.3×10^3	166.7×10^3	—
Carbon Molybdenum steels and chromemolybdenum steels (utpt 3% Cr).	206.9×10^3	206.9×10^3	203.0×10^3	197.1×10^3	190.3×10^3	180.4×10^3	168.7×10^3
Intermediate chromemolybdenum steels and austenitic stainless steels	189.3×10^3	189.3×10^3	186.3×10^3	182.4×10^3	176.5×10^3	169.7×10^3	157.0×10^3

Table 8.4 (b) Values of E* for Aluminium and its alloys, MN/m²

Material Grade	Design Temperature °C								
	-200	-100	0	50	75	100	125	150	200
1B, N3, X4	76.5×10^3	72.6×10^3	69.6×10^3	68.7×10^3	68.7×10^3	67.7×10^3	66.7×10^3	65.7×10^3	62.7×10^3
H9	72.6×10^3	69.6×10^3	66.7×10^3	64.7×10^3	64.7×10^3	63.7×10^3	61.8×10^3	60.8×10^3	58.8×10^3
H15	81.4×10^3	77.5×10^3	73.6×10^3	72.6×10^3	72.6×10^3	71.6×10^3	70.6×10^3	69.6×10^3	66.7×10^3
A6	87.3×10^3	83.4×10^3	80.4×10^3	79.4×10^3	78.5×10^3	77.5×10^3	76.5×10^3	75.5×10^3	72.6×10^3

* Values of E in Metric units (kgf/mm²) can be obtained by dividing the values given in Tables 8.4(a) and 8.4(b) with 9.807.

Table 8.4 (c) Values of E* for Nickel and Nickel alloys, MN/m²

Material	Design Temperature °C						
	20	300	400	500	600	700	750
Nickel							
70% Ni and 30% Cu alloy	206.9×10^3	200.0×10^3	184.4×10^3	161.8×10^3	146.1×10^3	114.7×10^3	106.9×10^3
75% Ni, 15% Cr and 10%	184.4×10^3	176.5×10^3	172.6×10^3	165.7×10^3	158.9×10^3	152.0×10^3	147.1×10^3
Ferrous alloy	213.8×10^3	203.0×10^3	196.1×10^3	172.6×10^3	156.9×10^3	127.5×10^3	116.7×10^3

Table 8.4 (d) Values of E* for Copper and its alloys, MN/m²

Material	Composition	Design Temperature °C								
		20	50	100	150	200	250	300	350	400
Copper	99.98% Cu	109.8×10^3	108.9×10^3	107.9×10^3	115.7×10^3	104.0×10^3	102.0×10^3	99.1×10^3	95.1×10^3	—
Commercial brass	66% Cu, 34% Zn	96.1×10^3	95.1×10^3	94.1×10^3	93.2×10^3	89.2×10^3	87.3×10^3	84.3×10^3	83.4×10^3	—
Leaded tin bronze	88% Cu, 6% Sn, 1.5% Pb, 4.5% Zn.	89.2×10^3	88.3×10^3	87.3×10^3	85.3×10^3	82.4×10^3	80.4×10^3	78.5×10^3	75.5×10^3	—
Phosphor bronze	85.5% Cu, 12.5% Sn, 10% Zn.	103.0×10^3	101.0×10^3	100.0×10^3	96.1×10^3	93.2×10^3	89.2×10^3	83.4×10^3	65.7×10^3	—
Muntz	59% Cu, 39% Zn	105.0×10^3	100.0×10^3	96.1×10^3	89.2×10^3	81.4×10^3	75.5×10^3	—	—	—
Cupro nickles	80% Cu, 20% Ni OR 70% Cu and 30% Ni.	130.4×10^3	128.5×10^3	126.5×10^3	123.6×10^3	121.6×10^3	118.7×10^3	115.7×10^3	112.8×10^3	100.0×10^3

Note: Intermediate values may be obtained by interpolation.

* Values of E in metric units (kgf/mm²) can be obtained by dividing the values given in tables 8.4(c) and 8.4(d) with 9.807.

Table 8.5 *Coefficients, c_1, c_2, c_3, c_4 and c_5*

Material of cover plate	Method of holding edges	Circular plate		Rectangular plate		Elliptical plate
		c_1	c_2	c_3	c_4	c_5
Cast iron	Supported, free	0.54	0.038	0.75	1.73	1.5
Cast iron	Fixed	0.44	0.010	0.62	1.4; 1.6*	1.2
Mild Steel	Supported, free	0.42	..	0.60	1.38	1.2
Mild Steel	Fixed	0.35	..	0.49	1.12; 1.28	0.9

Table 8.6 *Maximum Allowable Stresses in Stays and Stay Bolts*

Type of stay	Stress, MN/m² (kgf/mm²)	
	Forlengths between support	
	Not exceeding 120 dia.	Exceeding 120 dia.
a) Unwelded or flexible stays less than 20 diameters long, screwed through plates with ends riveted over	52.0 (5.3)	..
b) Hollow steel stays less than 20 dia. long screwed through plates with ends riveted over	55.0 (5.6)	..
c) Unwelded stays and unwelded portions of welded stays, except as specified in (a) and (b)	66.0 (6.7)	59.0 (6.0)
d) Steel through stays exceeding 40 mm diameter	71.5 (7.3)	62.0 (6.3)
e) Welded portions of stays	41.2 (4.2)	41.2 (4.2)

* With Gasket.

Table 8.7 Maximum Stresses and Deflection in Flat Plates

Form of plate	Type of loading	Type of Support	Eq.	Total load F	Maximum stress σ_{max}	Location of σ_{max}	Maximum deflection y_{max}
(circle, radius r_0)	Distributed over the entire surface	Edge supported	(1)	$\pi r_0^2 p$	$\sigma_r = \sigma_t = \dfrac{-3F(3m+1)}{8\pi m t^2}$	Center	$\dfrac{3F(m-1)(5m+1)r_0^2}{16\pi E m^2 t^3}$
		Edge fixed	(2)	$\pi r_0^2 p$	$\sigma_t = \dfrac{3F}{4\pi t^2}$	Edge	$\dfrac{3F(m^2-1)r_0^2}{16\pi E m^2 t^3}$
(diagram with r, r_0)	Distributed over a concentric circular area of radius r	Edge supported	(3)	$\pi r^2 p$	$\sigma_r = \sigma_t = \dfrac{-3F}{2\pi m t^2}\left[(m+1)\log_e\dfrac{r_0}{r} - (m-1)\dfrac{r^2}{4r_0^2} + m\right]$	Center	$\dfrac{3F(m^2-1)}{16\pi E m^2 t^3}\left[\dfrac{(12m+4)r_0^2}{m+1} - 4r^2\log_e\dfrac{r_0}{r} - \dfrac{(7m+3)r^2}{m+1}\right]$
		Edge fixed	(4)	$\pi r^2 p$	$\sigma_r = \dfrac{-3F}{2\pi t^2}\left(1 - \dfrac{r^2}{2r_0^2}\right)$ $\sigma_r = \sigma_t = \dfrac{-3F}{2\pi m t^2}\left[(m+1)\log_e\dfrac{r_0}{r} + (m+1)\dfrac{r^2}{4r_0^2}\right]$	Edge Center	$\dfrac{3F(m^2-1)}{16\pi E m^2 t^3}\left[4r_0^2 - 4r^2\log_e\dfrac{r_0}{r} - 3r^2\right]$ when r is very small (concentrated load) $\dfrac{3F(m^2-1)}{4\pi E m^2 t^3}$
(diagram with r, r_0)	Distributed on circumference of a concentric circle of radius r	Edge supported	(5)	$2\pi r p$	$\sigma_r = \sigma_t = \dfrac{-3F}{4\pi m t^2}\left[\dfrac{m+1}{2} + (m+1)\log_e\dfrac{r_0}{r} - (m-1)\dfrac{r^2}{2r_0^2}\right]$	All points inside the circle of radius r	$\dfrac{3F(m^2-1)}{2\pi E m^2 t^3}\left[\dfrac{(3m+1)(r_0^2-r^2)}{2(m+1)} - r^2\log_e\dfrac{r_0}{r}\right]$
		Edge fixed	(6)	$2\pi r p$	$\sigma_r = \sigma_t = \dfrac{-3F}{4\pi m t^2}\left[(m+1)\left(2\log_e\dfrac{r_0}{r} + \dfrac{r_0^2}{r^2} - 1\right)\right]$ $\sigma_r = \dfrac{3F}{2\pi t^2}\left(1 - \dfrac{r^2}{r_0^2}\right)$	Centre when $r < 0.31r_0$ Edge when $r > 0.31r_0$	$\dfrac{3F(m^2-1)}{2\pi E m^2 t^3}\left[\tfrac{1}{2}(r_0^2-r^2) - r^2\log_e\dfrac{r_0}{r}\right]$

Table 8.7 Maximum Stresses and Deflection in Flat Plates – (Contd..)

Description	Loading	No.	F	Stress	Location	Deflection
Distributed over a concentric circular area of radius r	Uniform pressure over entire lower surface	(7)	$F = \pi r^2 p$	$\sigma_r = \sigma_t = \dfrac{-3F}{2\pi mt^2}$ $\left[(m+1)\log_e\dfrac{r_0}{r} + \dfrac{m-1}{4}\left(1 - \dfrac{r^2}{r_0^2}\right)\right]$	Center	$\dfrac{3F(m^2-1)}{16\pi Em^2 t^3}\left[4r^2\log_e\dfrac{r_0}{r}\right.$ $+2r^2\left(\dfrac{3m+1}{m+1}\right) - r_0^2\left(\dfrac{7m+3}{m+1}\right)$ $+\dfrac{(r_0^2-r^2)r^4}{r^2 r_0^2} + \left.\dfrac{r^4}{r_0^2}\right]$ when r is very small (concentrated load) $\dfrac{3F(m-1)(7m+3)r_0^2}{16\pi Em^2 t^3}$
Distributed over the entire surface	Outer edge supported	(8)	$F = \pi(r_0^2 - r_i^2)p$	$\sigma_t = \dfrac{-3p}{4mt^2(r_0^2 - r_i^2)}$ $\left[r_0^4(3m+1) + r_i^4(m-1) - 4mr_0^2 r_i^2\right.$ $\left.-4(m+1)r_0^2 r_i^2\log_e\dfrac{r_0}{r}\right]$	Inner edge	$\dfrac{3F(m^2-1)}{2Em^2 t^3}\left[\dfrac{r_0^4(5m+1)}{8(m+1)} - \dfrac{r_0^2 r_i^2(3m+1)}{2(m+1)}\right.$ $+\dfrac{r_i^4(7m+3)}{8(m+1)} - \dfrac{r_0^2 r_i^2(3m+1)}{2(m-1)}$ $+\dfrac{r_0^2 r_i^2(3m+1)}{2(m-1)}\log_e\dfrac{r_0}{r_i}$ $\left.-\dfrac{2r_0^2 r_i^4(m+1)}{(r_0^2 - r_i^2)(m-1)}\left(\log_e\dfrac{r_0}{r}\right)^2\right]$
Distributed over the entire surface	Outer edge fixed and supported	(9)	$F = \pi(r_0^2 - r_i^2)p$	$\sigma_t = \dfrac{-3p(m^2-1)}{4mt^2}$ $\left[\dfrac{r_0^2 - r_i^4 - \frac{1}{2}r_i^2 r_0^2\log_e\frac{r_0}{r_i}}{r_0^2(m-1) + r_i^2(m+1)}\right]$	Inner edge	
Distributed over the entire surface	Outer edge fixed and supported, inner edge fixed	(10)	$F = \pi(r_0^2 - r_i^2)p$	$\sigma_r = \dfrac{3p}{4t^2}\left[(r_0^2 + r^2) - \right.$ $\left.\dfrac{4r_0^2 r^2}{r_0^2 - r^2}\left(\log_e\dfrac{r_0}{r}\right)^2\right]$	Inner edge	$\dfrac{3p(m^2-1)}{16Em^2 t^3}\left[r_0^4 + 3r_i^4 - 4r_0^2 r_i^2\right.$ $-4r_0^2 r_i^2\log_e\dfrac{a}{b}$ $\left.+\dfrac{16r_0^2 r_i^4}{r_0^2 - r_i^2}\left(\log_e\dfrac{r_0}{r_i}\right)^2\right]$

Table 8.7 Maximum Stresses and Deflection in Flat Plates – (Contd..)

			F =	σ		Inner edge
Distributed over the entire surface	Inner edge fixed and supported	(11)	$F = \pi(r_0^2 - r_i^2)p$	$\sigma_r = \dfrac{3p}{4t^2}\left[4r_0^4(m+1)\log_e\dfrac{r_0}{r} - \dfrac{r_0^4(m-1)+r_0^4(m-1)+4r_0^2 r_i^2}{r_0^2(m+1)+r_i^2(m-1)}\right]$	Inner edge	
Uniform over entire surface	All edges supported	(12)	$F = abp$	$\sigma_b = \dfrac{-0.75b^2 p}{t^2\left[1+1.61\frac{b^3}{a^3}\right]}$	Center	$\dfrac{0.1422b^4 p}{Et^3\left[1+2.21\frac{b^3}{a^3}\right]}$
Uniform over the entire surface	All edges fixed	(13)	$F = abp$	$\sigma_b = \dfrac{0.5b^2 p}{t^2\left[1+0.623\frac{b^6}{a^6}\right]}$	Center of long edge	$\dfrac{0.0284b^4 p}{Et^3\left[1+1.056\frac{b^5}{a^5}\right]}$
Uniform over the entire surface	Short edges fixed, long edges supported	(14)	$F = abp$	$\sigma_a = \dfrac{0.75b^2 p}{t^2\left[1+0.8\frac{b^4}{a^4}\right]}$	Center of short edge	
Uniform over the entire surface	Short edges supported, long edges fixed	(15)	$F = abp$	$\sigma_b = \dfrac{-b^2 p}{2t^2\left[1+0.2\frac{a^4}{b^4}\right]}$	Center of long edge	

Positive sign for σ indicates tension at upper surface and equal compression at lower surface; negative sign indicates reverse condition.

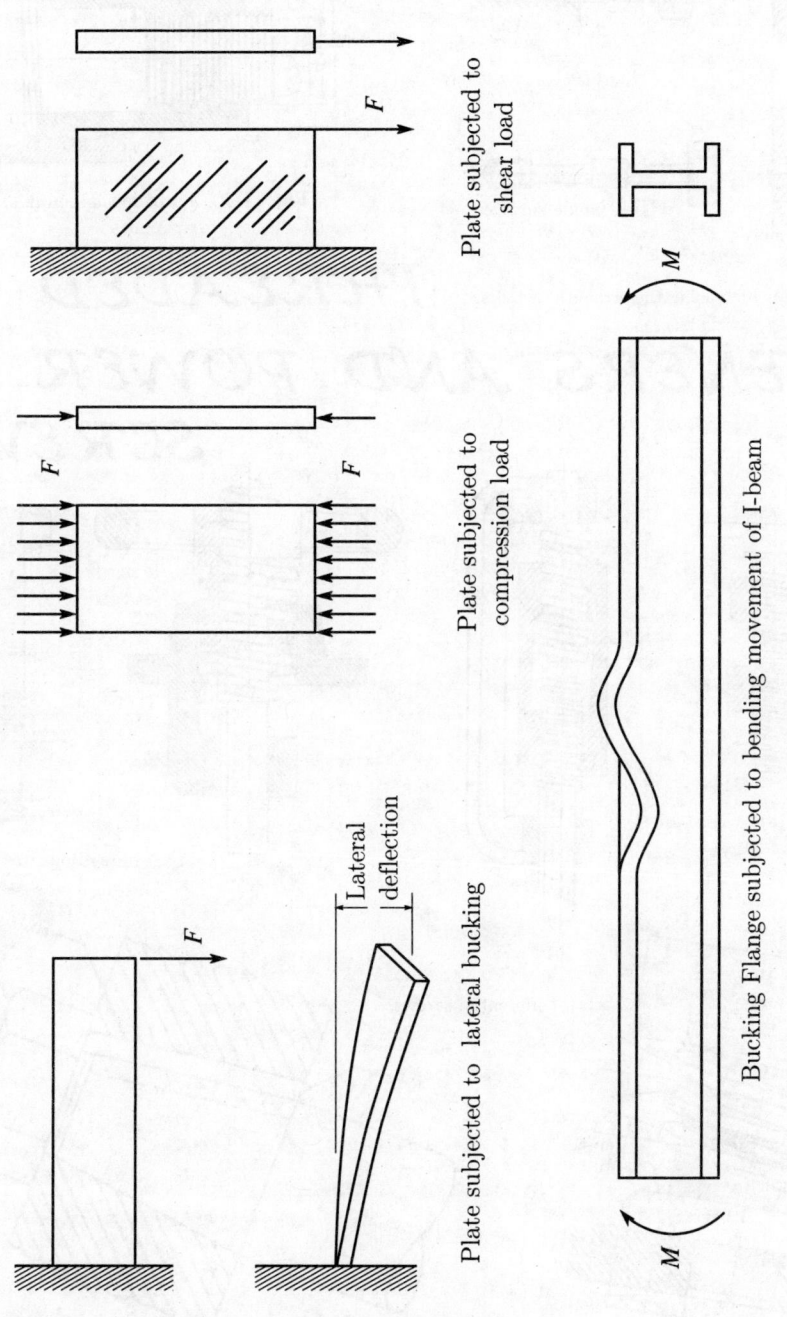

Plate subjected to shear load

Plate subjected to compression load

Plate subjected to lateral bucking

Lateral deflection

Bucking Flange subjected to bending movement of I-beam

Flat plates subjectd to different types of loads

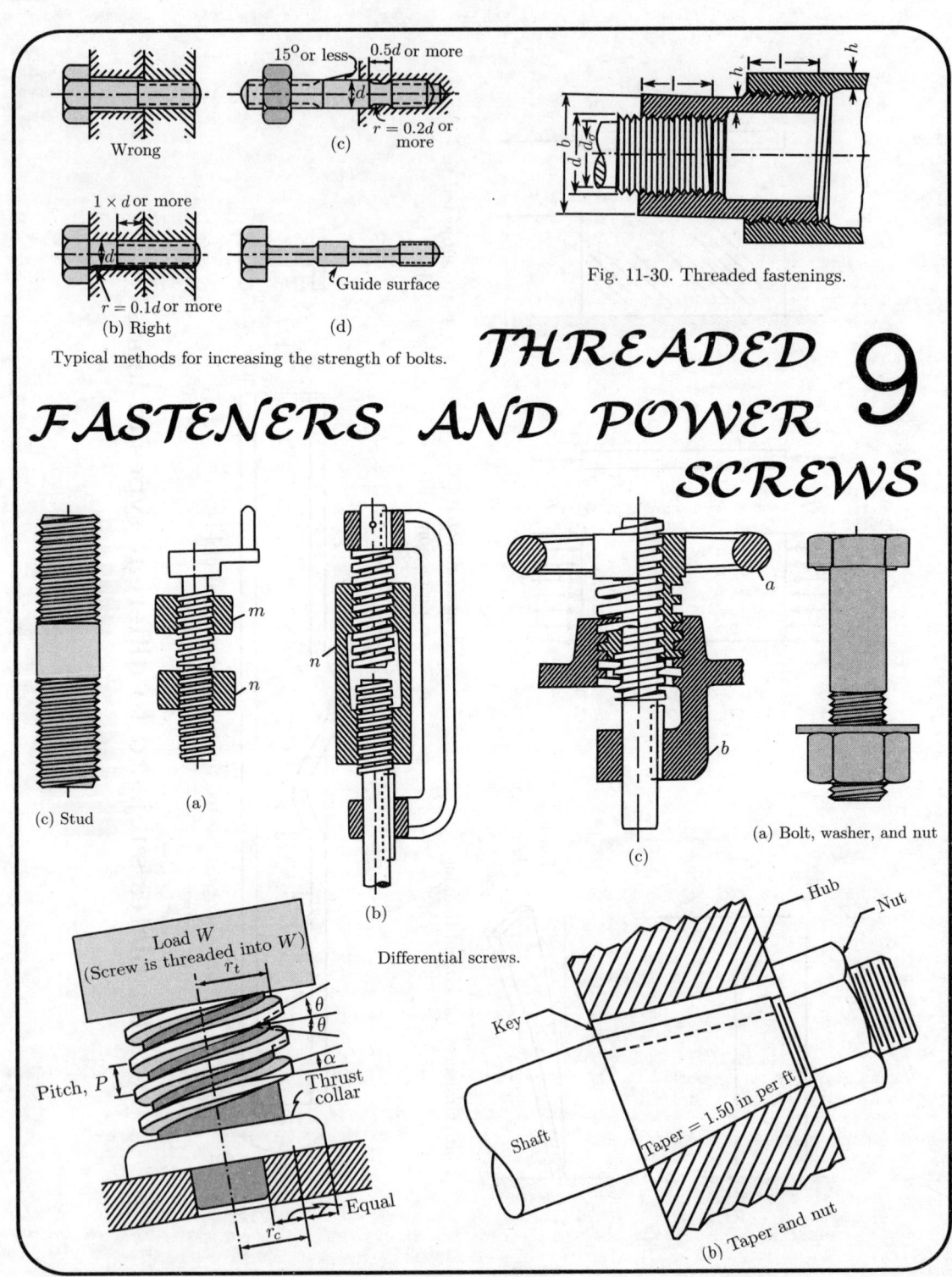

Wrong

15° or less   0.5d or more

$r = 0.2d$ or more

(c)

Fig. 11-30. Threaded fastenings.

$1 \times d$ or more

$r = 0.1d$ or more

(b) Right

Guide surface

(d)

Typical methods for increasing the strength of bolts.

THREADED FASTENERS AND POWER SCREWS

9

(c) Stud

m

n

n

a

b

(a)

(b)

(c)

(a) Bolt, washer, and nut

Differential screws.

Load W
(Screw is threaded into W)

r_t

θ
θ

α

Pitch, P

Thrust collar

Equal

r_c

Hub

Nut

Key

Shaft

Taper = 1.50 in per ft

(b) Taper and nut

9

Threaded Fasteners and Power Screws

Symbols	Description and Units
d, D	major diameters of external and internal threads respectively, mm
d_1, D_1	minor diameters of external and internal threads respectively, mm
d_2, D_2	pitch diameters of external and internal threads respectively, mm
l	lead, mm
n	number of threads in the nut
p	pitch, mm
p_b	allowable bearing pressure between threads of nut and screw, MN/m^2 (kgf/mm^2)
α	helix angle, deg
η	efficiency
ϕ	friction angle, deg
σ_d	working stress, MN/m^2 (kgf/mm^2)
θ	half apex angle, deg

Particular	Equation	Eqn. No.
Set Screws :		
The empirical formula to determine the proper size of set screw, mm	$d = \dfrac{d_s}{8} + 8.0$ mm where d = set screw diameter, mm d_s = shaft diameter, mm	9.1(a)
The maximum safe holding force of set screws, N (kgf)	F = 6.344 $(d)^{2.31}$ SI units = 0.6465 $(d)^{2.31}$ Metric units	9.1(b)
The initial tension load in a bolt (according to experiments conducted at Cornell University), N (kgf)	F_t = 2805d SI units = 286d Metric units	9.1(c)
The relation between the torque applied to the nut and the axial tension load in a bolt	$T = 0.2F_a \times$ (nominal diameter of bolt)	9.1(d)

Particular	Equation	Eqn. No.
Effect of Applied loads on Bolt Stresses: (Fig. 9.1)		
The final load on the bolt (gasket joint), N (kgf)	$F = KF_a + F_i$	9.2(a)
where $K = \left(\dfrac{E_b A_b}{L}\right) \Big/ \left(\dfrac{E_b A_b}{L} + \dfrac{E_g A_g}{t}\right)$		9.2(b)

($K = 0$ to 1 depending on the nature of the gasket Table 9.1)

A_b is the cross sectional area of bolt, mm^2

A_g is the loaded are of gasket, mm^2

L is the length of bolt from nut to head, mm

E_b, E_g are modulus of elasticity of bolt and gasket materials respectively,

F is the final load, N (kgf)

F_a is the external applied load, N (kgf)

F_i is the initial load due to tightening, N (kgf)

t is the gasket thickness

Stresses in tension bolts:		
According to Seaton and Routhwaite, the working stress for bolts made of steel containing from 0.08 to 0.25 percent carbon and with diameters of 20 mm and above.	$\sigma_d = C(A_r)^{0.418}$	9.3(a)

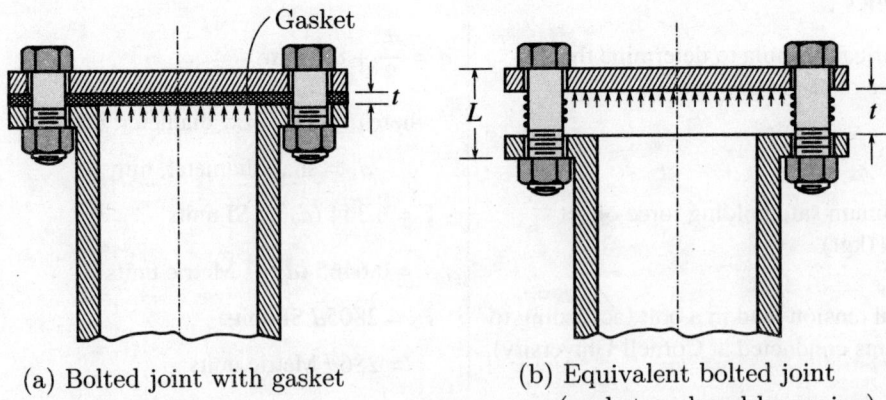

(a) Bolted joint with gasket   (b) Equivalent bolted joint
                                          (gasket replaced by spring)

Fig. 9.1: *Bolted Joint*

Particular	Equation	Eqn. No.
The total load capacity of the bolt	$F_a = \sigma_d A_r = C(A_r)^{1.418}$	9.3(b)

where A_r is the stress area of bolt, mm

$C = 2.29$ SI units

$\quad = 0.23$ Metric units $\quad\Big\}$ For low carbon steels

$C = 0.70$ SI units

$\quad = 6.87$ Metric units $\quad\Big\}$ For alloy steel bolts

$C = 0.460$ SI units

$\quad = 0.047$ Metric units $\quad\Big\}$ For bronze bolts

C is a coefficient (Table 9.2)

The allowable stress for fluid tight joints (Unwins formulas)		
a) For rough joint	$\sigma_d = 0.01711\ (d^2 + 645)$ SI Units.	9.3(c)
	$\quad = 0.001745\ (d^2 + 645)$ Metric units	
b) For faced joint	$\sigma_d = 0.03207\ (d^2 + 537.5)$ SI units	9.3(d)
	$\quad = 0.00327\ (d^2 + 537.5)$ Metric units	

Unstressed Bolt:

The root diameter of a bolt which is not stressed initially as in the case of lifting eye bolt, crane hook etc.	$d_3 = \left(\dfrac{4F}{\pi\sigma_d}\right)^{\frac{1}{2}}$	9.4

where F = load, N

$\sigma_d = 0.8\ \sigma_{yp}$, for unhardened bolts

$\quad = 0.6\ \sigma_{yp}$, for hardened bolts

Joint with axial load with subsequent tightening:

The root diameter of a bolt which is subjected to axial load with subsequent tightening as in the case of turn buckle etc.	$d_3 = \left(\dfrac{1.25F}{(\pi/4)\sigma_d}\right)^{\frac{1}{2}}$	9.5

where $\sigma_d = (0.25$ to $0.40)\ \sigma_{\gamma p}$, for $d = 16$ to 30 mm

$\quad = (0.40$ to $0.60)\ \sigma_{\gamma p}$, for $d = 30$ to 60 mm

Particular	Equation	Eqn. No.
Number of bolts:		
Empirical rule for the number of bolts in pipe joints is given by	$N = 0.024D_c + 2$	9.6(a)
Empirical rule for number of bolts in steam engine cylinder	$N = (0.026D_c)$ to $(0.028D_c)$	9.6(b)
Empirical rule for number of studs in gas engine	$N = (0.016D_c + 4)$ to $(0.024D_c + 4)$ where D_c = diameter of the cylinder, mm	9.6(c)
The maximum spacing of the bolts in any fluid tight joint	$S \leq 6d$	9.6(d)
Eccentric Loading on rectangular base: (Refer Fig. 9.2)		
The magnitude of the shear load	$F' = F/N$ where N is the number of bolts	9.7(a)
The maximum secondary tensile force due to turing	$F_{max} = F_1 = \dfrac{Fel_1}{2(l_1^2 + l_2^2 + l_3^2)}$	9.7(b)
The equivalent tensile load*	$F_{te} = \dfrac{1}{2}\left[F_1 + \sqrt{(F_1^2 + 4F'^2)}\right]$	9.7(c)
The equivalent shear load	$F_{se} = \dfrac{1}{2}\left(F_1^2 + F'^2\right)^{\frac{1}{2}}$	9.7(d)

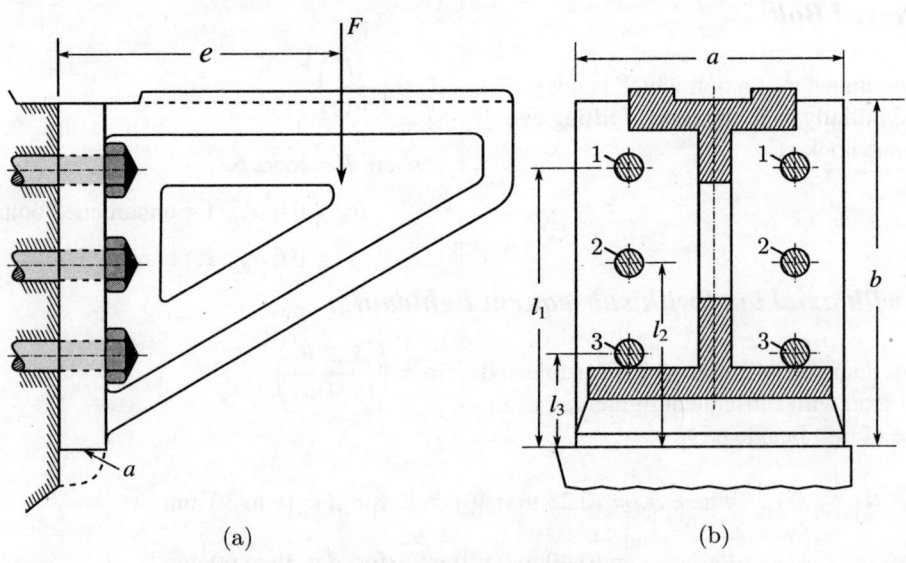

Fig. 9.2: *Eccentric loading on rectangular base*

*when there is lip the shear load is taken by it, and the bolt is to be designed for the tensile stress only, $F_{te} = F_1$

Particular	Equation	Eqn. No.
Eccentric Loading on Circular Base: **(Refer Fig. 9.3)**		
The magnitude of the shear load on the bolts (with no lip)	$F' = F/N$ where N is the number of bolts	9.8(a)
The magnitude of secondary tensile force due to turning on the bolt 1 (Fig. 9.3(a))	$F_1 = \dfrac{Fe\,l_1}{l_1^2 + l_2^2 + l_3^2 + l_4^2} = \dfrac{Fe(a - b\cos\alpha)}{4a^2 + 2b^2}$ where $l_1 = a - b\cos\theta$ $l_2 = a + b\sin\theta$ $l_3 = a + b\cos\theta$ $l_4 = a - b\sin\theta$	9.8(b)
The general expression for tensile force for N bolts	$F_{1-n} = \dfrac{2Fe(a - b\cos\theta)}{(2a^2 + b^2)N}$	9.8(c)
The maximum tensile force on the bolt	$F_{\max} = \dfrac{2Fe(a + b)}{(2a^2 + b^2)N}$	9.8(d)
When the direction of F is fixed and the bolts are so arranged that two of them are equally stressed (Fig. 9.3(b)), the maximum load in the bolts	$F_{\max} = 2Fe\left(\dfrac{a + b\cos(180/N)^\circ}{(2a^2 + b^2)N}\right)$	9.8(e)

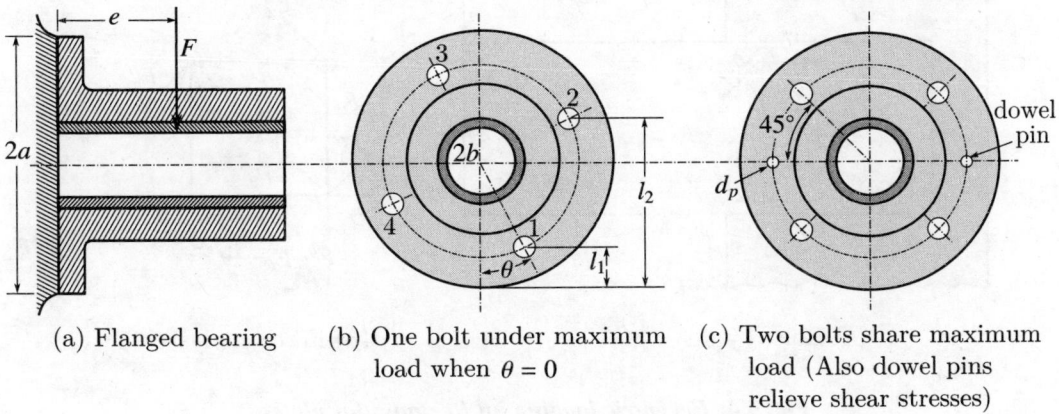

(a) Flanged bearing (b) One bolt under maximum load when $\theta = 0$ (c) Two bolts share maximum load (Also dowel pins relieve shear stresses)

Fig. 9.3: *Eccentric loading on circular base*

Particular	Equation	Eqn. No.
Eccentric Loading on Rectangular Plates (Fig. 9.4)		
The magnitude of the diret or shear force on the bolts	$F' = F/N$	9.9(a)
The direct or primary shear stress	$\tau' = \dfrac{F'}{A} = \dfrac{F}{NA}$	9.9(b)
The torsional moment	$T = Fe$	9.9(c)
The magnitude of the secondary shear force due to moment on any bolt	$F_n'' = \dfrac{Tc_n}{\Sigma c^2} = \dfrac{Fec_n}{\Sigma c^2}$	9.9(d)
The maximum secondary shear force	$F_{max}'' = F'' = \dfrac{Fec_{max}}{\Sigma c^2}$	9.9(e)
The maximum secondary shear stress	$\tau_{max}'' = \tau'' = \dfrac{F''}{A} = \dfrac{Fec_{max}}{Ac^2} = \dfrac{Tc_{max}}{J}$	9.9(f)

where $c_1, c_2, c_3 \ldots c_n$ are the radial distances from the c.g. to the centre of the bolt, mm

where $\Sigma Ac^2 = J$ the polar moment of inertia of the bolt areas about the centre of gravity, mm^4

Particular	Equation	Eqn. No.
The resultant shear force on the bolt	$F_R = \sqrt{F'^2 + F''^2 + 2F'F'' \cos\theta}$	9.9(g)
	where θ is the smallest angle between the primary and secondary shear forces	

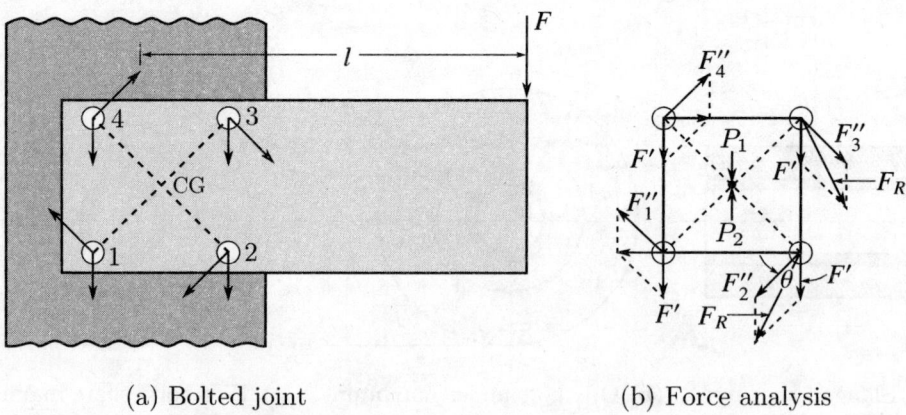

(a) Bolted joint   (b) Force analysis

Fig. 9.4: *Eccentric loading on Rectangular plates*

Particular	Equation	Eqn. No.
Efficiency of Triangular Threads:		
The relation between the applied torque (T) and the resisting load (W)	$T = \dfrac{Wl}{2\pi\eta}$	9.10(a)
The lead angle or helix angle of a V-thread	$\tan\alpha = (l/\pi d_2)$ where $l = pn$, lead of the screw, mm	9.10(b)
The tangential force for V-thread at mean radius of screw	$F_t = W\tan(\phi + \alpha) = W\dfrac{(\tan\alpha + f)}{(1 - f\tan\alpha)}$ where α is the helix angle ϕ is the angle of friction $f = \tan\phi$, coefficient of friction (Table 9.3)	9.10(c)
The tangential force for V-thread at mean radius without friction	$F_t' = W\tan\alpha$	9.10(d)
The efficiency of V-thread	$\eta = \dfrac{F_t'}{F_t} = \dfrac{\tan\alpha}{\tan(\alpha + \phi)} = \dfrac{\tan\alpha(1 - f\tan\alpha)}{(\tan\alpha + f)} = \dfrac{(1 - f\tan\alpha)}{(1 + f\cot\alpha)}$	9.10(e)

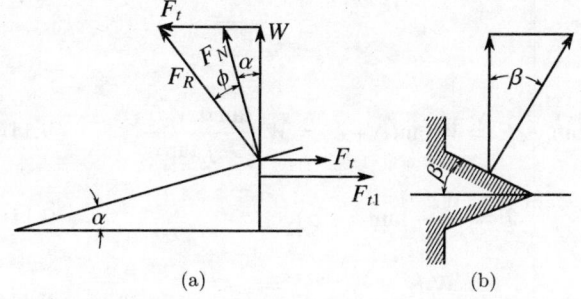 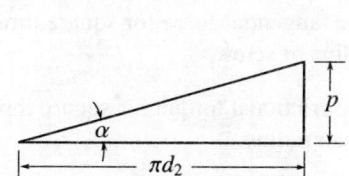

Fig. 9.5: *Forces acting on a V-thread*   **Fig. 9.6:** *Helix angle of a V-thread*

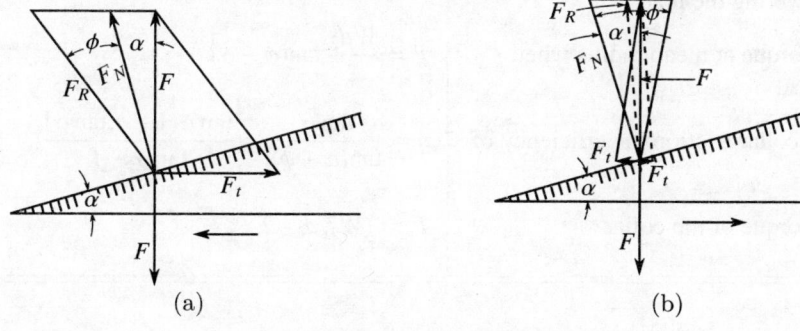

Fig. 9.7: *Forces acting on a square thread*

Particular	Equation	Eqn. No.
Taking into accout the triangularity of the thread the tangential force of V-thread at mean radius of screw	$F_{t1} = W\left(\dfrac{\tan\alpha + f\sec\beta}{1 - f\tan\alpha\sec\beta}\right)$	9.10(f)
Considering triangularity of the thread, the efficiency of V-thread	$\eta = \dfrac{F'_t}{F_{t1}} = \dfrac{\tan\alpha(1 - f\tan\alpha\sec\beta)}{(\tan\alpha + f\sec\beta)}$ $= \left(\dfrac{\cos\beta - f\tan\alpha}{\cos\beta + f\cot\alpha}\right)$	9.10(g)
For V-Thread the total frictional torque including collar friction	$T = \dfrac{W}{2}\left[d_2\left(\dfrac{\tan\alpha + f\sec\beta}{1 - f\tan\alpha\sec\beta}\right) + f_c d_c\right]$	9.10(h)
For V-thread the total frictional torque including collar friction torque	$T = \dfrac{W}{2}\left[d_2\left(\dfrac{\tan\alpha + f\sec\theta}{1 - f\tan\alpha\sec\theta}\right) + f_c d_c\right]$	9.10(i)
The efficiency formula for V-thread with half apex angle θ and an allowance for nut or end friction on a diameter d_c	$\eta = \dfrac{d_2\tan\alpha}{d_2\frac{\tan\alpha + f\sec\theta}{1 - f\tan\alpha\sec\theta} + f_c d_c}$	9.10(j)

Power Screws

Particular	Equation	Eqn. No.
The tangential force for square thread at mean radius of screw	$F_t = W\tan(\phi + \alpha) = W\dfrac{\tan\alpha + f}{1 - f\tan\alpha}$	9.11(a)
The frictional torque for square thread at mean radius	$T = \dfrac{Wd_2}{2}\tan(\phi + \alpha)$	9.11(b)
In the absence of friction the torque	$T' = \dfrac{Wd_2}{2}\tan\alpha$	9.11(c)
The tangential force for square thread at mean radius when lowering the load	$F_t = W\tan(\phi - \alpha) = \dfrac{W(f - \tan\alpha)}{1 + f\tan\alpha}$	9.11(d)
The frictional torque at mean radius when lowering the load	$T = \dfrac{Wd_2}{2}\tan(\phi - \alpha)$	9.11(e)
Neglecting the collar friction the efficiency of square thread	$\eta = \dfrac{\tan\alpha}{\tan(\alpha + \phi)} = \dfrac{\tan\alpha(1 - f\tan\alpha)}{\tan\alpha + f}$	9.11(f)
The frictional torque of the collar	$T_c = (Wf_c d_c)/2$	9.11(g)

Particular	Equation	Eqn. No.

where d_c = mean diameter of thrust collar, mm

$= (2/3)d'$ for flat pivot

$= \dfrac{2}{3}\dfrac{d'}{\sin \alpha_1}$ for conical pivot

$= \dfrac{2}{3}\left(\dfrac{d'^3 - d''^3}{d'^2 - d''^2}\right)$ for truncated conical pivot

d' is the outer diameter of the pivot, cone or collar, mm

d'' is the inner diameter of the truncated cone or collar, mm

α_1 is the semi-vertical angle of the cone, which is usually $60°$

W is the axial load, N (kg)

f_c is the coefficient of collar friction (Table 9.6)

Particular	Equation	Eqn. No.
For square threads the total frictional torque including collar friction torque.	$T = \dfrac{W}{2}\left[d_2 \tan(\phi + \alpha) + f_c d_c\right]$ $= \dfrac{W}{2}\left(d_2\left[\dfrac{\tan\alpha + f}{1 - f\tan\alpha}\right] + f_c d_c\right)$	9.12(a)

The efficiency formula for square thread considering collar friction

$$\eta = \dfrac{d_2 \tan\alpha}{d_2\dfrac{\tan\alpha + f}{1 - f\tan\alpha} + f_c d_c} = \dfrac{1}{\pi[d_2 \tan(\alpha + \phi) + f_c d_c]} \qquad 9.12(b)$$

Particular	Equation	Eqn. No.
The overhauling condition for square threads	$\tan\alpha \geq \left(\dfrac{f d_2 + f_c d_c}{d_2 - f f_c d_c}\right)$	9.12(c)
The number of threads necessary in the case of square threaded nut	$n = \dfrac{4W}{p_b \pi(d^2 - D_1^2)}$	9.13(a)
Length of the nut	$l_n = p_n = \dfrac{4W_p}{p_b \pi(d^2 - D_1^2)}$	9.13(b)

where p_b is the allowable bearing pressure (Table 9.5)

References

[1] Siegel M. J., Maleev V. L. Hartman, J. B., *"Mechanical Design of Machines"*, 4th edition, International Text Book Company, 1965.

[2] Vallance, A., Doughtie, V. L., *"Design of Machine Members"*, 3rd edition McGraw Hill Book Co., 1951.

[3] Shigley, J. E., *"Machine Design"*, McGraw Hill Book Company, Inc.

[4] Bhattacharya, S. C., Basu Mallik, J. R., *"Machine Design"*, Basu Mallik & Co., Calcutta, 1966.

Table 9.1 *Values of K for Equation 9.2(a)*

Type of Joint		K
Soft packing with studs	..	1.00
Soft packing with through bolts	..	0.75
Asbestos	..	0.60
Soft-copper gasket with long through bolts	..	0.50
Hard-copper gasket with long through bolts	..	0.25
Metal-to-metal joints with through bolts	..	0.00

Table 9.2 *Properties of some bolt Materials*

Material	Ultimate Strength MN/m^2 (kgf/mm^2)	Yield Point MN/m^2 (kgf/mm^2)	Elastic Limit MN/m^2 (kgf/mm^2)	Endurance Limit MN/m^2 (kgf/mm^2)	Constant C
Low Carbon Steel (Hot rolled) C-0.10 to 0.20	410 (42.0)	268 (27.3)	213 (21.7)	172 (17.5)	2.28 (0.232)
Low carbon Steel (Hot rolled) C-0.20 to 0.30	456 (46.9)	295 (30.1)	240 (24.5)	256 (26.1)	2.55 (0.260)
Medium Carbon Steel (Annealed) C-0.30 to 0.40	480 (49.0)	316 (32.2)	288 (29.4)	240 (24.5)	2.67 (0.272)
Ni-steel (Heat treated drawn at 540° C) Ni-3.25 to 3.75 C-0.35 to 0.45	865 (88.2)	714 (72.8)	652 (66.5)	343 (35.0)	4.79 (0.488)
Ni-Cr. Steel (Heat treated drawn at 540°C) Ni-1.00 to 1.5 C-0.35 to 0.45 Cr-0.45 to 0.75	1030 (105.0)	960 (98.0)	652 (66.5)	550 (56.0)	5.70 (0.581)
Cr.-Va Steel (Heat treated drawn at 425°C) Cr-0.80 to 1.10 C-0.45 to 0.55 Va-0.18	1565 (159.6)	1440 (147.0)	1170 (119.0)	550 (56.0)	8.62 (0.879)

Table 9.3 *Coefficient of friction*

Lubricant	Coefficient of friction (f)
Machine oil and graphite	0.17
Lard oil	0.11
Heavy machine oil	0.14

*Taken from 'Design of Machine Members,' by A. Vallance & V. L. Doughtie, Copyright 1951. McGraw Hill Book Co., With permission from McGraw Hill Book Co.

Table 9.4 *Working stress and load for Indian Metric coarse thread*

Major Dia, (mm)	Stress Area A_r mm^2	Design stress, MN/m^2 (kgf/mm^2)	Permissible Load, N (kgf)
16	157	19.0 (1.93)	2970 (303)
20	245	23.0 (2.33)	5590 (570)
24	353	27.2 (2.77)	9590 (978)
30	561	32.2 (3.28)	18040 (1840)
36	817	37.8 (3.85)	30890 (3150)
42	1120	43.2 (4.40)	48350 (4930)
48	1472	48.4 (4.93)	71100 (7250)
56	2030	55.2 (5.63)	111800 (11400)

Table 9.5 *Safe Bearing Pressures in power Screws*

Service	Material		Safe Bearing pressure MN/m^2 (kgf/mm^2)	Remarks
	Screw	Nut		
Hand Press	Steel	Bronze	17.2 to 24.0 (1.75 to 2.45)	Low speed, well lubricated
Jack Screw	Steel	C.I.	12.4 to 17.2 (1.26 to 1.75)	Low speed, not over 0.04 m/s
Jack Screw	Steel	Bronze	11.0 to 17.2 (1.12 to 1.75)	Low speed, not over 0.05 m/s
Hoisting Screw	Steel	C.I.	4.1 to 7.0 (0.42 to 0.70)	Medium speed, (0.1 to 0.2) m/s
Hoisting Screw	Steel	Bronze	5.5 to 9.6 (0.56 to 0.98)	Medium speed (0.1 to 0.2) m/s
Lead Screw	Steel	Bronze	1.0 to 1.6 (0.11 to 0.17)	High speed 0.25 m/s and over

Table 9.6 *Coefficient of Friction on Thrust Collar*

Material	Coefficient of running friction	Coefficient of starting friction
Soft steel on cast iron	0.121	0.170
Hardened steel on C.I.	0.092	0.147
Soft steel on bronze	0.084	0.101
Hardened steel on bronze	0.063	0.081

Table 9.7 *Pitch Diameter Combinations for ISO Metric Screw Threads All dimensions in millimeters*

| Nominal Diameters | | Pitches | | | | | | | | | | | |
| 1st Choice | 2st Choice | Series with Graded Pitches | | Series with Constant Pitches | | | | | | | | | |
		Coarse	Fine	3	2	1.5	1.25	1	0.75	0.5	0.35	0.25	0.2
1		0.25											0.2
	1.1	0.25											0.2
1.2		0.25											0.2
	1.4	0.3											0.2
1.6		0.35											0.2
	1.8	0.35											0.2
2		0.4										0.25	
	2.2	0.45										0.25	
2.5		0.45									0.35		
3		0.5									0.35		
	3.5	0.6									0.35		
4		0.7								0.5			
	4.5	0.75								0.5			
5		0.8								0.5			
6		1							0.75				
	7	1							0.75				
8		1.25	1					1	0.75				
10		1.5	1.25				1.25	1	1.75				
12		1.75	1.25			1.5	1.25	1					
	14	2	1.5			1.5	1.25*	1					
16		2	1.5			1.5		1					
	18	2.5	1.5		2	1.5		1					
20		2.5	1.5		2	1.5		1					
	22	2.5	1.5		2	1.5		1					
24		3	2		2	1.5		1					
	25	3**											
	27	3	2		2	1.5		1					
30		3.5	2	(3)	2	1.5		1					
	33	3.5	2	(3)	2	1.5							
	35***				2	1.5							
36		4	3	3	2	1.5							
	39	4	3	3	2	1.5							

NOTE:- Pitches given within brackets should be avoided as far as possible   *(Contd.)*

  * Pitch 1.25 mm for diameter 14 mm is to be used only for spark plugs for engines

  * 25 × 3 mm thread is to be used only for track bolts for railway purposes

*** Diameter 35 mm is to be used for locking nuts for ball bearing.

Table 9.7 *Pitch Diameter Combinations for ISO Metric Screw Threads All dimensions in millimeters – (Contd..)*

Nominal Diameters		Series with Graded Pitches		Series with Constant Pitches				
1st Choice	2st Choice	Course	Fine	6	4	3	2	1.5
42		4.5	3		4	3	2	1.5
	45	4.5	3		4	3	2	1.5
48		4	3		4	3	2	1.5
	52	5	3		4	3	2	1.5
56		5.5	4		4	3	2	1.5
	60	5.5	4		4	3	2	1.5
64		6	4		4	3	2	1.5
	68	6	4		4	3	2	1.5
72				6	4	3	2	1.5
	76			6	4	3	2	1.5
80				6	4	3	2	1.5
	85			6	4	3	2	
90				6	4	3	2	
	95			6	4	3	2	
100				6	4	3	2	
	105			6	4	3	2	
110				6	4	3	2	
	115			6	4	3	2	
	120			6	4	3	2	
125				6	4	3	2	
	130			6	4	3	2	
140				6	4	3	2	
	150			6	4	3	2	
160				6	4	3		
	170			6	4	3		
180				6	4	3		
	190			6	4	3		
200				6	4	3		
	210			6	4	3		
220				6	4	3		
	240			6	4	3		
250				6	4	3		
	260			6	4			
280				6	4			
	300			6	4			

IS: 4218 (Part II)–1967

Table 9.8 *Basic Dimensions for Design Profiles of ISO Metric Screw Threads*

Basic Diameter mm.	Pitch mm.	Major Diameter mm.	Pitch Diameter mm.	Minor Diameter, mm.		Lead Basic	Angle at Pitch dia	Tensile Stress Area mm^2
				External Threads	Internal Threads	deg	min	
(1)	(2)	(3)	(4)	(5)	(6)	(7)	(8)	(9)
	0.25	1.0	0.837620	0.693283	0.729367	5	27	0.46
1	0.2	1.0	0.870096	0.756426	0.783494	4	11	0.53
	0.25	1.1	0.937620	0.793283	0.829367	4	52	0.59
1.1	0.2	1.1	0.970096	0.854626	0.883494	3	45	0.67
	0.25	1.2	1.037630	0.893283	0.929367	4	24	0.73
1.2	0.2	1.2	1.070096	0.954626	0.983494	3	24	0.82
	0.3	1.4	1.205144	1.031939	1.075240	4	34	0.98
1.4	0.2	1.4	1.270096	1.154626	1.183494	2	52	1.17
1.6	0.35	1.6	1.372668	1.170596	1.221114	4	38	1.27
	0.2	1.6	1.470096	1.354626	1.383494	2	29	1.59
	0.35	1.8	1.572668	1.370596	1.421114	4	3	1.70
1.8	0.2	1.8	1.670096	1.554626	1.583494	2	11	2.66
	0.4	2.0	1.740192	1.509252	1.566987	4	11	2.07
2	0.25	2.0	1.837620	1.693283	1.729367	2	29	2.45
2.2	0.45	2.2	1.907716	1.647909	1.712861	4	17	2.48
	0.25	2.2	2.037620	1.893283	1.929367	2	14	3.03
	0.45	2.5	2.207716	1.947909	2.012861	3	43	3.39
2.5	0.35	2.5	2.272668	2.070596	2.121114	2	20	3.70
	0.5	3.0	2.675240	2.386565	2.458734	3	24	5.03
3	0.35	3.0	2.272668	2.570596	2.621114	2	18	5.61
	0.6	3.5	3.110289	2.763878	2.850481	3	31	6.78
3.5	0.35	3.5	3.272668	3.070596	3.121114	1	57	7.90
	0.7	4.0	3.545337	3.141191	3.242228	3	36	8.78
4	0.5	4.0	3.675240	3.386565	3.458734	2	29	9.79
	0.75	4.5	4.012861	3.579848	3.688101	3	24	11.3
4.5	0.5	4.5	4.175240	3.886565	3.958734	2	11	12.8
	0.8	5.0	4.480385	4.018505	4.133975	3	15	14.2
5	0.5	5.0	4.675240	4.386565	4.458734	1	57	16.1

(1)	(2)	(3)	(4)	(5)	(6)	(7)	(8)	(9)
	1	6.0	5.350481	4.773131	4.917468	3	24	20.1
6	0.75	6.0	5.512861	5.079848	5.188101	2	29	22.0
	1	7.0	6.350481	5.773131	5.917468	2	52	28.9
7	0.75	7.0	6.512861	6.079849	6.188101	2	6	31.3
	1.25	8.0	7.188101	6.466413	6.646835	3	10	36.6
8	1	8.0	7.350481	6.773131	6.917468	2	29	39.2
	0.75	8.0	7.512861	7.079848	7.188101	1	49	41.8
	1.5	10.0	9.025721	8.159696	8.376202	3	2	58.0
10	1.25	10.0	9.188101	8.466413	8.646835	2	29	61.2
	1	10.0	9.350481	8.773131	8.917468	1	57	64.5
	0.75	10.0	9.512861	9.079848	9.188101	1	26	67.9
	1.75	12.0	10.863342	9.852979	10.105569	2	56	84.3
	1.5	12.0	11.025721	10.159696	10.376202	2	29	88.1
12	1.25	12.0	11.188101	10.466413	10.646835	2	2	92.1
	1	12.0	11.350481	10.773131	10.917438	1	36	96.1
	2	14.0	12.700962	11.546261	11.834936	2	52	115
	1.5	14.0	13.025721	12.159696	12.376202	2	6	125
14	1.25	14.0	13.188101	12.466413	12.646835	1	44	129
	1	14.0	13.350481	12.773131	12.917468	1	22	134
	2	16.0	14.700962	13.546261	13.834936	2	29	157
16	1.5	16.0	15.025721	14.159696	14.376202	1	49	167
	1	16.0	15.350481	14.773131	14.917468	1	11	178
	2.5	18.0	16.376202	14.932827	15.293671	2	47	192
	2	18.0	16.700962	15.546261	15.834936	2	11	204
18	1.5	18.0	17.025721	16.159696	16.376202	1	36	216
	1	18.0	17.350481	16773131	19.917468	1	3	229
	2.5	20.0	18.376202	16.932827	17.293671	2	29	245
	2.0	20.0	18.700962	17.546261	17.834936	1	57	258
20	1.5	20.0	19.025721	18.159696	18.376202	1	26	272
	1	20.0	19.350481	18.773131	18.917468	0	57	285
	2.5	22.0	20.376202	18.932827	19.293671	2	14	303
	2	22.0	20.700962	19.546261	19.834936	1	46	318
22	1.5	22.0	21.025721	20.159696	20.376202	1	18	333
	1	22.0	21.350481	20.773131	20.917468	0	51	348

(1)	(2)	(3)	(4)	(5)	(6)	(7)	(8)	(9)
	3	24.0	22.051443	20.319392	20.752405	2	49	353
	2	24.0	22.700962	21.546261	21.834936	1	39	384
24	1.5	24.0	23.025721	22.159696	22.376202	1	11	401
	1	24.0	23.350481	22.773131	22.917468	0	47	418
25	3	25.0	23.051443	21.319392	21.752405	2	36	385
	3	27.0	25.051443	23.319392	23.752405	2	11	459
	2	27.0	25.700962	24.546261	24.834936	1	25	496
27	1.5	27.0	26.025721	25.159696	25.376202	1	3	514
	1	27.0	26.350481	25.773131	25.917468	0	41	553
	3.5	30.0	27.726683	25.705957	26.211139	2	18	561
	3	30.0	28.051443	26.319392	26.722405	1	57	581
30	2	30.0	28.700962	27.546261	27.834936	1	16	621
	1.5	30.0	29.025721	28.159696	28.376202	0	57	642
	1	30.0	29.350481	28.773131	28.917468	0	37	663
	3.5	33.0	30.726683	28.705957	29.211139	2	5	694
	3	33.0	31.051443	29.319392	29.752405	1	46	716
33	2	33.0	31.700962	30.546261	30.834936	1	9	761
	1.5	33.0	32.025721	31.159696	31.376202	0	51	785
35	1.5	35.0	34.025721	33.159696	33.376202	0	48	886
	4	36.0	33.401924	31.092523	31.669873	2	11	817
	3	36.0	34.051443	32.319392	32.752405	1	36	865
36	2	36.0	34.700962	33.546261	33.834936	1	3	915
	1.5	36.0	35.025721	34.159696	34.376202	0	47	940
	4	39.0	36.401924	34.092523	34.669873	2	0	976
	3	39.0	37.051443	35.319392	35.752405	1	29	1030
39	2	39.0	37.700962	36.546261	36.834936	0	58	1080
	1.5	39.0	38.025721	37.159696	37.376202	0	43	1110
	4.5	42.0	39.077164	36.479088	37.128607	2	6	1120
	4	42.0	39.401924	37.092523	37.669873	1	51	1150
42	3	42.0	40.051443	38.319392	38.752405	1	22	1210
	2	42.0	40.700962	39.546261	39.834936	0	52	1260
	1.5	42.0	41.025721	40.159696	40.376202	0	40	1290
	4.5	45.0	42.077164	39.479088	40.128607	1	57	1300
	4	45.0	42.401924	40.092523	40.669873	1	43	1340

(1)	(2)	(3)	(4)	(5)	(6)	(7)	(8)	(9)
45	3	45.0	43.051443	41.319392	41.752405	1	16	1400
	2	45.0	43.700962	42.546261	42.834936	0	50	1460
	1.5	45.0	44.025721	43.159696	43.376202	0	37	1490
	5	48.0	44.752405	41.865653	42.587341	2	2	1470
	4	48.0	45.401924	43.092523	43.569873	1	36	1540
48	3	48.0	46.051443	44.319392	44.752405	1	11	1600
	2	48.0	46.700962	45.546261	45.834936	0	47	1670
	1.5	48.0	47.025721	46.159696	46.376202	0	35	1710
	5	52.0	48.752405	45.865653	43.587341	1	52	1760
	4	52.0	49.401924	47.092523	47.669873	1	29	1830
52	3	52.0	50.051443	48.319392	48.752405	1	6	1900
	2	52.0	50.700962	49.546261	49.834936	0	43	1970
	1.5	52.0	51.025721	50.159696	50.376202	0	32	2010
	5.5	56.0	52.427645	49.252219	50.046075	1	55	2030
	4	56.0	53.401924	51.092523	51.669873	1	22	2140
56	3	56.0	54.051443	52.319392	52.752405	1	1	2220
	2	56.0	54.700962	53.546261	53.834936	0	40	2300
	1.5	56.0	55.025721	54.159696	54.376202	0	30	2340
	5.5	60.0	56.427645	53.252219	54.046075	1	47	2360
	4	60.0	57.401924	55.092523	55.669873	1	16	2490
60	3	60.0	58.051443	53.319392	56.752405	0	57	2570
	2	60.0	58.700962	57.546261	57.834936	0	37	2650
	1.5	60.0	59.025721	58.159696	58.376202	0	28	2700
	6	64.0	60.102886	56.638784	57.504809	1	49	2680
	4	64.0	61.401924	59.092523	59.669873	1	11	2850
64	3	64.0	62.051443	60.319392	60.752405	0	53	2940
	2	64.0	62.700962	61.546261	61.834936	0	35	3030
	1.5	64.0	63.025721	62.159696	62.376202	0	26	3080
	6	68.0	64.102886	60.638784	61.504809	1	42	3060
	4	68.0	65.401924	63.092523	63.669873	1	7	3240
68	3	68.0	66.051443	64.319392	64.752405	1	50	3340
	2	68.0	66.700962	65.546261	65.834936	1	33	3430
	1.5	68.0	67.025721	66.159696	66.376202	0	24	3480

(1)	(2)	(3)	(4)	(5)	(6)	(7)	(8)	(9)
	6	72.0	68.102886	64.638784	65.504809	1	36	3460
	4	72.0	69.401924	67.092523	67.669873	1	3	3660
72	3	72.0	70.051443	68.319392	68.752405	0	47	3760
	2	72.0	70.700962	69.546261	69.834936	0	31	3860
	1.5	72.0	71.025721	70.159696	70.372602	0	23	3910
	6	76.0	72.102886	68.638784	69.504809	1	31	3890
	4	76.0	73.401924	71.092523	71.669873	1	0	4100
76	3	76.0	74.051443	72.319392	72.752405	0	44	4210
	2	76.0	74.700962	73.546261	73.834936	0	29	4320
	1.5	76.0	75.025721	74.159696	74.376202	0	22	4370
	6	80.0	76.102886	72.638784	73.504809	1	26	4340
	4	80.0	77.401924	75.092523	75.669873	0	57	4570
80	3	80.0	78.051443	76.319392	76.752405	0	42	4680
	2	80.0	78.700962	77.546261	77.834936	0	28	4790
	1.5	80.0	79.025721	78.159696	78.376202	0	21	4850
	6	85.0	81.102886	77.638784	78.504809	1	21	4950
	4	85.0	82.401924	80.092523	80.669873	0	53	5190
85	3	85.0	83.051443	81.319392	81.752405	0	50	5310
	2	85.0	83.700962	82.546261	82.834936	0	26	5430
	6	90.0	86.102886	82.638784	83.504809	1	16	5590
	4	90.0	87.401924	85.092523	85.669873	0	50	5840
90	3	90.0	88.051443	86.319392	86.752405	0	37	5970
	2	90.0	88.700962	87.546261	87.834936	0	25	6100
	6	95.0	91.102886	87.638784	88.504809	1	12	6270
	4	95.0	92.401924	90.092523	90.669873	0	47	6540
95	3	95.0	93.051443	91.319392	91.752405	0	35	6670
	2	95.0	93.700962	92.546261	92.834936	0	23	6810
	6	100.0	96.102886	92.638784	93.504809	1	8	7000
	4	100.0	97.401924	95.092523	95.669873	0	45	7280
100	3	100.0	98.051443	96.319392	96.752405	0	33	7420
	2	100.0	98.700962	97.346261	97.834936	0	22	7560

IS: 4218 (Part III)–1967

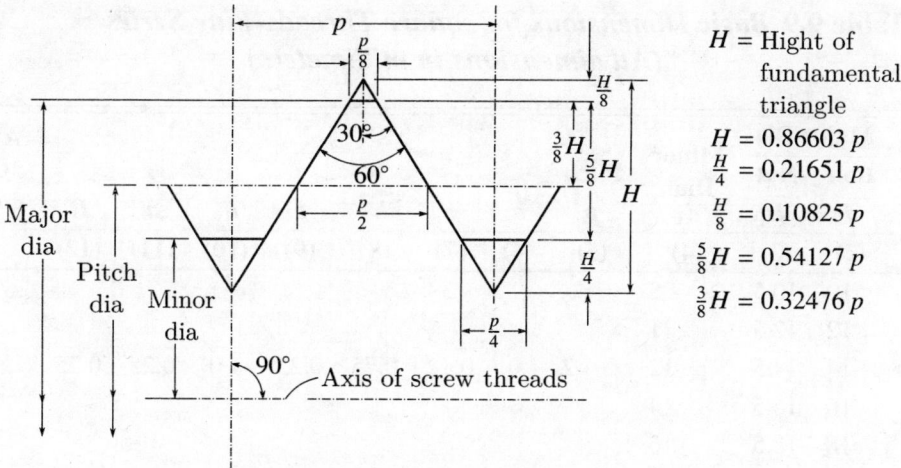

Fig. 9.8: *Basic Profile of ISO Metric Screw Threads*

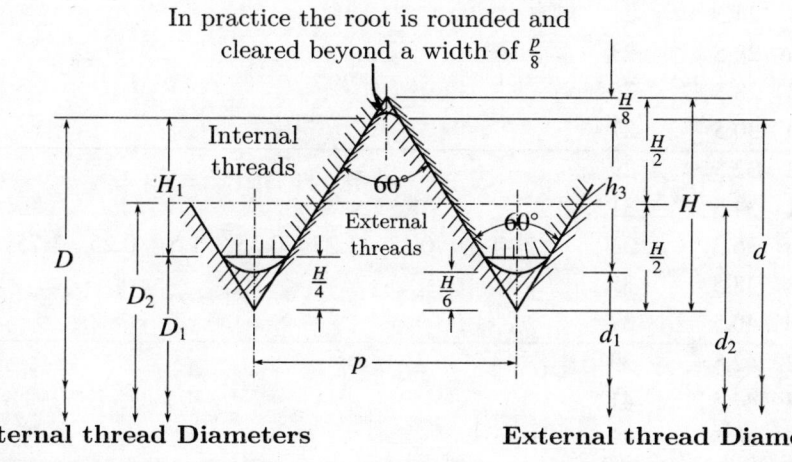

In practice the root is rounded and cleared beyond a width of $\frac{p}{8}$

Internal thread Diameters   **External thread Diameters**

p = Pitch

$H = 0.86603\,p$

$D = d$ – Major n diameter

$D_2 = d_2 = d - \dfrac{3}{4}H$

$\quad = d - 0.64952\,p$

$D_1 = d_2 - 2\left(\dfrac{H}{2} - \dfrac{H}{4}\right)$

$\quad = d - 2H_1 = d - 1.08253\,p$

$d_1 = d_2 - 2\left(\dfrac{H}{2} - \dfrac{H}{6}\right)$

$\quad = d - 1.22687\,p$

$H_1 = \dfrac{D - D_1}{2} = \dfrac{5}{8}H$

$\quad = 0.54127\,p$

$\quad$ = maximum depth of engagement

$h_3 = \dfrac{d - d_1}{2} = \left(\dfrac{17}{24}H\right)$

$\quad = 0.61343\,p$

$\quad$ = basic depth of
$\qquad$ extended thread

$r = \dfrac{H}{6} = 0.14434\,p$

Fig. 9.9: *ISO Metric Screw Thread–Design Profiles of External and Internal Threads*

IS: 4218 (Part I)-1967

Table 9.9 *Basic Dimensions for square Threads-Fine Series*
(All dimensions in millimeters)

Nom. Dia.	Major Dia		Minor Dia., d_1	Pitch								Area of Core, mm^2
	Bolt d	Nut D		p	e	r	h_2	b	h_1	a	H	
(1)	(2)	(3)	(4)	(5)	(6)	(7)	(8)	(9)	(10)	(11)	(12)	(13)
10	10	10.5	8									50.3
12	12	12.5	11									78.5
14	14	14.5	12	2	1.0	0.12	0.75	0.25	1.0	0.25	0.25	113.0
16	16	16.5	14									154.0
18	18	18.5	16									201.0
20	20	20.5	18									254.0
22	22	22.5	19									284.0
24	24	24.5	21									346.0
26	26	26.5	23									415.0
28	28	28.5	25									491.0
30	30	30.5	27									573.0
32	32	32.5	29									661.0
(34)	34	34.5	31									755.0
36	36	36.5	33	3	1.5	0.12	1.25	0.25	1.5	0.25	1.75	855.0
(38)	38	38.5	35									962.0
40	40	40.5	37									1075.0
42	42	42.5	39									1195.0
44	44	44.5	41									1320.0
(46)	46	46.5	43									1452.0
48	48	48.5	45									1590.0
50	50	50.5	47									1735.0
52	52	52.5	49									1886.0
55	55	55.5	52									2124.0
(58)	58	58.5	55	3	1.5	0.12	1.25	0.25	1.5	0.25	1.75	2376.0
60	60	60.5	57									2552.0
(62)	62	62.5	59									2734.0
65	65	65.5	61									2922.0
(68)	68	68.5	64									3217.0
70	70	70.5	66	4	2.0	0.12	1.75	0.25	2.0	0.25	2.25	3421.0
(72)	72	72.5	68									3632.0
75	75	75.5	71									3959.0

Table 9.9 *Basic Dimensions for square Threads-Fine Series (All dimensions in millimeters) – (Contd..)*

(1)	(2)	(3)	(4)	(5)	(6)	(7)	(8)	(9)	(10)	(11)	(12)	(13)
(78)	78	78.5	74									4301.0
80	80	80.5	76									4538.0
(82)	82	82.5	78	4	2.0	0.12	1.75	0.25	2.0	0.25	2.25	4778.0
85	85	85.5	81									5153.0
(88)	88	88.5	84									5542.0
90	90	90.5	86									5809.0
(92)	92	92.5	88									6082.0
95	95	95.5	91									6504.0
(98)	98	98.5	94	4	2.0	0.12	1.75	0.25	2.0	0.25	2.25	6940.0
100	100	100.5	96									7288.0
(105)	105	105.5	101									8018.0
110	110	110.5	106									8825.0
(115)	115	115.5	109									9331.0
120	120	120.5	114									10207.0
(125)	125	125.5	119	6	3.0	0.25	2.5	0.5	3.0	0.25	3.25	11122.0
130	130	130.5	124									12076.0
(135)	135	135.5	129									13070.0
140	140	140.5	135									14103.0
(145)	145	145.5	139									15175.0
150	150	150.5	144									16286.0
(155)	155	155.5	149									17437.0
160	160	160.5	154	6	3.0	0.25	2.5	0.5	3.0	0.25	3.25	18627.0
(165)	165	165.5	159									19856.0
170	170	170.5	164									21124.0
(175)	175	175.5	169									22432.0
180	180	180.5	172									23235.0
(185)	185	185.5	177									24606.0
190	190	190.5	182	8	4.0	0.25	3.5	0.5	4.0	0.25	4.25	26016.0
(195)	195	195.5	187									27465.0
200	200	200.5	192									28953.0
210	210	210.5	202									32047.0
220	220	220.5	212	8	4.0	0.25	3.5	0.5	4.0	0.25	4.25	35299.0
230	230	230.5	222									38708.0
240	240	240.5	232									42272.0
250	250	250.0	238									44488.0
260	260	260.5	248									48305.0

Table 9.9 *Basic Dimensions for square Threads-Fine Series*
(All dimensions in millimeters) – (Contd..)

(1)	(2)	(3)	(4)	(5)	(6)	(7)	(8)	(9)	(10)	(11)	(12)	(13)
270	270	270.5	258									52279.0
280	280	280.5	268									56410.0
290	290	290.5	278									60699.0
300	300	300.5	288	12	6.0	0.25	5.5	0.5	6.0	0.25	6.25	65144.0
320	320	320.5	308									74506.0
340	340	340.5	328									84496.0
360	360	360.5	348									95115.0
380	380	380.5	368									106362.0
400	400	400.5	388									118237.0
420	420	421.0	402									126923.0
440	440	441.0	422									139867.0
460	460	460.0	442	18	9.0	0.5	8.0	1.0	1.0	0.5	9.5	153439.0
480	480	481.0	462									167639.0
500	500	501.0	482									182467.0
520	520	521.0	496									193221.0
540	540	541.0	516	24	12.0	0.5	11.0	1.0	12.0	0.5	12.5	209117.0
560	560	561.0	536									225642.0
580	580	581.0	556									242795.0
600	600	601.0										
620	620	621.0										
640	640	641.0										

Note: Diameters indicated within brackets are of second preference.   IS: 4694–1968

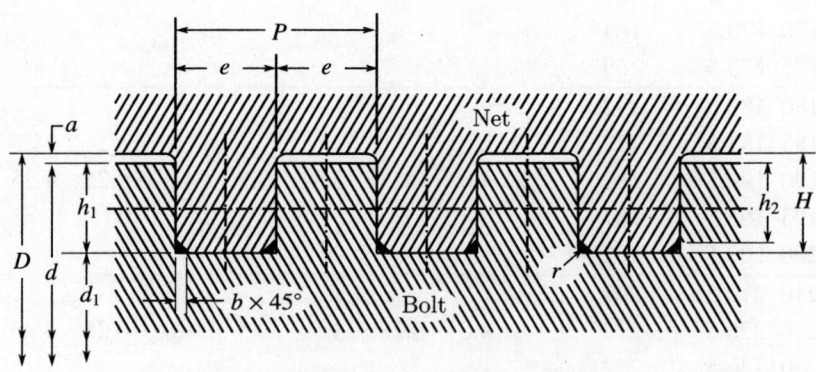

Fig. 9.10: *Basic profile of square threads*

$$h_1 = 0.5p \quad H' = 0.5p + a \quad h_2 = 0.5p - b \quad e = 0.5p \quad D = d + 2a \quad d_1 = d - 2h_1$$
$$\text{Area of core} = \frac{\pi}{4}d_1^2$$

Table 9.10 *Basic Dimensions for Square Threads-Normal Series* *(All dimensions in millimeters)*

Nom. Dia.	Major Dia		Minor Diameter	Pitch								Area of Core, mm²
	Bolt d	Nut D	d₁	p	e	r	h₂	b	h₁	a	H	
(1)	(2)	(3)	(4)	(5)	(6)	(7)	(8)	(9)	(10)	(11)	(12)	(13)
22	22	22.5	17									227
24	24	24.5	19	5	2.5	0.25	2.0	0.5	2.5	0.25	2.75	284
26	26	26.5	21									346
28	28	28.5	23									415
30	30	30.5	24									452
32	32	32.5	26	6	3.0	0.25	2.5	0.5	3.0	0.25	3.25	531
(34)	34	34.5	28									616
36	36	36.5	30									707
(38)	38	38.5	31									755
40	40	40.5	33	7	3.5	0.25	3.0	0.5	3.5	0.25	3.75	855
(42)	42	42.5	35									962
44	44	44.5	37									1075
(46)	46	46.5	38									1134
48	48	48.5	40	8	4.0	0.25	3.5	0.5	4.0	0.25	4.25	1257
50	50	50.5	42									1385
52	52	52.4	44									1521
55	55	55.5	46									1662
(58)	58	58.5	49	9	4.5	0.25	4.0	0.5	4.5	0.25	4.75	1886
60	60	60.5	51									2043
(62)	62	62.5	53									2206
65	65	65.5	55									2376
(68)	68	68.5	58									2642
70	70	70.5	60									2827
(72)	72	72.5	62	10	5.0	0.25	4.5	0.5	5.0	0.25	5.25	3019
75	75	75.5	65									3318
(78)	78	78.5	68									3632
80	80	80.5	70									3848
(82)	82	82.5	72									4072

Table 9.10 *Basic Dimensions for Square Threads-Normal Series*
(All dimensions in millimeters) – (Contd..)

(1)	(2)	(3)	(4)	(5)	(6)	(7)	(8)	(9)	(10)	(11)	(12)	(13)
85	85	85.5	73									4185
(88)	88	88.5	76									5436
90	90	90.5	78									4778
(92)	92	92.5	80									5027
95	95	95.5	83	12	6.0	0.25	5.5	0.5	6.0	0.25	6.25	5411
(98)	98	98.5	86									5809
100	100	100.5	88									6082
(105)	105	105.5	93									6793
110	110	110.5	98									7543
(115)	115	116.0	101									8012
120	120	121.0	106									8825
125	125	126.0	111									9677
130	130	131.0	116	14	7.0	0.5	6.0	1.0	7.0	0.5	7.5	70568
(135)	135	136.0	121									11499
140	140	141.0	126									12469
(145)	145	146.0	131									13478
150	150	151.0	134									14103
(155)	155	156.0	139									15175
160	160	161.0	144	16	8.0	0.5	7.0	1.0	8.0	0.5	8.5	16286
(165)	165	166.0	149									17437
170	170	171.0	154									18627
(175)	175	176.0	159									19856
180	180	181.0	162									20612
(185)	185	186.0	167									21904
190	190	191.0	172	18	9.0	0.5	8.0	1.0	9.0	0.5	9.5	23235
(195)	195	196.0	177									24606
200	200	201.0	182									26016
210	210	211.0	190									28353
220	220	221.0	200	20	10.0	0.5	9.0	1.0	10	0.5	10.5	31416
230	230	231.0	210									34636

Table 9.10 *Basic Dimensions for Square Threads-Normal Series*
(All dimensions in millimeters) – (Contd..)

(1)	(2)	(3)	(4)	(5)	(6)	(7)	(8)	(9)	(10)	(11)	(12)	(13)
240	240	241.0	218									37325
250	250	251.0	228	22	11.0	0.5	10	1.0	11.0	0.5	11.5	40828
260	260	261.0	238									44488
270	270	271.0	246									47529
280	280	281.0	256	24	12.0	0.5	11.0	1.0	12.0	0.5	12.5	51472
290	290	291.0	266									55572
300	300	301.0	274	26	13.0	0.5	12.0	1.0	13.0	0.5	13.5	58965

Note:- Diameters within brackets are of second preference

IS: 4694–1968

Table 9.11 *Basic Dimensions for Square Threads-Coarse Series*
(All dimensions in millimeters)

Nom. Dia.	Major Dia		Minor Dia-meter	Pitch								Area of Core, mm^2
	Bolt	Nut										
	d	D	d_1	p	e	r	h_2	b	h_1	a	H	
(1)	(2)	(3)	(4)	(5)	(6)	(7)	(8)	(9)	(10)	(11)	(12)	(13)
22	22	22.5	14									164
24	24	24.5	16	8	4	0.25	3.5	0.5	4	0.25	4.25	201
26	26	26.5	18									254
28	28	28.5	20									314
30	30	30.5	20									314
32	32	32.5	22									360
(34)	34	34.5	24	10	5	0.25	4.5	0.5	5	0.25	5.25	452
36	36	36.5	26									531
(38)	38	38.5	28									616
40	40	40.5	28									616
(42)	42	42.5	30									707
44	44	44.5	32									804
(46)	46	46.5	34	12	6	0.25	5.5	0.5	6	0.25	6.25	908
48	48	48.5	36									1018
50	50	50.5	38									1134

Table 9.11 *Basic Dimensions for Square Threads-Coarse Series*
(All dimensions in millimeters) – (Contd..)

(1)	(2)	(3)	(4)	(5)	(6)	(7)	(8)	(9)	(10)	(11)	(12)	(13)
52	52	52.5	40									1257
55	55	56.0	41									1320
(58)	58	59.0	44	14	7	0.5	6.0	1.0	7	0.5	7.5	1521
60	60	61.0	46									1662
(62)	62	63.0	48									1810
65	65	66.0	49									1886
(68)	68	69.0	52									2124
70	70	71.0	54									2290
(72)	72	73.0	56	16	8	0.5	7.0	1.0	8	0.5	8.5	2463
75	75	76.0	59									2734
(78)	78	79.0	62									3019
80	80	81.0	64									3217
(82)	82	83.0	66									3421
85	85	86.0	67									3526
(88)	88	89.0	70									3848
90	90	91.0	72	18	9	0.5	8.0	1.0	9	0.5	9.5	4072
(92)	92	93.0	74									4301
95	95	95.0	77									4657
(98)	98	99.0	80									5027
100	100	101.0	80									5027
(105)	105	106.0	85	20	10	0.5	9.0	1.0	10	0.5	10.5	5675
110	110	111.0	90									6362
(115)	115	116.0	93									6793
120	120	121.0	98	22	11	0.5	10.0	1.0	11	0.5	11.5	7543
(125)	125	126.0	103									8332
130	130	131.0	108									9161
(135)	135	136.0	111									9677
140	140	141.0	116									10568
(145)	145	146.0	121	24	12	0.5	11.0	1.0	12	0.5	12.5	11499
150	150	151.0	126									12469
(155)	155	156.0	131									13478

Table 9.11 *Basic Dimensions for Square Threads-Coarse Series (All dimensions in millimeters) – (Contd..)*

(1)	(2)	(3)	(4)	(5)	(6)	(7)	(8)	(9)	(10)	(11)	(12)	(13)
160	160	161.0	132									13685
(165)	165	166	137									14741
170	170	171	142	28	14	0.5	13.0	1.0	14	0.5	14.5	15837
(175)	175	176.0	147									16972
180	180	181.0	152									18146
(185)	185	186	153									18385
190	190	191	158									19607
(195)	195	196	163	32	16	0.5	15.0	1.0	16	0.5	16.5	20867
200	200	201	168									22167
210	210	211	174									23779
220	220	221	184									26590
230	230	231	194	36	18	0.5	17.0	1.0	18	0.5	18.5	29559
240	240	241	204									32685
250	250	251	210									34636
260	260	261	220									38013
270	270	271	230	40	20	0.5	19.0	1.0	20	0.5	20.5	41548
280	280	281	240									45239
290	290	291	246									47529
300	300	301	256									51472
320	320	321	276	44	22	0.5	21.0	1.0	22	0.5	22.5	59828
340	340	341	296									68813
360	360	361	312									76454
380	380	381	332	43	24	0.5	23.0	1.0	24	0.5	24.5	86570
400	400	401	352									97314

Note:- Diameters within brackets are of second preference.

IS: 4694–1968

Table 9.12 *Limits of Sizes for Fine Series Nut Threads-Tolerance Class 5H*

Size	Pitch p	Major Diameter D Min	Pitch Diameter D_2			Minor Diameter D_1		
			Max	*Min*	Tolerance	*Max*	*Min*	Tolerance
(1)	(2)	(3)	(4)	(5)	(6)	(7)	(8)	(9)
	mm	mm	mm	mm	μm	mm	mm	μm
M8 × 1	1	8.0	7.468	7.350	118	7.107	6.917	190
M10 × 1.25	1.25	10.0	9.313	9.188	125	8.859	8.647	212
M12 × 1.25	1.25	12.0	11.328	11.188	140	10.859	10.647	212
(M14 × 1.5)	1.5	14.0	13.176	13.026	150	12.612	12.376	236
M16 × 1.5	1.5	16.0	15.176	15.026	150	14.612	14.376	236
(M18 × 1.5)	1.5	18.0	17.176	17.026	150	16.612	16.376	236
M20 × 1.5	1.5	20.0	19.176	19.026	150	18.612	18.376	236
(M22 × 1.5)	1.5	22.0	21.176	21.026	150	20.612	20.376	236
M24 × 2	2	24.0	22.881	22.701	180	22.135	21.835	300
(M27 × 2)	2	27.0	25.881	25.701	180	25.135	24.835	300
M30 × 2	2	30.0	28.881	28.701	180	27.135	27.835	300
(M33 × 2)	2	30.0	28.881	28.701	180	28.135	27.835	300
(M33 × 2)	2	33.0	31.881	31.701	180	31.135	30.835	300
M36 × 3	3	36.0	34.263	34.051	212	33.152	32.752	400
(M39 × 3)	3	39.0	37.263	37.051	212	36.152	35.752	400

μm=0.001 mm

Note:- Second preference sizes are given in brackets in col 1.

IS: 4218 (Part VI)–1967

Table 9.13 *Limits of Sizes for Fine Series Bolt Threads-Tolerance Class 4h*

Size	Pitch p	Major Diameter d			Pitch Diameter d_2			Minor Diameter d_3		
		Max	Min	Tolerance	Max	Min	Tolerance	Max	Min	Tolerance
(1)	(2)	(3)	(4)	(5)	(6)	(7)	(8)	(9)	(10)	(11)
	mm	mm	mm	μm	mm	mm	μm	mm	mm	μm
M8 × 1	1	8.0	7.888	112	7.350	7.279	71	6.773	6.630	143
M10 × 1.25	1.25	10.0	9.868	132	9.188	9.113	75	8.466	8.301	165
M12 × 1.25	1.25	12.0	11.868	132	11.188	11.103	85	10.466	10.291	175
(M14 × 1.5)	1.5	14.0	13.850	150	13.026	12.936	90	12.160	11.962	198
M16 × 1.5	1.5	16.0	15.850	150	15.026	14.936	90	14.160	13.962	198
(M18 × 1.5)	1.5	18.0	17.850	150	17.026	16.936	90	16.160	15.962	198
M20 × 1.5	1.5	20.0	19.850	150	19.026	18.936	90	18.160	17.962	198
(M22 × 1.5)	1.5	22.0	21.850	150	21.026	20.936	90	20.160	19.962	198
M24 × 2	2	24.0	23.820	180	22.701	22.595	106	21.546	21.296	250
(M27 × 2)	2	27.0	26.820	180	25.701	25.595	106	24.546	24.296	250
M30 × 2	2	30.0	29.820	180	28.701	28.595	106	27.546	27.296	250
(M33 × 2)	2	33.0	31.820	180	31.701	31.595	106	30.546	30.296	250
M36 × 3	3	36.0	35.764	236	34.051	33.926	125	32.319	31.978	341
(M39 × 3)	3	39.0	38.764	236	37.051	36.926	125	35.319	34.978	341

μm=0.001 mm.

Second preference sizes are shown in brackets in Col. 1

IS: 4218 (Part VI)–1967

Table 9.14 *Limits of Sizes for Course Series Nut Threads-Tolerance Class 7H*

Size	Pitch p	Major Diameter D Min	Pitch Diameter D_2			Minor Diameter D_1		
			Max	Min	Tolerance	Max	Min	Tolerance
(1)	(2)	(3)	(4)	(5)	(6)	(7)	(8)	(9)
	mm	mm	mm	mm	μm	mm	mm	μm
M1	0.25	1.000	—	—	—	—	—	—
(M1.1)	0.25	1.100	—	—	—	—	—	—
M1.2	0.25	1.200	—	—	—	—	—	—
(M1.4)	0.3	1.400	—	—	—	—	—	—
M1.6	0.35	1.600	—	—	—	—	—	—
(M1.8)	0.35	1.800	—	—	—	—	—	—
M2	0.4	2.000	—	—	—	—	—	—
(M2.2)	0.45	2.200	—	—	—	—	—	—
M2.5	0.45	2.500	—	—	—	—	—	—
M3	0.5	3.000	2.800	2.675	125	2.639	2.459	180
(M3.5)	0.6	3.500	3.250	3.110	140	3.050	2.850	200
M4	0.7	4.000	3.695	3.545	150	3.466	3.242	224
(M4.5)	0.75	4.500	4.163	4.013	150	3.924	3.688	236
M5	0.8	5.000	4.640	4.480	160	4.384	4.134	250
M6	1	6.000	5.540	5.350	190	5.217	4.917	300
(M7)	1	7.000	6.540	6.350	190	6.217	5.917	300
M8	1.25	8.000	7.388	7.188	200	6.982	6.647	335
M10	1.5	10.000	9.250	9.026	224	8.751	8.376	375
M12	1.75	12.000	11.113	10.863	250	10.531	10.106	425
(M14)	2	14.000	12.966	12.701	265	12.310	11.835	472
(M16)	2	16.000	14.966	14.701	265	14.213	13.835	475
(M18)	2.5	18.000	16.656	16.376	280	15.854	15.294	560
M20	2.5	20.000	18.656	19.376	280	17.854	17.294	560
(M22)	2.5	22.000	20.656	20.376	280	19.854	19.294	560
M24	3	24.000	22.386	22.051	335	21.382	20.757	630
(M27)	3	27.000	25.386	25.051	335	24.383	23.752	630
M30	3.5	30.000	28.082	27.727	355	26.921	26.211	710
(M33)	3.5	33.000	31.082	30.727	355	29.921	29.211	710
M36	4	36.000	33.777	33.402	375	32.420	31.670	750
(M39)	4	39.000	36.777	36.402	375	35.420	34.670	750

μm=0.001 mm

Note:- Second preference sizes are shown in brackets in col. 1

IS: 4218 (Part VI)–1967

Table 9.15 *Limits of Sizes for Coarse Series Bolt Threads-Tolerance Class 8g*

Size	Pitch p	Major Diameter d			Pitch Diameter d_2			Minor Diameter d_3		
		Max	Min	Tolerance	Max	Min	Tolerance	Max	Min	Tolerance
(1)	(2)	(3)	(4)	(5)	(6)	(7)	(8)	(9)	(10)	(11)
	mm	mm	mm	μm	mm	mm	μm	mm	mm	μm
M1	0.25	—	—	—	—	—	—	—	—	—
(M1.1)	0.25	—	—	—	—	—	—	—	—	—
M1.2	0.25	—	—	—	—	—	—	—	—	—
(M1.4)	0.3	—	—	—	—	—	—	—	—	—
M1.6	0.35	—	—	—	—	—	—	—	—	—
(M1.8)	0.35	—	—	—	—	—	—	—	—	—
M2	0.4	—	—	—	—	—	—	—	—	—
(M2.2)	0.4	—	—	—	—	—	—	—	—	—
M2.5	0.45	—	—	—	—	—	—	—	—	—
M3	0.5	—	—	—	—	—	—	—	—	—
(M3.5)	0.6	—	—	—	—	—	—	—	—	—
M4	0.7	—	—	—	—	—	—	—	—	—
(M4.5)	0.75	—	—	—	—	—	—	—	—	—
M5	0.8	4.976	4.740	236	4.456	4.306	150	3.995	3.787	208
M6	1	5.974	5.694	280	5.324	5.144	180	4.747	4.495	252
(M7)	1	6.974	6.694	280	6.324	6.144	180	5.747	5.495	252
M8	1.25	7.972	7.637	335	7.160	6.970	190	6.438	6.158	280
M10	1.5	9.968	9.593	375	8.994	8.782	212	8.128	7.808	320
M12	1.75	11.966	11.541	425	10.829	10.593	236	9.819	9.457	362
(M14)	2	13.962	13.512	540	12.663	12.413	250	11.508	11.114	394
M16	2	15.962	15.512	450	14.663	14.413	250	13.508	13.114	394
(M18)	2.5	17.958	17.428	530	16.334	16.069	265	14.891	14.446	445
M20	2.5	19.958	19.428	530	18.334	18.069	265	16.891	16.446	445
(M22)	2.5	21.958	21.428	530	20.334	20.069	265	18.891	18.446	445
M24	3	23.952	23.352	600	22.003	21.688	315	20.271	19.740	531
(M27)	3	26.952	26.352	600	25.003	24.688	315	23.271	22.740	531
M30	3.5	29.947	29.277	670	27.674	27.339	335	25.653	25.066	587
(M33)	3.5	32.947	32.277	670	30.674	30.339	335	28.653	28.066	587
M36	4	35.940	35.190	750	33.342	32.987	355	31.033	30.390	643
(M39)	4	38.940	38.190	750	36.342	35.987	355	34.033	33.390	643

μm=0.001 mm

Note:- Second preference sizes are shown in brackets in col. 1.

IS: 4218 (Part V)–1967

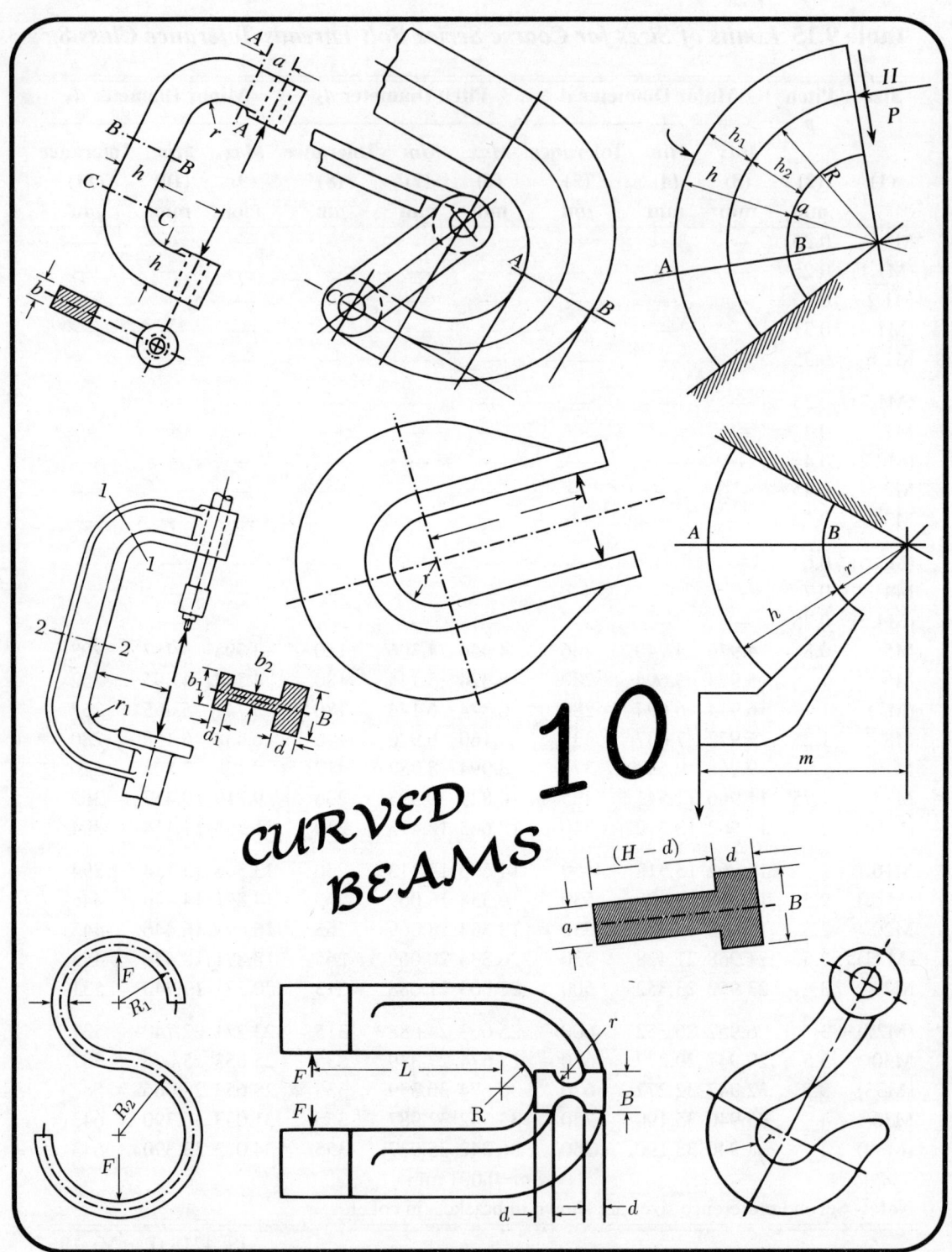

CURVED
BEAMS

10

Curved Beams

Symbols	Description and Units
A	area of section, mm^2
c_1, c_2	distances from centroidal axis to inner radius and outer radius respectively (Table 1.3), mm
c_i, c_o	distances from neutral axis to inner radius and outer radius respectively, mm
e	distance from the centroidal axis to neutral axis, mm
F	load, N (kgf)
M	Applied moment or bending moment, N mm (kgf-mm)
R	Radius to centroidal axis, mm
R_n	Radius to neutral aixs, mm
R_i, R_o	inner and outer radius of curvature respectively, mm
σ_i, σ_o	stresses at inner and outer radius respectively, MN/mm (kgf/mm^2)

Particular	Equation	Eqn. No.
General equation for the stress at any fiber at a distance y from the neutral axis (Fig. 10.1)	$\sigma = \dfrac{M}{Ae}\left(\dfrac{y}{R_n + y}\right)$	10.1(a)
At the inner fiber the maximum tensile stress due to bending (Fig. 10.1)	$\sigma_i = +\dfrac{Mc_i}{AeR_i}$	10.1(b)
At the outer fiber the maximum compressive stress due to bending (Fig.10.1)	$\sigma_o = -\dfrac{Mc_o}{AeR_o}$	10.1(c)
where $c_o = c_2 + e$, $c_i = c_1 - e$		10.1(d)
Chain links		
Bending moment at the section AA, i.e. 90° away from the point of application of load and in all the straight parts of the link (Fig. 10.3)	$M_A = \dfrac{FR}{2}\left[\dfrac{2R - \pi R}{\pi R + l}\right]$	10.2(a)
Bending moment at the section BB, i.e. at the point of application of load (Fig. 10.3)	$M_B = \dfrac{FR}{2}\left[\dfrac{2R + t}{\pi R + l}\right]$	10.2(b)

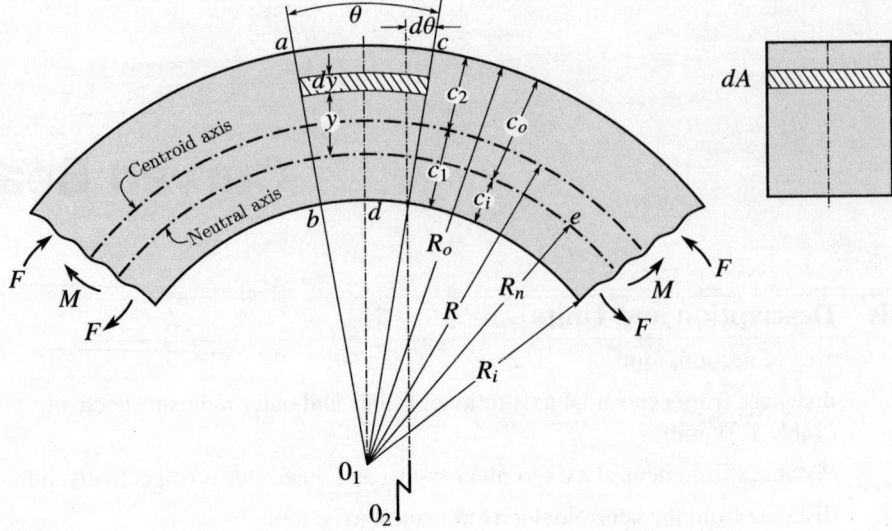

Fig. 10.1: *Analysis of stresses in curved beams*

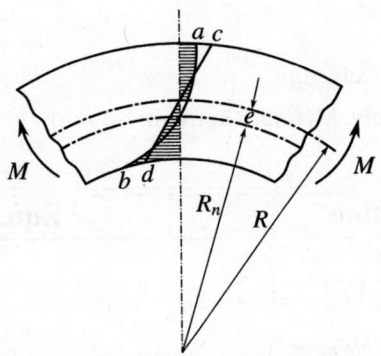

Fig. 10.2: *Bending stresses in curved beam*

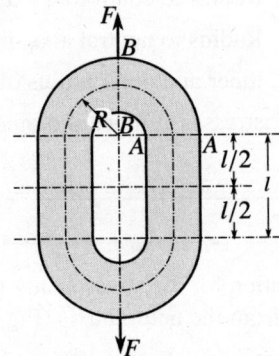

Fig. 10.3: *Chain link*

Particular	Equation		Eqn. No.
	Ring subjected to tension (Fig. 10.4)	**Ring subjected to compression (Fig. 10.5)**	
Closed Rings:			
Bending moment at any section of a closed ring	$M = M_A + \frac{1}{2}FR(1 - \sin\theta)$	$M = M_A - \frac{1}{2}FR(1 - \sin\theta)$	10.4
Maximum moment for a circular ring at the point of application of the load, i.e. when $\theta = 0$	$M_{\max} = 0.318FR$	$M_{max} = -0.318FR$	10.5

Particular	Equation		Eqn. No.
	Ring subjected to tension (Fig. 10.4)	**Ring subjected to compression (Fig. 10.5)**	
Another maximum moment for a circular ring at a point 90° away from the point of application of the load, i.e. when $\theta = 90°$	$M_{max} = -0.182FR$	$M_{max} = 0.182FR$	10.6
Where M_A is the bending couple at the section AA	$M_A = -0.182FR$	$M_A = 0.182FR$	10.7
The stress at any point in the section	$\sigma = \dfrac{\frac{1}{2}F\sin\theta}{A} + \dfrac{M}{Ae}\left(\dfrac{y}{R_n + y}\right);$	$\sigma = -\dfrac{\frac{1}{2}F\sin\theta}{A} + \dfrac{M}{Ae}\left(\dfrac{y}{R_n + y}\right)$	10.8

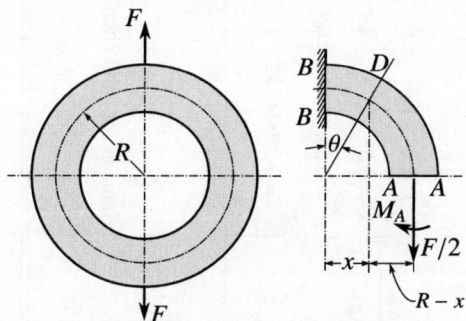

Fig. 10.4: *Closed ring (Tension)*

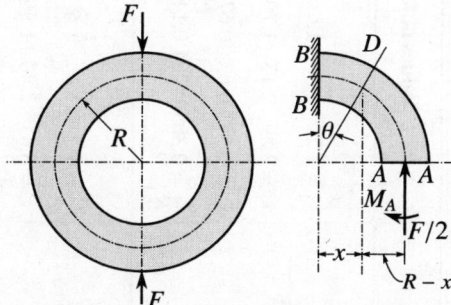

Fig. 10.5: *Closed ring (Compression)*

References

[1] Siegel M.J., Maleev, V. L. Hartman, J.B., *"Mechanical Design of Machines"* 4th edition, International Text Book Company, 1965.

[2] Hall, A. S., Holomenko, A. R., Laughlin, H. G., Schaum's Outline of *"Theory and Problems of Machine Design"*, Schaum Publishing Co., 1961.

[3] Roark, R. J., *"Formulas for stress and strain"*, McGraw Hill Book Company, 1954.

[4] Seely and Smith, *"Resistance of Materials"*.

[5] Arthur Morely, *"Strength of Materials"*, William Clomes & Sons Limited, London and Beccles, 1953.

Table 10.1 *Formulae for Curved Beams*

1. Solid rectangular section

Precise formula for e and approximate formula for k_i:

$$e = R - R_n = R - \frac{h}{\log_e\{(R+c)/(R-c)\}}$$

$$k_i = 1 + 0.5\frac{1}{bc^2}\left[\frac{1}{R-c} + \frac{1}{R}\right]$$

Values of k_i, k_o and e/R for various values of R/c.

R/c	1.2	1.4	1.6	1.8	2.0	3.0	4.0	6.0	8.0	10.0
k_i	2.89	2.13	1.79	1.63	1.52	1.30	1.20	1.12	1.09	1.07
k_o	0.57	0.63	0.67	0.70	0.73	0.81	0.85	0.90	0.92	0.94
$\dfrac{e}{R}$	0.305	0.204	0.149	0.112	0.090	0.041	0.021	0.009	0.0052	0.0033

2. Solid circular section

$$e = R - R_n = R - \frac{\frac{1}{2}c^2}{R - \sqrt{R^2 - c^2}}$$

$$k_i = 1 + 1.05\frac{I}{Dc^2}\left[\frac{1}{R-c} + \frac{1}{R}\right]$$

R/c	1.2	1.4	1.6	1.8	2.0	3.0	4.0	6.0	8.0	10.0
k_i	3.41	2.40	1.96	1.75	1.62	1.33	1.23	1.14	1.10	1.08
k_o	0.54	0.60	0.65	0.68	0.71	0.79	0.84	0.89	0.91	0.93
$\dfrac{e}{R}$	0.224	0.151	0.108	0.084	0.069	0.030	0.016	0.0070	0.0039	0.0025

3. Hollow circular section

(When $c = 2c_1$)

$$e = R - R_n = R - \frac{\frac{1}{2}(c^2 - c_1^2)}{\sqrt{R^2 - c_1^2} - \sqrt{R^2 - c^2}}$$

$$k_i = 1 + 1.05\frac{I}{D_1 c^2}\left[\frac{1}{R-c} + \frac{1}{R}\right]$$

R/c	1.2	1.4	1.6	1.8	2.0	3.0	4.0	6.0	8.0	10.0
k_i	3.28	2.31	1.89	1.70	1.57	1.31	1.21	1.13	1.10	1.07
k_o	0.58	0.64	0.68	0.71	0.73	0.81	0.85	0.90	0.92	0.93
$\dfrac{e}{R}$	0.269	0.182	0.134	0.104	0.083	0.038	0.020	0.0087	0.0049	0.0031

4. Solid elliptical section

$$e = R - R_n = R - \frac{\frac{1}{2}c^2}{R - \sqrt{R^2 - c^2}}$$

$$k_i = 1 + 1.05\frac{I}{bc^2}\left[\frac{1}{R-c} + \frac{1}{R}\right]$$

Same as for solid circular section.

Table 10.1 Formulae for Curved Beams – (Contd..)

5. Hollow elliptical section

$$e = R - R_n = R - \frac{\frac{1}{2}(bc - b_1c_1)}{\left[(R/c) - \sqrt{R/c^2 - 1}\right] - b_1\left[(R/c_1) - \sqrt{(R/c_1)^2 - 1}\right]}$$

$$k_i = 1 + 1.05\frac{I}{bc^2}\left[\frac{1}{R-c} + \frac{1}{R}\right]$$

(When $c = 1\frac{1}{4}c_1,\ b = c$)

$\dfrac{R}{c}$ =	1.2	1.4	1.6	1.8	2.0	3.0	4.0	6.0	8.0	10.0
k_i =	3.03	2.15	1.82	1.65	1.53	1.29	1.20	1.12	1.09	1.07
k_o =	0.58	0.64	0.68	0.71	0.73	0.81	0.85	0.90	0.92	0.93
$\dfrac{e}{R}$ =	0.295	0.195	0.146	0.114	0.085	0.041	0.021	0.0088	0.005	0.0032

6. Triangular section

$$e = R - R_n = R - \frac{\frac{1}{2}h^2}{(R+c_2)\log_e(R+c_2)/(R-c_1) - h}$$

$$k_i = 1 + 0.5\frac{I}{bc_1^2}\left[\frac{1}{R-c_1} + \frac{1}{R}\right]$$

(When $h = 0.6b$)

$\dfrac{R}{c_1}$ =	1.2	1.4	1.6	1.8	2.0	3.0	4.0	6.0	8.0	10.0
k_i =	3.26	2.39	1.99	1.78	1.66	1.37	1.27	1.16	1.12	1.09
k_o =	0.44	0.50	0.54	0.57	0.60	0.70	0.75	0.82	0.86	0.88
$\dfrac{e}{R}$ =	0.361	0.251	0.186	0.144	0.116	0.052	0.029	0.013	0.0060	0.0039

7. Trapezoidal section

$$e = R - R_n = R - \frac{A}{\dfrac{b_1(R+c_2) - b(R-c_1)}{h}\log_e\dfrac{R+c_2}{R-c_1} - (b_1 - b)}$$

$$k_i = 1 + 0.5\frac{I}{bc_1^2}\left[\frac{1}{R-c_1} + \frac{1}{R}\right]$$

(When $b_1 = 2b$ and $h = 3b$)

$\dfrac{R}{c_1}$ =	1.2	1.4	1.6	1.8	2.0	3.0	4.0	6.0	8.0	10.0
k_i =	3.09	2.25	1.91	1.73	1.61	1.37	1.26	1.17	1.13	1.11
k_o =	0.56	0.62	0.66	0.70	0.73	0.81	0.86	0.91	0.94	0.95
$\dfrac{e}{R}$ =	0.336	0.229	0.168	0.128	0.102	0.046	0.024	0.011	0.0060	0.0039

Table 10.1 Formulae for Curved Beams – (Contd..)

8. T-beam or channel section

$$e = R - R_n = R - \cfrac{A}{B\log_e\left[\frac{R+d-c_1}{R-c_1}\right] + a\log_e\left[\frac{R+c_2}{R+d-c_1}\right]}$$

(When $B = 4a$, $d = \frac{3}{2}a$, $H = 6a$)

$\frac{R}{c_1}$	1.2	1.4	1.6	1.8	2.0	3.0	4.0	6.0	8.0	10.0
k_i	3.63	2.54	2.14	1.89	1.73	1.41	1.29	1.18	1.13	1.10
k_o	0.58	0.63	0.67	0.70	0.72	0.79	0.83	0.88	0.91	0.92
$\frac{e}{R}$	0.418	0.299	0.229	0.183	0.149	0.069	0.040	0.018	0.010	0.0065

$$k_i = 1 + 0.5\,\frac{1}{bc_1^2}\left[\frac{1}{R-c_1} + \frac{1}{R}\right]$$

9. Symmetrical I-beam or hollow rectangular

$$e = R - R_n = R - \cfrac{A}{B\log_e\left[\frac{R+d-c}{R-c}\right] + B\log_e\left[\frac{R+d+c}{R+d-c}\right] + B\log_e\left[\frac{R+c}{R+c-d}\right]}$$

(When $B = 3d$, $(B - b) = d$, $H = 6d$)

$\frac{R}{c}$	1.2	1.4	1.6	1.8	2.0	3.0	4.0	6.0	8.0	10.0
k_i	2.52	1.90	1.63	1.50	1.41	1.23	1.16	1.10	1.07	1.05
k_o	0.67	0.71	0.75	0.77	0.79	0.86	0.89	0.92	0.94	0.95
$\frac{R}{e}$	0.408	0.285	0.208	0.160	0.127	0.058	0.030	0.013	0.0076	0.0048

$$k_i = 1 + 0.5\,\frac{I}{Bc^2}\left[\frac{1}{R-c} + \frac{1}{R}\right]$$

10. Unsymmetrical I-beam section

$$e = R - R_n = R - \cfrac{A}{B\log_e\left(\frac{R+d-c_1}{R-c_1}\right) + b_2\log_e\left(\frac{R+c_2-d}{R+d-c_1}\right) + b_1\log_e\left(\frac{R+c_2}{R+c_2-d_1}\right)}$$

(When $B = 6d_1$, $d = 2d_1$, $b_1 = 4d_1$, $H = 6d_1$, $b_2 = d_1$)

$\frac{R}{c_1}$	1.2	1.4	1.6	1.8	2.0	3.0	4.0	6.0	8.0	10.0
k_i	3.55	2.48	2.07	1.83	1.69	1.38	1.26	1.15	1.10	1.08
k_o	0.67	0.72	0.76	0.78	0.80	0.86	0.89	0.92	0.94	0.95
$\frac{e}{R}$	0.409	0.292	0.224	0.178	0.144	0.067	0.038	0.018	0.010	0.0065

$$k_i = 1 + 0.5\,\frac{I}{bc_1^2}\left[\frac{1}{R-c_1} + \frac{1}{R}\right]$$

Notation: $k_i = \sigma_i/\sigma$ and $k_o = \sigma_o/\sigma$ where σ is the fictitious unit stress in corresponding fiber as computed by ordinary flexure formula for a straight beam. A = area of section. c = distance from centroidal axis to extreme fibre on concave side of beam (Refer Table 1.3). I = moment of inertia of cross section about centroidal axis perpendicular to a plane of curvature.

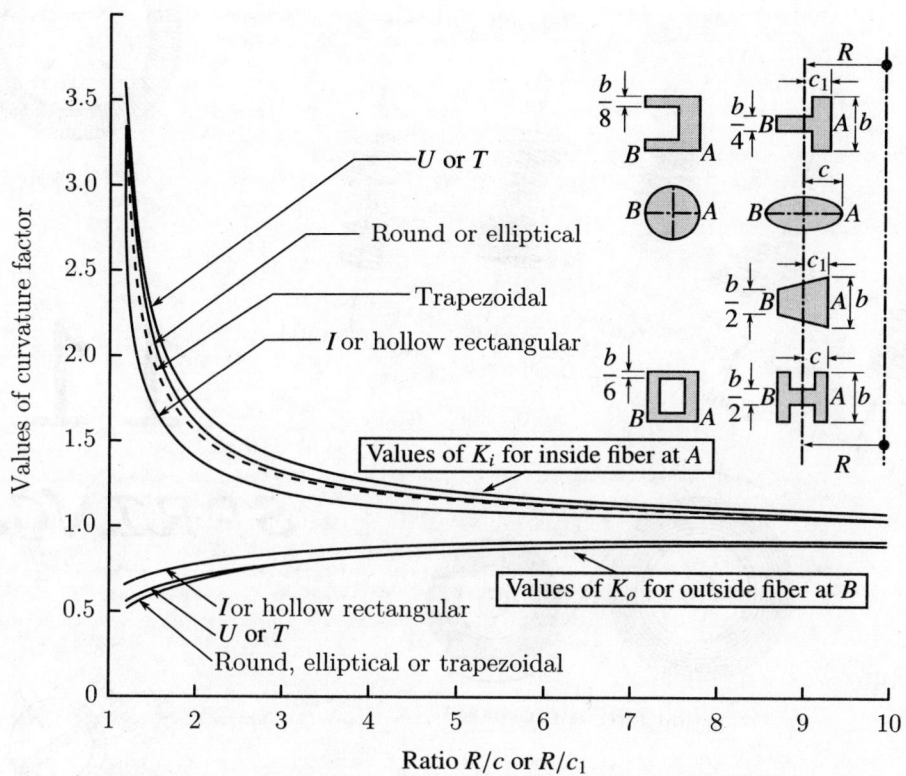

Effect of curvature on bending stresses

where
$$k_i = \sigma_i/\sigma,$$ Curvature factor at the inner fiber

$$\sigma_i = k_i\sigma,$$ Stress at the inner fiber

$$k_0 = \sigma_0/\sigma,$$ Curvature factor at the outer fiber

$$\sigma_0 = k_0\sigma,$$ Stress at the outer fiber

$$\sigma = Mc/I,$$ Fictitions unit stress as computed by ordinary flexure formula for a straight beam

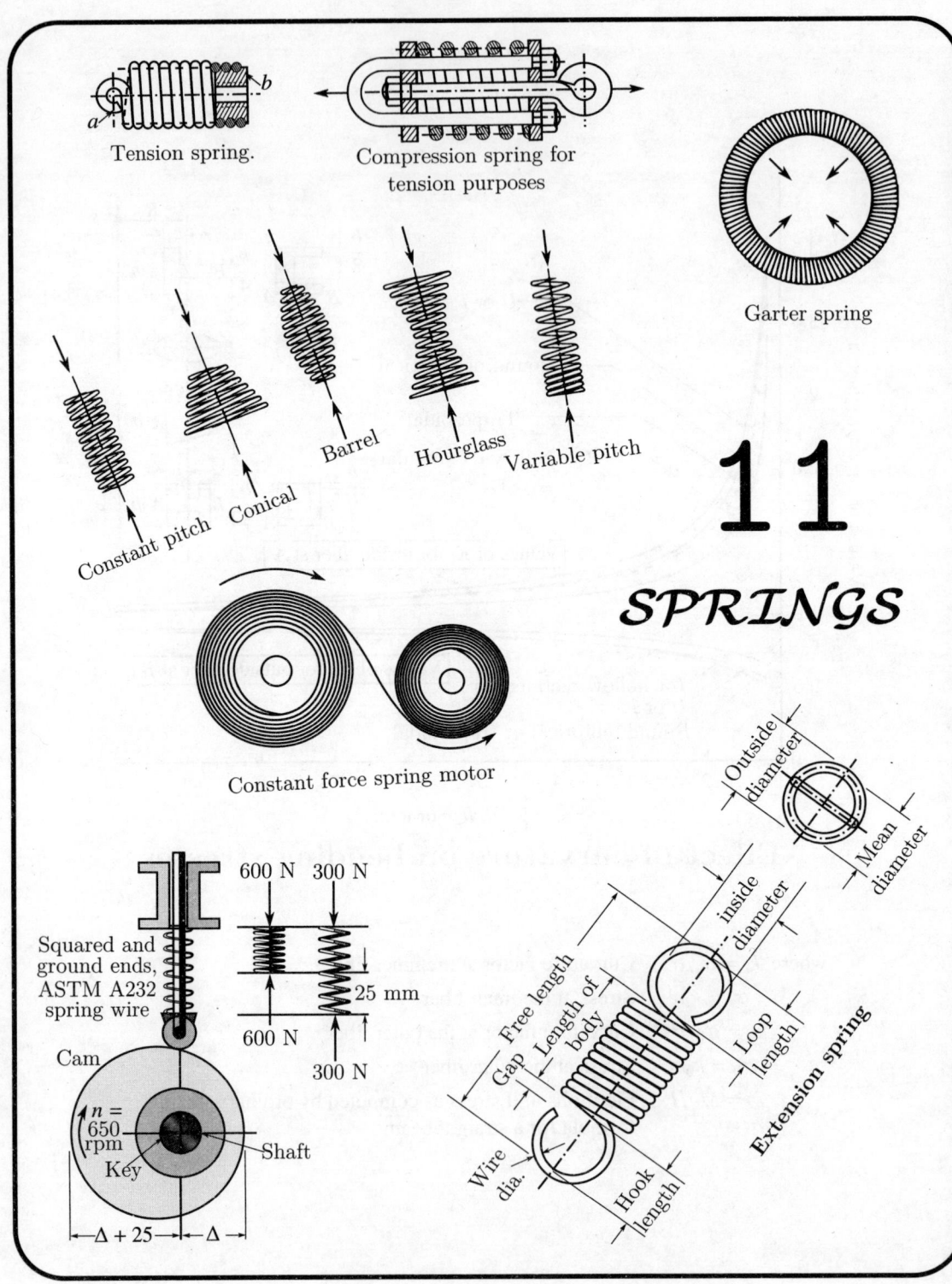

Tension spring.

Compression spring for
tension purposes

Garter spring

Constant pitch Conical Barrel Hourglass Variable pitch

Constant force spring motor

11

SPRINGS

Squared and
ground ends,
ASTM A232
spring wire

Cam

$n = 650$ rpm

Key

Shaft

$\Delta + 25$ Δ

600 N 300 N

25 mm

600 N

300 N

Outside
diameter

Mean
diameter

inside
diameter

Free length

Length of
body

Gap

Loop
length

Wire
dia.

Hook
length

Extension spring

11

Springs

Symbols	Description and Units
B	size factor
C	spring index
d	diameter of the wire, mm
D	pitch diameter or mean diameter of spring, mm
f	natural frequency of the spring, H_2
F	load on the spring, N (kgf)
F_a	variable load, N (kgf)
F_m	average or mean load, N (kgf)
F_o	spring scale or rate, N/mm (kgf/mm)
F_{cr}	critical axial load on the spring, N (kgf)
F_{max}	maximum load on the spring, N (kgf)
F_{min}	minimum load on the spring, N (kgf)
i	the number of active coils in the spring
K	stress correction factor
K_t	stress concentration factor
K_{tf}	fatigue stress concentration factor
R	reliability factor
U	resilence of the spring, N mm (kgf-mm)
V	volume of the spring, mm^3
y	axial deflection of the spring, mm
τ	maximum stress in the helical spring, MN/m^2 (kgf/mm^2)
τ_d	design stress for static loading, MN/m^2 (kgf/mm^2)
τ_{dr}	design stress for completely reversed loads, MN/m^2 (kgf/mm^2)
τ_e	Elastic limit stress in shear, MN/m^2 (kgf/mm^2)
σ	maximum stress in the leaf spring, MN/m^2 (kgf/mm^2)
σ_f	stress in the full length leaves, M/Nm^2 (kgf/mm^2)
σ_g	stress in the graduated leaves, MN/m^2 (kgf/mm^2)

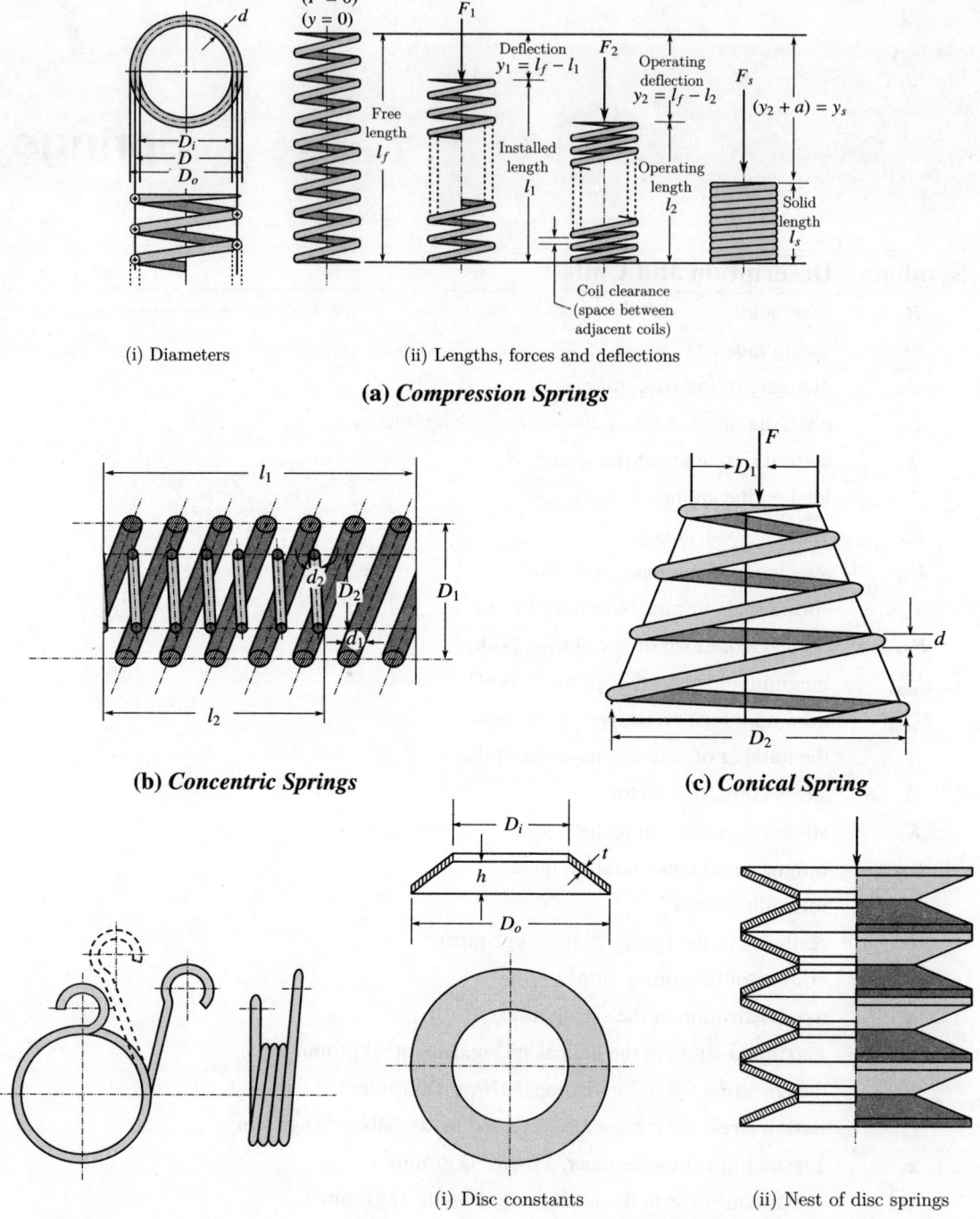

(i) Diameters   (ii) Lengths, forces and deflections

(a) Compression Springs

(b) Concentric Springs   **(c) Conical Spring**

(d) Torsion Spring   (i) Disc constants   (ii) Nest of disc springs   **(e) Disc Springs**

Fig. 11.1: *Notations for different types of springs*

Particular	Equation	Eqn. No.
Cylindrical compression spring: *(a) Round section springs:*		
Torsional moment produced in the spring (Fig. 11.2)	$T = \dfrac{1}{2}FD$	11.1(a)
The internal resisting moment	$T = Z_p\tau = \left(\dfrac{\pi d^3}{16}\right)\tau$	11.1(b)
The shear stress due to torque only	$\tau = \dfrac{8FD}{\pi d^3}$	11.1(c)
The shear stress in the helical spring (considering compressive stress acting along the coil and also direct shear stress)	$\tau = \dfrac{8FDK}{\pi d^3} = \dfrac{yGdK}{\pi i D^2}$	11.1(d)
The wire diameter, (Table 11.1 and 11.2)	$d = \sqrt[3]{\left(\dfrac{8FDK}{\pi \tau}\right)}$	11.1(e)
	where K is the stress correction factor	
According to Wahl, the stress correction factor (Fig. 11.3)	$K = \dfrac{4C-1}{4C-4} + \dfrac{0.615}{C}$	11.2(a)
The stress correction factor (*Bergstroessar*)	$K = \dfrac{4C+2}{4C-3}$	11.2(b)
	where $C = (D/d)$, the spring index	11.2(c)
Very close approximate equation for the stress factor ($2 \geq C \leq 12$)	$K = \dfrac{2}{C^{0.25}} = 2\left(\dfrac{d}{D}\right)^{0.25}$	11.2(d)

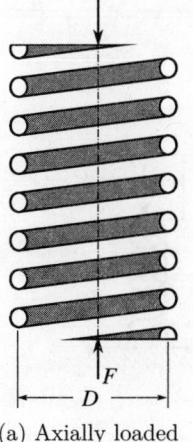
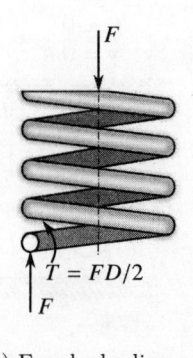

(a) Axially loaded   (b) Free-body diagram

$T = FD/2$

Fig. 11.2: *Helical Compression Spring*

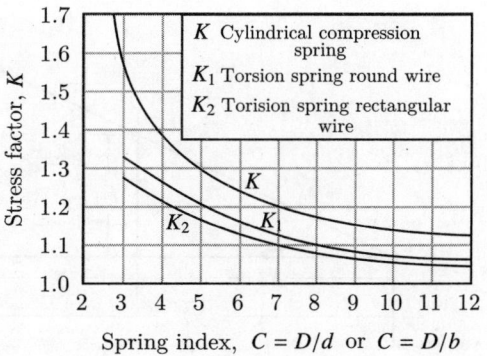

Spring index, $C = D/d$ or $C = D/b$

Fig. 11.3: *Stress factors for helical springs*

Particular	Equation	Eqn. No.
Taking the stress factor from Equation 11.2(d), the shear stress in the spring	$\tau = \dfrac{16FD^{0.75}}{\pi d^{2.75}} = \dfrac{5.1FC^{0.75}}{d^2}$	11.3
The angular deflection	$\theta = \dfrac{16FDl}{\pi Gd^4} = \dfrac{16FD^2 i}{Gd^4}$	11.4
	where $l = \pi Di$, length of the spring bar, mm	
The axial deflection of the spring	$y = \dfrac{8FD^3 i}{Gd^4} = \dfrac{8FC^3 i}{Gd}$	11.5(a)
The axial deflection of the spring in terms of the shear stress	$y = \dfrac{\pi i \tau D^2}{KGd} = \dfrac{\pi i \tau D^{2.25}}{2Gd^{1.25}}$	11.5(b)
The load acting along the axis of the spring	$F = \dfrac{yGd^4}{8D^3 i}$	11.5(c)
The shear stress in terms of deflection (y)	$\tau = \dfrac{yGdK}{\pi iD^2}$	11.5(d)
The number of active coils required	$i = \dfrac{yGd^4}{8FD^3} = \dfrac{yGd}{8FC^3} = \dfrac{yKGd}{\pi D^2 \tau}$	11.6
Spring scale or rate or stiffness	$F_o = F/y = \dfrac{d^4 G}{8iD^3}$	11.7(a)
Spring scale (Fig. 11.4)	$F_o = \dfrac{F_2 - F_1}{y'}$	11.7(b)

where deflections y_1 and y_2 are due to forces F_1 and F_2 respectively

$$y^1 = y_2 - y_1 \text{ and the total deflection } y_2 = \frac{F_2}{F_0} = \frac{y^1 F_2}{F_2 - F_1}$$

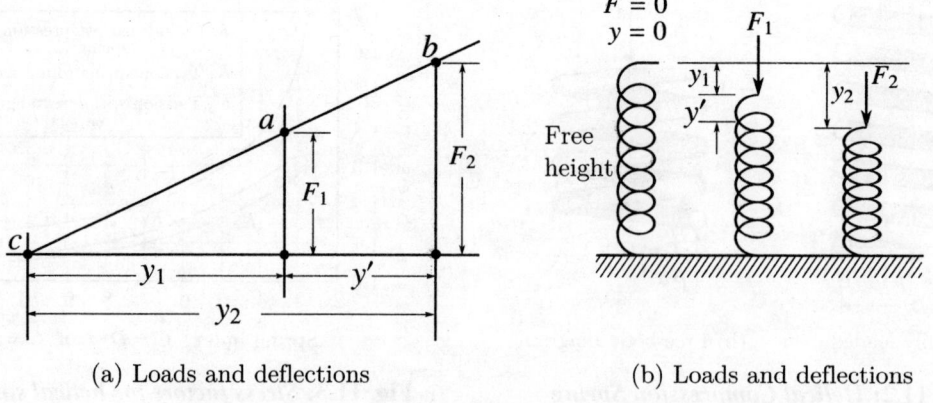

(a) Loads and deflections   (b) Loads and deflections

Fig. 11.4: *Loads and deflections in a helical spring*

Particular	Equation	Eqn. No.

The resilience of the spring or work done by the spring

$$U = \frac{Fy}{2} = \frac{4F^2D^3i}{Gd^4} = \frac{\pi^2d^2Di\tau^2}{16K^2G} = \frac{\pi^2d^{1.5}D^{1.5}i\tau^2}{64G} = \frac{0.155d^3C^{1.5}i\tau^2}{G}$$
$$= \frac{V\tau^2}{4K^2G} = \frac{V\tau^2C^{0.5}}{16G} = \frac{y^2d^4G}{16iD^3}$$

11.8

Volume of the spring

$$V = \pi Di \times \frac{\pi}{4}d^2$$

11.9

The size factor for sections above 12.5 mm wire diameter in section

$$B = \frac{d^{0.25}}{1.885}$$

11.10(a)

Note: For rectangular sections, the value of b or h whichever is smaller is used instead of d in the above Equation 11.10

Where b is the breadth of spring wire, mm and h is the thickness of spring wire, mm

Design or permissible shear stress (Table 11.3 and Fig. 11.8)

$$\tau_d = \frac{\tau_e}{RB} = \frac{1.885\tau_e}{Rd^{0.25}}$$

11.10(b)

Reliability factor

$$R = \frac{F((\text{compressed}))}{F(\text{working})} = \frac{y+a}{y}$$

11.11

where τ_e is the elastic limit stress in shear (Table 11.5 to 11.7)

y is the deflaction under the working load

a is the total clearance between the spring coils ($a \approx 25\%$ of y and then $R \approx 1.25$)

wire diameter for static loads

$$d = \left(\frac{6RF}{\tau_e}\right)^{0.4} \times D^{0.3}$$

11.12(a)

If there are no space limitations, then the diameter of the wire in terms of the spring index

$$d = \left(\frac{6RF}{\tau_e}\right)^{0.57} C^{0.43}$$

11.12(b)

Note: For good design, values of C between 8 and 10 are preferred

(b) Rectangular section springs:

The stress in the rectangular section spring

$$\tau = \frac{KFD(1.5h + 0.9b)}{b^2h^2} = \frac{KFD(1.5 + 0.9m)}{m^2h^3} \quad \text{where } K = \frac{4C-1}{4C-4} + \frac{0.615}{C}$$
$$= \frac{FD^{0.75}(3h + 1.8b)}{b^{1.75}h^2} = \frac{FD^{0.75}(3 + 1.81m)}{m^{1.75}h^{2.75}}$$

11.13(a)

$$\text{where } K = \frac{2}{C^{0.25}} = 2(d/D)^{0.25}, \quad C = \frac{D}{b} \text{ and } m = \frac{b}{h} \leq 1$$

Particular	Equation	Eqn. No.

The axial deflection in the rectangular section springs

$$y = \frac{2.83iFD^3(b^2 + h^2)}{b^3h^3G} = \frac{2.83iFD^3(1 + m^2)}{m^3h^4G}$$

11.13(b)

The spring rate $\qquad\qquad F_o = \dfrac{m^3h^4G}{2.83iD^3(1 + m^2)}$ 11.13(c)

According to IS; 7906

(Part VI)-1978, for springs made of
rectangular cross-section-Design Formulae

(i) Shear stress, MN/mm^2 (kgf/mm^2) $\qquad \tau = \dfrac{\psi D}{b^2h^2}F$ 11.14(a)

where, ψ = stress coefficient, dependent on ratio of cross-section side lengths b/h or h/b, and on coil ratio C (Fig. 11.5)

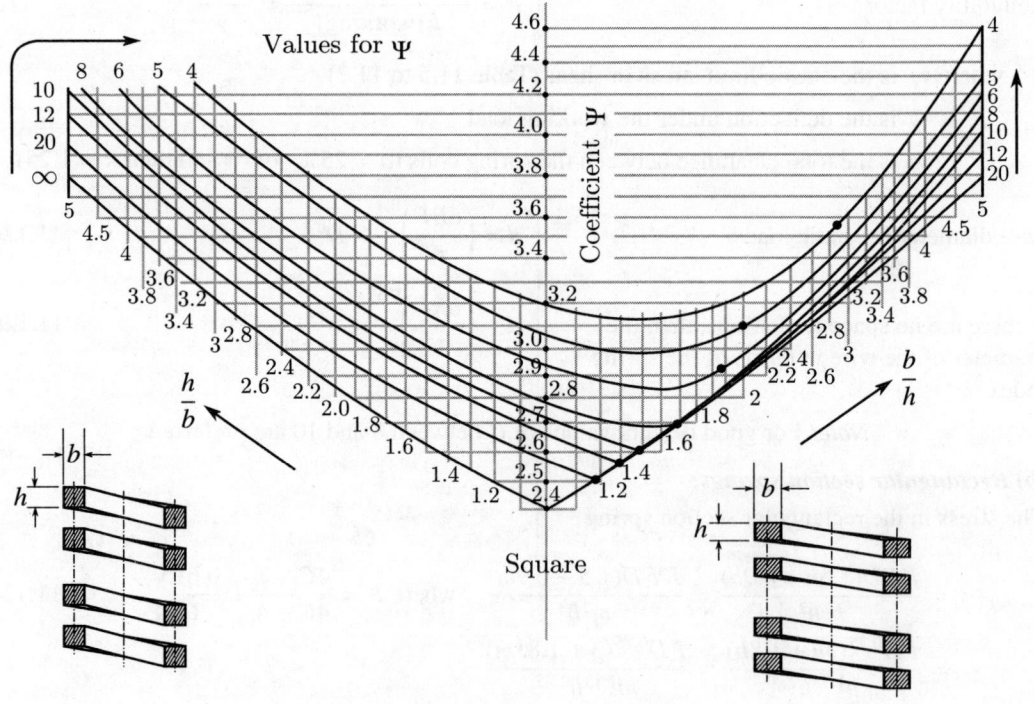

Fig. 11.5: *Stress Coefficient based on b/h or h/b*

Particular	Equation	Eqn. No.
(ii) Spring Deflection, mm	$y = \dfrac{\epsilon D^3 \times i}{b^2 h^2 G} F$	11.14(b)

where, ϵ Elasticity (resilience) coefficient, dependent on ratio of cross-section side lenghts b/h or h/b. (Table 11.8)

(iii) Number of active coils	$i = \dfrac{b^2 h^2 G}{\epsilon F_0 D^3}$	11.14(c)
(iv) Total No. of coils	$i_t = i + 2$	11.14(d)
(v) Spring rate (Fig. 11.4)	$F_0 = \dfrac{F}{y} = \dfrac{F_2 - F_1}{y_1 - y_2} = \dfrac{F_2 - F_1}{y^1}$	11.14(d)

(c) Square section springs:

Shear stress in square section springs ($b = h$)	$\tau = \dfrac{2.4KFD}{h^3} = \dfrac{4.8FD^{0.75}}{h^{2.75}}$	11.15(a)
Axial deflection in square section springs ($b = h$)	$y = \dfrac{5.66iFD^3}{h^4 G}$	11.15(b)

Repeated loading:

For cyclic loads in the springs, the most general equation for the equivalent static load	$F'_m = F_m + \dfrac{\tau_d}{\tau_{dr}} F_a$	11.16(a)
The design stress for static loading	$\tau_d = \dfrac{\tau_e}{RBK_t}$	11.16(b)
The design stress for completely reversed loads	$\tau_{dr} = \dfrac{\tau_{en}}{RBK_{tf}}$	11.16(c)

where τ_e is the elastic limit stress in shear, MN/m^2 (kgf/mm^2) (Table 11.5 to 11.7)

τ_{en} is the endurance limit stress in shear, MN/m^2 (kgf/mm^2)

$\tau_e \approx \tau_u$, for hardened brittle materials

For springs which ae carefully made to prevent scratches or other stress raisers, the general equation for the equivalent static load	$F'_m = F_m + \dfrac{\tau_e}{\tau_{en}} F_a$	11.6(d)
Springs made of with hardened meterials, the equation for the equivalent static load	$F'_m = F_m + 2F_a = \dfrac{1}{2}(3F_{max} - F_{min})$ where $\dfrac{\tau_e}{\tau_{en}} = \dfrac{\tau_u}{\tau_{en}} = \dfrac{\tau_u}{0.5\tau_u} = 2$	11.16(e)
The average load or mean load	$F_m = \dfrac{F_{max} + F_{min}}{2}$	11.16(f)
The variable load	$F_a = \dfrac{F_{max} - F_{min}}{2}$	11.16(g)

Particular	Equation	Eqn. No.

The wire diameter of the spring when it is subjected to cyclic loading

$$d = \left[\frac{3R(3F_{max} - F_{min})}{\tau_e}\right]^{0.4} \times (D^{0.3}) = \left[\frac{3R(3F_{max} - F_{min})}{\tau_e}\right]^{0.57} \times (C^{0.43}) \qquad 11.17(a)$$

| when a compression spring is subjected to alternating load, the wire diameter, mm | $d = \sqrt{\left\{\dfrac{4nKD(F_{max} - F_{min})}{\pi\tau_a}\right\}}$ | 11.17(b) |

where $\tau_r = 2\tau_a$, stress range corresponding the stroke h (amplitude of stress), MN/m^2 (kgf/mm^2)

h = Stroke (lift), that is, difference between two deflections or two load lengths mm.

$n = 2$ to 2.5, factor of safety

Minimum free length of the spring: (Table 11.4)

If the ends are bent before grinding	$l_o \geq (i + 2)d + y + a$	11.18(a)
If the ends are either ground or bent	$l_o \geq (i + 1)d + y + a$	11.18(b)
If the ends are neither ground nor bent	$l_o \geq (i)d + y + a$	11.18(c)

where $a = xdi$, total clearance between working coils, mm

i is the number of active coils (Table 11.4)

x is the constant (Fig. 11.6)

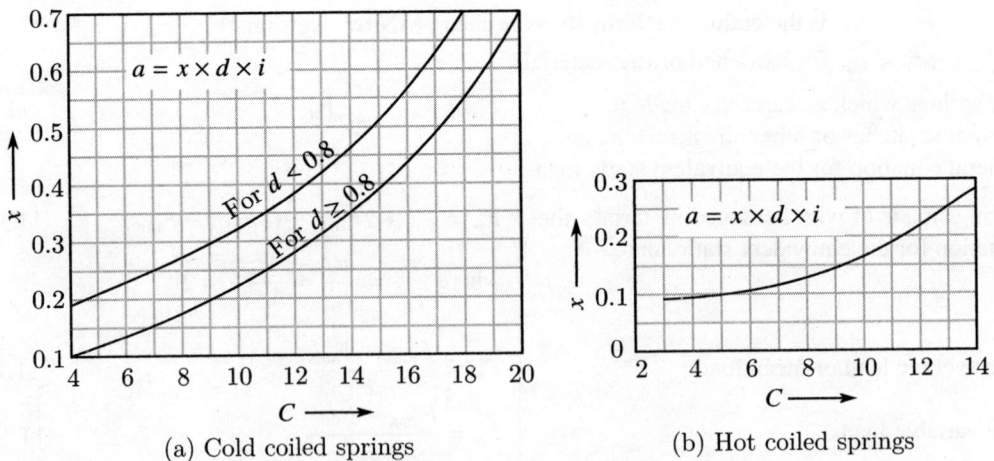

(a) Cold coiled springs   (b) Hot coiled springs

Fig. 11.6: *Value of x as a function of coil ratio (C)*

Particular	Equation	Eqn. No.
Buckling:		
The critical axial load that can cause buckling in a helical compression spring having a great length in proportion to its pitch diameter	$F_{cr} = F_o K_l l_o$ where F_o is the spring scale, N/mm $\quad K_l$ is a load factor depending on the ratio $\quad\quad l_o/D$ (Fig. 11.7(a)) $\quad l_o$ is the free length of the spring, mm.	11.19(a)
Resistance to Buckling: [*] Relative deflection in percent (Fig. 11.7(b))	$y\% = \dfrac{y}{l_0} \times 100$	11.19(b)
Degree of slendeness,	$k_0 = l_0/D$	11.19(c)
	when $k_0 \le 2.6$ - guide is not necessary $\quad\quad k_0 > 2.6$ - guide is necessary	
Concentric compression springs:		
The approximate relation between the sizes of two concentric springs wound from round wire of the same material (Fig. 11.1(b))	$\left(\dfrac{d_1}{d_2}\right)^{2.85} = \left(\dfrac{F_1}{F_2}\right)\left(\dfrac{D_1}{D_2}\right)$	11.20(a)
	$\dfrac{F_1}{F_2} = \left(\dfrac{D_2}{D_1}\right)\left(\dfrac{d_1}{d_2}\right)^{2.85}$	11.20(b)
The load on the inner spring	$F_2 = mF_1$	11.20(c)
The load on the outer spring	$F_1 = \dfrac{F}{(1 + m)}$	11.20(d)

where F_1 and F_2 are loads on outer and inner springs respectively
$\quad D_1$ and D_2 are pitch diameters of outer and inner spring respectively, mm
$\quad d_1$ and d_2 are wire diameters of outer and inner springs respectively, mm
$\quad F = F_1 + F_2$ the total maximum spring load and $m = F_2/F_1 \le 1$

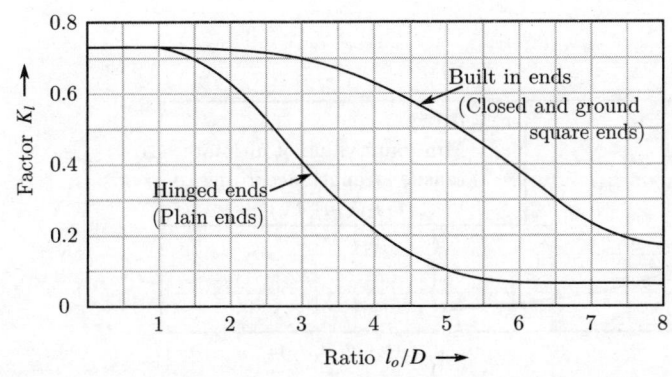

Fig. 11.7(a): *Backling factor for helical compression springs*

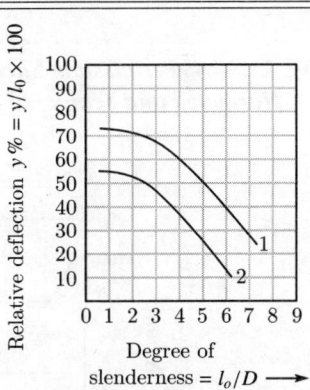

Fig. 11.7(b): *Limits of Resistance to Buckling of Compression Springs. Ends of which are Axially Guided*

[*]The point corresponding to the two co-ordinates $y\%$ and $k_0 = l_o/D$ lies below the curves (Fig. 11.7(b)), then the spring is buckie-proof.

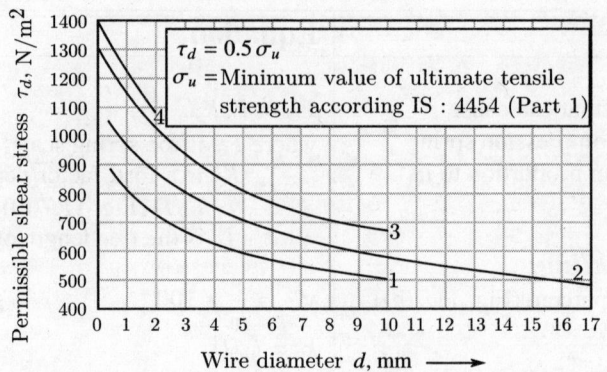

Fig. 11.8(a): *Permissible Shear Stress τ_d for Cold Coiled Compression Springs Made of Patented and Cold Drawn Spring Steel Wires - Unalloyed Grades 1, 2, 3 and 4*

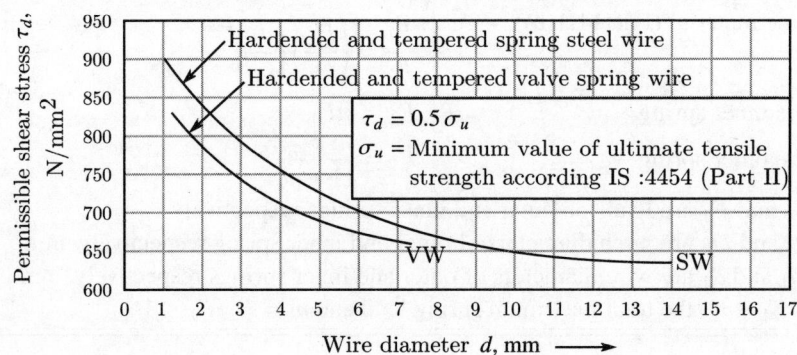

Fig. 11.8(b): *Permissible Shear Stress τ_d for Cold Coiled Compression Springs made from Oil Hardened and Tempered Spring Steel Wire and Valve Spring Wire - Unalloved Grades*

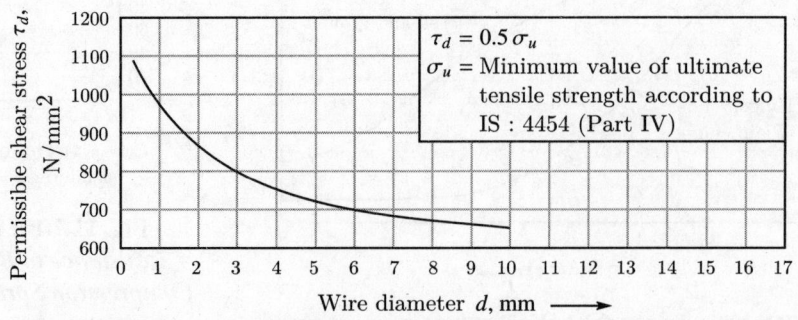

Fig. 11.8(c): *Permissible Shear Stress τ_d for Cold Coiled Compression Springs made of Stainless Spring Steel Wire for Normal Corrosion Resistance, Grades 1 and 2*

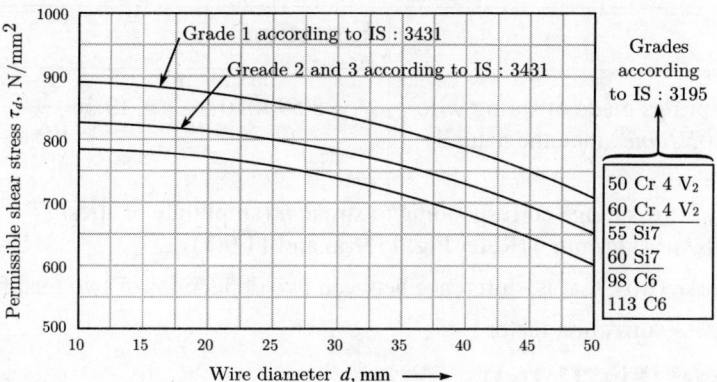

Fig. 11.8(d): *Permissible Shear Stress τ_d for Hot Coiled Compression Springs made from Grades 1, 2 and 3 Steel*

Particular	Equation	Eqn. No.
Vibration of cylindrical springs:		
The natural period of vibration, sec	$T = 2\pi \sqrt{W/F_o g}$	11.21

where W is the weight of the oscillating system, i.e., weight of the spring, N (kgf)

F_o is the force necessary to deflect the spring 1 mm, N/mm (kgf/m)

and g is the acceleration of gravity, 9.81×10^3 mm/sec^2

The natural frequency of the spring: (vibrations per second)

Note: When one end of the spring is at rest, the amplitude of the coils moving back and forth gradualy decreases toward the coil which is at rest. In this case the mass in motion is assumed as one-half the spring mass i.e. (W/2g).

Particular	Equation	Eqn. No.
(a) When one end of the spring is at rest (mass = W/2g)	$f = \dfrac{1}{T} = \dfrac{1}{2\pi}\sqrt{2F_o g/W} = 22.3\sqrt{F_o/W}$	11.22(a)
(b) when both ends of the spring are fixed (Force = $4F_o$ and mass = W/2g)	$f = \dfrac{1}{\pi}\sqrt{\dfrac{F_o g}{W}} = 31.5\sqrt{F_o/W}$	11.22(b)
In the case of a spring guided at both ends and periodically compressed by the stroke h, the natural frequency	$f = \dfrac{d}{2\pi i D^2}\sqrt{\dfrac{Gg}{2\gamma}}$	11.22(c)

where γ = specifie gravity

g = acceleration due to gravity

Particular	Equation	Eqn. No.
For commercial springs made of spring wire having $G = 81370 N/mm^2$, then the natural frequency	$f = 3.59 \times 10^5 \dfrac{d}{iD^2} = 13.56 \dfrac{\tau_r}{hK}$	11.22(d)

where $\tau_r = 2\tau_a$, stress range corresponding to stroke h (amplitude of stress),
MN/m² (kgf/mm²) (Refer Fig. 11.9(a) and 11.9(b))

h = stroke (lift), that is, difference between two deflections or two load lenghts, mm

K = Stress correction factor

Conical Springs: (Fig. 11.1(c))

The axial deflection of a spring made of round stock (Fig. 11.1c)

$$y = \frac{2iF(D_2^3 + D_2^2 D_1 + D_2 D_1^2 + D_1^3)}{d^4 G} = \frac{\pi i \tau (D_2^3 + D_2^2 D_1 + D_2 D_1^2 + D_1^3)}{4dD_2 KG} \qquad 11.23(a)$$

where D_1 and D_2 are the small and large pitch diameters of the conical spring, mm

d is the wire diameter of the spring, mm

i is the number of active coils

The axial deflection of Conical spring made of rectangular stock

$$y = \frac{0.71 iF(b^2 + h^2)(D_2^3 + D_2^2 D_1 + D_2 D_1^2 + D_1^3)}{b^3 h^3 G} \qquad 11.23(b)$$

where b = radial thickness, mm; h = axial thickness, mm

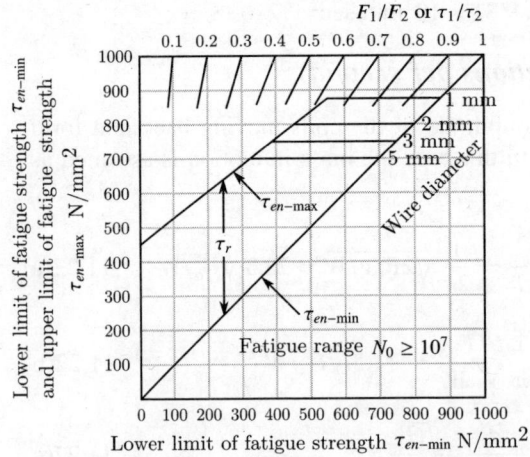

Fig. 11.9(a): *Fatigue Strength Diagram for Cold Coiled Compression Springs made of Oil Hardendened and Tempered Valve Spring Wire, Not Shot Peened*

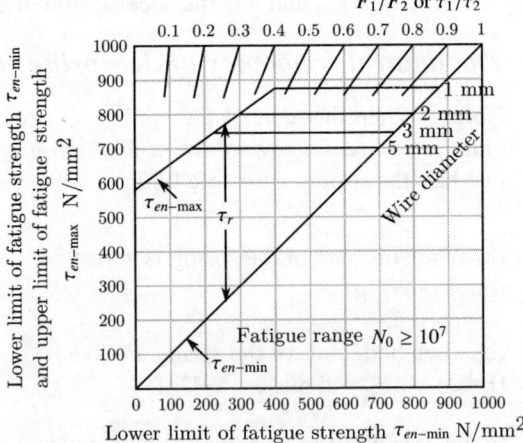

Fig. 11.9(b): *Fatigue Strength Diagram for Cold Coiled Compression Springs Made of Hardened and Tempered Valve Spring Wire Shot Peened*

Particular	Equation	Eqn. No.
***Torsion Springs:* (Fig. 11.1(d))**		
The maximum stress in torsion springs	$\sigma = \dfrac{KT}{Z} + \dfrac{2T}{DA}$	11.24(a)

where $K = K_1$ or K_2, the stress factor for torsion spring (Fig. 11.3)

M is the bending moment on the wire $\approx$ Torsional moment $(T) = \dfrac{FD}{2}$

$Z = \dfrac{\pi}{32}d^3$, section modulus, mm^3

D is the mean diameter of the coil, mm

A is the cross sectional area of the wire, mm^2

The deflection, measured by the distance travelled by a point on the pitch diameter of the end coil to which the pull is applied is approximately	$y = \dfrac{TLD}{2EI}$	11.24(b)

where $L = i\pi D$, length of the coil part of the spring

I is the moment of inertia of the wire, mm^4

(i) *Round wire spring:*		
The maximum stress in round wire torsion springs	$\sigma = \dfrac{8T(4K_1D + d)}{\pi d^3 D}$	11.25(a)
The stress factor for round wire torsion springs (Fig. 11.3) (according to Wahl)	$K_1 = \dfrac{4C - 1}{4C - 4}$ or $\dfrac{4C^2 - C - 1}{4C(C - 1)}$	11.25(b)
(ii) *Rectangular wire springs:*		
The maximum stress in rectangular wire torsion springs	$\sigma = \dfrac{6K_2T}{b^2h} + \dfrac{2T}{Dbh}$	11.26

where $C = D/b$; $Z = \dfrac{1}{6}hb^2$, section modulus, mm^3; $K_2 = K$, stress factor (Fig. 11.3)

b is the radial thickness, mm; h is the axial thickness, mm

***Leaf Springs:* (Fig. 11.10)**		
(a) *Flat Springs:*		
In the case of leaf springs the general expression for–		
(i) the maximum stress	$\sigma = \dfrac{C_1Fl}{bh^2}$	11.27(a)
(ii) the maximum deflection	$y = \dfrac{C_2Fl^3}{Ebh^3}$	11.27(b)
The thickness of the spring plate	$h = \dfrac{C_2\sigma l^2}{C_1Ey}$	11.27(c)

Particular	Equation	Eqn. No.
The width of the spring plate (Table 11.10)	$b = \dfrac{C_1 F l}{\sigma h^2}$ where the constants C_1 and C_2 can be taken from the Table 11.9 for different types of beams shown in Fig. 11.10	11.27(d)
(b) Multi-Leaf Springs: (Fig. 11.11)		
The width of the laminated spring	$b' = b/i$ where i is the number of springs or leaves	11.28(a)
The load carried by the laminated spring	$F = \dfrac{\sigma i b' h^2}{C_1 l}$	11.28(b)
The maximum deflection of the laminated spring under the load	$y = \dfrac{C_2 F l^3}{E i b' h^3}$	11.28(c)

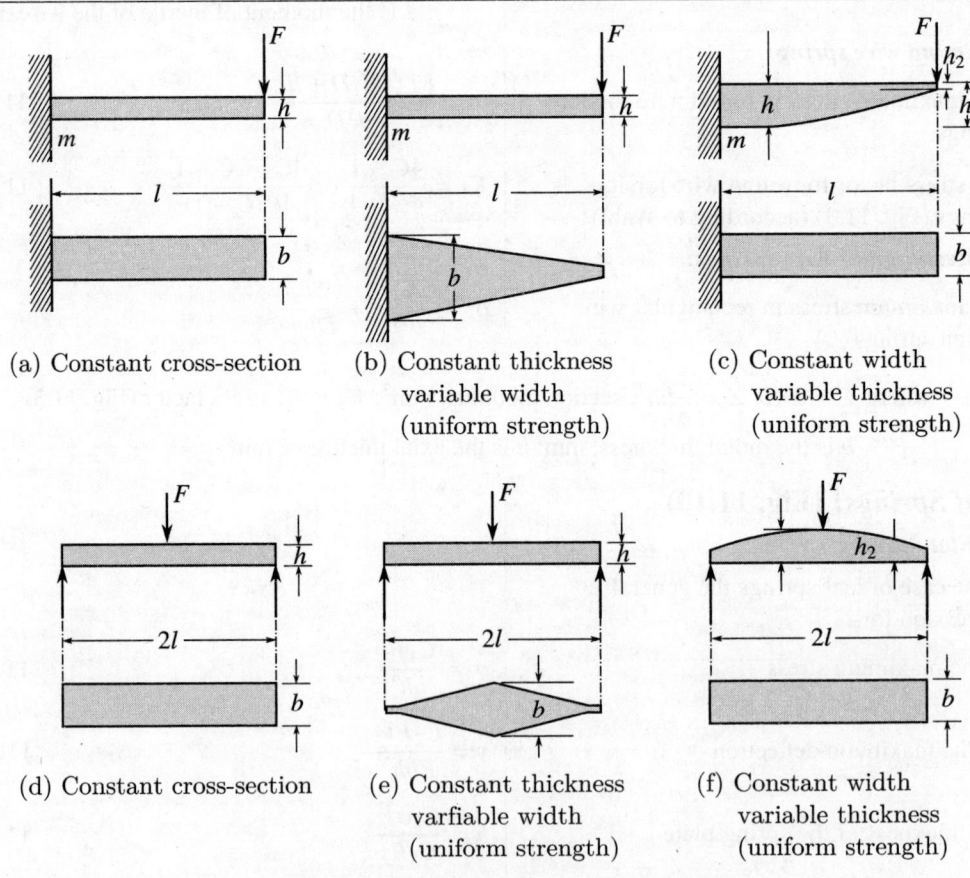

(a) Constant cross-section

(b) Constant thickness variable width (uniform strength)

(c) Constant width variable thickness (uniform strength)

(d) Constant cross-section

(e) Constant thickness varfiable width (uniform strength)

(f) Constant width variable thickness (uniform strength)

Fig. 11.10: *Beams with a rectangular section*

Particular	Equation	Eqn. No.
(c) Laminated leaf springs: (Fig. 11.12)		
The stress in the full length leaves	$\sigma_f = \dfrac{3}{2}\sigma_g$	11.29(a)
The load on the graduated leaves	$F_g = \dfrac{2i_g F_f}{2i_f} = \left(\dfrac{2i_g}{2i_g + 3i_f}\right)F$	11.29(b)
The load on the full length leaves	$F_f = \dfrac{3i_f}{(2i_g + 3i_f)}F$	11.29(c)
The total load on the spring	$F = F_g + F_f$	11.29(d)

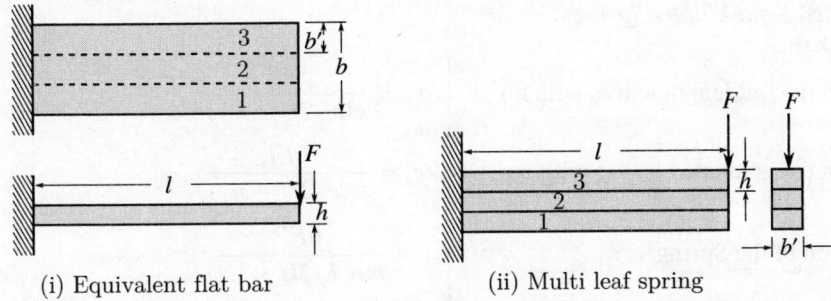

(i) Equivalent flat bar   (ii) Multi leaf spring

(a) Uniform cross-section cantilever leaf spring

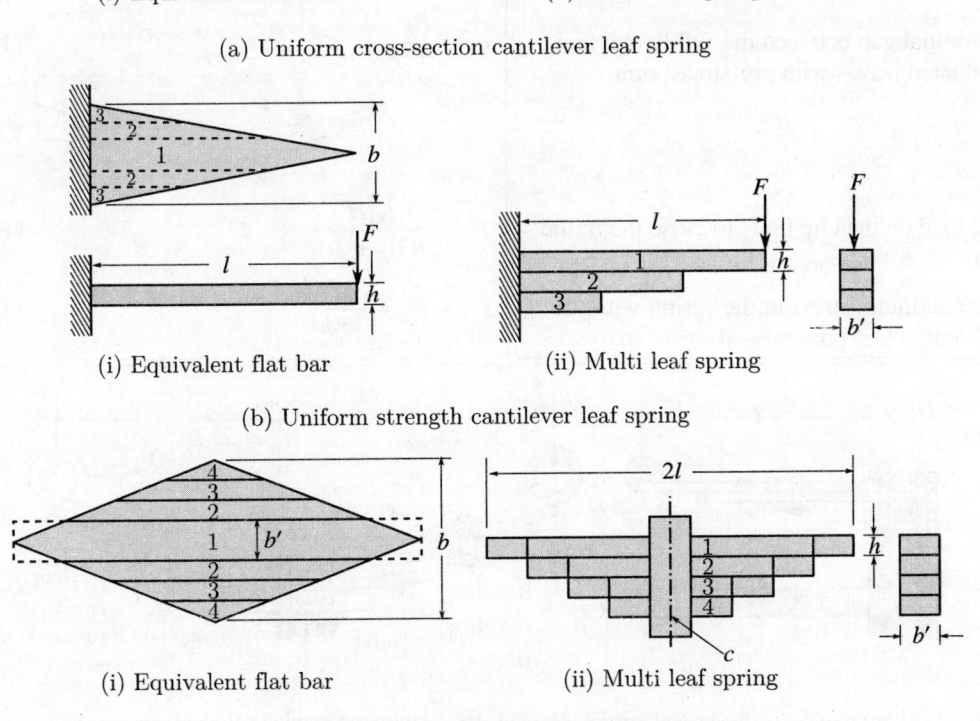

(i) Equivalent flat bar   (ii) Multi leaf spring

(b) Uniform strength cantilever leaf spring

(i) Equivalent flat bar   (ii) Multi leaf spring

Fig. 11.11: *Laminated Springs*

Particular	Equation	Eqn. No.
Bending stresses and deflection		
(i) Laminated cantilever Springs: *(Fig. 11.12(a))*		
The stress in the full length leaves	$\sigma_f = \dfrac{6Fl}{i_f b' h^2}\left(\dfrac{3i_f}{2i_g + 3i_f}\right) = \dfrac{18Fl}{b' h^2(2i_g + 3i_f)}$	11.30(a)
The stress in the graduated leaves	$\sigma_g = \dfrac{12Fl}{b' h^2(2i_g + 3i_f)}$	11.30(b)
The deflection of the spring	$y = \dfrac{12Fl^3}{b' h^3 E(2i_g + 3i_f)}$	11.30(c)
(ii) Laminated Semi-elliptic Springs: *(Fig. 11.12(b))*		
The stress in the full length leaves with no pre-stress	$\sigma_f = \dfrac{9Fl}{b' h^2(2i_g + 3i_f)}$	11.31(a)
The stress in the graduated leaves with no pre-stress	$\sigma_g = \dfrac{6Fl}{b' h^2(2i_g + 3i_f)}$	11.31(b)
The deflection of the Spring	$y = \dfrac{6Fl^3}{b' h^3 E(2i_g + 3i_f)}$	11.31(c)
The initial gap between the full length and graduated leaves with pre-stress, mm	$c = \dfrac{Fl^3}{i' h^3 E}$ 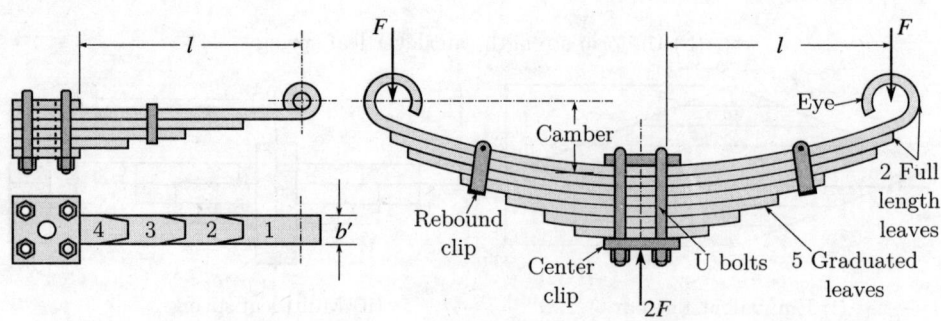	11.32(a)
The load on the clip bolts to close the initial gap	$F_b = \dfrac{i_g i_f F}{i(2i_g + 3i_f)}$	11.32(b)
The maximum stress in the spring with the full-length leaf pre-stressed	$\sigma_f = \sigma_g = \dfrac{3Fl}{ib' h^2}$	11.32(c)

(a) Laminated cantilever leaf spring   (b) Laminated semielliptic leaf spring

Fig. 11.12: *Laminated leaf springs*

Particular	Equation	Eqn. No.
The deflection of the spring using the correction factor	$y = \dfrac{C_2 F l^3 K_4}{E i b' h^3}$	11.32(d)

where $K_4 = 0.73 r^{0.1}$ for $2 < r < 20$; $K_4 = 1$ for $r > 20$

$r = i/i_f$; $i = i_g + i_f$, the total number of leaves

i_f is the number of full length leaves; i_g is the number of graduated leaves

Disc Springs or Belleville Springs: (Fig. 11.1(e))

The relation between the load F and the axial deflection y of each disc (Fig. 11.1(e))

when the load is applied uniformly around the edge

$$F = \frac{4Ey}{(1 - \mu^2)MD_0^2}\left[(h - y)\left(h - \frac{y}{2}\right)t + t^3\right] \qquad 11.33(a)$$

where μ is the Poisson's ratio; y is the axial deflection of each disc

M is a constant which depends on the ratio D_o/D_i (Fig. 11.13)

D_o and D_i are the outer and inner diameters of the disc

t is the thickness of the disc (Fig. 11.1(e)); h is the thickness of the spring (Fig. 11.1(e))

Particular	Equation	Eqn. No.
The maximum stress at the inner edge of the disc spring	$\sigma = \dfrac{4Ey}{(1 - \mu^2)MD_0^2}\left[C_1(h - \frac{y}{2}) + C_2 t\right]$	11.33(b)
The stress at the outer edge of the disc spring	$\sigma = \dfrac{4Ey}{(1 - \mu^2)MD_0^2}\left[C_1(h - \frac{y}{2}) - C_2 t\right]$	11.33(c)

where C_1 and C_2 are constants depending on the ratio D_o/D_i (Fig. 11.13)

$$M = \frac{6}{\pi \log_e(D_o/D_i)}\left[\frac{(D_o/D_i) - 1}{D_o/D_i}\right]^2 \qquad 11.33(d)$$

$$C_1 = \frac{6}{\pi \log_e(D_o/D_i)}\left[\frac{(D_o/D_i) - 1}{\log_e(D_o/D_i)} - 1\right] \qquad 11.33(e)$$

$$C_2 = \frac{6}{\pi \log_e(D_o/D_i)}\left[\frac{(D_o/D_i) - 1}{2}\right] \qquad 11.33(f)$$

Particular	Equation	Eqn. No.
Rubber Springs:-		
(a) Rubber in compression:		
The percentage deformation of rectangular members is given by equation (Fig. 11.14)	$y\% = 2.94 \dfrac{(LK_R)^{2/3}}{A^{\frac{1}{2}}E}(E_{55}y_{55})$	11.34(a)

where $y\%$ is the deformation percent

   K_R is the the form factor or ratio of the long side to the short side of rectangular members

   A is the loading area, mm^2

   E is the modulus of Elasticity of rubber, MN/m^2 (kgf/mm^2) (Fig. 11.17)

   E_{55} is the modulus of elasticity of 55 durometer rubber, MN/m^2 (kgf/mm^2)

   y_{55} is the deflection of a 25.4 mm cube of 55 durometer rubber, percent (Fig. 11.16)

The percentage deformation of cylindrical members in compression	$y\% = (24.5)\dfrac{K_c}{A^{1/2}E}(E_{55}y_{55})$	11.34(b)
	where K_c is the form factor for cylindrical rubber compression members (Fig. 11.18)	
The actual deflection	$y = \left(\dfrac{(y\%)}{(100)}\right)L$	11.34(c)

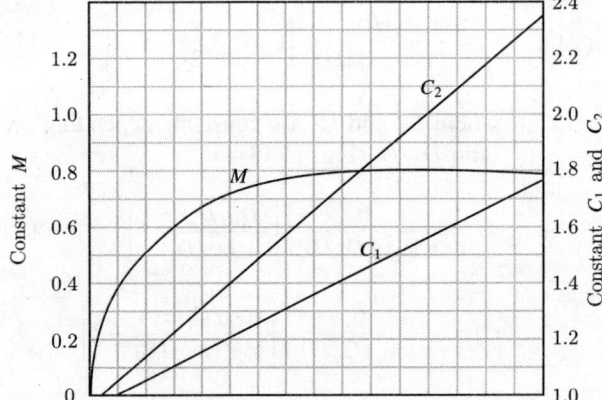

Fig. 11.13: *Disc Constants*

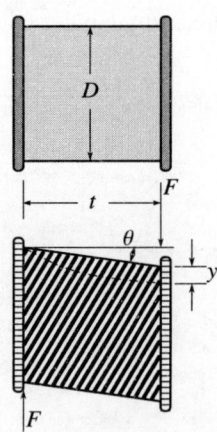

Fig. 11.14: *Rectangular Rubber Shear Mounting*

Particular	Equation	Eqn. No.
(b) Rubber in shear:		
The angular deformation in radians for a rectangular shear mounting (Fig. 11.14)	$\theta = \dfrac{F}{AG}$	11.35(a)

where F = applied load, N (kgf); A = cross-sectional area parallel to the applied load, mm^2

G = modulus of rigidity, MN/m^2 (kgf/mm^2) (Fig. 11.17)

When the angular deformation is less than 30°, the approximate equation to determine the linear deflection in mm	$y = t\theta = \dfrac{Ft}{AG}$	11.35(b)
	where t is the distance between the shearing forces, mm	
The linear deformation for cylindrical rubber shear member (Fig. 11.15(a))	$y = \dfrac{F}{2\pi G}\left(\dfrac{D_o - D_i}{L_o D - L_i D_o}\right) \log_e \dfrac{L_o D_i}{L_i D_o}$	11.35(c)
(c) Rubber in torsional shear:		
The angular deformation in radians of rubber bushings (Fig. 11.15(b))	$\theta = \dfrac{T}{\pi L G}\left(\dfrac{1}{D_i^2} - \dfrac{1}{D_o^2}\right)$	11.36(a)
	where T is the applied torque, N mm (kgf-mm)	
	L is the effective length of bushing, mm	
The radial deflection of the inner cylinder (Fig. 11.15) is approximately	$y = \dfrac{\sigma_c}{1.2E}$	11.36(b)

where y = radial deflection, mm

σ_c = compressive stress on projected area of inner cylinder, MN/m^2 (kgf/mm^2)

E = modulus of elasticity in compression, MN/m^2 (kgf/mm^2)

Note: Equation 11.36(b) applies to rubber bushings having a wall thickness lessthan $D_i/3$ and a length greater than $4D_i$

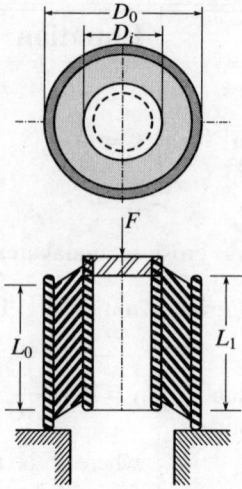

Fig. 11.15(a): *Cylinder Rubber Shear Member*

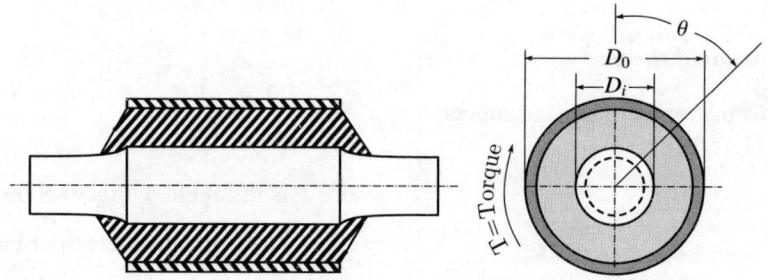

Fig. 11.15(b): *Torsion Bushing*

References

[1] Siegel, M. J., Maleev, V. L., Hartman J. B., *"Mechanical Design of Machines"* 4th edition, International Text Book Company, 1965.

[2] Vallance, A., Doughtie, V. L., *"Design of Machine Members"*, 3rd edition, McGraw Hill Book Co., 1951.

[3] Shigley, J. E., *"Machine Design"*, McGraw Hill Book Company, Inc.

[4] Black, P. H., *"Machine Design"*, 3rd edition, McGraw Hill Book Company, Inc.

[5] Spotts, M. E., *"Design of Machine Elements"*, 3rd edition, Prentice Hall, Inc., Maruzen Co., Ltd.

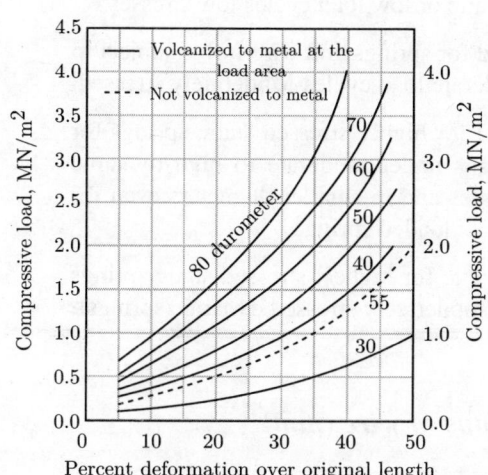

Fig. 11.16: *Load deformation curves for 12.5 mm cube of rubber*

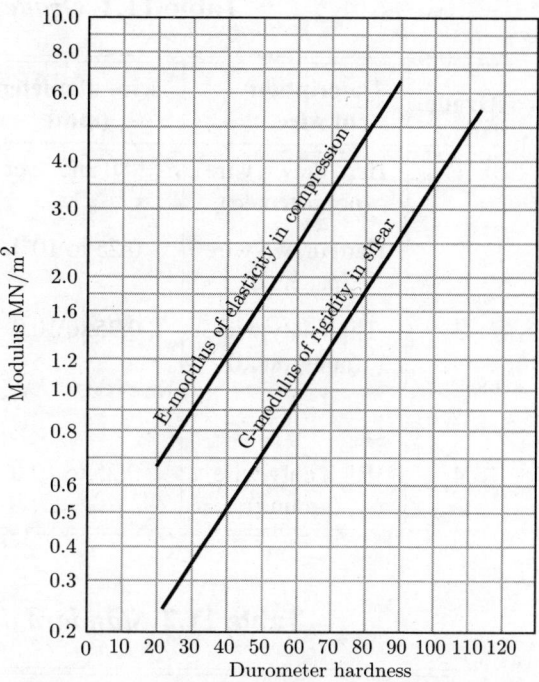

Fig. 11.17: *Variation of modulus of elasticity and rigidity of rubber*

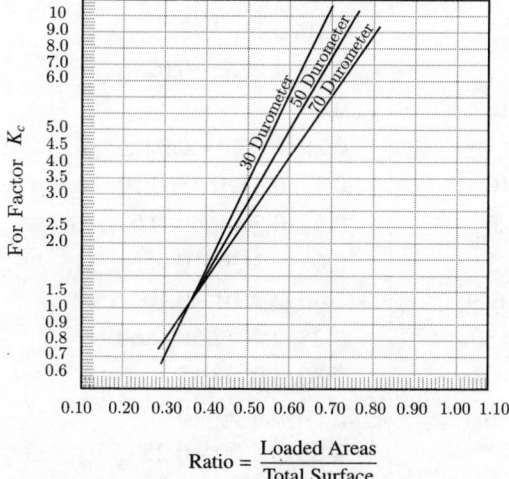

Fig. 11.18: *Form factor for cylindrical rubber compression members*

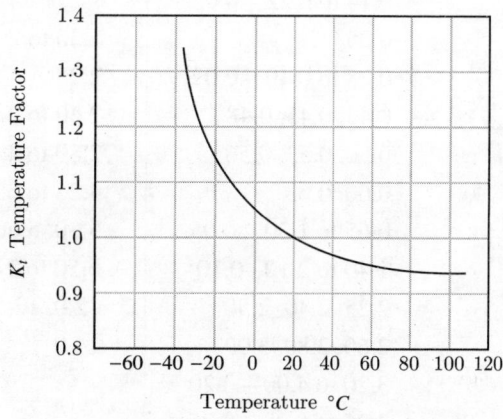

Fig. 11.19: *Temperature correction factor*

Table 11.1 *Grades and Sizes of wire*

Grade	Description of wire	wire diameter (mm)	Field of application
1	Hard drawn wire (not patented)	2.80 and over	Used for springs and wire forms subjected to static or low load cycles low stresses
2	Hard drawn wire (patented)	0.25 to 10.0	Used for springs and wire forms subject to moderate load cycles-Moderately stressed
3	High duty wire (not ground)	0.25 to 10.0	Used for highly stressed static springs for springs under moderate to high dynamic stresses and in smaller diameters even for impact loaded springs
4	High duty wire (ground)	0.25 to 10.0	Suitable for highest stressed static springs and moderately stressed dynamic springs

Table 11.2 *Standard dimensions of wire (mm)*

Cold drawn steel wire unalloyed	Hardened and tempered spring steel wire and value spring wire	Stainless steel wire for Normal corrosion resistance
increment	increment	increment
0.07 to 0.12 – 0.01	1.00 to 1.10 – 0.05	0.10, 0.11, 0.125
0.14 to 0.22 – 0.02	1.2, 1.25	0.14 to 0.22 – 0.02
0.25	1.30 to 2.10 – 0.10	0.25
0.28 to 0.40 – 0.02	2.25	0.28 to 0.40 – 0.02
0.43, 0.45, 0.48	2.40 to 2.60 – 0.10	0.43, 0.45, 0.48, 0.50
0.50, 0.53, 0.56	2.80 to 4.00 – 0.20	0.53, 0.56, 0.60, 0.63
0.60, 0.63	4.25 to 5.00 – 0.25	0.65 to 1.30 – 0.05
0.65 to 1.30 – 0.05	5.30, 5.60, 6.00, 6.30	1.40 to 2.10 – 0.10
1.40 to 2.10 –0.10	6.50 to 11.00 – 0.50	2.25, 2.40, 2.50, 2.60
2.25, 2.40, 2.50	12.0, 12.5, 13.0,	2.80, 3.00, 3.15
2.60, 2.80, 3.00	14.0	3.20 to 4.00 – 0.20
3.20 to 4.00 – 0.20		4.25 to 5.00 – 0.25
4.25 to 5.00 – 0.25		5.30, 5.60, 6.00, 6.30
5.30, 5.60, 6.00, 6.30		6.50 to 10.00 – 0.50
6.50 to 11.0 – 0.50		
12.0, 12.50		
13.00 to 17.00 – 1.00		

Table 11.3 *Spring Design stresses*

Wire diameter (mm)	Design Stress, MN/m^2 (kgf/mm^2)		
	Severe service	Average Service	Light service
Upto 2.10	414 (42.2)	517 (52.7)	640 (65.4)
2.10 – 4.50	380 (38.7)	476 (48.5)	586 (59.8)
4.50 – 8.00	330 (33.8)	414 (42.2)	510 (52.0)
8.00 – 13.00	290 (29.5)	360 (36.6)	448 (45.7)
13.00 – 25.00	248 (25.3)	310 (31.6)	386 (39.4)
25.00 – 38.00	220 (22.5)	276 (28.1)	345 (35.2)

Table 11.4 *Different types of spring coil ends*

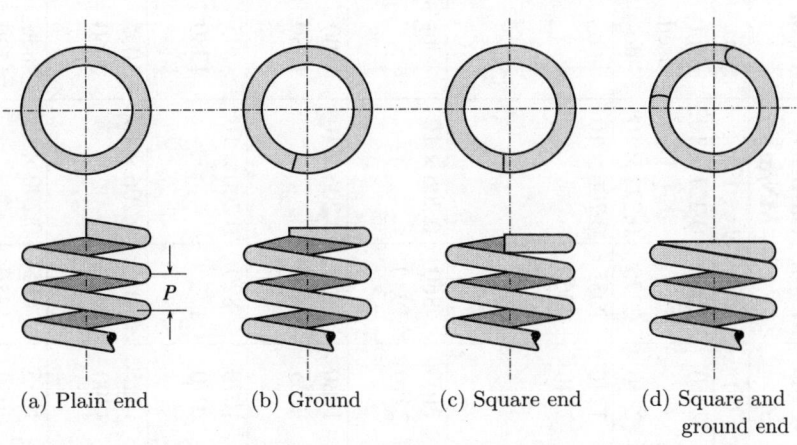

(a) Plain end   (b) Ground   (c) Square end   (d) Square and ground end

Type of Spring Coil Ends	Number of Coils			Length of Spring			Pitch (p) mm
	End Coils	Active Coils	Total	Solid (l_s) (mm)	Free (l_0) (mm)		
(a) Plain End	0	i	i	$(i+1)d$	$ip + d = ((i+1)d + y + a)$		$(l_0 - d)/i$
(b) Plain and Ground End	1	i	$(i+1)$	$(i+1)d$	$(i+1)p = (i+1)d + y + a$		$l_0/(i+1)$
(c) Square or Close End	2	i	$(i+2)$	$(i+3)d$	$(ip + 3d) = (i+3)d + y + a$		$(l_0 - 3d)/i$
(d) Square and Ground End	2	i	$(i+2)$	$(i+2)d$	$(ip + 2d) = (i+2)d + y + a$		$(l_0 - 2d)/i$

y = axial deflection; a = total clearance between working coils

Table 11.5 Physical Properties of Spring Materials

(1)	Material (2)	Element (3)	Percent (4)	Tensile properties* Ultimate strength, MN/m² (5)	Elastic limit, MN/m² (6)	Modulus of elasticity, MN/m² (7)	Torsional properties of wire* Ultimate strength, MN/m² (8)	Elastic limit, MN/m² (9)	Modulus in torsion, MN/m² (10)	Process of manufacture, chief uses, special properties (11)
Flat cold-rolled spring steel	Watch-Spring steel	C	1.10-1.19	2260	2060	0.221×10^6	Not used	Not used	Not used	Cold-rolled and heattreated before forming main springs for watches and similar uses
		Mn	0.15-0.25	2350	2275	0.221×10^6	-do-	-do-	-do-	
	Clock-spring steel	C	0.90-1.05	1240	1035	0.206×10^6	-do-	-do-	-do-	Cold rolled and heat-treated before forming clock and motor springs, miscellaneous flat springs for hish stress.
		Mn	0.30-0.50	2340	2060					
	Flat spring steel	C	0.65-0.80	1100	860	0.206×10^6	-do-	-do-	-do-	Cold-rolled or annealed or tempered, miscellaneous flat springs
		Mn	0.50-0.90	2210	1930					
Carbon steel wires	High Carbon wire	C	0.85-0.95	1380	1100	0.206×10^6	1100	760	0.07845×10^6	Cold-rolled or drawn high-grade helical springs or wire forms.
		Mn	0.25-0.60	1725	1450		1380	1035		
	Oil-tempered wire	C	0.60-0.70	1070	820	0.200×10^6	795	5515	0.07845×10^6	Cold-drawn and heat treated before coiling general spring use.
		Mn	0.60-0.90	2070	1725		1380	900		
	Music wire	C	0.70-1.00	1725	1035	0.206×10^6	1035	620	0.07845×10^6	Patented and cold-drawn misc. smal springs of various types high quality.
		Mn	0.30-0.60	3790	2410		2060	1240		
	Hard-drawn spring wire	C	0.60-0.70	1035	685	0.200×10^6	830	520	0.07845×10^6	Patented and cold-drawn same uses as music wire but lower quality wire
		Mn	0.90-1.20	2060	1380		1520	90		

* To obtain the values in metric Units (kgf/mm²), divide the given values by 9.8067

Table 11.5 Physical Properties of Spring Materials (Contd...)

(1)	(2)	(3)	(4)	(5)	(6)	(7)	(8)	(9)	(10)	(11)
Alloys and stainless spring materials	Hot-rolled bars-special steel	C Mn	0.90-1.05 0.25-0.50	1210 1380	725 965	0.196×10^6	758 965	520 758	0.07257×10^6	Hot-rolled heavy coil or flat springs.
	Chrome-vandium alloy steel 0.50% C	C Mn Cr V	0.45-0.55 0.50-0.80 0.80-1.10 0.15-0.18	1380 1725	1240 1590	0.206×10^6	965 1205	690 900	0.07845×10^6	Cold-rolled or drawn; special applications
	Silico Manganese alloy steel	C Mn Si	0.55-0.65 0.60-0.90 1.80-2.20	About the same as chrome vanadium					About the same as chrome vanadium	Hot-or cold-rolled or drawn; in some applications may be used as a lower cost material in place of chrome vanadium
	Type 18-8 stainless	Cr Ni C Mn	17-20 7-10 0.08-0.15 2 max	1100 2275	415 1795	0.193×10^6	830 1650	300 965	0.06865×10^6	Cold-rolled or drawn; best corrosion resistance; fair temperature resistance
	Cutlery type stainless	Si Cr C	0.30-0.75 12-14 0.25-0.40	1180 1725	900 1380	0.193×10^6	830 1240	550 830	0.07551×10^6	Cold-rolled or drawn; heat-treated after forming, resists corrosion when polished; good temperature resistance
Non-ferrous spring materials	Spring brass	Cu Zn	64-72 balance	690 900	275 414	0.103×10^6	310 620	206 414	0.03825×10^6	Cold-rolled or drawn for electrical conductivity at low stresses for corrosion resistance.
	Nickel Silver	Cu Zn Ni	56 25 18	900 1035	550 760	0.110×10^6	590 685	414 480	0.03825×10^6	Cold-rolled or drawn; better quality than brass corrosion resistance

* To obtain the values in metric Units (kgf/mm^2), divide the given values by 9.8067

Table 11.5 *Physical Properties of Spring Materials (Contd...)*

(1)	(2)	(3)	(4)	(5)	(6)	(7)	(8)	(9)	(10)	(11)
Non-ferrous spring materials	Phosphor bronze	Cu Sn or Cu Sn	91-93 7-9 94-96 4-6	690 1035	414 760	0.103×10^6	550 725	345 590	0.04315×10^6	Cold-rolled or drawn; used for corrosion resistance and electrical conductivity
	Silicon bronze	Si Sn or Mn Cu	2-3 small amounts balance	Properties similar to phosphor bronze						Cold-rolled or drawn; used as substitute for phosphor bronze where lower cost is necessary
	Monel	Ni Cu Mn Fe	64 26 2.5 2.25	690 965	550 830	0.180×10^6	520 760	310 480	0.06571×10^6	Cold-rolled or drawn; resists corrosion; moderate stresses to 200° C
	Inconel	Ni Ce Fe	80 14 balance	965 1210	760 930	0.210×10^6	660 830	380 550	0.07551×10^6	Cold-rolled or drawn; resists corrosion; high stresses to 340° C
	K-monel	Ni Cu Al Fe	66 29 2.75 0.90	1100 1240	795 1000	0.180×10^6	725 860	450 590	0.06571×10^6	Cold-rolled or drawn; precipitation hardened by heat-treatment resists corrosion high stresses to 230° C
	Z-nickel	Ni Cu Mn Fe Si	98 Small amounts	1240 1590	900 1180	0.206×10^6	830 1035	414 620	0.07551×10^6	Cold-rolled or drawn; precipitation hardened by heat-treatment; resists corrosion; high stresses to 290° C
	Beryllium copper	Cu Be	98 2	1100 1380	685 1035	0.100×10^6 0.128×10^6	690 900	450 660	0.04120×10^6 0.04805×10^6 subject to heat treatment	Cold-rolled or drawn; corrosion resistance like copper, high physicals for electrical work; low hysteresis.

* To obtain the values in metric Units (kgf/mm²), divide the given values by 9.8067

Table 11.6 *(a) Chemical Composition of Steel for Patented and Cold Drawn Steel Wire–Unalloyed*

Grade	Carbon percent	Silicon percent	Manganese Max. percent	Sulphur max. percent	Phosphorus max. percent	Sulphur +Phosphorus max. percent	Copper max. percent
1.	0.50 – 0.70	0.15 – 0.35	1.0	0.050	0.040	–	0.20
2.	0.60 – 0.85	0.15 – 0.35	0.8	0.040	0.040	–	0.15
3.	0.75 – 1.0	0.15 – 0.35	0.8	0.030	0.030	0.050	0.12
4.	0.75 – 1.0	0.15 – 0.35	0.8	0.025	0.025	0.040	0.12

Table 11.6 *(b) Chemical Composition of Steel for Oil Hardened and Tempered Spring Steel wire and Value Spring Wire-Unalloyed*

Quality	Grade	Constituent					
		Carbon percent	Silicon percent	Manganese percent	Sulphur max. percent	Phosphorus max percent	Copper max. percent
Oil hardened and tempered spring steel wire	SW	0.55 to 0.75	0.10 to 0.35	0.60 to 0.90	0.040	0.040	0.15
Oil hardened and tempered value spring wire	VW	0.60 to 0.70	0.10 to 0.25	0.60 to 0.90	0.020	0.025	0.06

Table 11.6 *(c) Chemical Composition of Stainless Spring Steel Wire for Normal Corrosion Resistance*

Grade	Constituent, percent by weight							
	C max.	si max.	Mn max.	p max.	s max.	Cr	A1	Ni
1 (18/8)	0.15	1.00	2.00	0.045	0.030	17.0	–	8.0
2 (17/7 A1)	0.09	1.00	1.00	0.040	0.030	16 to 18	0.75 to 1.25	6.75 to 7.75

Table 11.6 *(d) Physical Properties of Oil Hardened and Tempered Spring Steel Wire and Valve Spring Wire-Unalloyed*

Wire Dia. (Nominal) mm	Tensile strength,	N/mm² (kfg/mm²)
1	SW	VW
	2	3
1.00 to 1.10	1760 to 1960 (180 to 200)	1670 to 1810 (170 to 185)
1.20 to 1.40	1720 to 1910 (175 to 195)	1620 to 1760 (165 to 180)
1.50 to 1.90	1670 to 1860 (170 to 190)	1570 to 1690 (160 to 172)
2.00 to 2.40	1620 to 1760 (165 to 180)	1520 to 1620 (155 to 165)
2.50 to 2.80	1570 to 1720 (160 to 175)	1470 to 1570 (150 to 160)
3.00 to 3.40	1520 to 1670 (155 to 170)	1430 to 1530 (146 to 156)
3.60 to 4.00	1480 to 1630 (151 to 166)	1400 to 1500 (143 to 153)
4.25 to 5.00	1440 to 1590 (147 to 162)	1370 to 1470 (140 to 150)
5.30 to 6.30	1400 to 1550 (143 to 158)	1340 to 1440 (137 to 147)
6.50 to 7.50	1360 to 1510 (139 to 154)	1300 to 1400 (133 to 143)
8.00 to 9.50	1290 to 1400 (132 to 147)	—
10.0 to 14.0	1250 to 1400 (128 to 143)	—

IS: 4454 (Part II) 1975

Modulus of Elasticity, E = 205880 N/mm²
Modulus of rigidity, G = 81370 N/mm²

Table 11.6 *(e) Physical Properties of Stainless Steel Wire for Normal Corrosion Resistance*

Wire Dia. (Nominal), mm	Tensile strength, N/mm² (kgf/mm²)
0.10	2060 (210)
0.11 to 0.20	2010 (205)
0.22 to 0.32	1960 (200)
0.34 to 0.50	1910 (195)
0.64 to 0.80	1860 (190)
0.85 to 1.25	1760 (180)
1.30 to 2.00	1670 (170)
2.10 to 3.15	1570 (160)
3.20 to 5.00	1470 (150)
5.30 to 8.00	1320 (135)
8.50 to 10.00	1270 (130)

IS:4454 (Part IV) - 1975

Modulus of Elasticity, E N/mm²		Modulus of Rigidity, G N/mm²	
Grade Tempered Untempered		Tempered	Untempered
1 190200 ± 4900 180390 ± 3920		73530 ± 1960	69610 ± 1960
2 295100 ± 4900 190200 ± 3920		78430 ± 1960	73530 ± 1960

Table 11.7 *Physical Properties of Patented and Cold Drawn Steel Wire-Unalloyed*

Uncoated wire dia (Nominal mm)	Tensile strength, N/mm² (kgf/mm²)			
(1)	Grade 1 (2)	Grade (3)	Grade 3 (4)	Grade 4 (5)
0.07	—	—	2550 (260)	—
0.08	—	—	2540 (259)	—
0.09	—	—	2530 (258)	—
0.10	—	—	2530 (258)	—
0.11	—	—	2520 (257)	—
0.12	—	—	2520 (257)	—
0.14	—	—	2510 (256)	—
0.16	—	—	2500 (255)	—
0.18	—	—	2500 (255)	—
0.20	—	—	2490 (254)	2700 (275)
0.22	—	—	2480 (253)	2680 (273)
0.25	—	—	2470 (252)	2670 (272)
0.28	—	—	2460 (251)	2660 (271)
0.30	1720 (175)	2060 (210)	2460 (251)	2660 (271)
0.32	1710 (174)	2050 (209)	2450 (250)	2650 (270)
0.34	1710 (174)	2050 (209)	2450 (250)	2640 (269)
0.36	1700 (173)	2040 (208)	2440 (249)	2630 (268)
0.38	1700 (173)	2040 (208)	2430 (248)	2620 (267)
0.40	1700 (173)	2040 (208)	2430 (248)	2620 (267)
0.43	1690 (172)	2030 (207)	2420 (247)	2610 (266)
0.45	1680 (171)	2020 (206)	2410 (246)	2600 (265)
0.48	1680 (171)	2020 (206)	2400 (245)	2590 (264)
0.50	1670 (170)	2010 (205)	2390 (244)	2580 (263)
0.53	1660 (169)	2000 (204)	2380 (243)	2570 (262)
0.56	1660 (169)	2000 (204)	2370 (242)	2560 (261)
0.60	1650 (168)	1990 (203)	2360 (241)	2550 (260)
0.63	1640 (167)	1980 (202)	2340 (239)	2540 (259)
0.65	1640 (167)	1980 (292)	2330 (238)	2540 (258)

Table 11.7 *(Contd....)*

(1)	Grade 1 (2)	Grade (3)	Grade 3 (4)	Grade 4 (5)
0.70	1630 (166)	1970 (201)	2320 (237)	2530 (258)
0.75	1620 (165)	1960 (200)	2300 (235)	2500 (255)
0.80	1610 (164)	1950 (199)	2280 (233)	2480 (253)
0.85	1610 (163)	1930 (197)	2260 (231)	2460 (251)
0.90	1590 (162)	1920 (196)	2250 (230)	2440 (249)
0.95	1580 (161)	1910 (195)	2250 (229)	2420 (247)
1.00	1570 (160)	1900 (194)	2240 (228)	2400 (245)
1.05	1560 (159)	1890 (193)	2210 (225)	2380 (243)
1.10	1550 (159)	1880 (192)	2120 (223)	2370 (242)
1.20	1540 (157)	1860 (190)	2170 (221)	2340 (239)
1.25	1530 (156)	1850 (189)	2140 (218)	2320 (237)
1.30	1520 (155)	1840 (188)	2130 (217)	2300 (335)
1.40	1500 (153)	1820 (186)	2110 (215)	2290 (234)
1.50	1490 (152)	1800 (184)	2100 (214)	2260 (231)
1.60	1470 (150)	1780 (182)	2080 (212)	2250 (229)
1.70	1460 (149)	1760 (180)	2050 (209)	2220 (226)
1.80	1440 (147)	1750 (178)	2030 (207)	2190 (224)
1.90	1430 (146)	1730 (176)	2010 (205)	2180 (222)
2.00	1420 (145)	1720 (175)	1990 (203)	2160 (220)
2.10	1410 (144)	1700 (173)	1960 (200)	2130 (217)
2.25	1400 (143)	1680 (171)	1940 (198)	2100 (214)
2.40	1380 (141)	1660 (169)	1910 (195)	2070 (211)
2.50	1370 (140)	1640 (167)	1890 (193)	2050 (209)
2.60	1360 (139)	1620 (165)	1860 (190)	2030 (207)
2.80	1340 (137)	1600 (163)	1840 (188)	2000 (204)
3.00	1320 (135)	1570 (160)	1830 (187)	1980 (202)
3.20	1310 (134)	1550 (158)	1790 (183)	1960 (200)
3.40	1290 (132)	1530 (156)	1760 (180)	1920 (196)
3.60	1270 (130)	1510 (154)	1750 (178)	1890 (193)
3.80	1260 (129)	1490 (152)	1720 (175)	1860 (190)

Table 11.7 *(Contd....)*

(1)	Grade 1 (2)	Grade (3)	Grade 3 (4)	Grade 4 (5)
4.00	1250 (128)	1480 (151)	1700 (173)	1840 (188)
4.25	1250 (127)	1460 (149)	1680 (171)	1820 (186)
4.50	1230 (125)	1440 (147)	1660 (169)	1800 (184)
4.75	1210 (123)	1420 (145)	1620 (165)	1770 (181)
5.00	1190 (121)	1390 (142)	1600 (163)	1750 (178)
5.30	1170 (119)	1370 (140)	1570 (160)	1720 (175)
5.60	1150 (117)	1350 (138)	1550 (158)	1690 (172)
6.00	1130 (115)	1320 (135)	1530 (156)	1670 (170)
6.30	1120 (114)	1310 (134)	1500 (153)	1640 (167)
6.50	1110 (113)	1290 (132)	1480 (151)	1620 (165)
7.00	1090 (111)	1260 (129)	1460 (149)	1610 (164)
7.50	1070 (109)	1250 (127)	1430 (146)	1570 (160)
8.00	1050 (107)	1220 (124)	1400 (143)	1540 (157)
8.50	1020 (104)	1200 (122)	1370 (140)	1500 (153)
9.00	1000 (102)	1180 (120)	1350 (138)	1480 (151)
9.50	990 (101)	1150 (117)	1310 (134)	—
10.0	980 (100)	1130 (115)	1290 (132)	—
10.5	—	1100 (112)	—	—
11.0	—	1080 (110)	—	—
12.0	—	1040 (106)	—	—
12.5	—	1030 (105)	—	—
13.0	—	1020 (104)	—	—
14.0	—	990 (101)	—	—
15.0	—	970 (99)	—	—
16.0	—	960 (98)	—	—
17.0	—	950 (97)	—	—

IS: 4454 (Part I)–1981

Modulus of Elasticity, $E = 210790$ N/mm^2

Modulus of rigidity, $G = 88370$ N/mm^2.

Table 11.8 *Values of* ϵ

b/h or h/b	1.0	1.1	1.2	1.3	1.4	1.5	1.6	1.7	1.8	1.9	2.0	
ϵ	5.59	5.61	5.67	5.77	5.88	6.02	6.17	6.33	6.50	6.68	6.87	
b/h or h/b	2.2	2.4	2.6	2.8	3.0	3.2	3.4	3.6	3.8	4.0	4.5	5.0
ϵ	7.26	7.67	8.09	8.51	8.95	9.39	9.83	10.28	10.73	11.19	12.33	13.48

Table 11.9 *Constants in beam equations 11.27 and 11.28*

Constant	Cantilever beam (Fig. 11.10)			Simple beam (Fig. 11.10)		
	a	b	c	d	e	f
C_1–for the stress	6	6	6	3	3	3
C_2–for the deflection	4	6	8	2	3	4
Unit resilience per unit volume	$\dfrac{\sigma^2}{18E}$	$\dfrac{\sigma^2}{6E}$	$\dfrac{\sigma^2}{6E}$	$\dfrac{\sigma^2}{18E}$	$\dfrac{\sigma^2}{6E}$	$\dfrac{\sigma^2}{6E}$

Table 11.10 *(a) The normal sizes of flats (Laminated springs for automotive suspension)*

Width *(mm)*	40	45	50	55	60	65	70	75	90	100	120	150
Thickness *(mm)*	4	5	6	7	8	10	12	14	16			

Table 11.10 *(b) Standard Sections of Flat (Laminated springs–Railway Rolling Stock) All dimensions in mm*

Width (mm)	50	50	63	63	63	63	63	75	75	75	75	75	75
Thickness (mm)	10	13	6	8	10	11	13	6	8	10	11	13	16

Width (mm)	90	90	90	90	90	90	90	100	100	100	100	100	100
Thickness	6	8	10	11	13	16	19	8	10	11	13	16	19

Width (mm)	115	115	115	115	115	120	120	125	125	125	140	140	150	150	150
Thickness (mm)	10	11	13	16	19	16	19	10	13	16	11	13	11	13	16

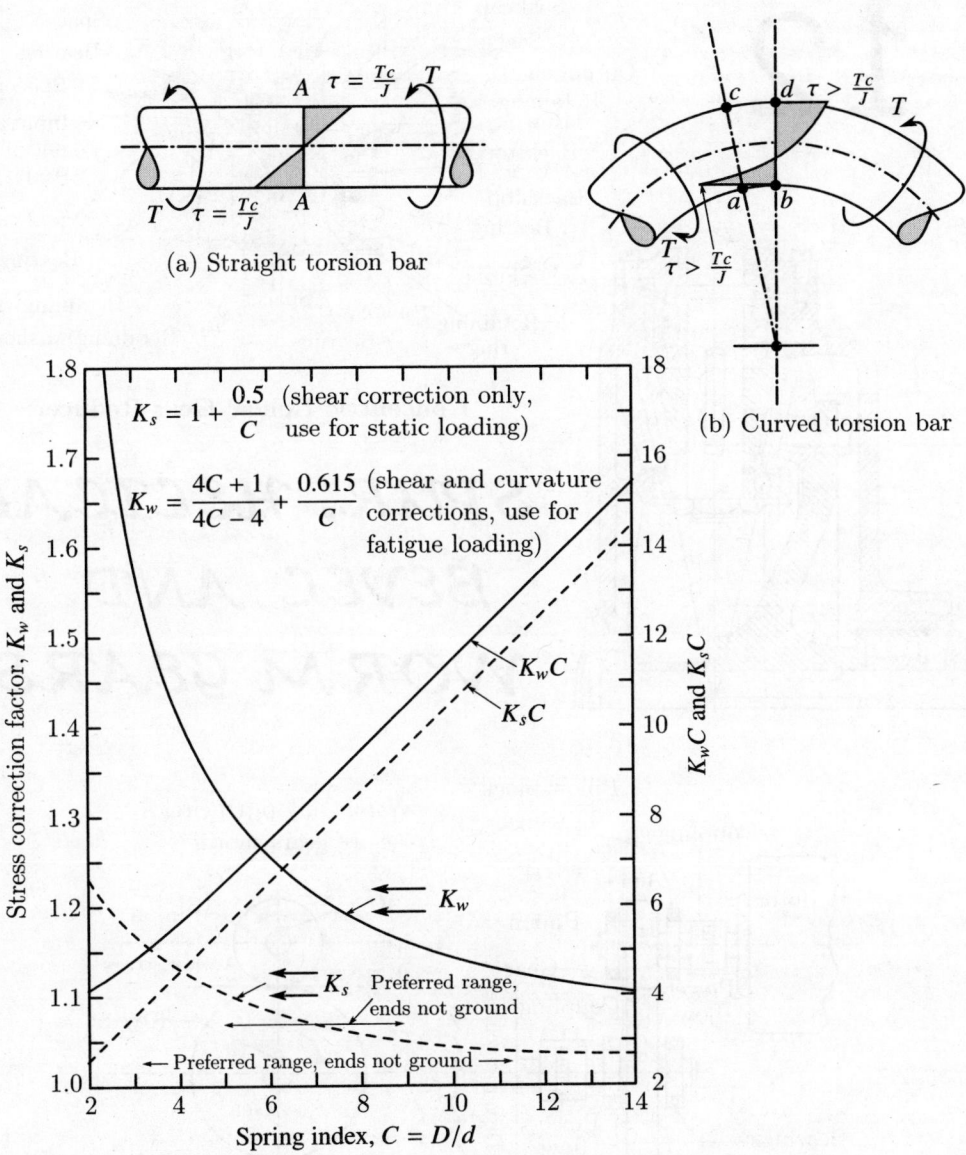

(a) Straight torsion bar

(b) Curved torsion bar

$$K_s = 1 + \frac{0.5}{C} \quad \text{(shear correction only, use for static loading)}$$

$$K_w = \frac{4C + 1}{4C - 4} + \frac{0.615}{C} \quad \text{(shear and curvature corrections, use for fatigue loading)}$$

Stress correction factors for Helical springs

12

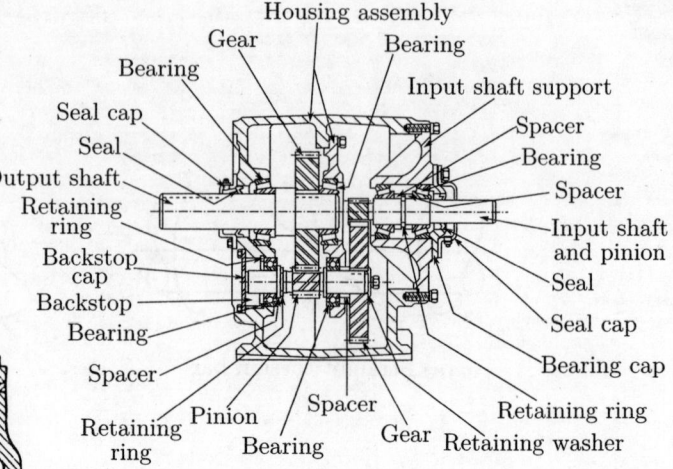

Housing assembly
Gear
Bearing
Bearing
Seal cap
Seal
Output shaft
Retaining ring
Backstop cap
Backstop
Bearing
Spacer
Retaining ring
Pinion
Bearing
Spacer
Gear
Input shaft support
Spacer
Bearing
Spacer
Input shaft and pinion
Seal
Seal cap
Bearing cap
Retaining ring
Retaining washer

Concentric Helical Gear Reducer

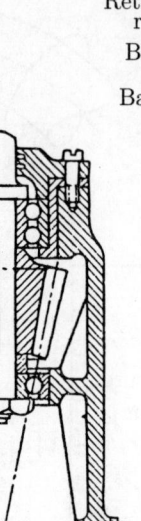

SPUR, HELICAL, BEVEL AND WORM GEARS

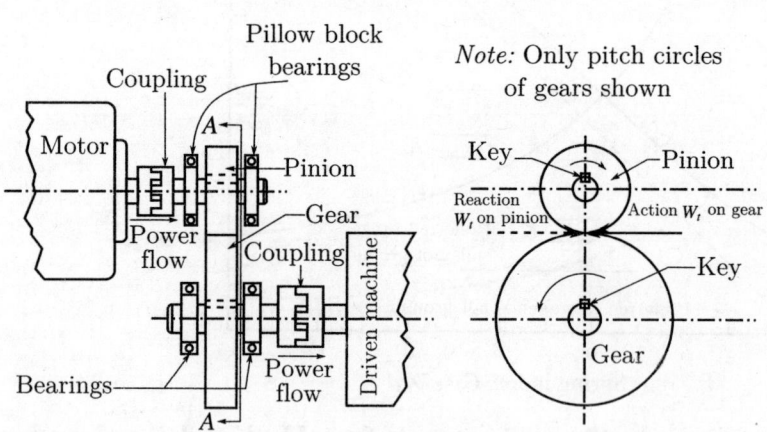

Pillow block bearings
Coupling
Motor
Power flow
Bearings
Pinion
Gear
Coupling
Power flow
Driven machine

Note: Only pitch circles of gears shown

Key — Pinion
Reaction W_t on pinion
Action W_t on gear
Key
Gear

(a) Side view

(b) View $A - A$ showing tangential forces on bearings

12

Spur, Helical, Bevel and Worm Gears

Symbols	Description and Units
a	centre distance, mm
b	face width, mm
C_v	velocity factor
d_1, d_2	pitch diameters of the pinion and the gear respectively, mm
E_1, E_2	modulus of elasticity of the pinion and gear respectively, MN/m^2 (kgf/mm^2)
F_t	Driving force or tangential load at pitch line, N (kgf)
F_d	dynamic load, N (kgf)
F_w	the limiting load for wear, N (kgf)
F_s	The dynamic strength of the gear, N (kgf)
i	gear ratio
K	load stress factor
K_w	wear load factor
m	module, mm
m_n	the normal module, mm
n	speed, rev/s
p	circular pitch, mm
p_d	diametral pitch
p_{dn}	normal diametral pitch
p_n	normal circular pitch, mm
v	pitch line velocity, m/s
y	Lewis form factor
Y	form factor
z_1, z_2	number of teeth on pinion and gear respectively
α	pressure angle, deg
β	helix angle, deg
γ	lead angle, deg
σ_{en}	endurance limit stress, MN/m^2 (kgf/mm^2)

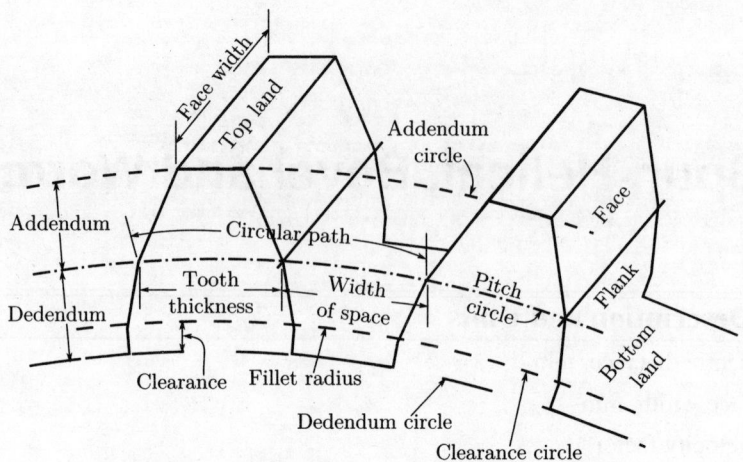

Fig. 12.1(a): *Nomenclature of Spur-gear Teeth*

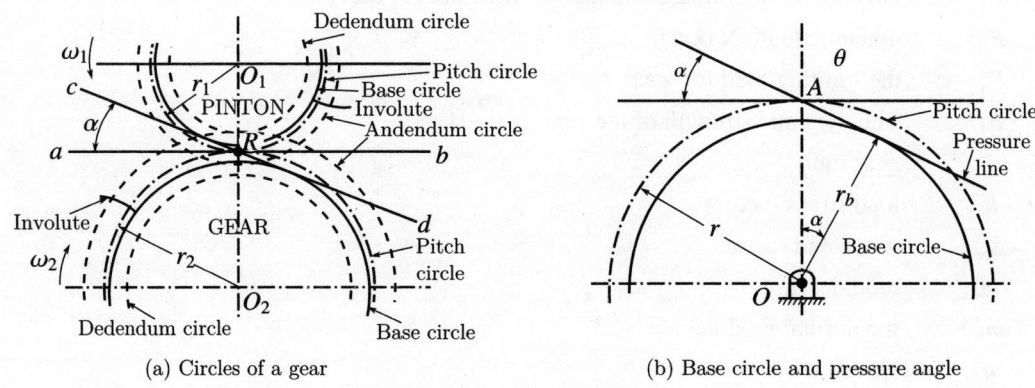

(a) Circles of a gear   (b) Base circle and pressure angle

Fig. 12.1(b): *Gear layout*

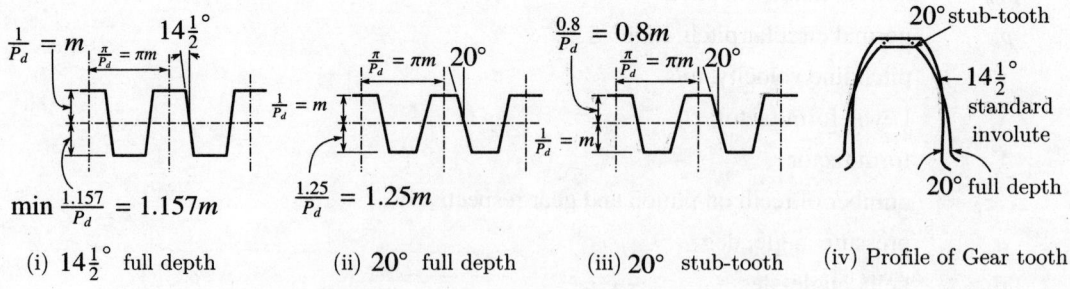

(i) $14\frac{1}{2}°$ full depth   (ii) $20°$ full depth   (iii) $20°$ stub-tooth   (iv) Profile of Gear tooth

Fig. 12.1(c): *Basic rack for involute system*

Particular	Equation	Eqn. No.
Spur Gears: (Fig. 12.1)		
The circular pitch	$p = \pi d/z = \pi/p_d = \pi m$	12.1(a)
The diametral pitch (Table 12.1)	$p_d = z/d = 1/m$	12.1(b)
The relation between the circular pitch and diametral pitch	$pp_d = \pi$	12.1(c)
The module (Table 12.2)	$m = d/z = 1/p_d$	12.1(d)
The pitch diameter (Table 12.3)	$d = mz = (pz/\pi) = (z/p_d)$	12.1(e)
The base circle diameter (Fig. 12.1(b))	$d_b = d \cos \alpha$	12.2(a)
The dedendum circle or root diameter	$d_r = d - 2(t_f + t_c - K')m$	12.2(b)

where $t_f = 1$, tooth factor for standard tooth

$t_c = 0.15$ to 0.25, tooth clearance factor

K' is correction factor or shift factor

Addendum circle or outside diameter	$d_o = d_r + 2h$	12.2(c)

where h = height of tooth = $(2t_f + t_c)m$, when $K'_p = K'_g$ or $K'_p = -K'_g$

or $h = \dfrac{2t_f + t_c}{2(t_f + t_c)} \left(a - \dfrac{d_1 + d_2}{2}\right)$ when K'_p is not equal to K'_g.

The centre distance in an uncorrected gear or in a gear with height correction ($K'_p = -K'_g$)	$a = \left(\dfrac{d_1 + d_2}{2}\right) = \left(\dfrac{z_1 + z_2}{2}\right)m$	12.3(a)
Relation between z_1 and z_2 to determine the minimum number of teeth on pinion of involute gears without interference (Table 12.4(b))	$z_1^2 + 2z_1 z_2 = \dfrac{4K_1(z_2 + K_1)}{\mathrm{Sin}^2 \alpha}$	12.3(b)
Relation to determine the minimum number of teeth on pinion without interference in the case of rack and pinion	$z_1 = \dfrac{2K_1}{\sin^2 \alpha}$	12.3(c)

where $K_1 = 1$, for $14\frac{1}{2}^\circ$ and 20° full depth system. Fig. 12.1(c)

$= 0.8$, for stub teeth system. Fig. 12.1(c)

The theoretical length of the line of action of any pair of true involute gears is given by the equation

$$L_a = \left[\sqrt{(r_1 + mK_{1p})^2 - r_1^2 \cos^2 \alpha} + \sqrt{(r_2 + mK_{1g})^2 - r_2^2 \cos^2 \alpha} - (R_1 + R_2)\sin \alpha\right] \qquad 12.3(d)$$

where r_1, r_2 are pitch radii of pinion and gear respectively, mm

The maximum number of teeth in action at one time is given by the relation.	$z_a = \dfrac{L_a}{\pi m \cos \alpha}$	12.3(e)

Particular	Equation	Eqn. No.
Power transmitting capacity P of spur gears:		
(i) in kW (SI Units)	$P = \dfrac{F_t v}{1000}$	12.4(a)
(ii) in MHP (Metric Units)	$P = \dfrac{F_t v}{75}$	12.4(b)

where F_t is the driving force or tangential load at pitch line

v is the pitch line velocity, m/s (Table 12.4(c))

Lewis equation (Fig. 12.2)	$F_t = \sigma byp = \sigma_d C_v byp = \pi \sigma_d C_v bym$ $= (\sigma_d C_v bY)/p_d = \sigma_d C_v bYm$	12.5(a)
Lewis equation for beam strength of tooth	$m = \sqrt{F_t/(\sigma_d C_v kY)} = \left\{ \dfrac{2M_t}{\sigma_d C_v kYz} \right\}^{\frac{1}{3}}$	12.5(b)

where $k = b/m$

$y = \dfrac{t^2}{6\pi hm}$, Lewis form factor (Table 12.5 and 12.6)

$Y = \pi y$, form factor

σ_d is the allowable static stress (Table 12.7)

M_t is the transmitted torque, N mm (kgf-mm)

Lewis form factor (Table 12.5)

$$y = \left(0.124 - \frac{0.684}{z}\right) \text{ for } 14\tfrac{1}{2}^{\circ} \text{ involute system} \qquad 12.5(c)$$

$$= \left(0.154 - \frac{0.912}{z}\right) \text{ for } 20^{\circ} \text{ involute system} \qquad 12.5(d)$$

$$= \left(0.175 - \frac{0.95}{z}\right) \text{ for } 20^{\circ} \text{ stub teeth system} \qquad 12.5(e)$$

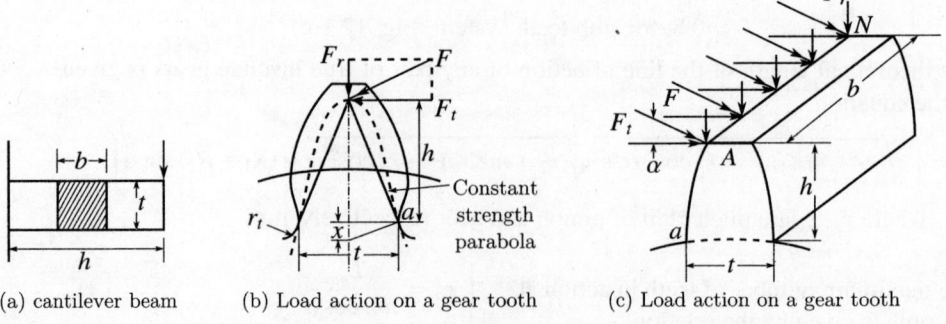

(a) cantilever beam   (b) Load action on a gear tooth   (c) Load action on a gear tooth

Fig. 12.2: *Forces on Gear Teeth*

Particular	Equation	Eqn. No.
The face width of gear in terms of module	$9.5m \leq b \leq 12.5m$	12.5(f)

Under certain conditions where there are space limitations the face width can be taken from 6m to 20m

The velocity factors:

(a) For ordinary cut gears, running with a pitch line velocity upto 8 m/s (Barth's formula)	$C_v = \dfrac{3.05}{3.05 + v}$	12.6(a)
(b) Barth's formula for carefully cut gears with a pitch line velocity upto 13 m/s	$C_v = \dfrac{4.58}{4.58 + v}$	12.6(b)
(c) Barth's formula for very accurately cut and ground metallic gears having a pitch line velocity from 6 m/s to 20 m/s	$C_v = \dfrac{6.1}{6.1 + v}$	12.6(c)
(d) For hardened steel, ground, and lapped in precision gears made for speeds over 20 m/s	$C_v = \dfrac{5.55}{5.55 + \sqrt{v}}$	12.6(d)
(e) For non-metallic gears as recommended by AGMA	$C_v = \dfrac{0.7625}{1.0167 + v}$	12.6(e)

The tangential tooth load

$$F_t = \frac{1000PC_s}{v} \quad \text{when } P \text{ is in } kW \text{ (S.I. Units)} \qquad 12.7(a)$$

$$= \frac{75PC_s}{v} \quad \text{when } P \text{ is in } MHP \text{ (Metric Units)} \qquad 12.7(b)$$

where C_s is the service factor (Table 12.8)

Bach's formula for beam strength of tooth	$m = 0.88 \sqrt[3]{\left(\dfrac{M_t}{K_2 kz}\right)}$	12.8

where K_2 = strength coefficient

= 5.88 to 7.85 MN/m^2 (0.60 to 0.80 Kgf/mm^2) for steel

= 4.90 MN/m^2 (0.50 kgf/mm^2) for bronze

= 3.92 MN/m^2 (0.40 kgf/mm^2) for cast iron

= 1.47 to 1.96 MN/m^2 (0.15 to 0.20 kgf/mm^2) for plastic materials

$k = b/m$

Particular	Equation	Eqn. No.
Forces acting in a spur gear: (Fig. 12.3)		
Tangential force or peripheral force	$F_t = 2M_t/d$	12.8(a)
Radial force	$F_r = F_t \tan \alpha$	12.8(b)
The normal force acting on the tooth	$F_n = \dfrac{F_t}{\cos \alpha} = \dfrac{2M_{t2}}{d_2 \cos \alpha} = \dfrac{M_{t2}(i+1)}{ai \cos \alpha}$	
	$F_n = \dfrac{F_t}{\cos \alpha} = \dfrac{2M_{t1}}{d_1 \cos \alpha} = \dfrac{M_{t1}(i+1)}{a \cos \alpha}$	12.8(c)
The pitch diameter of pinion	$d_1 = 2a/(i+1)$	12.9(a)
The pitch diameter of gear	$d_2 = 2ai/(i+1)$	12.9(b)

where $i = (z_2/z_1) = (d_2/d_1) \geq 1$, gear ratio (Table 12.9)

F_r is the radial force, N(kg)

F_n is the normal force, N(kg)

Strength of teeth considering load concentration, dynamic load and wear factors: (Dobrovolsky)

The load on a unit length along the face width (unit load)	$F_{nu} = \dfrac{F_n}{b} = \dfrac{M_{t_2}(i+1)}{abi \cos \alpha} = \dfrac{M_{t_1}(i+1)}{ab \cos \alpha}$	12.10(a)
The maximum unit load	$F_{nu-max} = K_c F_{nu}$	12.10(b)

where K_c is the load concentration factor from Table 12.10

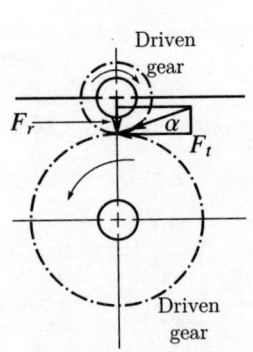

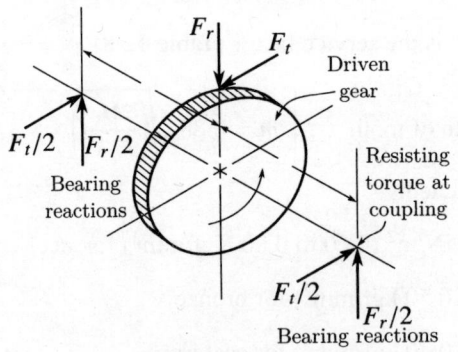

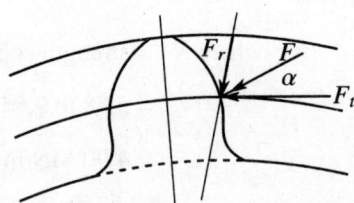

Fig. 12.3(a): *tangential and radial forces on the driven gear*

Fig. 12.3(b): *Forces on a shaft carrying a spur gear*

Fig. 12.3(c): *Forces on gear tooth*

Particular	Equation	Eqn. No.
The dynamic load (Dobrovolsky)	$F_d = F_n + F_i$	12.11(a)

where F_n is the normal load due to the torque and

F_i is the increment load due to dynamic action

Particular	Equation	Eqn. No.
Dynamic load factor (Dobrovolsky refer Table 12.11)	$K_d = \dfrac{F_d}{F_n} = \dfrac{F_n + F_i}{F_n}$	12.11(b)
Unit design load considering load concentration, dynamic load and wear factors	$F_{nu} = \dfrac{F_n}{b} K_c K_d K_w = \dfrac{M_{t_2}(i+1)K_c K_d K_w}{abi \cos \alpha}$	12.11(c)
Allowable bending stress, considering load concentration, dynamic load and wear factors	$\sigma_b = \dfrac{M_{t_2}(i+1)K_c K_d K_w}{abi \cos \alpha}$	12.11(d)
	$= \dfrac{(1.26)^3 M_{t_2} K_c K_d K_w}{z_1 ikYm^3 \cos \alpha} \leq \sigma_d$	12.11(e)

where $K_w = 1.25$ to 1.50 wear factor and $k = b/m$

K_d is the dynamic factor (Table 12.11)

Dynamic load: (Buckingham)

Particular	Equation	Eqn. No.
The approximate Buckingham equation to determine the maximum dynamic load on the gear tooth	$F_d = F_t + F_i = F_t + \dfrac{K_3 v(Cb + F_t)}{K_3 v + \sqrt{Cb + F_t}}$	12.12

where $C = \dfrac{e}{k_1(1/E_1 + 1/E_2)}$, Dynamic factor depending upon machining errors (Table 12.12)

e is the measured error in action between gears in mm (Table 12.13, Fig. 12.4)*

$k_1 = 9.345$ for $14\frac{1}{2}^\circ$ full depth teeth; $k_1 = 9.00$ for 20° full depth teeth

$k_1 = 8.70$ for 20° stub teeth

$K_3 = 20.67$ in SI units; $k_3 = 6.60$ in Metric Units

E_1, E_2 are modulus of elasticity of pinion and gear respectively.

Particular	Equation	Eqn. No.
The beam strength of teeth or the endurance strength of gear	$F_{en} = \sigma_{en} bYm$	12.13(a)

where σ_{en} is the endurance limit, MN/m² (kgf/mm²) (Table 12.15)

---

*The probable error (Table 12.13 and Fig. 12.4) must be less than the permissible error (Table 12.14 and Fig. 12.5)

Particular	Equation	Eqn. No.
Margin of safety of beam strength		
(a) For steady loads	$F_{en} = 1.25F_d$	12.13(b)
(b) For pulsating loads	$F_{en} = 1.35F_d$	12.13(c)
(c) For shock loads	$F_{en} = 1.50F_d$	12.13(d)
Margin of safety	$MS = \dfrac{F_{en}}{F_d} - 1$	12.14
The limiting load for wear	$F_w = d_1bQK = mz_1bQK \geq F_d$	12.15(a)

where $K = \dfrac{\sigma_{es}^2 \sin\alpha}{1.4}\left[\dfrac{1}{E_1} + \dfrac{1}{E_2}\right]$, the load stress factor (Table 12.16 and 12.17)   12.15(b)

$\qquad Q = $ the ratio factor $= 2d_2/(d_2 + d_1) = 2z_2/(z_2 + z_1)$ 12.15(c)

The surface endurance limit of a gear pair for steels may be approximately estimated   12.15(d)
by the relation MN/m² (kgf/mm²) $\sigma_{es} = [2.75(\text{BHN}) - 70]$

where (BHN) is the average Brinall hardhness number of gear and pinion for the steels

The dynamic strength of the gear	$F_s = \sigma_d bYm \geq F_d$	12.16

Cast teeth:

The tooth load

$$F_t = 0.054\sigma_d C_v bp = \dfrac{0.17\sigma_d C_v d}{p_d} = 0.17\sigma_d C_v bm \qquad \text{12.17(a)}$$

$$\text{where } C_v = \dfrac{3.05}{3.05 + v}, \text{ The velocity factor} \qquad \text{12.17(b)}$$

The face width	$b = 6m$ to $8m$	12.17(c)

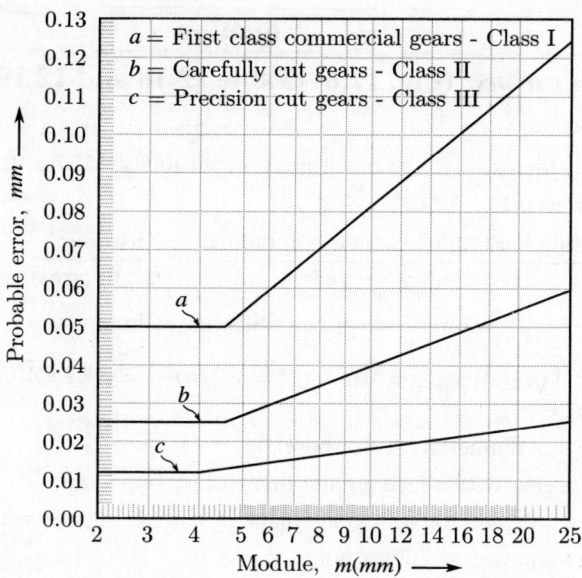

Fig. 12.4: *Probable errors in tooth profiles and spacing*

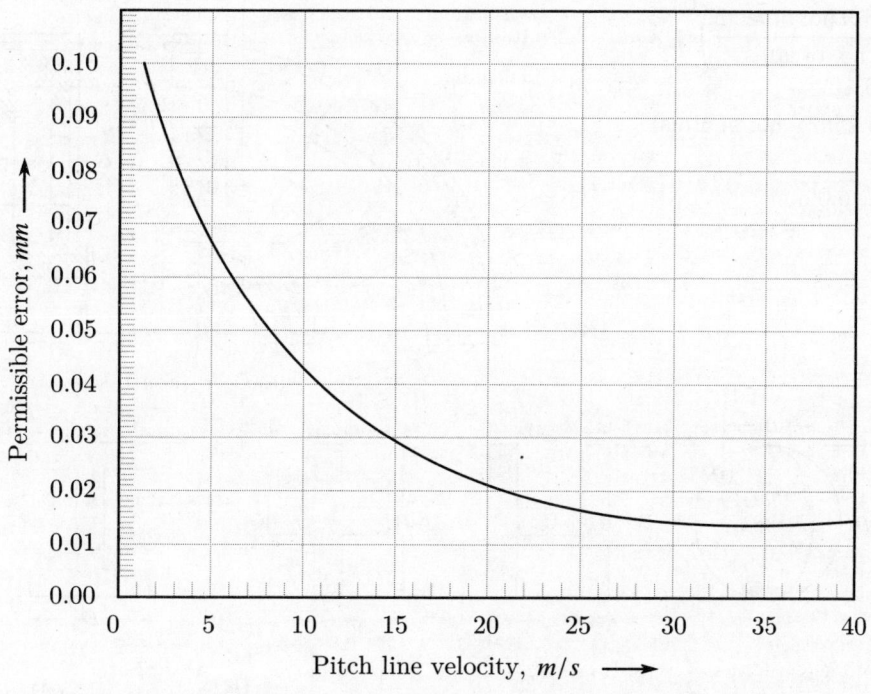

Fig. 12.5: *Permissible error in tooth profiles for quiet operation of gears*

Particular	Equation	Eqn. No.

Proportions for Gear arms: (Fig. 12.6) (Table 12.18 and 12.19)

Stalling load $\qquad$ $F = \pi \sigma_d bym$ $\qquad\qquad\qquad$ 12.18(a)

where σ_d is the stress in the material at zero velocity, MN/m^2 (kgf/mm^2)

The section modulus of arm (Fig. 12.6)

$$Z = \frac{\text{Stalling load (pitch radius–hub radius)}}{\text{no. of arms} \times \text{stress}} = \frac{\pi byma_1}{\text{no. of arms}} \qquad 12.18(b)$$

where a_1 = (pitch radius-hub radius)

The width of an elliptical or oval section arm (Fig. 12.6(b) at the hub) $\qquad$ $D = 4(Z/\pi)^{1/3} = 2.73 \sqrt[3]{Z}$ $\qquad$ 12.18(c)

$A = 0.4 \times$ bore, hence hub diameter = $1.8 \times$ bore

$B = 1.25 \times$ bore, (For a gear with a face greater than $1.25 \times$ bore, make B

$\qquad$ equal to the face width, and for split gears make B, large enough to accommodate bolts)

$C = 0.55A$, hence bead diameter = $2.24 \times$ bore

$E = (D-60)$mm taper per m

$E_1 = 0.5E$ (for split gears and oval arms)

$I = 0.25\ G$ (for split gears)

$J = \left(\dfrac{0.5 \times \text{no. of teeth}}{\text{no. of arms}}\right)^{1/3} \times m = 2.5m$ to $4m$

$K = 1.25J.$

$L = 1/(4.25m \times \text{no. of arms})$

$M = 2A$

$N = E_1 + 6.0$ mm

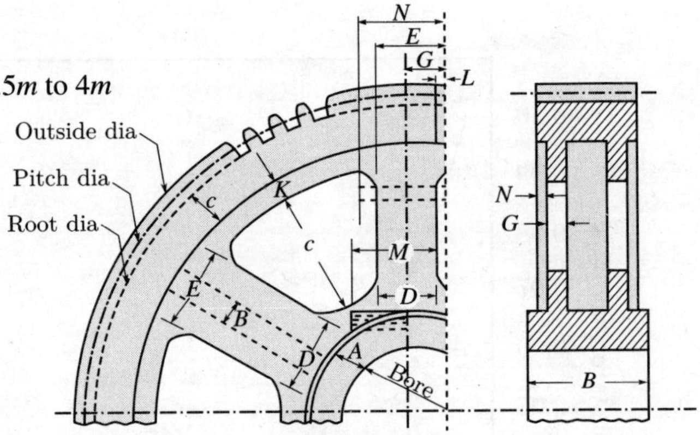

(a) Gear wheel

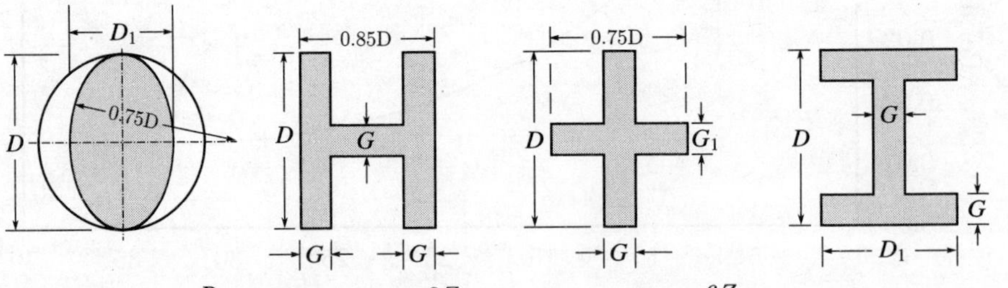

(b) Oval arm $D_1 = \dfrac{D}{2}$ (c) H arm $G = \dfrac{3Z}{D^2}$ (d) Cross arm $G = \dfrac{6Z}{D^2}$ (e) I arm

$\qquad\qquad\qquad\qquad\qquad\qquad\qquad\qquad\qquad\qquad\qquad\qquad\qquad\qquad\qquad\qquad$ $G_1 = 0.75G$ $\qquad$ $D_1 = 0.5$D to 0.6D

H=(0.1)(Face) for H-arm and cross arm $\qquad\qquad\qquad\qquad\qquad\qquad\qquad\qquad\qquad\qquad$ $G = 3Z/D^2$

Fig. 12.6: *Proportions for Gear Arms*

Particular	Equation	Eqn. No.
Helical Gears (Fig. 12.17 and 12.8)		
In case of helical gears the (transverse) circular pitch (same as spur gears)	$p = \pi d/z = p_n/\cos\beta$	
The normal circular pitch	$p_n = p\cos\beta = \dfrac{\pi d}{z}\cos\beta$ $= \pi m\cos\beta = \pi m_n$	12.19(a)
The diametral pitch	$p_d = \dfrac{\pi}{p} = \dfrac{z}{d} = \dfrac{1}{m} = \dfrac{\cos\beta}{m_n}$	
The normal diametral pitch	$p_{dn} = \dfrac{p_d}{\cos\beta} = \dfrac{z}{d\cos\beta} = \dfrac{1}{m\cos\beta} = \dfrac{1}{m_n}$	12.19(b)
The normal module (Table 12.2)	$m_n = m\cos\beta = \dfrac{d}{z}\cos\beta$	12.19(c)
The number of teeth	$z = \dfrac{d\cos\beta}{m_n} = d p_{dn}\cos\beta$	12.19(d)
Pitch circle diameter	$d = \dfrac{z}{p_d} = zm = \dfrac{z}{p_{dn}\cos\beta} = \dfrac{zm_n}{\cos\beta}$	12.19(e)
The dedendum circle diameter or root diameter	$d_r = d - 2(t_{fn} + t_{cn} - K'_n)m_n$	12.19(f)

where $t_{fn} = t_f/\cos\beta$; $t_{cn} = t_c/\cos\beta$; $K'_n = K'/\cos\beta$

The addendum circle or outside diameter	$d_o = d_r + 2h$	12.19(g)

where h = height of tooth;

$K'_{np} = K'_{ng} = 0$ for uncorrected gears; $(K'_{np}) = (-K'_{ng})$ with height correction

The center distance in an uncorrected gear or in a gear with height correction ($K'_{np} = K'_{ng}$)	$a = \left(\dfrac{z_1 + z_2}{2}\right)\dfrac{m_n}{\cos\beta}$	12.20
The axial thrust (Fig. 12.17(b))	$F_a = F_t\tan\beta$	12.21
The virtual number of teeth in the equivalent spur gear or the formative number of teeth	$z_e = \dfrac{z}{\cos^3\beta}$	12.22(a)
The relation between the pressure angle in the normal plane (α_n) and the pressure angle in the transverse plane α (Table 12.20)	$\tan\alpha_n = (\tan\alpha\cos\beta)$	12.22(b)

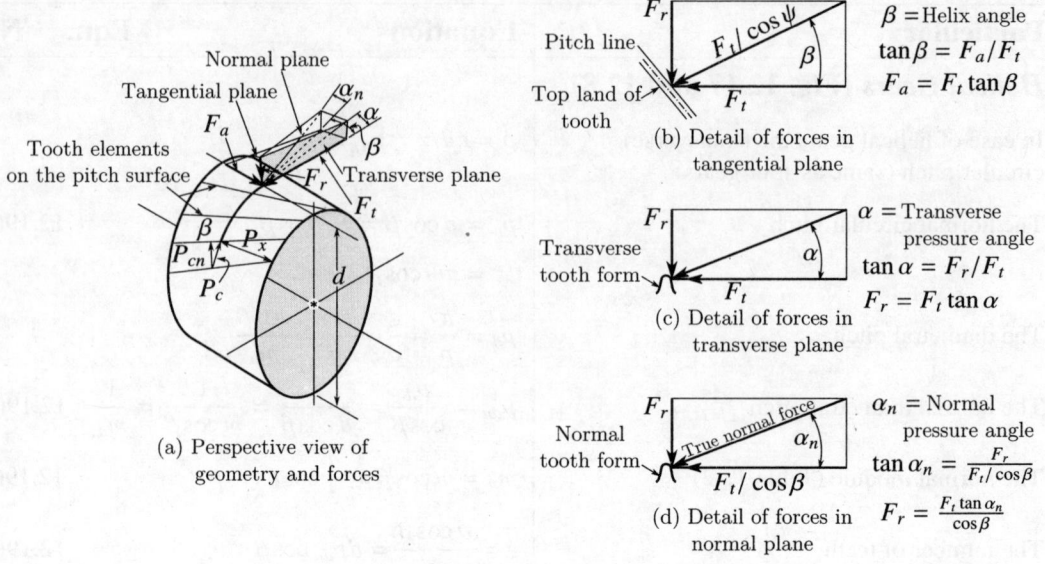

β = Helix angle

$\tan \beta = F_a / F_t$

$F_a = F_t \tan \beta$

(b) Detail of forces in tangential plane

α = Transverse pressure angle

$\tan \alpha = F_r / F_t$

$F_r = F_t \tan \alpha$

(c) Detail of forces in transverse plane

α_n = Normal pressure angle

$\tan \alpha_n = \dfrac{F_r}{F_t / \cos \beta}$

$F_r = \dfrac{F_t \tan \alpha_n}{\cos \beta}$

(d) Detail of forces in normal plane

(a) Perspective view of geometry and forces

Fig. 12.7: *Helical Gear Geometry and Forces*

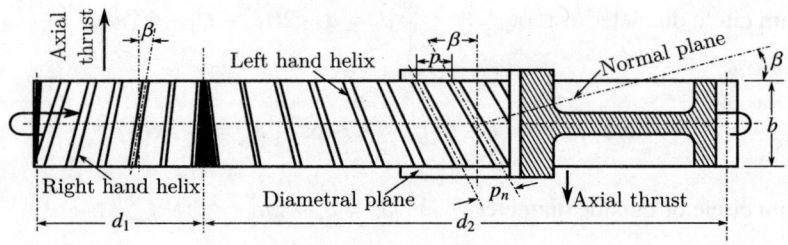

Fig. 12.7(e): *Helical Gear*

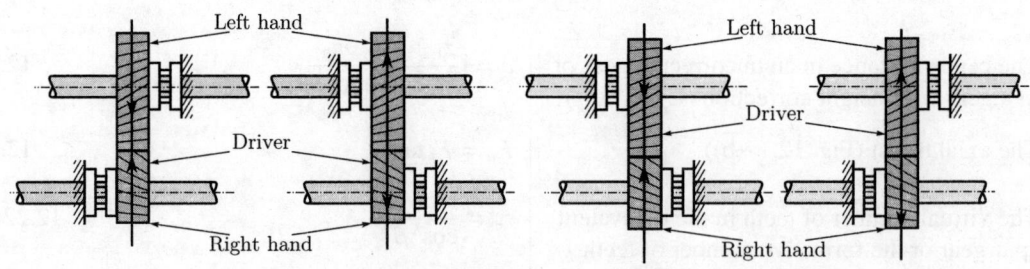

Fig. 12.7(f): *Directions of rotation and thrust for helical gears*

Particular	Equation	Eqn. No.
Helix angle and face width:		
According to Fellows practice, the minimum face width	$b = \dfrac{(1.1)\pi m}{\tan\beta} = \dfrac{1.1\pi m_n}{\sin\beta}$	12.23(a)
According to AGMA, the minimum face width	$b = \dfrac{(1.15)\pi m}{\tan\beta} = \dfrac{1.15\pi m_n}{\sin\beta}$	12.23(b)
The maximum value of face width	$b \le \dfrac{20m}{\tan\beta} \le \dfrac{20m_n}{\sin\beta}$	12.23(c)
According to AGMA the minimum value of face width for herringbone gears	$b \ge \dfrac{(2.3)\pi m}{\tan\beta} \ge \dfrac{2.3\pi m_n}{\sin\beta}$	12.23(d)
The maximum value of face width for herringbone gears, given by AGMA.	$b \le \dfrac{30m}{\tan\beta} \le \dfrac{30m_n}{\sin\beta}$	12.23(e)
For helical gears, face width	$b = 12.5m_n$ to $20m_n$	12.23(f)
For herringbone gears, face width	$b = 20m_n$ to $30m_n$	12.23(g)

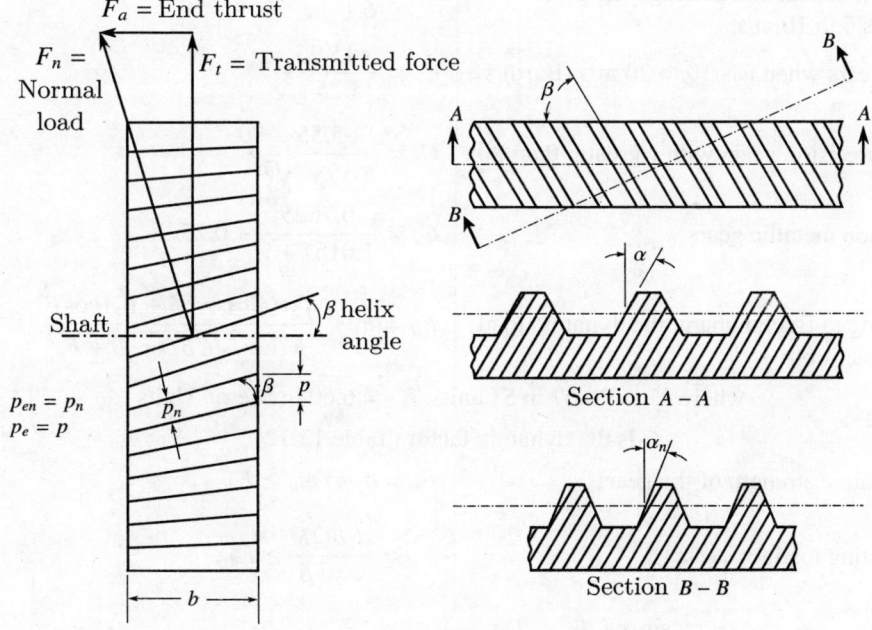

Fig. 12.8

Particular	Equation	Eqn. No.
Strength of Helical gears:		
Lewis equation for the helical or herringbone gears	$F_t = \dfrac{\sigma_d C_v bY}{P_{dn} C_w} = \dfrac{\sigma_d C_v bY m_n}{C_w}$	12.24(a)
Lewis equation for beam strength of tooth	$m_n = \left(\dfrac{F_t C_w}{\sigma_d C_v kY}\right)^{1/2} = \left(\dfrac{2M_t C_w \cos\beta}{\sigma_d C_v kYz}\right)^{\frac{1}{3}}$	12.24(b)

where σ_d is the allowable static stress (Table 12.22)

$\qquad$ C_w is the wear and lubrication factor (Table 12.21)

$\qquad$ $Y = \pi y$, form factor

$\qquad$ y is the Lewis form factor from Table 12.5 (Based on virtual number of teeth)

$\qquad$ $k = b/m_n$; m_n is the normal module (Table 12.2)

Velocity factor for Helical gears:		
(a) For low-angle helical gears when v is less than 5 m/s	$C_v = \dfrac{4.58}{4.58 + v}$	12.25(a)
(b) For all helical and herringbone gears when v is 5 to 10 m/s	$C_v = \dfrac{6.1}{6.1 + v}$	12.25(b)
(c) For gears when v is 10 to 20 m/s (Barth's formula)	$C_v = \dfrac{15.25}{15.25 + v}$	12.25(c)
(d) For precision gears with v greater than 20 m/s	$C_v = \dfrac{5.55}{5.55 + \sqrt{v}}$	12.25(d)
(e) For non metallic gears	$C_v = \dfrac{0.7625}{1.0167 + v} + 0.25$	12.25(e)
According to Buckingham, the dynamic load on the gear tooth	$F_d = F_t + \dfrac{K_3 v(Cb\cos^2\beta + F_t)\cos\beta}{K_3 v + \sqrt{Cb\cos^2\beta + F_t}}$	12.26(a)

$\qquad$ where $K_3 = 20.67$ in SI units; $K_3 = 6.60$ in Metric Units

$\qquad$ C is the dynamic factor (Table 12.12)

The dynamic strength of the gear	$F_s = \sigma_d bY m_n \geq F_d$	12.26(b)
The limiting load for wear	$F_w = \dfrac{d_1 bQK}{\cos^2\beta} \geq F_d$	12.26(c)

where $K = \dfrac{\sigma_{es}^2 \sin\alpha}{1.40}\left(\dfrac{1}{E_1} + \dfrac{1}{E_2}\right)$, load stress factor (Table 12.16 and 12.17)

$Q = 2d_2/(d_2 + 1) = 2z_2/(z_2 + z_1)$, ratio factor

Particular	Equation	Eqn. No.

Helical Gear Calculation for surface strength:

Surface compressive stress (Dobrovolsky)

$$\sigma_{sur} = 0.418 \left[\frac{M_t(i+1)^3 K_c K_n K_d E \cos\beta}{a^2 i^2 b \in \lambda \cos\alpha \sin\alpha} \right]^{\frac{1}{2}}$$

12.27

where $K_n = K_t/K_c$, load concentration factor in the pitch point

K_t is the maximum load concentration factor along the line of contact

K_c is the load concentration factor (Table 12.10)

K_d is the dynamic load factor (Table 12.11)

ϵ is the overlap factor in the circumferential cross-section

λ is the factor of variation in total length of the lines of contact

Gear calculation for beam strength:

The allowable bending stress (Dobrovolsky)

$$\sigma_d = \frac{C' M_t K_c K_d(i+1)}{aibm_n Y}$$

12.28

where $C' = 0.75$ to 0.50 for helix angle $\beta = 8°$ to $45°$

Bevel Gears (Fig. 12.9 and 12.10)
Angle relations:

(a) Acute angle Bevel gears: (Fig. 12.10)

The pitch angle of pinion

$$\tan\delta_1 = \frac{d_1 \sin\theta}{d_1 + d_1 \cos\theta} = \frac{\sin\theta}{\frac{z_2}{z_1} + \cos\theta}$$
$$= \frac{\sin\theta}{i + \cos\theta}$$

12.29(a)

The pitch angle of gear

$$\tan\delta_2 = \frac{d_2 \sin\theta}{d_1 + d_2 \cos\theta} = \frac{\sin\theta}{\frac{z_1}{z_2} + \cos\theta}$$
$$= \frac{\sin\theta}{\frac{1}{i} + \cos\theta}$$

12.29(b)

The addendum angle

$$\tan\delta_a = \frac{2h_{a1} \sin\delta_1}{d_1} = \frac{2h_{a2} \sin\delta_2}{d_2}$$

12.29(c)

The dedendum angle

$$\tan\theta_d = \frac{2h_{f1} \sin\delta_1}{d_1} = \frac{2h_{f2} \sin\delta_2}{d_2}$$

12.29(d)

where h_{a1}, h_{a2} are addendum of the pinion and gear respectively, mm (Table 12.23)

h_{f1}, h_{f2} are dedendum of pinion and gear respectively, mm (Table 12.23)

The outside diameter of the pinion

$$d_{o1} = d_1 + 2h_{a1} \cos\delta_1$$

12.30(a)

The outside diameter of the gear

$$d_{o2} = d_1 + 2h_{a2} \cos\delta_2$$

12.30(b)

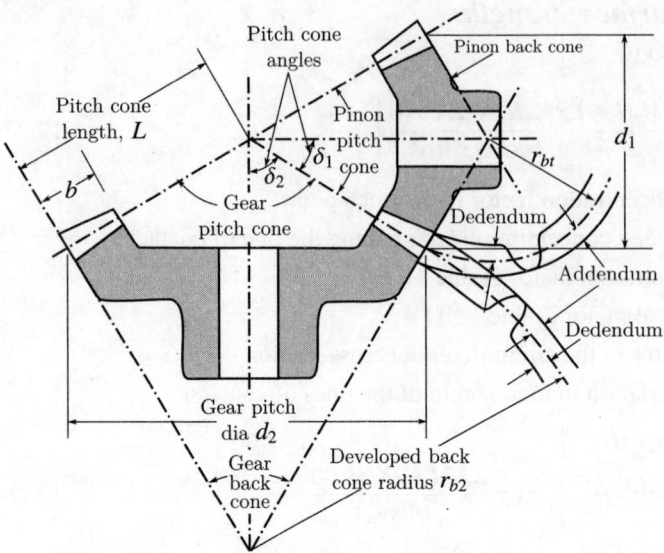

Fig. 12.9(a): *Bevel gear terminology and definitions*

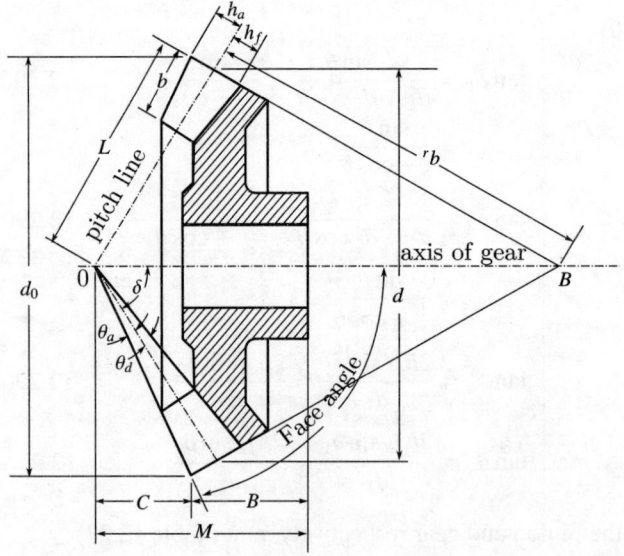

Fig. 12.9(b): *Bevel gear terminology and definitions*

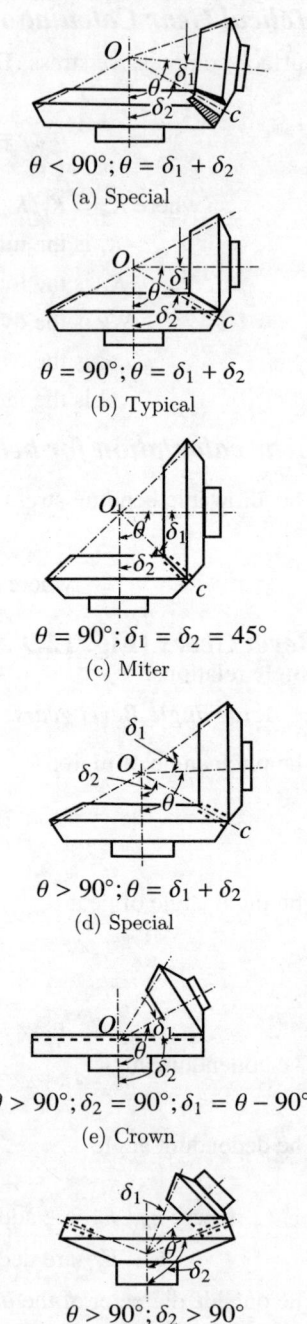

$\theta < 90°; \theta = \delta_1 + \delta_2$

(a) Special

$\theta = 90°; \theta = \delta_1 + \delta_2$

(b) Typical

$\theta = 90°; \delta_1 = \delta_2 = 45°$

(c) Miter

$\theta > 90°; \theta = \delta_1 + \delta_2$

(d) Special

$\theta > 90°; \delta_2 = 90°; \delta_1 = \theta - 90°$

(e) Crown

$\theta > 90°; \delta_2 > 90°$

(f) Internal

Fig. 12.9(c): *Types of bevel gears*

Particular	Equation	Eqn. No.
(b) Obtuse angle bevel gears:		
The pitch angle of pinion	$\tan \delta_1 = \dfrac{\sin(180 - \theta)}{\dfrac{z_2}{z_1} - \cos(180 - \theta)}$	12.31(a)
The pitch angle of the gear	$\tan \delta_2 = \dfrac{\sin(180 - \theta)}{\dfrac{z_1}{z_2} - \cos(180° - \theta)}$	12.31(b)
(c) Right angle bevel gears:		
The pitch angle of pinion	$\tan \delta_1 = \dfrac{d_1}{d_2} = \dfrac{z_1}{z_2} = \dfrac{1}{i}$	12.32(a)
The pitch angle of the gear	$\tan \delta_2 = \dfrac{d_2}{d_1} = \dfrac{z_2}{z_1} = i$	12.32(b)
The cone distance (Fig. 12.9)	$L = \dfrac{1}{2} \sqrt{d_1^2 + d_2^2} = \dfrac{d_2}{2 \sin \delta_2} = \dfrac{d_1}{2 \sin \delta_1}$	12.33
	where d_1 and d_2 are the pitch circle diameters on the larger diameter of pinion and gear respectively	
The pitch circle diameter	$d = mz$	12.34(a)
The mean diameter	$d_m = \left(1 - \dfrac{0.5}{k_2}\right) d$	12.34(b)
The mean module	$m_m = \left(1 - \dfrac{0.5}{k_2}\right) m$ where $k_2 = L/b$	12.34(c)

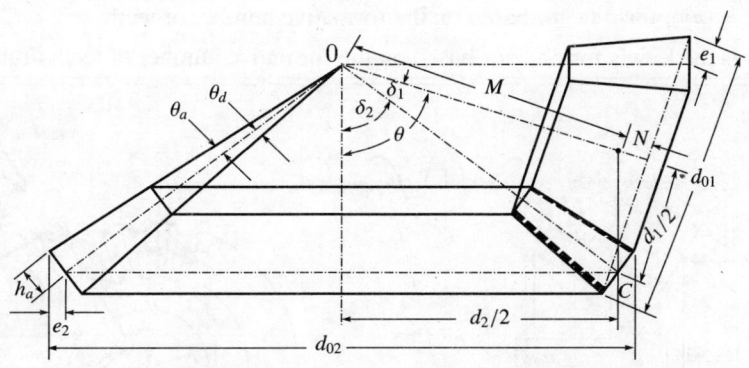

Fig. 12.10: *Acute-angle bevel gears*

Particular	Equation	Eqn. No.

Proportions of Bevel gears in terms of equivalent spur gears (Fig. 12.11)

The equivalent pitch circle diameter	$d_e = d/\cos\delta$	12.35(a)
The equivalent outside circle diameter	$d_{oe} = d_o/\cos\delta$	12.35(b)
The equivalent gear ratio	$i_e = i^2$	12.35(c)
The equivalent teeth or the formative number of teeth for straight bevel gears	$z_e = z/\cos\delta$	12.35(d)
The equivalent teeth for spiral bevel gears	$z_e = \dfrac{z}{\cos\delta\cos^3\beta_m}$	12.35(e)

where β_m = angle of tooth inclination at the middle of the face width

$$= \beta\left(1 + \frac{0.5}{k_2}\right) \quad \text{and} \quad \tan\beta \geq \frac{\pi m}{v}\left(1 - \frac{1}{k_2}\right)$$

Width of Bevel gear face:

The width of bevel gear face	$b \geq 6m;\ b \leq 10m$	12.36(a)
	$b \leq L/3$	12.36(b)
The width of gear face as per the practice of Gleason Works	$b = 6m$ to $7m$ if $L < 30m$	12.36(c)
	$b = 7m$ to $10m$ if $L > 30m$	12.36(d)

Strength of cut teeth:

The equivalent tangential force at large end as per Lewis equation for bevel gears (Fig. 12.12)

$$F_t = \frac{\sigma_d C_v bY}{p_d}\left(\frac{L-b}{L}\right) = \sigma_d C_v bYm\left(\frac{L-b}{L}\right) \tag{12.37}$$

where σ_d = allowable static stress (Table 12.7)

p_d = diametral pitch at large end (Table 12.25)

m = module at large end (Table 12.24)

$Y = (\pi y)$, form factor based on the formative number of teeth

y is the Lewis form factor based on the formative number of teeth (Table 12.5)

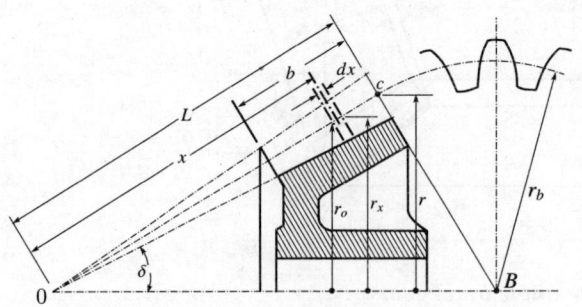

Fig. 12.11: *Strength determination of a bevel gear tooth*

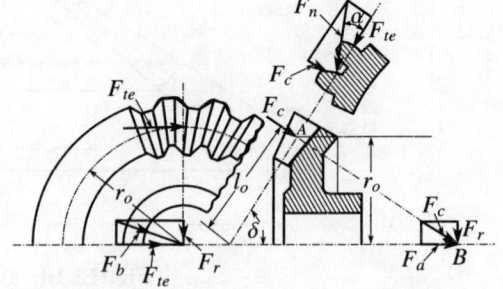

Fig. 12.12: *Tooth-loads on bevel gears*

Particular	Equation	Eqn. No.
The velocity factor for bevel gears		
(a) when the teeth are cut by form cutters	$C_v = \dfrac{3.05}{3.05 + v}$	12.38(a)
(b) For generated teeth	$C_v = \dfrac{6.1}{6.1 + v}$	12.38(b)
The beam or Endurance strength of bevel gear teeth	$F_{en} = \sigma_{en} b Y m \left(\dfrac{L - b}{L} \right)$	12.39
The dynamic load equation for bevel gears (same as spur gear (Eqn. 12.12))	$F_d = F_t + \dfrac{K_3 v (Cb + F_t)}{K_3 v + \sqrt{Cb + F_t}}$	12.40
The limit load for wear	$F_w = \dfrac{d_1 b Q_e K}{\cos \delta_1}$ where $Q_e = 2z_{e2}/(z_{e2} + z_{e1})$, the ratio factor	12.41
The allowable bending stress (Dobrovolsky)	$\sigma = \dfrac{k_2^2 M_t K_c K_d (\sqrt{i^2 + 1})}{n i Y (k_2 - 0.5)^2 L^2 \cos \alpha} < \sigma_d$ where $k_2 = L/b$	12.42
The normal power transmitted		

$$P(kW) = \frac{F_t v}{1000} = \frac{F_t \pi d_o n}{1000 \times 1000} \quad \text{(S.I. Units)} \qquad \text{12.43(a)}$$

$$P(MHP) = \frac{F_t v}{75} = \frac{F_t \pi d_o n}{75 \times 1000} \quad \text{(Metric Units)}$$

Surface Strength of Bevel Gear

Surface compressive stress (Dobrovolsky)	$\sigma_{sur} = \dfrac{1050}{(L - 0.5b)i} \sqrt{\dfrac{(L^2 + 1)^{3/2}}{b} M_t K_c K_d}$	12.44
Bearing loads on straight bevel gears: (Fig. 12.12)		
The effective tooth load	$F_{te} = \dfrac{T}{r_0} = \dfrac{F_t l}{l - 0.5b}$	12.45(a)

where $r_0 = r\left(\dfrac{l - 0.5b}{l}\right)$ is the radius of the application of the effective tooth load

The effetive normal tooth load,	$F_n = F_{te}/\cos \alpha$	12.45(b)
The load along pitch cone line AB (Fig. 12.12)	$F_c = F_n \sin \alpha = Fte \tan \alpha$	12.45(c)
The lateral or radial load	$F_r = F_c \cos \delta = F_{te} \tan \alpha \cos \delta$	12.45(d)
The axial load or thrust	$F_a = F_c \sin \delta = F_{te} \tan \alpha \sin \delta$	12.45(e)
The total lateral load on the bearings	$F_b = \sqrt{F_{te}^2 + F_r^2} = F_{te} \sqrt{1 + (\tan \alpha \cos \delta)^2}$	12.45(f)

Particular	Equation	Eqn. No.

Worm Gears (Fig. 12.13) (Table 12.26 and 12.27)

The linear or axial pitch of the worm (Fig. 12.14)

$$p_c = p_2 \qquad \qquad 12.46(a)$$

where $p_2 = \dfrac{\pi}{p_{d_2}} = \dfrac{\pi d_2}{z_2} = \pi m_2$, Circular pitch of the worm gear, mm

p_{d2} is the diametral pitch of worm gear

The lead, mm $\qquad l = z_1 p_c = z_1 p_2 = \pi m_2 z_1 = \pi m_1 z_1 \tan r \qquad \qquad 12.46(b)$

where $l = p_2 = \pi m_2$, for single-thread worm

$\qquad = 2p_2 = 2\pi m_2$, for double-thread worm

$\qquad = 3p_2 = 3\pi m_2$, for triple-thread worm etc.

z_1 is the numbe threads of the worm

z_2 is the number of teeth on worm gear

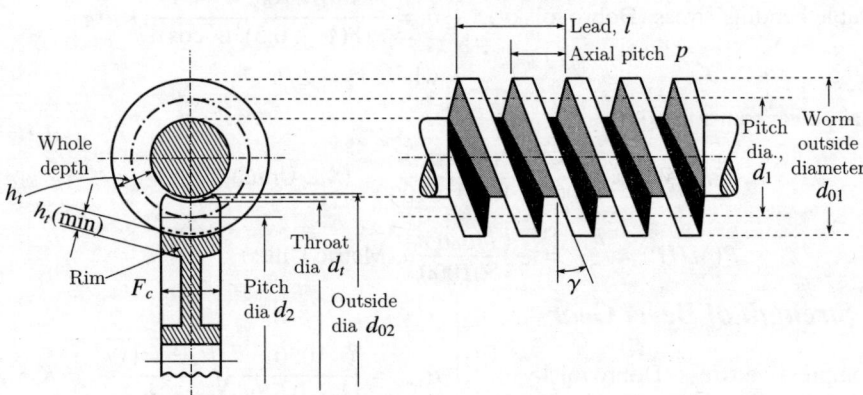

Fig. 12.13(a): Worm and Worm gear terminology

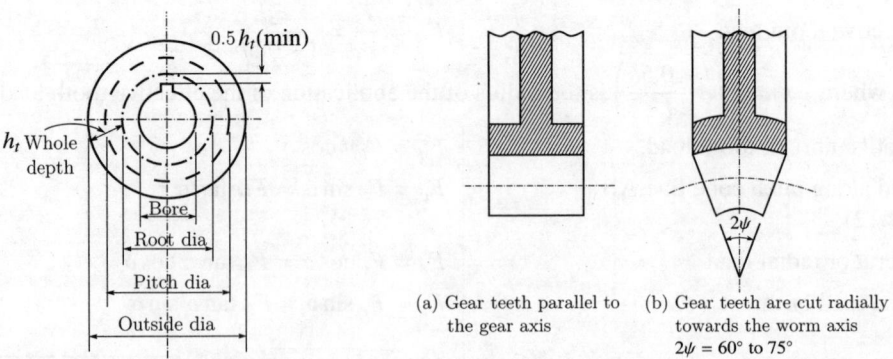

Fig. 12.13(b): Shell worm

(a) Gear teeth parallel to the gear axis

(b) Gear teeth are cut radially towards the worm axis $2\psi = 60°$ to $75°$

Fig. 12.13(c): Types of worm gear teeth

Particular	Equation	Eqn. No.
The normal circular pitch (Fig. 12.14)	$p_n = p_1 \sin \gamma = p_2 \cos \gamma$ $= \pi m_1 \sin \gamma = \pi m_2 \cos \gamma$	12.46(c)
The normal lead (Fig. 12.14)	$l_n = l \cos \gamma = \pi m_2 z_1 \cos \gamma$	12.46(d)
The lead angle (Table 12.28(a))	$\tan \gamma = \dfrac{l}{\pi d_1} = \dfrac{z_1 p_c}{z_1 p_1} = \dfrac{z_1 p_2}{z_1 p_1} = \dfrac{p_2}{p_1} = \dfrac{V_2}{V_1}$	12.46(e)
The normal diametral pitch	$p_{dn} = \dfrac{\pi}{p_n} = \dfrac{\pi}{p_1 \sin \gamma} = \dfrac{\pi}{p_2 \cos \gamma}$	12.46(f)
The module of worm	$m_1 = m_2 / \tan \gamma$	12.46(g)
Pitch diameter of worm		
	$d_1 = \dfrac{z_1 p_1}{\pi} = \dfrac{z_1 p_n}{\pi \sin \gamma} = \dfrac{z_1}{p_{dn} \sin \gamma} = \dfrac{z_1 p_2}{\pi \tan \gamma} = \dfrac{z_1 m_2}{\tan \gamma}$	12.46(h)
Pitch diameter of gear		
	$d_2 = \dfrac{z_2 p_2}{\pi} = \dfrac{z_2 p_n}{\pi \cos \gamma} = \dfrac{z_2}{p_{dn} \cos \gamma} = z_2 m_2$	12.46(i)

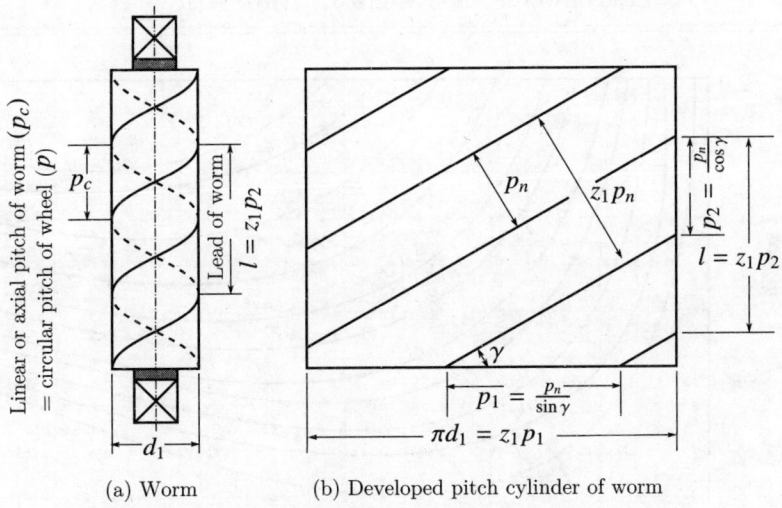

(a) Worm   (b) Developed pitch cylinder of worm

Fig. 12.14: *Geometry of the worm*

Particular	Equation	Eqn. No.
The centre distance (Fig. 12.15)	$a = \left(\dfrac{d_1 + d_2}{2}\right)$	12.47(a)
	$= \left(\dfrac{1}{2p_{dn}}\right)\left\{\dfrac{z_1}{\sin\gamma} + \dfrac{z_2}{\cos\gamma}\right\}$	12.47(b)
	$= \left(\dfrac{m_2\cos\gamma}{2}\right)\left\{\dfrac{z_1}{\sin\gamma} + \dfrac{z_2}{\cos\gamma}\right\}$	12.47(c)
from the above equation 12.47(b) and (c)	$\left(\dfrac{2p_{dn}}{z_2}\right)a = \left\{\dfrac{(z_1/z_2)}{\sin\gamma} + \dfrac{1}{\cos\gamma}\right\}$ or	12.47(d)
	$\left(\dfrac{2}{z_2 m_2\cos\gamma}\right)a = \left\{\dfrac{(z_1/z_2)}{\sin\gamma} + \dfrac{1}{\cos\gamma}\right\}$	12.47(e)

where p_1 and p_2 are the circular pitches of worm and worm gear respectively, mm

m_1 and m_2 are the modules of worm and worm gear respectively, mm

d_1 and d_2 are the pitch diameters of worm and worm gear respectively, mm

The pitch line velocity of the worm, m/s	$v_1 = \dfrac{\pi d_1 n_1}{1000} = \dfrac{n_1 z_1 p_1}{1000}$	12.48(a)
The pitch line velocity of the gear, m/s	$v_2 = \dfrac{\pi d_2 n_2}{1000} = \dfrac{n_2 z_2 p_2}{1000} = \dfrac{n_1 z_1 p_2}{1000}$	12.48(b)

where n_1 and n_2 are the speeds of worm and gear respectively, m/s

Velocity ratio

$$v_r = \frac{\text{pitch circumference of gear}}{\text{Lead of worm}} = \frac{\pi d_2}{z_1 p_c} = \frac{z_2 p_2}{z_1 p_c} = \frac{z_2 p_2}{z_1 p_2} = \frac{z_2}{z_1} \qquad 12.48(c)$$

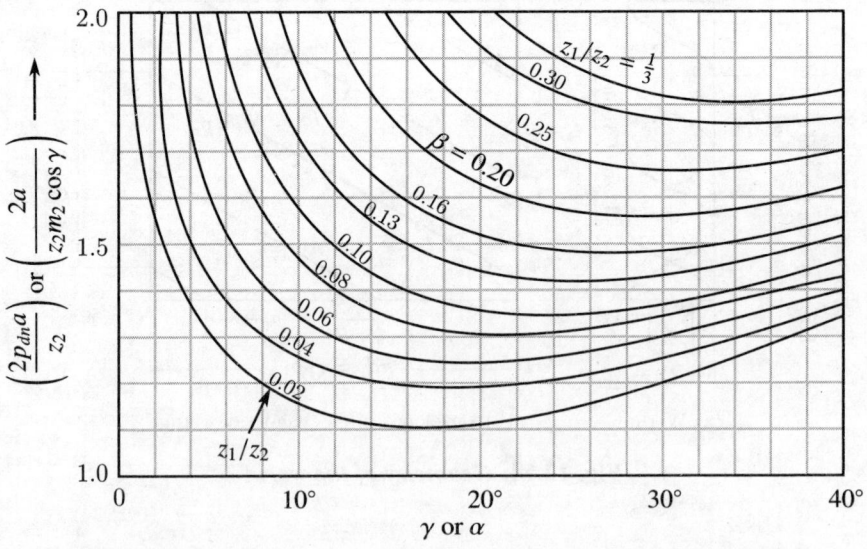

Fig. 12.15: *Design chart for worm and helical gears for* 90° *shafts*

Particular	Equation	Eqn. No.
The module	$$m = \frac{2a}{q + z_2}$$ where $q = d_1/m = 6$ to 13, number of modules in the pitch diameter of the worm	12.49
The centre distance (Dobrovolsky)	$$a = \left[\frac{z_2}{q} + 1\right]\left[\left(\frac{540}{\frac{z_2}{q}\sigma_{sur}}\right)^2 M_t K_c K_d\right]^{\frac{1}{3}}$$ where σ_{sur} is the allowable surface stress	12.50
For speed reducers with integral worms, the AGMA recommends a mean (pitch) worm diameter	$$d_1 = \frac{a^{0.875}}{1.466}$$	12.51(a)
For maximum power transmitting capacity, the pitch diameter of worm	$$\frac{a^{0.875}}{3.0} \leq d_1 \leq \frac{a^{0.875}}{1.6}$$	12.51(b)
The recommended value for the face angle or width angle (Fig. 12.13(c))	$$\tan\psi \leq \frac{\tan\alpha}{\tan\gamma}$$	12.52(a)
For a compact design the lead angle may be selected approximately from the relation	$\tan\gamma = \sqrt[3]{n_2/n_1}$ where ψ is the face angle, deg	12.52(b)

Strength of worm gear teeth:

Particular	Equation	Eqn. No.
The permissible tooth load according to Lewis equation	$$F_t = \frac{\sigma_d C_v bY}{p_d} = \sigma_d C_v bYm$$ where $Y = \pi y$, is the form factor; y is the Lewis form factor (from Table 12.5 and 12.6)	12.53(a)
If the number of the teeth in the worm gear plus the number of threads in 25 mm length in the worm is greater than 40, Y may be determined from the equation	$Y = 0.314 + 0.015(\alpha - 14.5°)$	12.53(b)
The velocity factor	$C_v = (3.05)/(3.05 + v)$ $= (6.1)/(6.1 + v)$ which takes into account the dynamic load	12.53(c)
The permissible tooth load	$$F_t = \frac{2M_{te}}{d_2}$$ where $M_{te} = M_t K_l$, the effective torque K_l is the load factor from Table 12.33	12.53(d)
The dynamic strength of gears	$F_s = \sigma_d bYm$	12.54
The allowable bending stress (Dobrovolsky)	$$\sigma_b = \frac{1.9 M_t K_c K_d \cos\gamma}{m^3 q z_2 Y} \leq \sigma_d$$ where $q = 6$ to 13, the number of modulus in the pitch diameter of worm	12.55

Particular	Equation	Eqn. No.

Forces acting between worm thread and worm gear tooth (Fig. 12.16)

Neglecting frictional resistance,

Normal reaction along (Fig. 12.16)

(i) The axis-OX	$F_{Nx} = F_N \cos\theta \cos\gamma$	12.56(a)
(ii) The axis-OY	$F_{Ny} = F_N \sin\theta$	12.56(b)
(iii) The axis-OZ	$F_{Nz} = F_N \cos\theta \sin\gamma$	12.56(c)

where θ is the angle between F_n and the plane X-Z

$$\tan\theta = \tan\alpha \cos\gamma \qquad \text{12.56(d)}$$

When the worm turns the worm gear

(a) The force due to friction between the worm and the gear teeth acting along the tangent to the helix	$F'_N = \mu F_N$	12.56(e)
(b) The friction force along		
(i) the axis-OX	$F'_{Nx} = \mu F_N \sin\gamma$	12.56(f)
(ii) the axis-OY	$F'_{Ny} = 0$	12.56(g)
(iii) the axis-OZ	$F'_{Nz} = \mu F_N \cos\gamma$	12.56(h)

$R = F_y$, the magnitude of the downward pressure upon the worm staft or the upward pressure upon the worm-gear shaft

$Q = F_z$, the turning force on a worm

$F_t = F_x$, the tangential load on the worm gear

x-axis is parallel to the axis of the worm

y-axis is in the radial direction on the worm

z-axis is in the tangential direction for the worm normal to the plane X-Y

F_N is the normal reaction between the worm and a gear tooth at the point of contact '0'

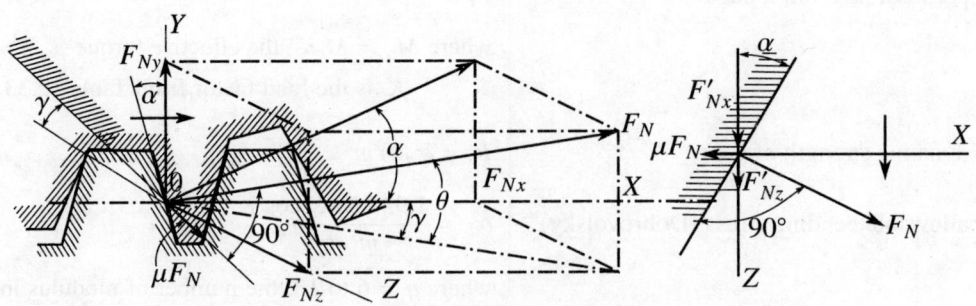

Fig. 12.16: *Forces for worm gearing*

Particular	Equation	Eqn. No.

The magnitude of the tangential driving force exerted by the worm upon the worm-gear teeth

$$F_t = F_x = F_{Nx} - F'_{Nx} = F_N(\cos\theta\cos\gamma - \mu\sin\gamma) = Q\frac{\cos\theta\cos\gamma - \mu\sin\gamma}{\cos\theta\sin\gamma + \mu\cos\gamma} \qquad 12.56(i)$$

The magnitude of the turning force required at the pitch radius of the worm

$$Q = F_z = F_{Nz} + F'_{Nz} = F_N(\cos\theta\sin\gamma - \mu\cos\gamma) = F_t\frac{\cos\theta\sin\gamma + \mu\cos\gamma}{\cos\theta\cos\gamma - \mu\sin\gamma} \qquad 12.56(j)$$

The downward pressure (separating force) upon the worm shaft or the upward pressure upon the worm-gear shaft

$$R = F_y = F_{Ny} = F_N\sin\theta = F_t\frac{\sin\theta}{\cos\theta\cos\gamma - \mu\sin\gamma} \qquad 12.56(k)$$

Efficiency of worm gearing:

Particular	Equation	Eqn. No.
The magnitude of the turning force when there is no friction ($\mu = 0$)	$Q' = F_t\dfrac{\cos\theta\sin\gamma}{\cos\theta\cos\gamma} = F_t\tan\gamma$	12.57(a)
The efficiency when the worm drives the worm wheel (Fig. 12.16)	$\eta = \dfrac{Q'}{Q} = \dfrac{\cos\theta - \mu\tan\gamma}{\cos\theta + \mu\cot\gamma}$	12.57(b)
The efficiency when the worm gear drives the worm	$\eta = \dfrac{\cos\theta - \mu\cot\gamma}{\cos\theta + \mu\tan\gamma}$	12.57(c)
Barr's formula for the efficiency of worm gearing	$\eta = \dfrac{\tan\gamma(1 - \mu\tan\gamma)}{\mu + \tan\gamma}$	12.57(d)

Conditions for maximum efficiency:

The lead angle which gives the best efficiency:

Particular	Equation	Eqn. No.
(a) when worm drives the wheel	$\gamma = 45 - \dfrac{1}{2}\tan^{-1}(\mu/\cos\theta)$	12.58(a)
(b) when wheel drives the worm	$\gamma = 45 + \dfrac{1}{2}\tan^{-1}(\mu/\cos\theta)$	12.58(b)

Losses in the thrust bearing:

Taking into consideration the losses in the thrust bearing:

(a) Resulting turning force on the worm

$$F_z = F_x\left[\frac{\left(\cos\theta(\sin\gamma + \frac{\mu'D'}{d_1}\cos\gamma)\right)}{\cos\theta\cos\gamma - \mu\sin\gamma} + \frac{\left(\mu(\cos\gamma - \frac{\mu'D'}{d_1}\sin\gamma)\right)}{\cos\theta\cos\gamma - \mu\sin\gamma}\right] \qquad 12.59(a)$$

(b) Resulting turning force on the worm wheel

$$F_x = F_z\frac{\cos\theta\cos\gamma + \mu\sin\gamma}{\cos\theta\left(\sin\gamma - \frac{\mu'D'}{d_1}\cos\gamma\right) - \mu\left(\cos\gamma + \frac{\mu'D'}{d_1}\sin\gamma\right)} \qquad 12.59(b)$$

Particular	**Equation**	**Eqn. No.**

(c) Efficiency when the worm drives the wheel

$$\eta = \frac{(\cos\theta - \mu\tan\gamma)}{\cos\theta\left(1 + \dfrac{\mu'D'}{d_1}\cot\gamma\right) + \mu\left(\cot\gamma - \dfrac{\mu'D'}{d_1}\right)}$$ 12.59(c)

(d) Efficiency when the wheel drives the worm

$$\eta = \frac{\cos\theta\left(1 - \dfrac{\mu'D'}{d_1}\cot\gamma\right) - \mu\left(\cot\gamma + \dfrac{\mu'D'}{d_1}\right)}{(\cos\theta + \mu\tan\gamma)}$$ 12.59(d)

where μ = coefficient of friction between worm and worm wheel

μ' = coefficient of friction in thrust bearing

F_n = N = Normal force acting on tooth at the pitch point, N (kgf)

F_x = Resulting turning force on the worm wheel, N (kgf)

F_z = Resulting turning force on the worm, N (kgf)

F_y = The force which tends to separate the axes, N (kgf)

The coefficient of friction

$$\mu = \frac{0.0422}{(v_r)^{0.28}}, \text{ for } 0.2 \text{ m/s} < v < 2.75 m/s$$ 12.60(a)

$$= 0.025 + \frac{3.281}{1000}v_r, \text{ for speeds greater than 2.75 m/s}$$ 12.60(b)

Note: (1) Using best materials for the worm and the worm gear, with precision machining, and with good lubrication, $\mu \approx 0.025$

with (2) load speeds with indifferent lubrication $\mu \approx 0.10$

where $v_r = \dfrac{\pi d_1 n_1}{1000\cos\gamma}$, rubbing velocity, m/s

$v_r \ngtr 6$ m/s, for ordinary industrial worms

$\ngtr 15$ m/s, for well-designed, hardered and ground worms

With best load angle, the lowest friction coefficient,

the best thrust bearing and the best lubrication,

the empirical equation given by De Lavas for $\eta = 1 - 0.005 r_v$ 12.61

the efficiency of worm gearing ($r_v > 8$)

where r_v is the speed ratio of the worm and the gear

Particular	Equation	Eqn. No.

Wear load and heat Dissipation:

The limiting load for wear

$$F_w = d_2 b K$$ 12.62(a)

where K is the load stress factor from Table 12.30

Another formula for the limiting wear load, which takes into account the various gear data and assumes the use of the proper grade of lubricant

$$F_w = \frac{A \cos \gamma C_v \sigma_c}{C_s}$$ 12.62(b)

where $A = \dfrac{h d_1 \psi}{57.3}$, projected tooth area of contact, mm^2

h is the depth of tooth, mm from Table 12.26

ψ is the one half of the face angle, deg

C_s is the Service factor form Table 12.31

σ_c is the allowable surface pressure, MN/m^2, (kgf/mm^2) (Table 12.32)

$C_v = \dfrac{3.05}{3.05 + v}$, Barth's velocity factor for the worm

Heat dissipation:

The amount of heat generated, J/s (kgf m/s)

$$Q = \frac{\mu F_n v_r}{\cos \gamma}$$ 12.63(a)

where F_n is the force normal to the tooth surface, N (kgf)

The heat to be dissipated, J/s

$$Q = 1000(kW)(1 - \eta)$$ 12.63(b)

Another form of equation for heat to be dissipated, J/s

$$Q = \frac{0.407}{10^3}(A_g + A_w)(t_2 - t_1)$$ 12.63(c)

where $A_w = L_w d_1$, projected area of the worm, mm^2; $A_g = \dfrac{\pi}{4} d_2^2$, area of the worm gear, mm^2

t_2 is the gear temperature, °C; t_1 is the room temperature, °C

For speed reducers with integral worms, the AGMA recommends a face, mm

$$b = \frac{a^{0.875}}{2.0}$$ 12.64

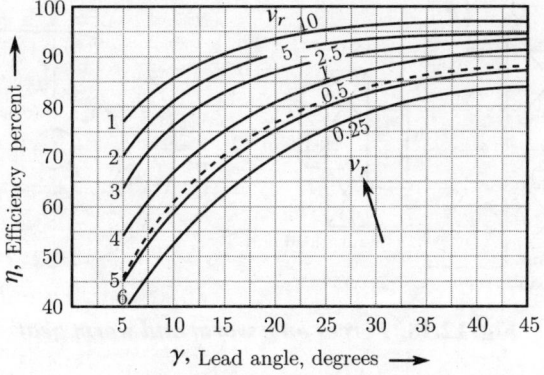

Fig. 12.17: *Efficiencies of worm drives*

Particular	Equation	Eqn. No.

Bearing loads in worm gearing: (Fig. 12.18)   *

(1) Worm gear shaft:

The resultant radial load at bearing D

$$R_D = \left[\frac{F_x^2}{4} + \left(\frac{F_y}{2} + \frac{F_z d_2}{2L} \right)^2 \right]^{\frac{1}{2}}$$ 12.65(a)

The resultant radial load at bearing C

$$R_C = \left[\frac{F_x^2}{4} + \left(\frac{F_y}{2} - \frac{F_z d_2}{2L} \right)^2 \right]^{\frac{1}{2}}$$ 12.65(b)

where L = distance between bearings C and D

(2) Worm shaft:

The resultant radial load at bearing B

$$R_B = \left[\frac{F_z^2}{4} + \left(\frac{F_y}{2} - \frac{F_x d_1}{2L'} \right)^2 \right]^{\frac{1}{2}}$$ 12.66

The resultant radial load at bearing A

$$R_A = \left[\frac{F_z^2}{4} + \left(\frac{F_y}{2} + \frac{F_x d_1}{2L'} \right)^2 \right]^{\frac{1}{2}}$$ 12.67

where L' = distance between the bearings A and B

The limiting input Power rating of a plain worm gear unit from the stand point of heat dissipation, for worm gear speeds up to 2,000 rpm

$$P(kW) = 0.02905 \frac{a^{1.7}}{i' + 5} \quad \text{(SI units)}$$ 12.68(a)

$$P(MHP) = 0.0395 \frac{a^{1.7}}{i' + 5} \quad \text{(Metric units)}$$ 12.68(b)

where a = center distance, mm

$i' = \dfrac{n_1}{n_2}$, transmission ratio

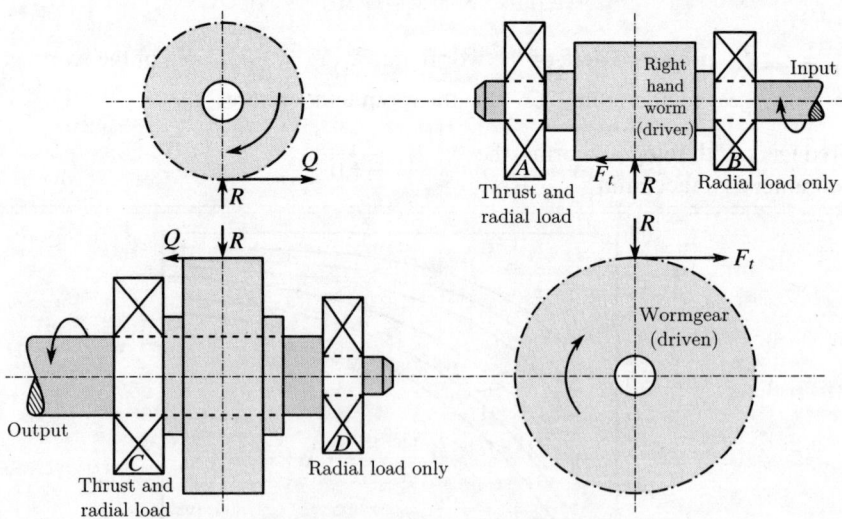

Fig. 12.18: *Forces on a worm and worm gear*

*It is assumed that the bearings C and D, Fig. 12.18, are located symmetrically with respect to the middle plane of the gear

Table 12.1 *Recommended Series of Diametral Pitches*

p_d	20 (18) 16 (14) 12 (11) 10 (9) 8 (7) 6 (5.5) 5 (4.5) 4 (3.5) 3 (2.75) 2.50
	(2.25) 2.0 (1.75) 1.50 1.25 1.00 (0.875) 0.625 0.50

Note: The diametral pitches given in Table 12.3 applies to straight and helical gears. The diametral pitches with in the brackets are of second preference.

Table 12.2 *Recommended Series of Modules (mm)*

Preferred (1)	Choice 2 (2)	Choice 3 (3)	Preferred (1)	Choice 2 (2)	Choice 3 (3)
1			8	7	(6.5)
1.25	1.125		10	9	
1.5	1.375		12	11	
2	1.75		16	14	
2.5	2.25		20	18	
3	2.75	(3.25)	25	22	
4	3.5		32	28	
5	4.5	(3.75)	40	36	
6	5.5		50	45	

Note: The modules given in the above table apply to spur and helical gears. In case of helical gears and double helical gears, the modules represent normal modules
Modules with in brackets are of second preference

IS:2535–1969

Table 12.3 *Standard Tooth Proportions of Involute Spur Gears*

Gear Terms	Proportions of Machine cut teeth		
	Circular pitch p	Diametral pitch P	Module m
Addendum (h_a)	0.3183 p	1/P	m
Dedendum (h_f)	0.3977 p	1.25/P	1.25 m
Tooth thickness (t)	0.5 p	1.5708/P	1.5708 m
Tooth space	0.5 p	1.5708/P	1.5708 m
Working depth	0.6366 p	2/P	2 m
Whole depth	0.7160 p	2.25/P	2.25 m
Clearance	0.0794 p	0.25/P	0.25 m
Pitch diameter (d)	zp/π	z/P	zm
Outside diameter (d_o)	$(z+2)p/\pi$	$(z+2)/P$	$(z+2)m$
Root diameter (d_r)	$(z-2.5)p/\pi$	$(z-2.5)/P$	$(z-2.5)m$
Fillet radius (r)	0.1273 p	0.4/P	0.4 m

Table 12.4 (a) *Properties of Involute Teeth (American Standard)*

Tooth characteristics	Cast teeth	$14\frac{1}{2}°$ system	Full depth 20° system	Stub teeth system
Pressure angle (deg)	15	$14\frac{1}{2}$	20	20
Addendum (mm)	0.943m	m	m	0.8m
Minimum dedendum (mm)	1.257m	1.157m	1.157m	m
Minimum total depth (mm)	2.2m	2.157m	2.157m	1.8m
Minimum clearance (mm)	0.314m	0.157m	0.157m	0.2m
Thickness of the tooth (mm)	1.493m	1.571m	1.571m	1.571m
Backlash (mm)	0.157m	0	0	0
Outside diameter (mm)	$(z + 2)m$	$(z + 2)m$	$(z + 2)m$	$(z + 1.6)m$
Approximate fillet radius (mm)	0.209m	0.209m	0.209m	0.209m

m = module, mm

Table 12.4 (b) *Guide to Selection of Gear-Tooth System*

Interchangeable tooth system	Smallest no. of teeth that mesh with rack without interference	Smallest number of teeth in equal pinion that will give continuous driving	Comments
$14\frac{1}{2}°$ full-depth involute system	32	20 teeth with contact ratio of 1.080 (24 gives contact ratio of 1.469)	Recommended to use when the pinion has 40 or more teeth
20° full-depth involute system	18	12 teeth with contact ratio of 1.049 (14 gives contact ratio of 1.415)	Recommended for general use
20° stub-tooth involute system	14	12 teeth gives contact ratio of 1.185	Recommended to use when the number of teeth in pinion is too small for satisfactory use of 20° full-depth teeth

Table 12.4 (c) *Peripheral Speeds of Gears*

Accuracy	Cutting method	Finishing operation for tooth contact surface	Nature of service	Peripheral velocities		Efficiency
				spur gear	Bevel gear	
Low	Form cut or generated	None	Ordinary power transmission with moderate load and low speed.	Upto 2 m/s	Upto 4 m/s	94%
Medium	Form cut or generated	Machine cut, run in or lapped in pairs	General use requiring no special accuracy. Example: Gears for unimportant industrial machinery, tractors, agricultural equipment haulage machinery etc.	Upto 6 m/s	Upto 10 m/s	96%
High	Teeth generated on precision machines	Teeth ground, shaved or lapped after machining depending on nature of service	Gear wheels operating at high velocity and medium load or high load at moderate velocity. Example: Gear wheels of machine tools, reduction gears, automobiles, aircraft etc.	Upto 10 m/s	Upto 15 m/s	98%
Very high	Teeth generated on high precision machines	Precision ground or shaved	Gear wheels for smooth and noiseless operation or for operations at high velocities under heavy loads. Example: Gear wheels of machine tools, automobiles, air crafts, high speed reduction gears, indexing or dividing gears, turbine gears etc.	Upto 15 m/s	Upto 30 m/s	99%

Table 12.5 ***Values of Tooth-Form Factor (Lewis), Load at Tip of Tooth***

z	y					
	$14\frac{1}{2}°$-deg form	$14\frac{1}{2}$-deg variable centre distance	20-deg full depth form	20-deg stubtooth form	Internal Gears	
					Spur pinion	Internal gear
12	0.067	0.125	0.078	0.099	0.104	*
13	0.071	0.123	0.083	0.103	0.104	*
14	0.075	0.121	0.088	0.108	0.105	*
15	0.078	0.120	0.092	0.111	0.105	*
16	0.081	0.120	0.094	0.115	0.106	*
17	0.084	0.120	0.096	0.117	0.109	*
18	0.086	0.120	0.098	0.120	0.111	*
19	0.088	0.119	0.100	0.123	0.114	*
20	0.090	0.119	0.102	0.125	0.116	*
21	0.092	0.119	0.104	0.127	0.118	*
22	0.093	0.119	0.105	0.129	0.119	*
24	0.095	0.118	0.107	0.132	0.122	*
26	0.098	0.117	0.110	0.135	0.125	*
28	0.100	0.115	0.112	0.137	0.127	0.220
30	0.101	0.114	0.114	0.139	0.129	0.216
34	0.104	0.112	0.118	0.142	0.132	0.210
38	0.106	0.110	0.122	0.145	0.135	0.205
43	0.108	0.108	0.126	0.147	0.137	0.200
50	0.110	0.110	0.130	0.151	0.139	0.195
60	0.113	0.113	0.134	0.154	0.142	0.190
75	0.115	0.115	0.138	0.158	0.144	0.185
100	0.117	0.117	0.142	0.161	0.147	0.180
150	0.119	0.119	0.146	0.165	0.149	0.175
300	0.122	0.122	0.150	0.170	0.152	0.170
Rack	0.124	0.124	0.154	0.175		

* Internal gears with less than 28 teeth must be designed specially for the particular application, and their values of v must be determined for each one individually.

Table 12.6 *Values of y when the Load is near the Middle of the Tooth*

z	$14\frac{1}{2}°$-deg form	20-deg full depth form	20-deg stubtooth form	Internal Gears* Spur pinion	Internal Gears* Internal gear
12	0.113	0.132	0.158	0.207	
13	0.120	0.141	0.164	0.208	
14	0.127	0.149	0.172	0.209	
15	0.132	0.156	0.177	0.210	
16	0.137	0.160	0.184	0.211	
17	0.142	0.163	0.187	0.215	
18	0.146	0.166	0.192	0.218	
19	0.150	0.170	0.196	0.222	*
20	0.153	0.173	0.200	0.225	
21	0.156	0.176	0.203	0.228	
22	0.158	0.178	0.206	0.230	
24	0.162	0.182	0.211	0.233	
26	0.166	0.187	0.216	0.236	
28	0.170	0.190	0.219	0.239	0.400
30	0.172	0.193	0.222	0.242	0.395
34	0.176	0.200	0.227	0.246	0.387
38	0.180	0.207	0.232	0.250	0.380
43	0.183	0.214	0.235	0.253	0.372
50	0.187	0.221	0.241	0.256	0.364
60	0.192	0.227	0.246	0.260	0.356
75	0.195	0.234	0.252	0.264	0.348
100	0.198	0.241	0.257	0.268	0.340
150	0.202	0.248	0.264	0.272	0.332
300	0.207	0.255	0.272	0.276	0.325
Rack	0.210	0.262	0.280		

*Internal gears with less than 28 teeth must be designed specially for their particular application; their values of y must be determined for each one individually.

Table 12.7 *Allowable Static Stresses σ_d to use in Lewis formulae*

Material	Allowable static stress σ_d, MN/m^2 (kgf/mm^2)	BHN
Cast Iron Grade 20 ..	47.1 (4.80)	200
Cast Iron Grade 25 ..	56.4 (5.75)	220
Cast Iron Grade 35 ..	56.4 (5.75)	225
Cast Iron Grade 35 (Heat treated) ..	78.5 (8.00)	300
Cast steel, 0.20%C, untreated ..	138.3 (14.10)	180
Cast steel, 0.20%C, heat treated ..	193.2 (19.70)	250
Bronze ..	68.7 (7.00)	80
Phosphor gear bronze ..	82.4 (8.40)	100
Manganese bronze ..	138.3 (14.10)	100
Aluminium bronze ..	152.0 (15.50)	180
Forged steel, about 0.30%C (untreated) ..	172.6 (17.60)	150
Forged steel, about 0.30%C (heat treated) ..	220.0 (22.40)	200
Steel, C30 (heat treated) ..	220.6 (22.50)	300
Steel, C40, untreated ..	207.0 (21.10)	150
Steel, C45, untreated ..	233.4 (23.80)	200
Alloy steel, case hardened ..	345.2 (35.20)	650
Cr-Ni Steel, about 0.45%C heat treated ..	462.0 (47.10)	400
Cr-Va steel, about 0.45%C, heat treated ..	516.8 (52.70)	450
Rawhide, Fabroil, etc. ..	41.2 (4.20)	—
Plastic ..	58.8 (6.00)	—
Laminated phenolic materials (Bakelite, Micarta, Celoron) ..	41.2 (4.20)	—
Laminated steel (silent material) ..	82.4 (8.40)	—

Table 12.8 *Service factor C_s for gears in equation 12.7*

Type of load	Type of service		
	Intermittent or 3 h per day	8 to 10 h per day	Continuous 24 h/day
Steady	0.80	1.0	1.25
Light shocks	1.00	1.25	1.50
Medium shocks	1.25	1.50	1.80
Heavy shocks	1.50	1.80	2.00

Table 12.9 *Standard Gear Ratio $\left(i = \dfrac{Z_2}{Z_i} \right)$*

Stage reduction					
Single	Double	Triple	Single	Double	Triple
1.25	8.0	40	4.0	22.4	125
1.40	9.0	45	4.5	25.0	140
1.60	10.0	50	5.0	28.0	160
1.80	11.0	56	5.6	31.5	180
2.00	12.0	63	6.3	35.5	200
2.24	12.5	71	7.1	40.0	250
2.50	14.0	80	8.0	45.0	280
2.80	16.0	90	9.0	50.0	315
3.15	18.0	100	—	—	355
3.55	20.0	112	10.0	—	400

Table 12.10 *Load Concentration Factor K_c*

Ratio Face width to pitch diameter	Symmetrical bearings close to the gear	Pinion with non symmetrical bearings on		Cantilever pinion
		rigid shaft	less rigid shaft	
0.1 to 0.5	1.00	1.025	1.075	1.19
0.6 to 1.0	1.07	0.140	1.230	1.40
1.1 to 1.5	1.18	1.280	1.440	should not be used

Table 12.11 *Dynamic Load Factors, K_d*

Accuracy of teeth	Hardness BHN	Peripheral velocity m/s											
		Upto 1.0		> 1 to 3		> 3 to 8		> 8 to 12		> 12 to 18		> 18 to 25	
		1*	2*	1*	2*	1*	2*	1*	2*	1*	2*	1*	2*
Very high	Upto 350	—	—	—	—	1.2	1.0	1.3	1.1	—	1.2	—	1.4
	> 350	—	—	—	—	1.2	1.0	1.3	1.0	—	1.1	—	1.2
High	Upto 350	—	—	1.25	1.1	1.45	1.0	1.55	1.2	—	1.3	—	1.5
	> 350	—	—	1.2	1.0	1.3	1.0	1.4	1.1	—	1.2	—	1.3
Medium	Upto 350	1.0	—	1.35	1.1	1.55	1.3	—	1.4	—	—	—	—
	> 350	1.0	—	1.3	1.1	1.4	1.2	—	1.4	—	—	—	—
Low	Upto 350	1.1	—	1.45	1.2	—	1.4	—	—	—	—	—	—
	> 350	1.1	—	1.4	1.2	—	1.3	—	—	—	—	—	—

1* Straight or spur gears
2* Helical gears

Table 12.12 *Values of the Dynamic Factor C*

Materials	Tooth form	Error in gears (mm)								
		0.01	0.02	0.03	0.04	0.06	0.08	0.10	0.12	0.15
Cast Iron and Cast Iron	$14\frac{1}{2}$ deg	55.2 (5.63)	110.4 (11.26)	165.6 (16.89)	220.9 (22.52)	331.3 (33.78)	441.7 (45.04)	552.1 (56.30)	662.5 (67.56)	828.2 (84.45)
Cast Iron and Steel	$14\frac{1}{2}$ deg	75.8 (7.73)	151.6 (15.46)	227.4 (23.19)	303.2 (30.97)	454.8 (46.38)	606.4 (61.84)	758.1 (77.30)	909.7 (92.76)	1137.1 (115.95)
Steel and Steel	$14\frac{1}{2}$ deg	110.3 (11.95)	220.6 (22.50)	330.9 (33.75)	441.3 (45.00)	662.0 (67.50)	882.6 (90.00)	1103.2 (112.5)	1323.9 (135.0)	1654.9 (168.75)
Cast Iron and Cast Iron	20-deg	57.3 (5.84)	114.5 (11.68)	171.8 (17.52)	229.1 (23.39)	343.6 (35.04)	458.2 (46.72)	572.7 (58.40)	687.3 (70.00)	859.1 (87.60)
Cast Iron and Steel	20-deg	78.6 (8.02)	157.3 (16.04)	235.9 (24.06)	314.6 (32.08)	471.9 (48.12)	629.2 (64.16)	786.5 (80.2)	943.8 (96.24)	1180.0 (120.30)
Steel and Steel	20-deg	114.4 (11.67)	228.9 (23.34)	343.3 (35.01)	457.8 (46.68)	686.7 (70.02)	915.6 (93.30)	1144.4 (116.7)	1373.3 (140.0)	1716.7 (175.05)
Cast Iron and Cast Iron	20-deg, stub	59.3 (6.05)	118.7 (12.10)	178.0 (18.15)	237.3 (24.20)	356.0 (36.30)	474.6 (48.40)	593.3 (60.5)	712.0 (72.6)	890.0 (90.75)
Cast Iron and Steel	20-deg, stub	81.4 (8.30)	162.8 (16.60)	244.2 (24.90)	325.6 (33.20)	488.4 (49.80)	651.2 (66.40)	814.0 (83.0)	976.7 (99.6)	1221.0 (124.50)
Steel and Steel	20-deg, stub	118.7 (12.10)	237.3 (24.20)	356.0 (36.30)	474.6 (48.40)	712.0 (72.60)	949.3 (96.8)	1186.6 (121.0)	1423.9 (145.2)	1780.0 (181.50)

Table 12.13 *Maximum of probable Error in Action between Gears (Fig. 12.4)*

Module, m (mm)	error, e (mm)		
	Class I Industrial or commercial gears	Class II Accurate or carefully cut gears	Class III precision gears
25	0.1217	0.0607	0.0304
20	0.1168	0.0580	0.0290
15	0.1080	0.0537	0.0272
12	0.0987	0.0492	0.0245
10	0.0891	0.0445	0.0221
8	0.0778	0.0386	0.0198
7	0.0712	0.0353	0.0186
6	0.0652	0.0316	0.0172
5	0.0555	0.0277	0.0150
4	0.0508	0.0254	0.0127

Table 12.14 *Maximum allowable or permisssible error in action between gears (Fig. 12.5)*

Velocity m/s	Error (mm)	Velocity m/s	Error (mm)
1.0	0.0960	8.0	0.0500
2.0	0.0880	10.0	0.0386
2.5	0.0840	12.0	0.0330
3.0	0.0785	15.0	0.0230
4.0	0.0710	20.0	0.0155
5.0	0.0640	25.0	0.0130
6.0	0.0590	26.0 and over	0.0127

Note: Probable error (Fig. 12.4) or maximum error (Table 12.13) should be less than permissible error (Fig. 12.5) or Maximum allowable error (Table 12.14)

Table 12.15 *Endurance limits for checking the beam strength of the teeth*

Material	Core (BHN)	σ_{en} MN/m^2 (kgf/mm^2)
Gray cast iron ..	160	83.5 (8.50)
Semi steel (High grade 1) ..	200	124.5 (12.70)
Manganese bronze ..	100	118.0 (12.00)
Gear bronze ..	100	165.5 (16.90)
Non-metallic ..	—	41.0 (4.20)
Cast steel (soft) ..	110	178.5 (18.20)
Cast steel (Medium) ..	120	206.0 (21.00)
Steel ..	150	259.0 (26.40)
Steel ..	200	345.0 (35.20)
Steel, normalised ..	240	414.0 (42.40)
Steel ..	250	429.0 (43.70)
	280	480.5 (49.00)
	300	515.0 (52.50)
	320	549.0 (56.00)
	350	583.5 (59.50)
	360	618.0 (63.00)
	400	686.5 (70.00)
	450	686.5 (70.00)
	500	686.5 (70.00)
	550	686.5 (70.00)
	600	686.5 (70.00)
Cr-Ni Steel, about 1% Ni and 0.40%C, heat treated	280	482.5 (49.20)
Cr-Ni Steel, about 2% Ni and 0.40%C, heat treated	320	552.0 (56.30)
Steel, Oil tempered	360	621.0 (63.30)
Steel, nitralloy	400	70.00 (70.30)

Table 12.16 *Values of load stress factor for computing limiting wear load*

Pinion		Gear		Endurance limit σ_{es} MN/m² (kgf/mm²)	K	
Material	BHN	Material	BHN		$14\frac{1}{2}°$	20°
Steel	150	Steel	150	343.2 (35.00)	0.205 (0.021)	0.284 (0.029)
Steel	200	Steel	150	412.0 (42.0)	0.294 (0.030)	0.402 (0.041)
"	250	"	150	480.5 (49.0)	0.402 (0.041)	0.539 (0.055)
"	200	"	200	480.5 (49.0)	0.402 (0.041)	0.539 (0.055)
"	250	"	200	549.0 (56.0)	0.520 (0.053)	0.706 (0.072)
"	300	"	300	617.8 (63.0)	0.657 (0.067)	0.902 (0.092)
"	250	"	250	617.8 (63.0)	0.657 (0.067)	0.902 (0.092)
"	300	"	250	686.5 (70.0)	0.814 (0.083)	1.108 (0.113)
"	350	"	250	755.0 (77.0)	0.990 (0.101)	1.344 (0.137)
"	300	"	300	755.0 (77.0)	0.990 (0.101)	1.344 (0.137)
"	350	"	300	823.8 (84.0)	1.177 (0.120)	1.599 (0.163)
"	400	"	300	858.0 (87.5)	1.275 (0.130)	1.746 (0.178)
"	350	"	350	892.5 (91.0)	1.383 (0.141)	1.893 (0.193)
"	400	"	350	961.0 (98.0)	1.598 (0.163)	2.189 (0.223)
"	450	"	350	995.0 (101.5)	1.716 (0.175)	2.344 (0.239)
"	450	"	450	1167.0 (119.0)	2.363 (0.241)	3.226 (0.329)
"	500	"	450	1201.5 (122.5)	2.500 (0.255)	3.413 (0.348)
"	600	"	450	1235.5 (126.0)	2.648 (0.270)	3.609 (0.368)
"	500	"	500	1304.5 (133.0)	2.952 (0.301)	4.040 (0.412)
"	600	"	600	1569.0 (160.0)	4.325 (0.441)	5.913 (0.603)
"	150	C.I.	180	343.0 (35.0)	0.304 (0.031)	0.412 (0.042)
"	200	C.I.	180	392.5 (40.0)	0.598 (0.061)	0.814 (0.083)
"	250	C.I.	180	617.8 (63.0)	0.990 (0.101)	1.344 (0.137)
"	150	phosphor bronze	100	343.0 (35.0)	0.314 (0.032)	0.422 (0.043)
"	200	"	100	392.5 (40.0)	0.628 (0.064)	0.853 (0.087)
"	250	"	100	583.5 (59.5)	0.932 (0.095)	1.265 (0.129)
C.I.	180	C.I.	180	617.8 (63.0)	1.324 (0.135)	1.814 (0.185)
Steel	150	Nickel C.I.	—	343.0 (35.0)	0.304 (0.031)	0.412 (0.042)
"	200	"	—	480.5 (49.0)	0.598 (0.061)	0.814 (0.083)
"	250	"	—	617.8 (63.0)	0.990 (0.101)	1.344 (0.137)
"	300	"	—	638.5 (65.1)	1.059 (0.108)	1.442 (0.147)
Hot-quenched Nickel C.I.	—	Hot-quenched Nickel C.I.	—	641.5 (65.4)	1.422 (0.145)	1.942 (0.198)
"	—	Phosphor bronze	—	572.5 (58.4)	1.187 (0.121)	1.618 (0.165)

Table 12.17 *Values of load stress factor K for gears made of hardened steels*

BHN for pinion and Gear	Endurance limit σ_{es} MN/m^2(kgf/mm^2)	Load stress factor K	
		$14\frac{1}{2}°$ deg	20° deg
10 × 10^6 repetitions of stress			
450	1294.5 (132.0)	2.903 (0.296)	3.972 (0.405)
500	1451.5 (148.0)	3.629 (0.370)	4.962 (0.506)
550	1608.5 (164.0)	4.472 (0.456)	6.100 (0.622)
600	1765.0 (180.0)	5.354 (0.546)	7.306 (0.745)
20 × 10^6 repetitions of stress			
450	1176.8 (120.0)	2.373 (0.242)	3.246 (0.331)
500	1314.0 (134.0)	2.962 (0.302)	4.060 (0.414)
550	1451.5 (148.0)	3.629 (0.370)	4.962 (0.506)
600	1588.5 (162.0)	4.354 (0.444)	5.943 (0.606)
50 × 10^6 repetitions of stress			
450	1015.0 (103.5)	1.775 (0.181)	2.422 (0.247)
500	1137.5 (116.0)	2.236 (0.228)	3.060 (0.312)
550	1255.5 (128.0)	2.726 (0.278)	3.756 (0.383)
600	1382.5 (141.0)	3.285 (0.335)	4.492 (0.458)
100 × 10^6 repetitions of stress			
450	902.0 (90.0)	1.432 (0.146)	1.961 (0.200)
500	1020.0 (104.0)	1.804 (0.184)	2.452 (0.250)
550	1128.0 (115.0)	2.177 (0.222)	2.981 (0.304)
600	1235.5 (126.0)	2.638 (0.269)	3.609 (0.368)

Table 12.18 *Number of arms of Gear*

Pitch circle diameter (mm)	No. of arms
Upto 500 mm	4-5
500 to 1500 mm	5
1500 to 2000 mm	8
Above 2000 mm	10

Table 12.19 *Dimensions of Gear Hubs*

| Type of Service | Hub diameter | | Length |
	Cast Iron	Steel Costing	
(1) Light load no shock	1.75d	1.6d	$l \geqq 1.5d$
(2) Medium load and shock	1.85d	1.7d	$l \geqq 1.75d$
(3) Heavy load with shock	2d	1.8d	$l \geqq 2d$

Table 12.20 *Helical Gear Proportions*

		Maximum	Minimum
Pressure angle in the plane of rotation, α		25°	15° 23′
Helix angle, β	..	45°	20°
The normal pressure angle, α_n	..	40° 30′	18° 15′
Abdendum, h_a	..	m	0.7m
Clearance, c	..	0.3m	0.157m

Table 12.21 *Wear and Lubrication Factor*

Nature of lubrication	C_w
For enclosed gears continuously lubricated with oil of the proper viscosity and character	1.15
For scant lubrication but regular, frequent inspection	1.25
For indifferent lubrication	1.35

Table 12.22 *Allowable static stress for Helical and Herringbone gears*

Material	Elastic limit MN/m^2	Allowable static stress MN/m^2 (kgf/mm^2)
Cast Iron, ordinary ...	84	28
Cast Iron, better grade ...	110	30
Laminated phenolic materials ...	70	28
Bronze, SAE65 ...	165	40
Cast steel, class B, medium ...	240	50
0.4 to 0.5% carbon steel, not treated ...	275	70
0.4 to 0.5% carbon steel, heat treated ...	345	85
High-carbon or alloy steels, heat treated ...	620	105

Table 12.23 (a) *Proportions of Bevel Teeth*

Elements	Symbol	Gear	Pinion
Normal depth of addendum	h_a	m	m*
Normal depth of dedendum	h_f	1.157m	1.157m*
Whole depth of tooth	h	2.157 m	2.157m
Normal addendum angle	θ_a	m/L	m/L
Normal dedendum angle	θ_d	$\dfrac{1.157m}{L}$	$\dfrac{1.157m}{L}$

*The dedendum of the gear equals the addendum of the pinion and the addendum of the gear equals the dedendum of the pinion for a common pitch line. The pinion addendum being greater than its dedendum.

Table 12.23 *(b) Proportions of Large and Short Addendum Bevel Gears*

		Pinion	Gear
Addendum	..	1.4m	0.6m
Dedendum	..	0.7571m	1.5571m
Tooth thickness on the pitch line	..		
with $14\frac{1}{2}°$	..	1.778m	1.364m
with 20°	..	1.862m	1.280m

Table 12.24 *Recommended Series of Modules (Bevel Gears)*

m	1.00 (1.125) 1.25 (1.375) 1.50 (1.75) 2.00 (2.25) 2.50 (2.75) 3.00 (3.25) 3.5 (3.75) 4.00 (4.50) 5.00 (5.50) 6.00 (6.50) 7.00 8.00 (9.00) 10.00 (11.00) 12.00 (14.00) 16.00 (18.00) 20.00 (22.00) 25.00 (28.00) 32.00 (36.00) 40.00 (45.00) 50.00

IS:5037–1969

Note: Modules within the brackets are of second preference

Table 12.25 *Recommended Series of Diametral Pitches (Bevel Gears)*

p_d	20.00 (18.00) 16.00 (14.00) 12.00 (11.00) 10.00 (9.00) 8.00 (7.00) 6.00 (5.50) 5.00 (4.50) 4.00 (3.50) 3.00 (2.75) 2.50 (2.25) 2.00 (1.75) 1.50 1.25 1.00 (0.875) 0.75 0.625 0.50

IS:5037–1969

Note: Within the brackets are of second preference

Table 12.26 *Proportions of Worms (American Gear Manufacturers Association)*

Dimension	Symbol (Fig. 12.11)	Single and double threads	Triple and quadruple threads
Normal pressure angle (deg)	α	$14\frac{1}{2}°$	$20°$
Pitch diameter, bored for shaft, mm	d_1	$2.40p_c+28$ mm $7.54m+28$ mm	$2.40p_c+28$ mm $7.54m+28$ mm
Pitch diameter, integral with shaft, mm	d_1	$2.35p_c+10$ mm $7.39m+10$ mm	$2.35p_c+10$ mm $7.39m+10$ mm
Face length, mm	L_w	$(4.5+0.02z_1)p_c$ $(14.14+0.063z_1)m$	$(4.5+0.02z_1)p_c$ $(14.14+0.063z_1)m$
Depth of tooth, mm	h	$0.686p_c$ $2.16m$	$0.623p_c$ $1.96m$
Addendum, mm	h_a	$0.318p_c$ m	$0.286p_c$ $0.9m$
Top radius, mm	r	$0.05p_c$ $0.157m$	$0.05p_c$ $0.157m$
Hub diameter, mm	d_k	$1.66p_c+25$ mm $5.21m+25$ mm	$1.726p_c+25$ mm $5.425m+25$ mm
Maximum bore for shaft, mm	d_s	$p_c+15.9$ mm $3.14m+15.9$ mm	$p_c+15.9$ mm $3.14m+15.9$ mm
Outside diameter of worm, mm	d_{01}	$d_1+0.636p_c$ d_1+2m	$d_1+0.572p_c$ $d_1+1.8m$

$p_c = (\pi_m)$ axial pitch, mm

m =module, mm

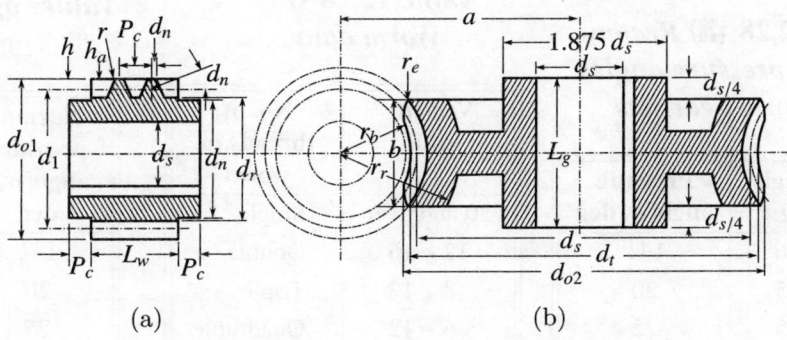

(a)   (b)

Fig. 12.19: *Proportions of worms and worm gears*

Table 12.27 *Proportions of Worm Gears*

Dimensions	Symbol (Fig. 12.14)	Single and double threads	Triple and quadruple threads
Normal pressure angle (deg)	α	$14\frac{1}{2}^\circ$	20
Outside diameter, mm	d_{o2}	$d_2 + 1.0135 p_c$ $d_2 + 3.1854\,m$	$d_2 + 0.890 p_c$ $d_2 + 2.7982\,m$
Throat diameter, mm	d_t	$d_2 + 0.636 p_c$ $d_2 + 2\,m$	$d_2 + 0.572 p_c$ $d_2 + 1.7978\,m$
Face width, mm	b	$2.38 p_c + 6.35$ mm $7.48\,m + 6.35$ mm	$2.15 p_c + 5.08$ mm $6.758\,m + 5.08$ mm
Radius of gear face, mm	r_b	$0.882 p_c + 14$ mm $2.772\,m + 14$ mm	$0.914 p_c + 14$ mm $2.873\,m + 14$ mm
Radius of gear rim, mm	r_r	$2.2 p_c + 14$ mm $6.915\,m + 14$ mm	$2.1 p_c + 14$ mm $6.6\,m + 14$ mm
Radius of edge, mm	r_e	$0.25 p_c$ $0.7858\,m$	$0.25 p_c$ $0.7858\,m$

p_c=axial pitch, mm; m=module, mm

Table 12.28 *(a) Recommended pressure angles for worm gear sets*

Lead angle γ, deg	Pressure angle α, deg
0 – 16	$14\frac{1}{2}$
16 – 25	20
25 – 35	25
35 – 45	30

Table 12.28 *(b) Worm data*

Velocity ratio	No. of threads in worm
20 and over	Single
12 – 16	Double
8 – 12	Triple
6 – 12	Quadruple
4 – 10	Sextuple

Table 12.28 *(c) Values of y for worm gears*

Normal pressure angle α_n, deg	form factor, y
$14\frac{1}{2}$	0.100
20	0.125
25	0.150
30	0.175

Table 12.29 *Dimensions of Worms (All dimensions in milli-metres)*

Module	Axial pitch	No. of starts	Diametral quotient	Reference diameter	Tip diameter	Root diameter	Lead Angle
m	p_c	z_1	q	d_1	d_{o1}	d_r	γ
(1)	(2)	(3)	(4)	(5)	(6)	(7)	(8)
1.0	3.142	1	16	16.00	18.00	13.60	3° − 35′
1.25	3.927	1	(18)	22.50	25.00	19.50	3° − 11′
1.5	4.712	1	16	24.00	27.00	20.40	3° − 35′
1.5	4.712	1	(18)	27.00	30.00	23.40	3° − 11′
2.0	6.283	1	(11)	22.00	26.00	17.20	5° − 12′
2.0	6.283	1	(18)	36.00	40.00	31.20	3° − 11′
2.0	6.283	2	(11)	22.00	26.00	17.20	10° − 18′
2.0	6.283	4	(11)	22.00	26.00	17.00	19° − 59′
2.5	7.854	1	(11)	27.00	32.50	21.50	5° − 12′
2.5	7.854	1	16	40.00	45.00	34.00	3° − 35′
2.5	7.854	2	(11)	27.50	32.50	21.50	10° − 18′
2.5	7.854	4	(11)	27.50	32.50	21.50	19° − 59′
2.5	7.854	6	(11)	27.50	32.50	22.84	28° − 37′
3	9.425	1	(11)	33.00	39.00	25.80	5° − 12′
3	9.425	1	(18)	54.00	60.00	46.80	3° − 11′
3	9.425	2	(11)	33.00	39.00	25.80	10° − 18′
3	9.425	4	(11)	33.00	39.00	25.80	19° − 59′
3	9.425	6	(11)	33.00	39.00	27.41	28° − 37′
4	12.566	1	10	40.00	48.00	30.40	5° − 43′
4	12.566	1	(18)	72.00	80.00	62.40	3° − 11′
4	12.566	2	10	40.00	48.00	30.40	11° − 19′
4	12.566	4	10	40.00	48.00	30.40	21° − 48′
4	12.566	6	(11)	44.00	52.00	36.55	28° − 37′
5	15.708	1	10	50.00	60.00	38.00	5° − 43′
5	15.708	1	(18)	90.00	100.00	78.00	3° − 11′
5	15.708	2	10	50.00	60.00	38.00	11° − 19′
5	15.708	4	10	50.00	60.00	38.00	21° − 48′
5	15.708	6	(11)	55.00	65.00	45.69	28° − 37′
6	18.850	1	10	60.00	72.00	45.60	5° − 43′
6	18.850	1	(18)	108.00	120.00	93.60	3° − 11′
6	18.850	2	10	60.00	72.00	45.60	11° − 19′
6	18.850	4	10	60.00	72.00	45.60	21° − 48′
6	18.850	6	10	60.00	72.00	49.36	30° − 58′
8	25.133	1	10	80.00	96.00	60.80	5° − 43′
8	25.133	1	(18)	144.00	160.00	124.80	3° − 11′
8	25.133	2	10	80.00	96.00	60.80	11° − 19′
8	25.133	4	10	80.00	96.00	60.80	21° − 48′

Table 12.29 *Dimensions of Worms (All dimensions in milli-metres) (Contd...)*

(1)	(2)	(3)	(4)	(5)	(6)	(7)	(8)
8	25.133	4	8	64.00	80.00	48.52	26° – 34′
8	25.133	7	(9)	72.00	88.00	58.71	33° – 41′
8	25.133	8	(11)	88.00	104.00	75.53	36° – 02′
10	31.416	1	10	100.00	120.00	76.00	4° – 43′
10	31.416	1	(18)	180.00	200.00	156.00	3° – 11′
10	31.416	2	10	100.00	120.00	76.00	11° – 19′
10	31.416	4	10	100.00	120.00	76.00	21° – 48′
10	31.416	8	(11)	110.00	130.00	94.42	36° – 02′
12	37.699	1	(9)	108.00	132.00	79.20	6° – 20′
12	37.699	1	(18)	216.00	240.00	187.00	3° – 11′
12	37.699	2	(9)	108.00	132.00	79.20	12° – 32′
12	37.699	4	(9)	108.00	132.00	79.20	23° – 58′
12	37.699	8	(11)	132.00	156.00	113.30	36° – 02′
16	50.266	1	(9)	144.00	176.00	105.60	6° – 20′
16	50.266	2	(9)	144.00	176.00	105.60	12° – 32′
16	50.266	4	(9)	144.00	176.00	105.60	23° – 58′
16	50.266	8	(11)	176.00	208.00	151.06	36° – 02′
20	62.832	1	(9)	180.00	220.00	132.00	6° – 20′
20	62.832	2	(9)	180.00	220.00	132.00	12° – 32′
20	62.832	4	(9)	180.00	220.00	132.00	23° – 58′
20	62.832	8	(11)	220.00	260.00	188.83	36° – 02′

IS:3734–1966

Table 12.30 *Load Stress Factor for worm gears for use in Equation 12.53(d)*

Material		Load stress factor, K		
Worm	Gear	$\gamma = 0 - 10°$	$\gamma = 10° - 25°$	$\gamma = 25°$ and up
Steel, 250 BHN	Phosphor bronze	0.412 (0.042)	0.515 (0.0525)	0.618 (0.063)
Hardened Steel	Phosphor bronze	0.549 (0.056)	0.687 (0.070)	0.824 (0.084)
Hardened Steel	Chilled bronze	0.824 (0.084)	1.030 (0.105)	1.236 (0.126)
Hardened Steel	Antimony bronze	0.824 (0.084)	1.030 (0.105)	1.236 (0.126)
Cast Iron	Phosphor bronze	1.030 (0.105)	1.285 (0.131)	1.746 (0.178)

Table 12.31 *Service factor C_s, for use in the wear formula 12.62(b)*

Type of load	Type of service		
	Intermittent or 3 h per day	8 to 10 h per day	Continuous 24 h/day
Steady	1.0000	1.2500	1.5625
Light shocks	1.2500	1.5625	1.8750
Medium shocks	1.5625	1.8750	2.2500
Heavy shocks	1.8750	2.2500	2.5000

Table 12.32 *Allowable Surface pressure σ_c in the wear load formula 12.62(b) MN/m^2 (kgf/mm^2)*

Material		Number of teeth in gear							
Worm	Gear	10	20	30	40	50	60	70	80 and more
C20 Steel, untreated	Cast iron	0.52 (0.053)	1.55 (0.158)	2.94 (0.30)	5.20 (0.53)	6.18 (0.63)	7.45 (0.76)	8.63 (0.88)	9.32 (0.95)
C40 Steel, untreated	bronze, sand cast	0.79 (0.08)	2.35 (0.24)	4.32 (0.44)	7.45 (0.76)	9.32 (0.95)	11.28 (1.15)	13.14 (1.34)	13.83 (1.41)
C40 Steel, Heat-treated, ground	bronze, sand cast	1.18 (0.12)	3.53 (0.36)	6.47 (0.66)	11.08 (1.13)	13.83 (1.41)	16.77 (1.71)	19.61 (2.00)	20.70 (2.11)
0.1%C, alloy steel, Carburizec, hardened and ground	bronze, sand cast	1.55 (0.158)	4.71 (0.48)	8.63 (0.88)	15.51 (1.58)	18.63 (1.90)	22.46 (2.29)	26.18 (2.67)	27.56 (2.81)
	bronze, chill cast	2.16 (0.22)	6.37 (0.65)	11.87 (1.21)	20.70 (2.11)	25.50 (2.60)	31.00 (3.16)	36.20 (3.69)	37.95 (3.87)
	Ni-bronze, sand cast	2.55 (0.26)	7.75 (0.79)	14.81 (1.51)	24.80 (2.53)	31.00 (3.16)	37.56 (3.83)	43.74 (4.46)	46.20 (4.71)
	Ni-bronze, chill cast	3.14 (0.32)	9.32 (0.95)	17.26 (1.76)	29.62 (3.02)	37.30 (3.80)	44.82 (4.57)	51.37 (5.34)	55.11 (5.62)

The values of allowable pressures, in the above table are given for a $14\frac{1}{2}^\circ$ pressure angle. For pressure angles of 20°, they can be increased by 5% and for 30° by 10 percent.

Table 12.33 *Load Factors for Various Machines*

Driver	Driver Machinery	Factor K_l
Steam turbine	Electric generator, steady load turbine blower ..	1.00
	Electric generator, uneven load; centrifugal pump ..	1.25
	Induced-draft fan; line shaft, gear drive ..	1.50
	Rolling mill, gear drive ..	2.00
Electric motor	Turbine blower; metal working machinery ..	1.25
	Centrifugal pump; woodworking machinery ..	1.50
	Line shaft; ship propeller; double-acting pump ..	1.75
	Triplex single-acting 'pump; elevator; crane ..	1.75
	Compressor, air or ammonia ..	1.75
	Rolling mill; rubber mill ..	2.50
Steam engine	Values for electric-motor drive multiplied by 1.2 to 1.5	
Gas and oil engines	Values for electric-motor drive multiplied by 1.3 to 1.6, the factor depending on the coefficient of steadiness of the flywheel	

References

[1] Siegel, M. J., Maleev, V. L., Hartman, J. B., *"Mechanical Design of Machines"* 4th edition, International Text Book Company, 1965.

[2] Vallance, A., Doughtie, V. L., *"Design of Machine Members"*, 3rd edition McGraw Hill Book Co., 1951.

[3] Black P. H., *"Machine Design"*, 3rd edition, McGraw-Hill Book Company, Inc., 19.

[4] Shigley, J. E., *"Machine Design"*, McGraw Hill Book Company, Inc.

[5] Hall A. S., Holowenko A. R., Laughlin, H. G., *"Theory and Problems of Machine Design"*, Schaum Publishing Co., 1961.

[6] Dobovolsky, V., Zablonsky, K., Mak, S., Radchick A., Erlikh, L., *"Machine Elements"*, Foreign Languages Publishing House, Moscow.

[7] Bhattacharya, S. C., Basu Mallik, J. R., *"Machine Design"*, Basu Mallik & Co., Calcutta, 1966.

[8] Ghosh, A. K., *"Practical Machine Design"*, S. Bhattacharya & Co., Calcutta, 1969.

[9] Berard, S. J., Waters E. O., Phelps, C. W., *"Principles of Machine Design"*, The Ronald Press Company, New York.

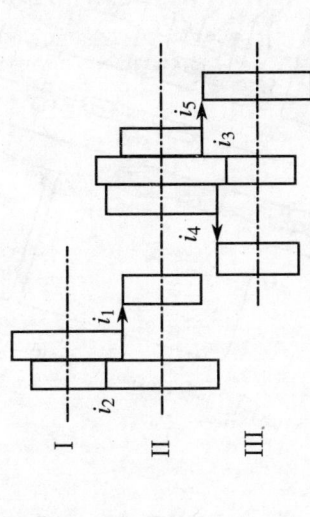

Gear layout 2×3 arrangement

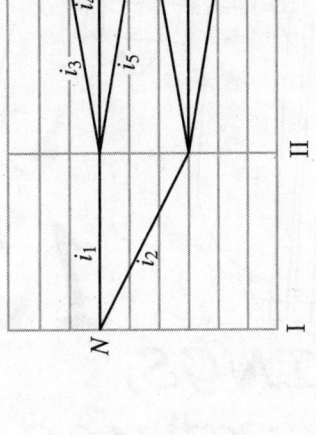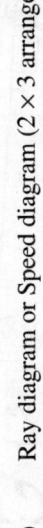

Ray diagram or Speed diagram (2×3 arrangement)

Gear layout 3×2 arrangement

Ray diagram or Speed diagram (3×2 arrangement)

Gear layout and Ray diagram or Speed diagram for six speed Gear Box

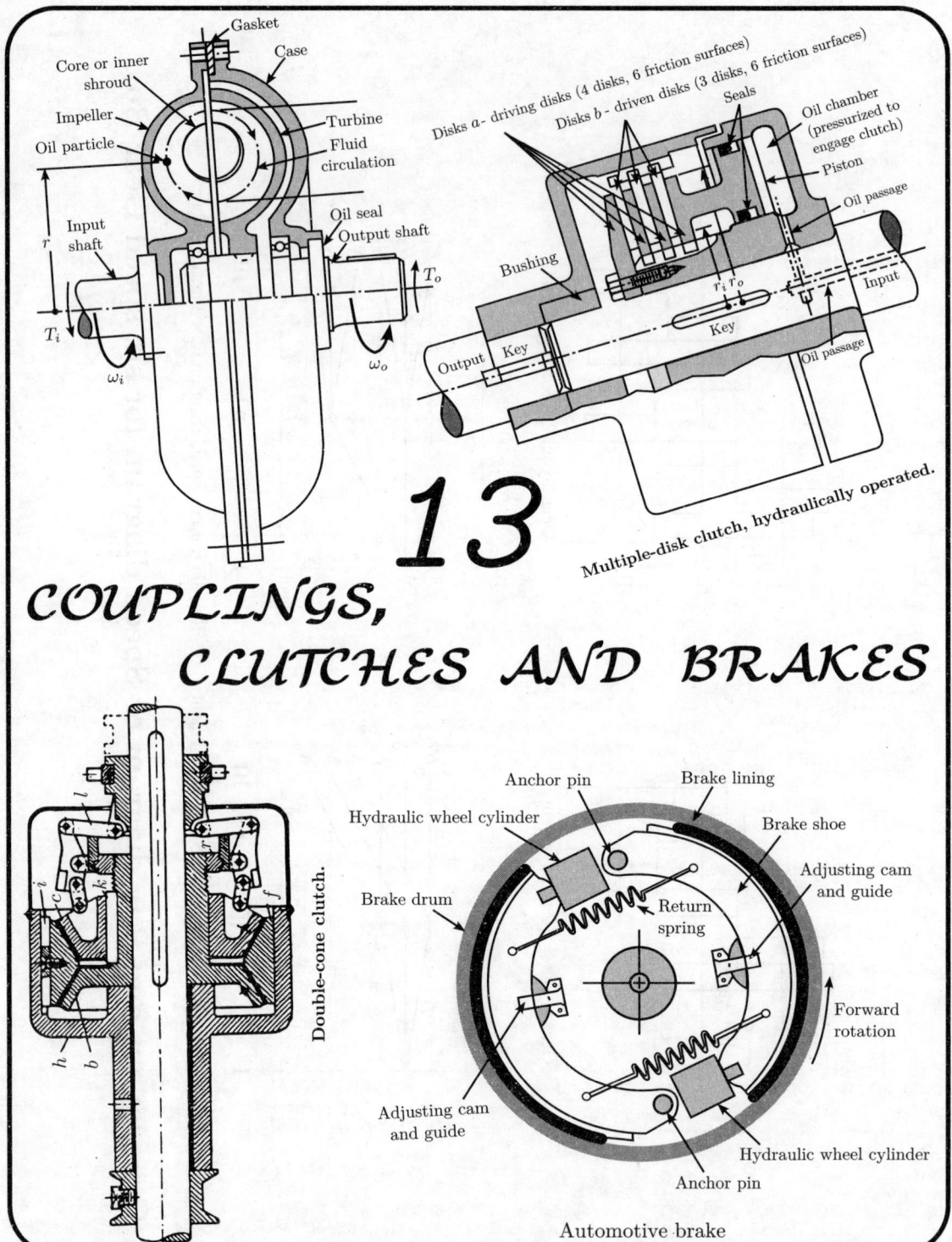

Gasket

Core or inner shroud

Case

Impeller

Turbine

Oil particle

Fluid circulation

Input shaft

r

Oil seal

Output shaft

T_o

T_i

ω_i

ω_o

Disks a - driving disks (4 disks, 6 friction surfaces)

Disks b - driven disks (3 disks, 6 friction surfaces)

Seals

Oil chamber (pressurized to engage clutch)

Piston

Oil passage

Bushing

$r_i\, r_o$

Input

Output

Key

Key

Oil passage

Multiple-disk clutch, hydraulically operated.

13

COUPLINGS,
CLUTCHES AND BRAKES

Double-cone clutch.

l

r

c

i

k

f

h

b

Anchor pin

Brake lining

Hydraulic wheel cylinder

Brake shoe

Adjusting cam and guide

Brake drum

Return spring

Forward rotation

Adjusting cam and guide

Hydraulic wheel cylinder

Anchor pin

Automotive brake

13

Couplings, Clutches and Brakes

Symbols	Description and Units
d	diameter of bolt, mm
D	diameter of shaft, mm
D_1	hub diameter, mm
D_2	diameter of the bolt circle, mm
D_3	outside diameter or flange, mm
i	number of bolts
t	thickness of flange, mm
T	torque, N mm (kgf mm)

Particular	Equation	Eqn. No.
Cast Iron Flange Coupling: (Fig. 13.1(a)) and Pulley Coupling. (Fig. 13.1(b))		
An empirical rule to determine the approximate number of bolts*	$i = \dfrac{1}{40} D + 2$ to $\dfrac{3}{80} D + 2$ (or)	13.1(a)
	$i = 0.02D + 3$	13.1(b)
The preliminary bolt diameter may be determined by the empirical formula	$d = \dfrac{0.423D}{\sqrt{i}} + 7.5$ mm (or) $d = \dfrac{0.5D}{\sqrt{i}}$	13.1(c)

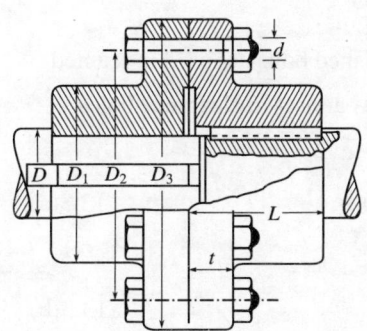

Fig. 13.1(a): *Cast iron flange coupling*

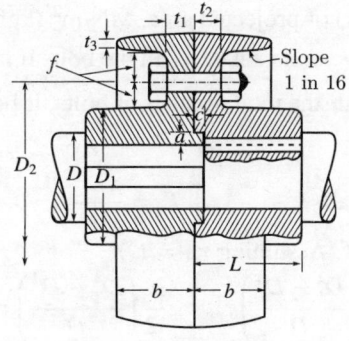

Fig. 13.1(b): *Cast iron pulley coupling*

$b = 0.5D + 25$ mm
$\quad > 0.3D + 1.3d + 7.55$ mm
$c = 0.1D + 2.5$ mm
$f = 1.5d$
$t_1 = 0.25D + 6.35$ mm
$t_2 = 0.30D + 7.50$ mm
$t_3 = 0.10D + 5.00$ mm
$a = 0.20D + 5.00$ mm

the nearest larger even number must be selected.

251

Particular	Equation	Eqn. No.
The hub diameter	$D_1 = 1.5D + 25$ mm (or) $2D$	13.1(d)
The diameter of the bolt circle	$D_2 = D_1 + 3.2d$ (or) $2D + 50$mm (or) $3D$	13.1(e)
The outside diameter of flange	$D_2 = D_1 + 6d$ (or) $2.5D + 75$ (or) $4D$	13.1(f)
The hub length		
	$L = 1.2D + 20$ mm (or) $1.25D + 20$mm (or) $125D$ to $1.5D$	13.1(g)
The flange thickness (CI Flange coupling)	$t = 0.35D + 9$ mm	13.1(h)
The maximum power capacity based upon friction such that slip occurs between faces of contact.	$P(kW) = \left(\dfrac{\pi}{0.5 \times 10^6}\right) Tn$ SI Units	13.2(a)
	$P(MHP) = \left(\dfrac{2\pi}{75000}\right) Tn$ Metric units	13.2(b)

where $T = \mu FR$, torque capacity based on friction, N mm (kgf mm)

F is the axial force caused by bolt loading, N (kgf); μ is the coefficient of friction

$R = \dfrac{1}{3}\left(\dfrac{D_o^3 - D_i^3}{D_o^2 - D_i^2}\right)$, friction radius assuming the pressure is uniformly distributed, mm

D_o = Outer diameter of contact, mm; D_i = Inner diameter of contact, mm

The torque capacity based on shear of bolts	$T = \dfrac{\tau \pi i d^2 D_2}{8}$	13.2(c)
The torque capacity based on bearing of bolts and flange	$T = \dfrac{\sigma_b i t d D_2}{2}$	13.2(d)
The torque capacity based on shear of flange	$T = \dfrac{\tau \pi D_1^2 t}{2}$	13.2(e)

where τ is the allowable shear stress, MN/m^2 (kgf/mm^2)

σ_b is the allowable bearing pressure for the bolt or web
    (whichever is weaker) of projected area, MN/m^2 (kgf/mm^2)

i = the number of effective bolts, taken as all the bolts if finished bolts are used in reamed
    holes and taken as half the total number of bolts, if bolts are set in clearance holes

Muff Coupling

Torque transmitted by the steel shaft	$T_s = \dfrac{\pi D^3}{16}\tau_s$	13.3(a)

Torque transmitted by the CI Muff (Assuming $\tau_{CI} = \tau_s$)

$$T_m = \dfrac{\pi}{16}\left(\dfrac{D_1^4 - D^4}{D}\right)\tau_{CI} = \dfrac{\pi}{32}\left(\dfrac{D_1^4 - D^4}{D}\right)\tau_s \qquad 13.3(b)$$

where τ_{CI} and τ_s are allowable shear stresses for cast iron and steel respectively

Hub diameter of Muff Coupling	$D_1 \approx 1.5D$	13.3(c)

Particular	Equation	Eqn. No.
Marine or Sold Flange Coupling (Fig. 13.3)		
The number of bolts	$i = 0.0132D + 2$	13.4(a)
The diameter of bolt circle	$D_2 = D + 1\frac{1}{2}d$ to $D + 2.5d$	13.4(b)
The average diameter of bolt circle	$D_2 = D + 2d$	13.4(c)

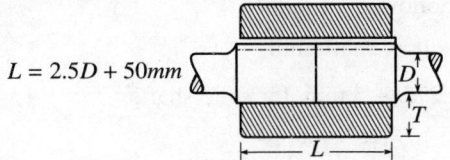

$L = 2.5D + 50mm$

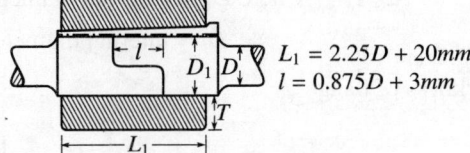

$L_1 = 2.25D + 20mm$
$l = 0.875D + 3mm$

(a) Ordinary muff coupling   (b) Fairbairn's halp-lap coupling

Fig. 13.2: *Muff Couplings*

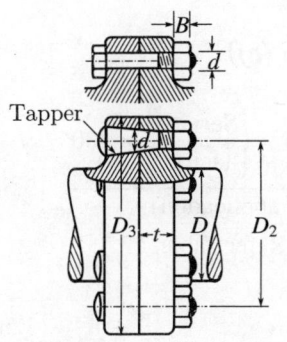

Fig. 13.3: *Marine or solid flange couplings*

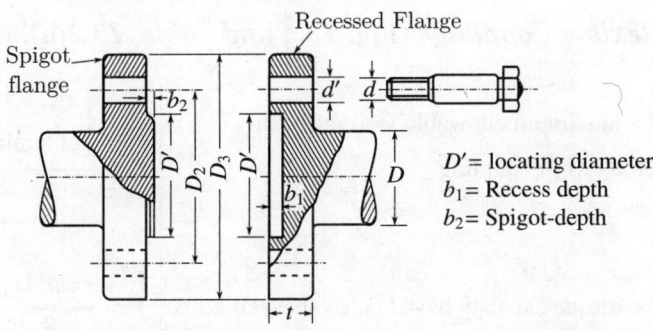

D' = locating diameter
b_1 = Recess depth
b_2 = Spigot-depth

Fig. 13.4: *Forged end type rigid coupling (Table 13.1)*

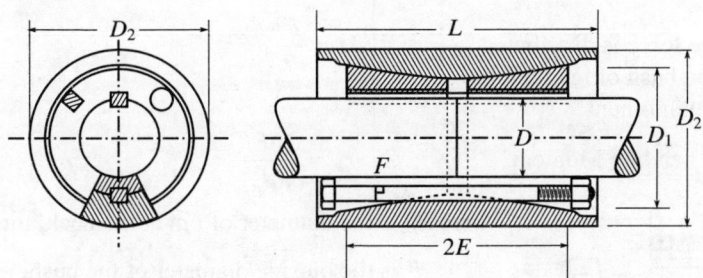

Length of box, $L = 4D$
Inside diameter of conical sleeve $D_1 = 2D + 12.5mm$
Outside diameter of box $D_2 = 3D$
Length of conical sleeve $E = 1.5D$

Fig. 13.5: *Sellers cone coupling*

Particular	Equation	Eqn. No.
If the bolts are made of the same material as the shaft, the diameter of bolt	$d = \left(\dfrac{D^3}{2iD_2}\right)^{\frac{1}{2}}$ for solid shafts	13.4(d)
	$= \left[\left(\dfrac{D_o^4 - D_i^4}{D_o}\right)\left(\dfrac{1}{2iD_2}\right)\right]^{\frac{1}{2}}$ for hollow shafts	13.4(e)

where D_o = external diameter of hollow shaft, mm

D_i = internal diameter of hollow shaft, mm

Thickness of flange	$t = 0.27D + 5$ mm for solid shafts	13.4(f)
	$= 0.29\left(\dfrac{D_o^4 - D_i^4}{D_o}\right)^{\frac{1}{3}}$ for hollow shafts	13.4(g)
Diameter of flange	$D_3 = (D_2 + 1.9d)$ to $(D_2 + 3.9d)$	13.4(h)

Flexible Couplings (Fig. 13.6 and Table 13.2(a), (b) and (c))

The maximum allowable load rating at 100 RPM of coupling	$P = \dfrac{\left\{\begin{array}{l} \text{kW of power} \\ \text{of application} \end{array}\right\} \times \left\{\begin{array}{l} \text{Service} \\ \text{factor} \end{array}\right\} \times 100}{(\text{RPM of application})}$ Service factor - Refer Table. 13.3	13.5(a)
The torque capacity based on so shear of bolts	$T = \dfrac{\tau \pi i d_p^2 D_2}{8}$	13.5(b)
The torque capacity based on bearing of pins and flange	$T = \dfrac{p_b i l d' D_2}{2}$	13.5(c)
Assuming that the force is distributed uniformly over the bush of length l, the maximum bending moment	$M = \dfrac{Fl}{2}$	13.5(d)
The stress due to bending Moment	$\sigma_b = \dfrac{16Fl}{\pi d_p^3}$	13.5(e)

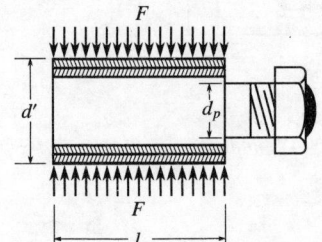

where d_p is the diameter of pin at the neck, mm

d' is the outside diameter of the bush, mm

p_b is the bearing pressure on the projected area of the bronze bushing, ($p_b = 0.2$ MN/m^2)

σ_b is the allowable bending stress

Particular	Equation	Eqn. No.
Oldham Flexible Coupling (Fig. 13.7)		
The total pressure on each side of the tongue of oldham flexible coupling	$F = \dfrac{1}{4}pD_3h$	13.6(a)
where p is the maximum pressure at the periphery of the coupling		
Distance to the pressure-area centroid from the centre line	$l = \dfrac{2}{3} \times \left(\dfrac{1}{2}D_3\right) = \dfrac{1}{3}D_3$	13.6(b)
Torque transmitted by both sides of the tongue	$T = 2Fl = \dfrac{1}{6}pD_3^2h$	13.6(c)
Power in kW which can be transmitted	$P = \dfrac{2\pi nT}{10^6} = \dfrac{\pi npD_3^2h}{3 \times 10^6}$	13.6(d)

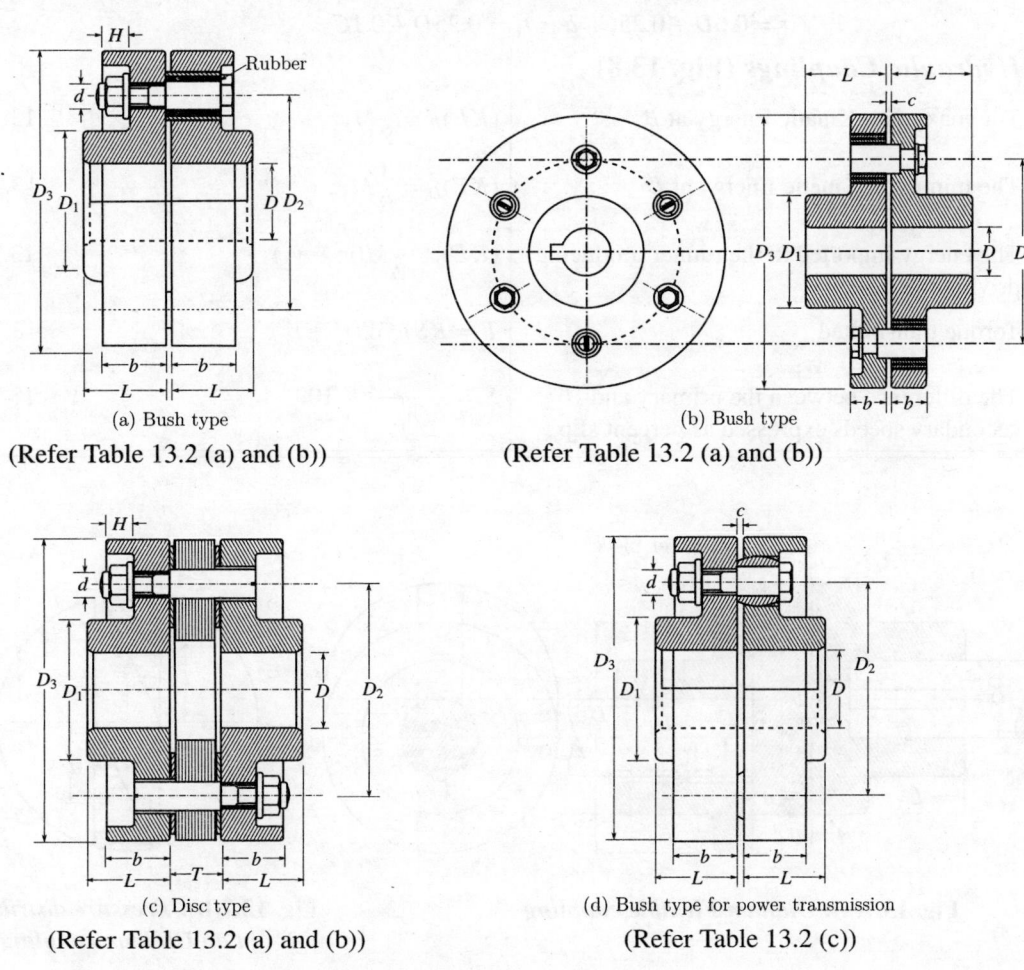

(a) Bush type
(Refer Table 13.2 (a) and (b))

(b) Bush type
(Refer Table 13.2 (a) and (b))

(c) Disc type
(Refer Table 13.2 (a) and (b))

(d) Bush type for power transmission
(Refer Table 13.2 (c))

Fig. 13.6: *Flexible Couplings*

Particular	Equation	Eqn. No.
where $p \not> 8.5$ MN/m^2, the allowable pressure between the faces of the grooves $\not> 7$ MN/m^2, for a considerable misalignment		

n is the speed, rev/s (rps)

$h = 0.25D + 0.1C$, axial dimension of the contact area

$c \not> 0.003D$, parallel shaft eccentricity, mm

$D_1 = 1.8D + 20$ mm, the hub diameter, mm

$D_3 = (3D + C)$ or $(3D$ to $4D)$, the flange diameter, mm

$L = (0.75D + 12.5\text{mm})$, the length of hub

$b = 0.45D$, the tongues of the centre piece, mm

$t = 0.6D + 0.25C; \quad a = t_1 = 0.25D + 0.1C$

Hydraulic Couplings (Fig. 13.8)

Particular	Equation	Eqn. No.
The maximum Kinatic Energy at B	$(KE)_B = \dfrac{1}{2}Mv_1^2$	13.7(a)
The minimum Kinetic Energy at D	$(KE)_D = \dfrac{1}{2}Mv_2^2$	13.7(b)
The energy imported to the runner producing driving torque	$(KE) = \dfrac{1}{2}M(v_1^2 - v_2^2)$	13.7(c)
Torque transmitted	$T = KSn^2W(r_o^2 - r_i^2)$	13.7(d)
The difference between the primary and secondary speeds expressed as percent slip	$S = \dfrac{n_p - n_s}{n_p} \times 100$	13.7(e)

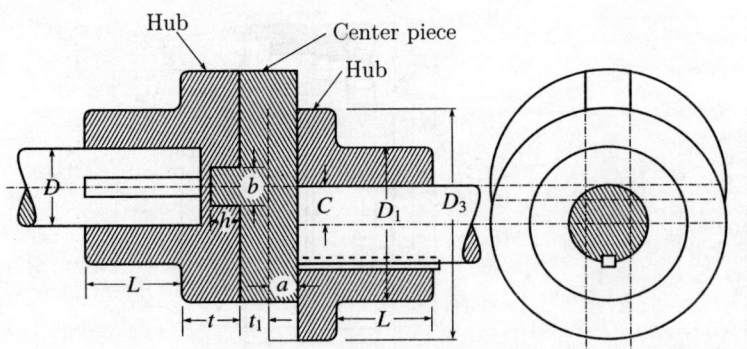

Fig. 13.7(a): *Oldham Flexible coupling*

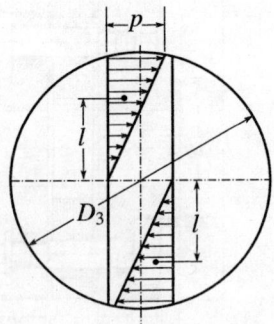

Fig. 13.7(b): *Pressure distribution in an Oldham coupling*

Particular	Equation	Eqn. No.
The percentage efficiency	$\eta = \dfrac{\text{power output}}{\text{power input}} \times 100 = 100 - S$	13.7(f)

where T is the torque transmitted, N mm (kgf mm); $K \approx 8.52 \times 10^{-6}$, a coefficient;

$S = 3$ to 6, percent slip; n is the impeller speed, rev/s

W is the weight of fluid circulating in operating portion of coupling, N/s (Kg./s)

$$r_i = \frac{2}{3}\left(\frac{r_2^3 - r_1^3}{r_2^2 - r_1^2}\right), \text{ mean radius of the inner passage, mm}$$

$$r_o = \frac{2}{3}\left(\frac{r_4^3 - r_3^3}{r_4^2 - r_3^2}\right), \text{ mean radius of the outer passage, mm}$$

r_1, r_2, r_3 and r_4 are as shown in Fig. 13.8.

Clutches

Positive Clutch: (Jaw clutch) (Fig. 13.9)

The tangential force acting on jaws	$F_t = 2T/d_m$	13.8(a)
	where d_m = mean diameter, mm	
Proportions of cast iron jaw clutch: (Fig. 13.9)		13.8(b)

$$D_3 = 2.2D + 25 \text{ mm} \quad H = 0.3D + 12.5 \text{ mm}$$
$$C = 1.2D + 30 \text{ mm} \quad E = 0.4D + 6.0 \text{ mm}$$
$$D_c = 1.4D + 8 \text{ mm} \quad J = 0.2D + 4.0 \text{ mm}$$
$$G = D + 5 \text{ mm} \quad L = 1.7D + 60.0 \text{ mm}$$
$$K = 1.2D + 20 \text{ mm}$$

The area in shear	$A_s = \dfrac{1}{2}\dfrac{(D_3 - B)H}{\sin \alpha}$	13.8(c)

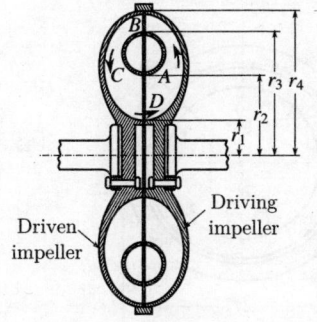

Fig. 13.8: *Hydraulic coupling*

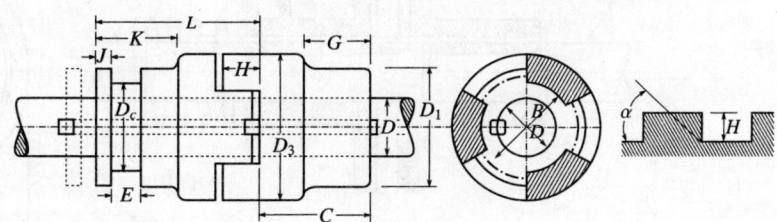

Fig. 13.9: *Cast iron square jaw clutch*

Particular	Equation	Eqn. No.
Assuming that only one half of the total number of jaws (*i*) are in actual contact, the shear stress	$\tau = \dfrac{F_t \sin \alpha}{\frac{1}{2}\cos\alpha(D_3 - B)H \times \frac{1}{2}i}$ $= \dfrac{2.8F_t}{(D_3 - B)Hi}$ for $\tan\alpha = 0.7$	13.8(d)

where α is the angle made by the shearing plane with the direction of pressure

$i = 2$ or 3, the number of square jaws.

A factor of safely of 2 should be used for the allowable shear stress.

p is the allowable bearing pressure (20 to 40 MH/m²)

Friction Clutches:

(a) Plate friction or Disc clutches: **(Fig. 13.10)**

(i) For uniform pressure distribution:

The axial force	$F_{ap} = \dfrac{1}{4}\pi p(D_0^2 - D_i^2)$	13.9(a)
Torque transmitted by one pair of friction surfaces	$T = \dfrac{1}{2}F_t D_m = \dfrac{1}{2}\mu F_{ap}D_{mp}$	13.9(b)
Torque transmitted by n' pairs of friction surfaces	$T = \dfrac{1}{2}\mu n' F_{ap}D_{mp} = \dfrac{\pi}{12}\mu n' p(D_0^3 - D_i^3)$	13.9(c)

where $D_{mp} = \dfrac{2}{3}\left\{\dfrac{D_0^3 - D_i^3}{D_0^2 - D_i^2}\right\}$, mean diameter, mm

μ is the coefficient of friction (Table 13.4)

(ii) For uniform wear:

The axial force	$F_{aw} = \dfrac{1}{2}\pi p_{\max}D_i(D_o - D_i)$	13.9(d)
Torque transmitted by one pair of friction surfaces	$T = \dfrac{1}{2}F_t D_{mw} = \frac{1}{2}\mu F_{aw}D_{mw}$	13.9(e)

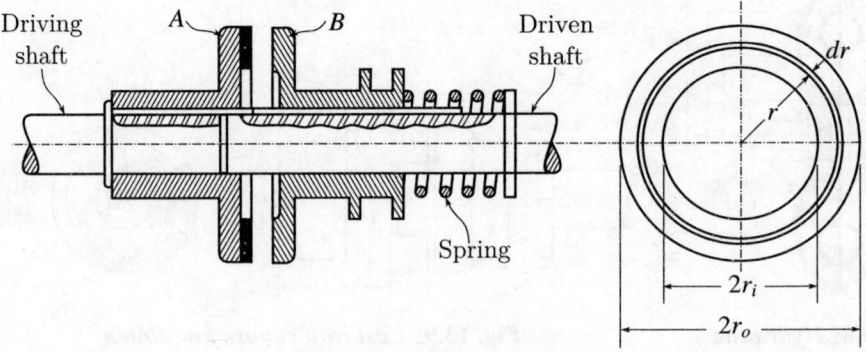

Fig. 13.10: *Plate friction clutch*

Particular	Equation	Eqn. No.
Torque transmitted by n' pairs of friction surfaces	$T = \dfrac{1}{2}\mu n' F_{aw} D_{mw} = \dfrac{\pi}{8}\mu n' p_{max} D_i(D_0^2 - D_i^2)$	13.9(f)

$$\text{where } D_{mw} = \left(\frac{D_0 + D_i}{2}\right), \text{ mean diameter, mm}$$

The friction torque, Nmm	$T_f = \beta$ (Design Torque)	13.9(g)

where β = engagement factor;

= 1.25 – 1.50 for machine tools; β = 1.20 – 1.50 for automobiles

= 2.00 – 2.50 for Tractors; $\beta > 1.50$ for crane machines

(b) Cone clutches: (Fig. 13.11)

The axial force in terms of normal force	$F_a = F_n \sin \alpha$	13.10(a)
The friction force or tangential force	$F_t = \mu F_n = \dfrac{\mu F_a}{\sin \alpha}$	13.10(b)
The relation between the axial force and the clutch dimensions	$F_a = \pi D_m b p \sin \alpha$	13.10(c)
The torque transmitted through friction	$T = \dfrac{F_t D_m}{2} = \dfrac{\mu F_a D_m}{2 \sin \alpha} = \dfrac{\pi}{2}\mu b p D_m^2$	13.10(d)

where $D_m \approx \frac{1}{2}(D_1 + D_2)$, mean diameter

α = one half of the cone angle, deg.

= 12.5° for cone clutches faced with leather

= 15° to 25°, for industrial clutches faced with wood

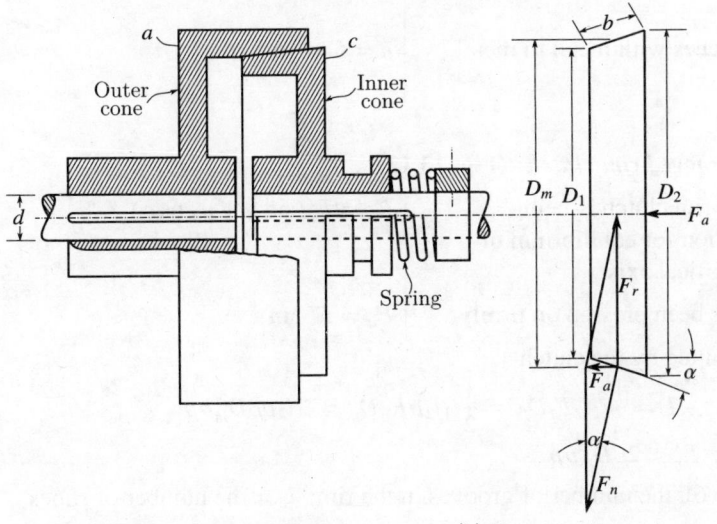

(a) Cone clutch coupling   (b) Forces acting on inner cone

Fig. 13.11: *Cone clutch coupling*

Particular	Equation	Eqn. No.

The power transmitted (taking into account the load factor)

$$P(kW) = \frac{\pi \mu F_a D_m n}{10^6 \sin \alpha K_l} = \frac{\pi^2 \mu p D_m^2 b n}{10^6 K_l} \qquad \text{13.10(e)}$$

$$P(MHP) = \frac{\pi \mu F_a D_m n}{75 \times 1000 \times K_l} = \frac{\pi^2 \mu p D_m^2 b n}{75 \times 1000 \times K_l} \qquad \text{13.10(f)}$$

where K_l = load factor (Table 12.33)

| The force necessary to engage the clutch when one member rotating | $F_a' = F_n(\sin \alpha + \mu \cos \alpha)$

 $= \pi D_m b p(\sin \alpha + \mu \cos \alpha)$ | 13.10(g) |

where μ = coefficient of friction

   = 0.15 for cast iron on cast iron

   = 0.20 for a surface faced with leather or wood

μ = 0.30 for a surface faced with asbestos; μ = 0.25 for cone surfaces with cork inserts

   p is the unit normal pressure at the contact surface

The ratio (D_m/b)	$q = D_m/b = 4.5$ to 8	13.10(h)
The mean diameter of clutch, mm	$D_m = 10^3 \sqrt[3]{\dfrac{PK_l q}{\pi^2 \mu p n}}$	13.10(i)
The mean diameter in case of commercial clutches	$D_m = 5D$ to $10D$	13.10(j)
The peripheral velocity for high speed, leather faced couplings	$v = 13$ to 25 m/s	13.10(k)
The speed for clutches with metal to metal contact surfaces	$n = 5$ to 16.5 rps	13.10(l)

Rim Clutches:

Block clutch or Grooved rim clutch: (Fig. 13.12)

| When the grooved rim clutch is being engaged, the equation for equilibrium of forces along the vertical axis | $F_n = F_n'(\sin \alpha + \mu \cos \alpha)$ | 13.11(a) |
| After the block has been pressed on firmly | $F_n = F_n' \sin \alpha$ | 13.11(b) |

The Torque transmitted by the clutch

$$T = \frac{1}{2} i_1 i_2 F_t D_m = \frac{1}{2} i_1 i_2 \mu F_n' D_m = i_1 i_2 \mu \beta D_m^2 b p \qquad \text{13.11(c)}$$

where $F_t = \mu F_n'$; $F_n' = 2\beta D_m b p$

   i_1 = (3 to 6), the number of grooves in the rim; i_2 = the number of shoes

   β is the angle of block or shoe in radians

   p is the normal pressure over the whole contact area of each block (Table 13.4)

   $b = 0.01 D_m + 6$mm, width of inclined face

Particular	Equation	Eqn. No.
Torque transmitted by flat rim clutch ($i_2 = 1$ and the number of sides b is only one half that of a grooved rim)	$T = \dfrac{1}{2}i_2\mu\beta D_m^2 bp$	13.11(d)

Expansion ring Clutch or Slip ring Clutch: (Fig. 13.13(a) and (b))

If the pressure is uniformly distributed over the contact surface, torque transmitted	$T = 2\mu pbr^2\theta = \dfrac{1}{2}\mu\pi pbd^2$	13.12(a)
Power transmitted by the clutch	$P(kw) = \dfrac{\pi^2\mu pb^n d^2}{1000k_l}$	13.12(b)

where θ = one half of the total arc of contact in rad ($\theta \approx \pi$ radians)

$\mu = 0.125$, for cast iron on cast iron; $\mu = 0.25$ for asbestos lined rings on cast iron

b = width of ring, mm; n is the speed, rps; p is the average pressure

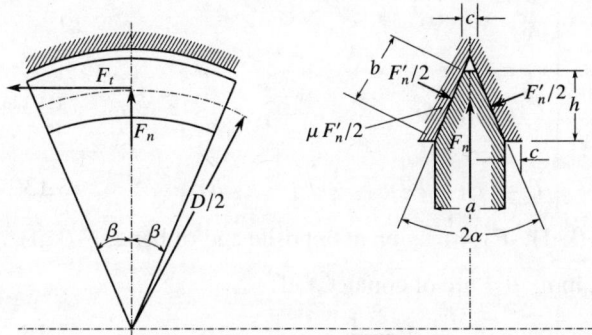

$b = 0.01D_m + 6mm$

$c = 0.15h$ to $0.25h$

2β = angle of contact, rad

2α = V-groove angle, deg

$2\alpha > 15°$ for cast iron blocks

$> 20°$ for wood or asbestos blocks

Fig. 13.12: *Grooved*

Note: (1) Total arc of contact, $2L_2\beta = 180°$ or one-half the circumference

(2) Angle α greater than 25° decreases the torque very much.

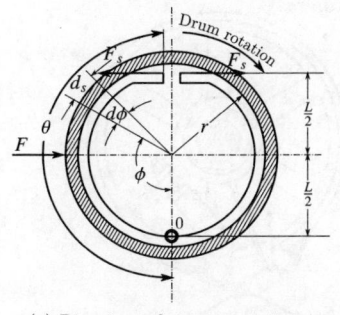
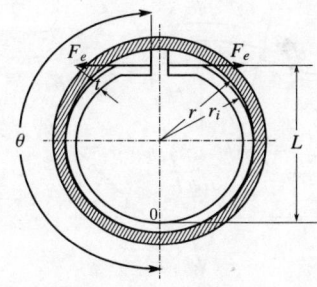

d_1 = original diameter of ring, mm

d = inner diameter of drum, mm

t = thickness of ring, mm

b = width of ring, mm

(a) Ring is made in two sections   (b) Ring is made in one piece

Fig. 13.13: *Expanding ring clutches*

Note: The outside diameter of a cast iron ring is usually made 0.4 mm to 0.8 mm smaller than the inner diameter of drum. If an asbestos-lined ring of flat steel is bent, the difference is 0.8mm for a small clutch and up to 5mm for a large clutch.

Particular	Equation	Eqn. No.
The moment of the normal forces for each half of the band (Fig. 13.13(a))	$M = pbrL = \frac{1}{2}pbd^2$	13.12(c)
The force F applied to the ends of the split ring to expand the ring (Fig. 13.13(a))	$F = pbr = \frac{1}{2}pbd = \frac{T}{\mu\pi d}$	13.12(d)
If the ring is made in one piece (Fig. 13.13(b), then the additional force required to expand the inner ring before contact is made with the inner surface of the shell	$F_e = \frac{Ebt^3}{6L}\left(\frac{1}{d_1} - \frac{1}{d}\right)$	13.12(e)
If the ring is made of one piece, the total force required to expand the ring and to produce the necessary pressure between the contact surfaces	$F_t = F + F_e = pbr + \frac{Ebt^3}{6L}\left(\frac{1}{d_1} - \frac{1}{d}\right)$	13.12(e)

Band Clutches: (Fig. 13.14)

The ratio of tensions on the two ends of the band	$F_1/F_2 = e^{\mu\theta}$	13.13(a)
The torque transmitted	$T = (F_1 - F_2)r = \frac{1}{2}(F_1 - F_2)d$	13.13(b)

where F_1 = maximum tension in band, N (kgf); F_2 = tension at opposite end of band, N (kgf)

$r = (d/2)$, radius of friction drum, mm; θ = arc of contact, rad

The maximum normal pressure	$P_{max} = \frac{F_1}{br} = \frac{2F_1}{bd}$	13.13(c)
	where b = width of band, mm	

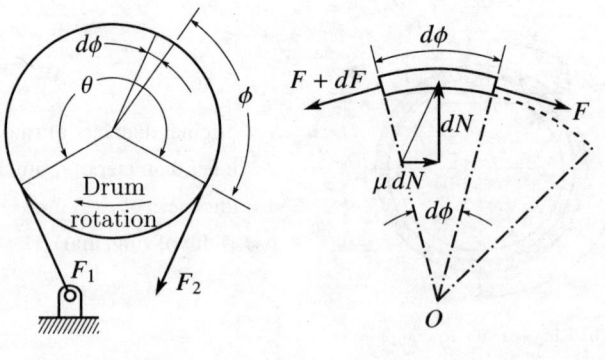
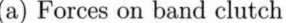
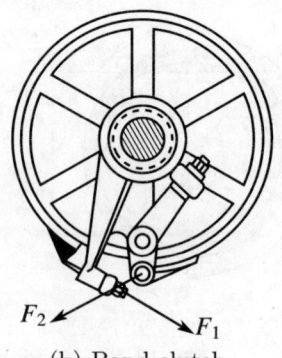

(a) Forces on band clutch   (b) Band clutch

Fig. 13.14: *Band clutch*

Particular	Equation	Eqn. No.
Roller Clutches: (Fig. 13.15)		
The force crushing the roller	$F = F_t / \tan \alpha$	13.14(a)
Torque transmitted	$T = \dfrac{1}{2} F_t D_2$	13.14(b)

where F_t = the tangential force necessary to transmit the torque at a pitch diameter D_2

α = angle between the tangents to the curves of the cam and the shell at points of roller contact ($\alpha < 2\phi$)

ϕ is the angle of friction

$\tan \phi = \mu = 0.03$ to 0.05 (varies between hardened and polished surfaces)

The allowable load for i' rollers	$F \leq i' \sigma_b k' l d$	13.14(c)

where l = length of the roller, mm

σ_b = allowable crushing stress, MN/m^2 (kgf/mm^2)

= 1030 (105) for high grade hardened chrome steel of about 0.85%C

$k' = \dfrac{4.64 \sigma_b}{E}$, coefficient of the flattening of the roller

$d = 0.1\,D$ to $0.25\,D$, roller diameter, mm

Single Block Clutch (Fig. 13.16)		
The torque transmitted by the single block clutch (Nm)	$T = \mu \left(\dfrac{4 \sin \theta}{2\theta + \sin 2\theta} \right) \dfrac{FD}{2}$	13.14(d)
The tangential frictional force on the block, N	$F_t = \dfrac{2T}{D} = \mu \left(\dfrac{4 \sin \theta}{2\theta + \sin 2\theta} \right) F = \mu' F$	13.14(e)

where F is the operating force on the block in a radial direction, N(kgf)

D is the diameter of the wheel, m; $\mu = \tan \phi$, the friction coefficient

θ is the one-half the angle of contact surfae of the block; ϕ is the angle of friction

$\mu' = \mu \left(\dfrac{4 \sin \theta}{2\theta + \sin 2\theta} \right)$, equivalent coefficient of friction

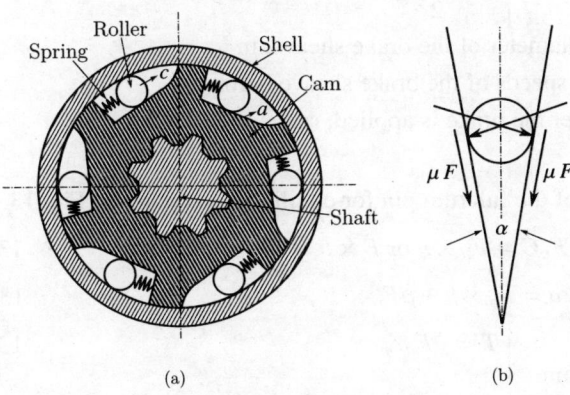

Fig. 13.15: *Roller Clutches*

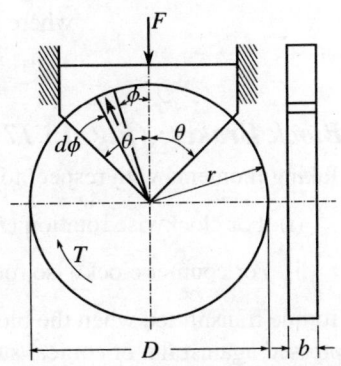

Fig. 13.16: *Single Block Clutch*

Particular	Equation	Eqn. No.
Brakes		
Energy equations:		
The decrease of kinetic energy for a change of the speed of the live load from v_1 to v_2, J (kgf m)	$E_k = \dfrac{Q(v_1^2 - v_2^2)}{2g}$	13.15(a)
The change of the potential energy absorbed by the brake during the time t, J (kgf m)	$E_p = \dfrac{1}{2}Q(v_1 + v_2)t$	13.15(b)
The change of the kinetic energy of all rotating parts such as the hoist drum and various gears and sheaves, absorbed by the brake, J (kgf m)	$E_r = \sum \dfrac{Wk_o^2(\omega_1^2 - \omega_2^2)}{2g}$	13.15(c)

where W is the weight of each of these part, N (kgf)

k_o is the radius of gyration of each of these part, m

g = acceleration due to gravity, 9.81 m/s^2

v_1, v_2 are the speeds of the live load before and after

the brake is applied, respectively, m/s

ω_1, ω_2 are the angular velocities of the rotating parts, rad/s

t is the duration of the brake application, s; Q is the load, N(kgf)

The work to be done by the tangential force F_t at the brake sheave surface in t sec, J (kgf m)	$W_k = \dfrac{F_t \pi D(n_1 + n_2)t}{2}$	13.15(d)
The work to be done by tangential force F_t is also equal to	$W_k = (E_k + E_p + E_r)$	13.15(e)
The tangential force at the brake sheave surface, N (kgf) (from Eqn. 13.15 (d) and (e))	$F_t = \dfrac{2(E_k + E_p + E_r)}{\pi D(n_1 + n_2)t}$	13.15(f)
The torque which the brake must absorb (Nm)	$T = \dfrac{1}{2}F_t D$	13.15(g)

where D is the diameter of the brake sheave, m

n_1, n_2 are the speeds of the brake sheave before

and after the brake is applied, rps

Block Brakes: (Fig. 13.17)

Taking moments with respect to the axis of the fulcrum pin for equilibrium condition (Fig. 13.17)

(i) For clockwise rotation $(F \times a) + \mu F_n C = F_n \times b$ or $F \times a = F_n b - \mu F_n c$		13.16(a)
(ii) For counter clockwise rotation $F \times a = F_n \times b + \mu F_n \times c$		13.16(b)
Torque transmitted when the blocks are pressed against flat or conical surface, N mm (kgf mm)	$T = \mu F_n r_m$	13.16(a)

Particular	Equation	Eqn. No.
The force (F) needed to operate the brake		
(i) For clockwise rotation	$F = \dfrac{F_n b - \mu F_n c}{a}$	13.16(c)
(ii) For counter clockwise rotation	$F = \dfrac{F_n b + \mu F_n c}{a}$	13.16(d)

where F is the applied force, N(kgf)

F_n is the normal reaction between the sheave and block, N(kgf)

(μF_n) is the friction force between the sheave and block, N(kgf)

F_n is the pin reaction between the sheave and block, N(kgf)

$F_t = (\mu F_n)$, the tangential force, N(kgf)

The torque transmitted or the torque absorbed by the brake	$T = \dfrac{1}{2} F_t D = \dfrac{1}{2} \mu F_n D$	13.16(e)

where D is the sheave or drum diameter (Table 13.6(a))

The normal force	$F_n = \dfrac{2T}{\mu D}$	13.16(f)
Required area of brake shoes	$A_{bs} = F_n / p$	13.16(g)

where A_{bs} is the projected area normal to the direction of F_n

p is the allowable specific pleassure, MN/m^2

For wooden or molded asbestos blocks, the product of prssure (MN/m^2) and rubbing velocity (v in m/s)   13.16(h)

$pv \leq 1.0$ for continuous operation

≤ 2.0 intermittent operation with comperatively long periods of rest

≤ 3.0 for continuous application of load and good dissipation of heat as in on oil bath

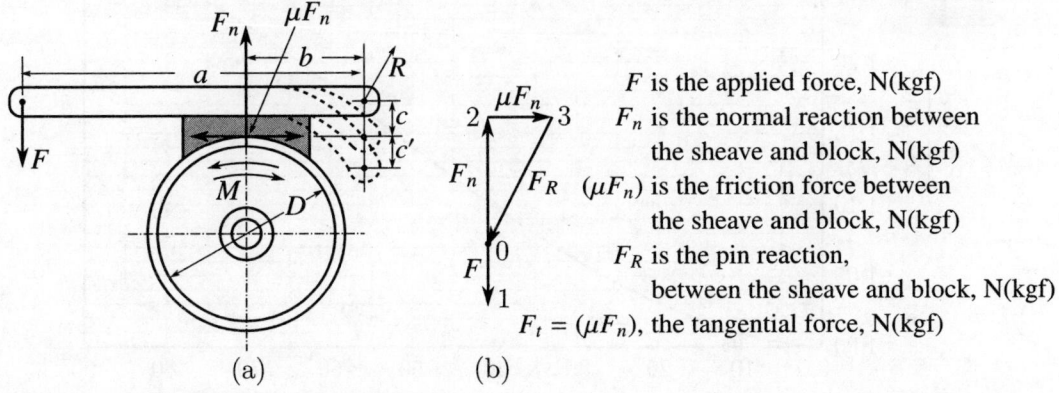

(a)   (b)

F is the applied force, N(kgf)

F_n is the normal reaction between the sheave and block, N(kgf)

(μF_n) is the friction force between the sheave and block, N(kgf)

F_R is the pin reaction, between the sheave and block, N(kgf)

$F_t = (\mu F_n)$, the tangential force, N(kgf)

Fig. 13.17: *Single-lever block brake*

Note : The magnitude of force F depends on the direction of rotation. It is smaller for clockwise rotation, zero if $b = \mu c$ and negative if $b < \mu c$. If $c = 0$, F does not depend on the direction of rotation.

Particular	Equation	Eqn. No.
The width of brake lining, mm	$B_l = B_d - (5 \text{ to } 10)\,\text{mm}$	13.16(i)

where B_d is the width of brake drum, mm (Table 13.6(a))

The projected length of the lining	$L_l = \dfrac{A_{bs}}{B_l}$	13.16(j)
The simi block angle of contact surface of the block	$\theta = 2\sin^{-1}\left(\dfrac{L}{D}\right)$	13.16(k)
Torque applied at the braking surface, when the blocks are pressed radially against the outer or inner surface of a cylindrical drum	$T = \mu F_n \dfrac{D}{2}\left(\dfrac{4\sin\theta}{2\theta + \sin 2\theta}\right)$	13.16(l)

where F_n is the operating force on the block in a radial direction, N (kgf)

D is the diameter of wheel, mm

θ is one-half the angle of contact surface of the block, deg

The tangential frictional force on the block	$F_t = \dfrac{2T}{D} = \mu F_n\left(\dfrac{4\sin\theta}{2\theta + \sin 2\theta}\right) = \mu' F_n$	13.16(m)

$$\text{where } \mu' = \mu\left(\dfrac{4\sin\theta}{2\theta + \sin 2\theta}\right)$$

$$= \text{equivalent coefficient of friction}$$

Torque applied when θ is less than 30°	$T = b\mu F_n r^2 \theta = \mu F_n R = \dfrac{\mu F_n D}{2}$	13.16(n)

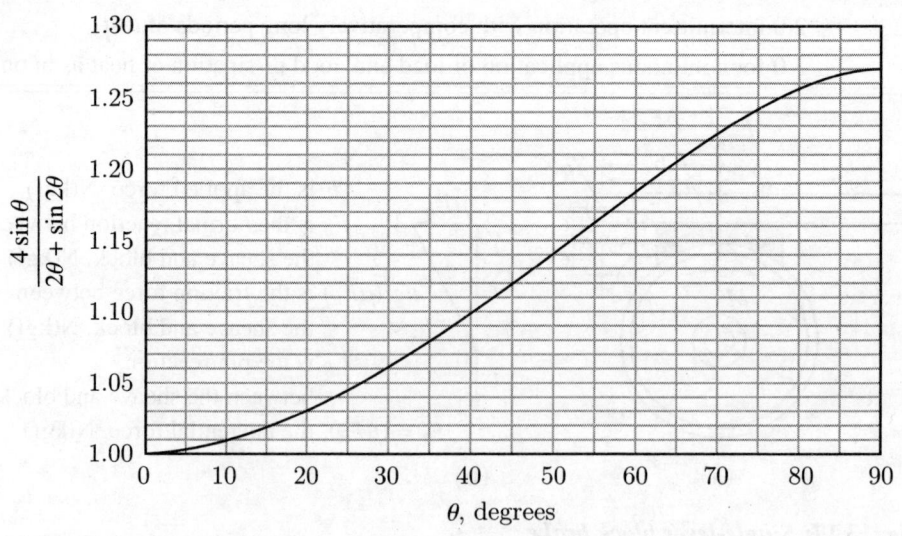

Fig. 13.17(c): $(4\sin\theta)/(2\theta + \sin 2\theta)$ plotted against the semiblock angle θ

Particular	Equation	Eqn. No.

Block Brakes:

F = Force at end of brake handle N (kgf)

F_t = Tangential force at rim of brake wheel, N (kgf)

μ = coefficient of friction between the brake block and brake wheel

Fig. a

(a) For rotation in either direction:

$$F = F_t \left[\frac{b}{a+b} \right] \frac{1}{\mu}$$

13.17(a)

Fig. b

(b) For clockwise rotation

$$F = \frac{F_t b}{a+b} \left(\frac{1}{\mu} - \frac{c}{b} \right)$$

13.17(b)

For counter-clockwise direction

$$F = \frac{F_t b}{a+b} \left(\frac{1}{\mu} + \frac{c}{b} \right)$$

13.17(c)

Fig. c

(c) For clockwise rotation

$$F = \frac{F_t b}{a+b} \left(\frac{1}{\mu} + \frac{c}{b} \right)$$

13.17(d)

For counter-clockwise rotation

$$F = \frac{F_t b}{a+b} \left(\frac{1}{\mu} - \frac{c}{b} \right)$$

13.17(e)

Simple and Differential Band Brakes:

Band Brakes : (13.18 (a))

The ratio of tensions	$\dfrac{F_1}{F_2} = e^{\mu\theta}$	13.18(a)
The tangential braking force	$F_t^* = F_1 - F_2$	13.18(b)
Force on high-tension side	$F_1 = (F_t e^{\mu\theta})/(e^{\mu\theta} - 1)$	13.18(c)
Force on low-tension side	$F_2 = F_t/(e^{\mu\theta} - 1)$	13.18(d)

*Note: For a required net tension F_t the magnitudes of F_1 and F_2 decrease with an increse of friction coefficient μ and also the angle of contact θ.

Particular	Equation	Eqn. No.
Force at the end of brake handle (Fig. 13.18)		
(i) For clockwise rotation	$$F = \frac{F_t(b_2 - e^{\mu\theta}b_1)}{(e^{\mu\theta} - 1)a}$$	13.18(e)
(ii) For counter clockwise rotation	$$F = \frac{F_t(e^{\mu\theta}b_2 - b_1)}{(e^{\mu\theta} - 1)a}$$	13.18(f)
In case of simple band brake (Fig. 13.18(b)		
(i) Force F for clockwise rotation	$$F = \frac{F_t b}{(e^{\mu\theta} - 1)a}$$	13.18(g)
(ii) Force F for counter clockwise rotation	$$F = \frac{F_t e^{\mu\theta} b}{(e^{\mu\theta} - 1)a}$$	13.18(h)
Force F of band brake for rotation in both directions	$$F = \frac{F_t b(e^{\mu\theta} + 1)}{(e^{\mu\theta} - 1)a}$$	13.18(i)
For a stationary sheave the pressure around the sheave	$$p = \frac{2F}{DB}$$ where B is the band width, mm	13.18(j)
The average pressure between the band and the brake sheave	$$p = \frac{F_1 + F_2}{DB}$$ where b = band width, mm	13.18(k)

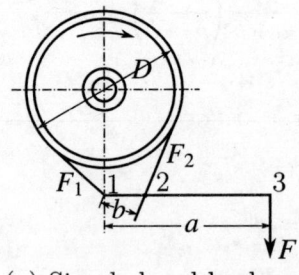

(a) Simple band brake.

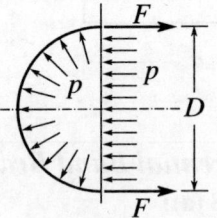

(b) Forces acting on a brake band.

Fig. 13.18: *Band Brake*

Note : For a required net tension F_t the magnitudes of F_1 and F_2 decrease with an increase of friction coefficient μ and also the angle of contact.

Particular	Equation	Eqn. No.
Pressure at the high tension end of the band	$p_1 = \dfrac{2F_1}{DB}$	13.18(l)
Pressure at the low-tension end of the band	$p_2 = \dfrac{2F_2}{DB}$	13.18(m)
The band thickness	$h = 0.005D$	13.18(n)
The width of band	$b = F_1/h\sigma_d$	13.18(o)

where σ_d = design stress of band (in selecting the design stress,

a reliability factor of 4 should be used)

Suitable drum diameter according to Hagen mm	$\left(\dfrac{T}{0.4335}\right)^{\frac{1}{3}} < D < \left(\dfrac{T}{0.3472}\right)^{\frac{1}{3}}$	13.18(p)

where T = design braking torque, N mm

$$\left(\frac{T}{0.0442}\right)^{\frac{1}{3}} < D < \left(\frac{T}{0.0354}\right)^{\frac{1}{3}} \qquad \text{13.18(q)}$$

when T is in kgf mm

F = Force at end of brake handle, N (kgf);

F_t = tangential force at rim of brake wheel, N (kgf)

θ = angle of contact of brake band with the brake wheel, rad

$F_1 = F_t \dfrac{e^{\mu\theta}}{e^{\mu\theta} - 1}$ Force on high-tension side, N (kgf);

$F_2 = F_t \left[\dfrac{1}{e^{\mu\theta} - 1}\right]$ Force on low-tension side, N (kgf);

$\dfrac{F_1}{F_2} = e^{\mu\theta}; \quad T = (F_1 - F_2)r = (F_1 - F_2)D/2$

Particular	Equation	Eqn. No.
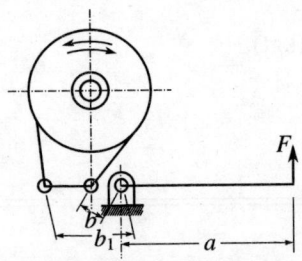 **Fig. d:** *Simple band brake*	**(a) Simple band brake:** For clockwise rotation $$F = \frac{bF_1}{a} = \frac{F_t b}{a}\left(\frac{e^{\mu\theta}}{e^{\mu\theta}-1}\right)$$ For counter-clockwise rotation: $$F = \frac{bF_2}{a} = \frac{F_t b}{a}\left(\frac{1}{e^{\mu\theta}-1}\right)$$	13.19(a) 13.19(b)
Fig. e: *Simple band brake*	**(b) Simple band brake:** For clockwise rotation $$F = \frac{bF_2}{a} = \frac{F_t b}{a}\left(\frac{1}{e^{\mu\theta}-1}\right)$$ For counter-clockwise rotation $$F = \frac{bF_1}{a} = \frac{F_t b}{a}\left(\frac{e^{\mu\theta}}{e^{\mu\theta}-1}\right)$$	13.19(c) 13.19(d)
Fig. f: *Differential band brake*	**(c) Differential band brake:** For clockwise rotation $$F = \frac{b_2 F_1 - b_1 F_2}{a} = \frac{F_t}{a}\left(\frac{b_2 e^{\mu\theta} - b_1}{e^{\mu\theta}-1}\right)$$ For counter-clockwise rotation $$F = \frac{(b_2 F_2 - b_1 F_1)}{a} = \frac{F_t}{a}\left(\frac{b_2 - b_1 e^{\mu\theta}}{e^{\mu\theta}-1}\right)$$	13.19(e) 13.19(f)

In equation 13.19(f), if b_2 is equal to or less than $b_1 e^{\mu\theta}$, force F will be zero or negative and the band brake works automatically.

Particular	Equation	Eqn. No.
Fig. g: *Differential band brake*	**(d) Differential band brake:** For clockwise direction $$F = \frac{b_2 F_1 + b_1 F_2}{a} = \frac{F_t}{a}\left(\frac{b_2 e^{\mu\theta} + b_1}{e^{\mu\theta}-1}\right)$$ For counter-clockwise rotation $$F = \frac{b_1 F_1 + b_2 F_2}{a} = \frac{F_t}{a}\left(\frac{b_1 e^{\mu\theta} + b_2}{e^{\mu\theta}-1}\right)$$ if $b_2 = b_1$, the formulae 13.19(g) and (h) reduce to $F = \dfrac{F_t b_1}{a}\left(\dfrac{e^{\mu\theta}+1}{e^{\mu\theta}-1}\right)$ In this case the same force F is required for rotation in either direction	13.19(g) 13.19(h) 13.19(i)

Particular	Equation	Eqn. No.
Cone Brakes: (Fig. 13.19)		
The normal force at the cone surface	$F_n = F_a / \sin \alpha$	13.20(a)
The radial force at the cone surface	$F_r = F_a / \tan \alpha$	13.20(b)
The tangential force or braking force	$F_t = \mu F_n = \mu F_a / \sin \alpha$	13.20(c)
The braking torque	$T = \mu F_a D_m / 2 \sin \alpha$	13.20(d)
where D_m is the mean diameter of the cone, mm		
The axial force	$F_a = F\, a/b$	13.20(e)
The relation between the operating force F and the braking force F_t	$F = \dfrac{F_t b \sin \alpha}{\mu a}$	13.20(f)
The area of the contact surfaces	$A = \pi D B / \cos \alpha$	13.20(g)
The average pressure between the contact surface	$p = F_n / A = \dfrac{F_a}{\pi D B \tan \alpha}$	13.20(b)
where $\alpha = 10$ to $18°$, half of the cone angle; $B = 0.12D$ to $0.22\,D$, axial width, mm		
The torsional resistance of n' pairs of friction surfaces	$T = \dfrac{\pi n' \mu p_i D_i (D_o^2 - D_i^2)}{4}$	13.20(i)
The axial force transmitted	$F_a = \frac{1}{2}\pi p_i D_i (D_o - D_i)$	13.20(j)
where p_i is the intensity of pressure at inner radius, MN/m^2 (kgf/mm^2)		

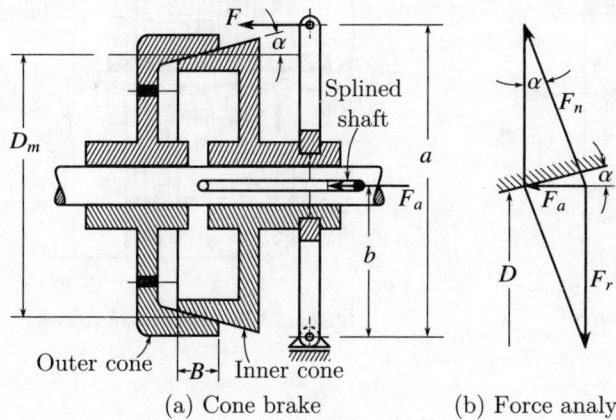

F is the operating force
F_a is the axial force
F_n is the normal force
F_r is the radial force
F_t is the tangential or braking force
D_m is the mean diameter of cone
B is the axial width

(a) Cone brake   (b) Force analysis

Fig. 13.19: *Cone brake*

Particular	Equation	Eqn. No.
Disk Brakes: (Fig. 13.20)		
Assuming Uniform wear, the relation between pressure and radius	$PR = p_i R_i = p_0 R_0$	13.21(a)
The pressure between the disks	$P = \dfrac{p_i R_i}{R} = \dfrac{p_0 R_0}{R}$	13.21(b)

where p_i, p_o are the pressures at inner and outer radii respectively

The axial force transmitted to the disks from the flange by one pair	$F_a = \dfrac{1}{2}\pi p_i D_i(D_0 - D_i)$	13.21(c)
The torsional resistance of n' pairs of friction surfaces	$T = \dfrac{1}{2}F_t n' D_m = \dfrac{1}{2}\mu n' F_a D_m{}^*$ $= \pi n' \mu p_i D_i(D_o^2 - D_i^2)/8$	13.21(d)

where p_i is the intensity of pressure at inner radius

$$D_m{}^* = \left(\frac{D_0 + D_i}{2}\right), \text{ mean diameter; } \quad n' \text{ is the number of pairs of friction surfaces}$$

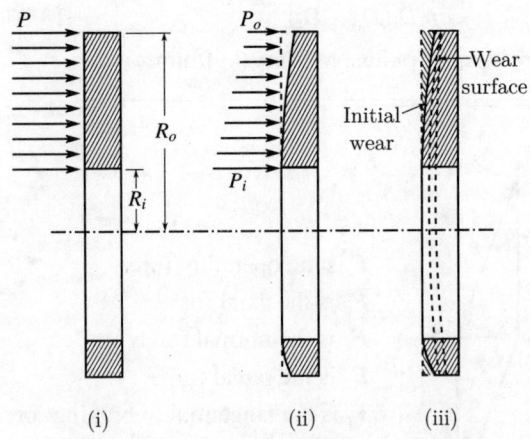

Fig. 13.20(a): *Disk pressure and wear*

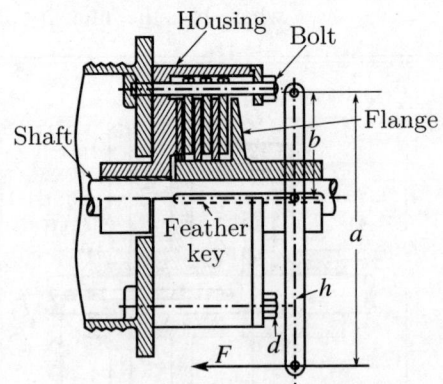

Fig. 13.20(b): *Multidisk break*

---

*More accurate value for D_m may be taken as $D_m = \dfrac{2}{3}\left(\dfrac{D_0^3 - D_i^3}{D_0^2 - D_i^2}\right)$

Particular	**Equation**	**Eqn. No.**

Forces on the brake shoe:

(a) internal expanding shoe:

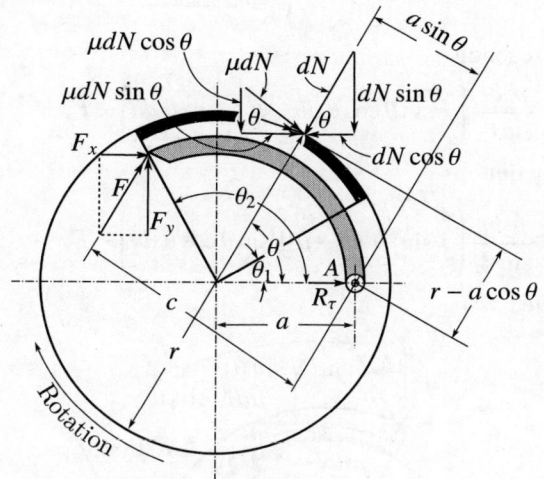

Fig. 13.21: *Forces on the shoe*

The maximum pressure located at the angle θ_a from the hinge pin

$$p = p_a \frac{\sin \theta}{\sin \theta_a}$$

13.22(a)

The moment of the frictional forces

$$M_f = \frac{\mu p_a br}{\sin \theta_a} \int_{\theta_1}^{\theta_2} \sin \theta (r - a \cos \theta) d\theta$$

13.22(b)

The moment of the normal forces

$$M_n = \frac{p_a bra}{\sin \theta_a} \int_{\theta_1}^{\theta_2} \sin^2 \theta \, d\theta$$

13.22(c)

For clockwise direction:

The actuating force

$$F = \frac{M_n - M_f}{c}$$

13.22(d)

Torque applied to the drum by the brake shoe

$$T = \frac{\mu p_a br^2 (\cos \theta_1 - \cos \theta_2)}{\sin \theta_a}$$

13.22(e)

The horizontal hinge-pin reaction

$$R_x = \frac{p_a br}{\sin \theta_a} \left(\int_{\theta_1}^{\theta_s} \sin \theta \cos \theta \, d\theta - \mu \int_{\theta_1}^{\theta_2} \sin^2 \theta \, d\theta \right) - F_x$$

13.22(f)

The vertical hinge-pin reaction

$$R_y = \frac{p_a br}{\sin \theta_a} \left(\int_{\theta_1}^{\theta_2} \sin^2 \theta \, d\theta + \mu \int_{\theta_1}^{\theta_2} \sin \theta \cos \theta \, d\theta \right) - F_y$$

13.22(g)

Particular	Equation	Eqn. No.
For counter-clockwise direction:		
The actuating force	$$F = \frac{M_n + M_f}{c}$$	13.22(h)
The horizontal hinge-pin reaction	$$R_x = \frac{p_a br}{\sin \theta_a} \left(\int_{\theta_1}^{\theta_2} \sin \theta \cos \theta \, d\theta + \mu \int_{\theta_1}^{\theta_2} \sin^2 \theta \, d\theta \right) - F_x$$	13.22(i)
The vertical hinge-pin reaction	$$R_y = \frac{p_2 br}{\sin \theta_a} \left(\int_{\theta_1}^{\theta_2} \sin^2 \theta \, d\theta - \mu \int_{\theta_1}^{\theta_2} \sin \theta \cos \theta \, d\theta \right) - F_y$$	13.22(j)

External-contracting shoe:

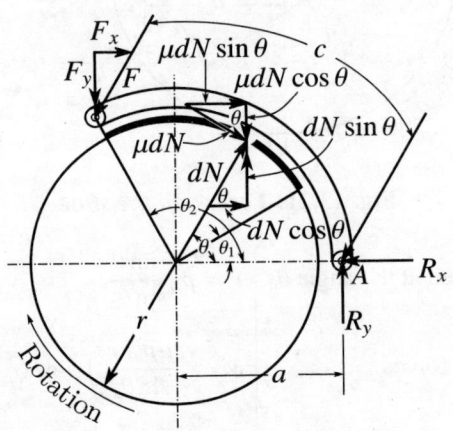

Fig. 13.22: *Notation for External-Contracting Shoe*

For clockwise rotation:		
The moment of the friction force	$$M_f = \frac{\mu p_a br}{\sin \theta_a} \int_{\theta_1}^{\theta_2} \sin \theta (r - a \cos \theta) d\theta$$	13.23(a)
The moment of the normal force	$$M_n = \frac{p_a bra}{\sin \theta_a} \int_{\theta_1}^{\theta_2} \sin^2 \theta d\theta$$	13.23(b)
The actuating force	$$F = \frac{M_n + M_f}{c}$$	13.23(c)
The horizontal hinge-pin-reaction	$$R_x = \frac{p_a br}{\sin \theta_a} \left(\int_{\theta_1}^{\theta_2} \sin \theta \cos \theta \, d\theta + \mu \int_{\theta_1}^{\theta_2} \sin^2 \theta \, d\theta \right) - F_x$$	13.23(d)
The vertical hinge-pin reaction	$$R_y = \frac{p_a br}{\sin \theta_a} \left(\mu \int_{\theta_1}^{\theta_2} \sin \theta \cos \theta \, d\theta - \int_{\theta_1}^{\theta_2} \sin^2 \theta \, d\theta \right) - F_y$$	13.23(e)

Particular	Equation	Eqn. No.
For counter-clockwise direction: The actuating force	$$F = \dfrac{M_n - M_f}{c}$$	13.23(f)
The horizontal hinge-pin reaction	$$R_x = \dfrac{p_a b r}{\sin \theta_a} \left(\int_{\theta_1}^{\theta_2} \sin\theta \cos\theta \, d\theta - \mu \int_{\theta_1}^{\theta_2} \sin^2\theta \, d\theta \right) - F_x$$	13.23(g)
The vertical hinge-pin reaction	$$R_y = \dfrac{p_a b r}{\sin \theta_a} \left(-\mu \int_{\theta_1}^{\theta_2} \sin\theta \cos\theta \, d\theta - \int_{\theta_1}^{\theta_2} \sin^2\theta \, d\theta \right) + F_y$$	13.23(h)

Heat dissipation:

The energy absorbed or heat to be radiated by a brake per second	$$H = \mu p A_f v$$	13.24(a)

Where μ is the friction coefficient depends on the nature of the friction surfaces, the specific pressure, and the rubbing velocity. (Table 13.11)

p is the specific pressure, MN/m^2 (kgf/mm^2) (Table 13.11)

A_f is the contact area of the friction surfaces, mm^2

v is the relative velocity of the friction surfaces, m/s (Fig. 13.23)

The capacity of the brake to dissipate the heat of friction	$$H_d = k A_d$$	13.24(b)

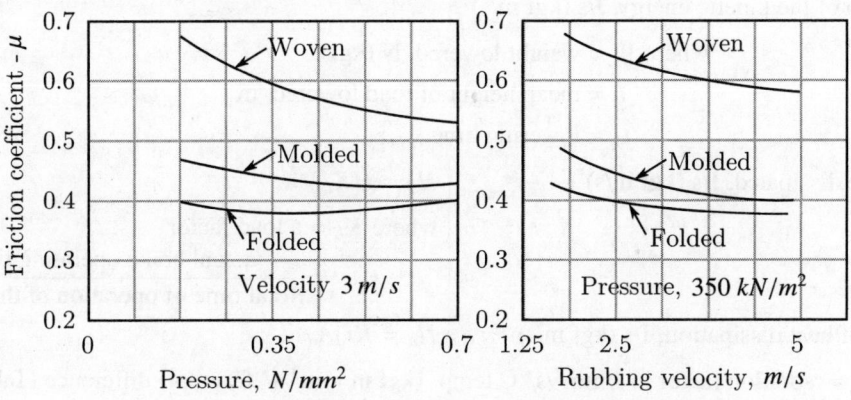

Fig. 13.23: *Friction coefficients of brake linings*

Particular	Equation	Eqn. No.
Heat energy absorbed	$H \leq H_d$ or $\mu p A_f v \leq k A_d$	13.24(c)

Where A_d is the area that dissipates the heat, mm^2

k = a factor which is a function of the service conditions

= 0.04 for continuous operations, lowering brakes, wood on cast iron

= 0.08 for intermittent operation, stopping brakes, wood on cast iron

= 0.12 for good heat dissipation, metal on cast iron in an oil both

= 0.08 for continuous operation, woven asbestos on steel

= 0.12 for intermittent operation, woven asbestos on steel

Particular	Equation	Eqn. No.
The coefficient of friction between steel wheels and cast iron blocks for rubbing velocities from 0 to 25 m/s is expressed by the relation	$\mu = 0.4/\sqrt[3]{v}$	13.24(d)
The tangential force	$F_t = \mu p A_f$	13.24(e)
The area that dissipates the heat	$A_d \geqq \dfrac{\mu p A_f v}{k} \geqq \dfrac{F_t v}{k}$	13.24(f)
The torque which the brake has to absorb	$T = \dfrac{1}{2}\mu p A_f D$	13.24(g)

Lowering the Load:

Particular	Equation	Eqn. No.
The heat to be radiated, J/s (kgf m/s)	$H = \mu F_n v$	13.24(h)
The amount of heat to be dissipated due to absorption of the kinetic energy, J/s (kgf m/s)	$H = \dfrac{Wh}{t_1}$	13.24(i)

where W = weight lowered, N (kgf)

h = mean height of load lowered, m

t_1 = lowering time, s

Particular	Equation	Eqn. No.
Heat to be dissipated, J/s (kgf m/s)	$H_d = HK_L$	13.24(j)
	where K_L = a load factor $= \dfrac{\text{actual brake operating time}}{\text{total time of operation of the cycle}}$	
The rate of heat dissipation, J/s (kgf m/s)	$H_d = Kt_d A_d$	13.24(k)

where K = radiation factor in J/mm^2/s/°C temp. (kgf m/mm^2/s/°C temp.) difference (Table 13.9)

A_d = radiating surface in mm^2

t_d = difference between the temperature of the radiating surface and the surrounding air, °C

Particular	Equation	Eqn. No.
The radiating surface	$A_d = \dfrac{HK_L}{Kt_d}$	13.24(l)

References

[1] Siegel, M. J., Maleev, V. L., Hartman, J. B., *"Mechanical Design of Machines"* 4th edition, International Text Book Company, 1965.

[2] Vallance. A., Doughtie, V. L., *"Design of Machine Members"*, 3rd edition, McGraw Hill Book Company, 1951.

[3] Spotts, M. E., *"Design of Machine Elements"*, 3rd edition, Prentice Hall, Inc., Maruzen Co., Ltd.

[4] Black, P. H., *"Machine Design"*, 3rd edition, McGraw Hill Book Company, Inc.

[5] Shigley, J. E., *"Machine Design"*, McGraw Hill Book Company, Inc.

[6] Hall, A. S., Holowenko, A. R., Laughlin, H. G., *"Theory and Problems of Machine Design"*, Schaum Publishing Co., 1961.

[7] Low D. A., *"A Pocket Book for Mechanical Engineers"*, Longmans, Green & Co., Ltd., London, 1955.

Table 13.1 Dimensions for Forged end Type Rigid Coupling (Refer Fig. 13.4) All Dimensions mm

Coupling number		For Shaft Dia D		Coupling Dimensions								
Recessed Flange	Spigot Flange	Max	Min	Flange Outside Dia D_3	Flange Width t'	Locating Dia D'	Recess Depth b_1	Spigot Depth	Pitch Circle Dia D_2	Bolt* Siez d	Bolt Hole Dia d' HB	Number of Bolts
(1)	(2)	(3)	(4)	(5)	(6)	(7)	(8)	(9)	(10)	(11)	(12)	(13)
R 1	S 1	35	—	100	17	50	6	4	70	M 10	11	4
R 2	S 2	45	36	120	22	60	6	4	85	M 12	13	4
R 3	S 3	55	46	140	22	75	7	5	100	M 14	15	4
R 4	S 4	70	56	175	27	95	7	5	125	M 16	17	6
R 5	S 5	80	71	195	32	95	7	5	140	M 18	19	6
R 6	S 6	90	81	225	32	125	7	5	160	M 20	21	6
R 7	S 7	110	91	265	36	150	9	7	190	M 24	25	6
R 8	S 8	130	111	300	46	150	9	7	215	M 30	32	6
R 9	S 9	150	131	335	50	195	9	7	240	M 32	34	6
R10	S10	170	151	375	55	195	10	8	265	M 36	38	8
R11	S11	190	171	400	55	240	10	8	290	M 36	38	8
R12	S12	210	191	445	65	240	10	8	315	M 42	44	8
R13	S13	230	211	475	70	280	10	8	340	M 45	46	8
R14	S14	250	231	500	70	280	10	8	370	M 45	46	10
R15	S15	270	251	560	80	330	10	8	400	M 52	55	10
R16	S16	300	271	600	85	330	10	8	440	M 56	60	10
R17	S17	330	301	650	90	400	10	8	480	M 60	65	10
R18	S18	360	331	730	100	400	10	8	520	M 68	72	10
R19	S19	390	361	775	105	480	11	9	570	M 72	76	10
R20	S20	430	391	875	110	480	11	9	620	M 76	80	12
R21	R21	470	431	900	115	560	11	9	670	M 80	85	12
R22	S22	520	471	925	120	560	12	10	730	M 90	95	12
R23	S23	570	521	1000	125	640	12	10	790	M100	105	12
R24	S24	620	571	1090	130	720	12	10	850	M110	115	12

*The dimension of the bolt shall be according to IS:3640

IS: 3653-1966

Table 13.2 (a) Dimensions of Flexible Couplings, Bush and Disc Types (Fig. 13.6(a), (b) and (c))

All dimensions in millimeters

	BUSH							DISC								
Coupling No.	Bore D		Outside Dia D_3 min	Hub Dia D_1 min	Hub Length L min	Flange Width b	Maximum Rating per 100 rev/min	Coupling No.	Bore D		Outside Dia D_3 min	Hub Dia D_1 min	Hub Length L min	Flange Width b	Thickness of Disc T	Maximum Rating per 100 ted/min	
	min	max							min	max						kW	kW
(1)	(2)	(3)	(4)	(5)	(6)	(7)	(8)	(9)	(10)	(11)	(12)	(13)	(14)	(15)	(16)	(17)	(18)
B_1	12	16	80	28	28	18	0.4	D_1	12	16	82	28	28	18	15,16	0.4	0.43
B_2	16	22	100	35	30	20	0.6	D_2	16	22	100	35	30	20	16,18	0.6	0.67
B_3	22	30	112	45	32	22	0.8	D_3	22	30	110	45	32	22	18,25	0.8	1.1
B_4	30	45	132	65	40	30	2.5	D_4	30	45	132	65	40	30	25,30	2.5	3.0
B_5	45	56	170	80	45	35	4.0	D_5	45	56	165	80	45	35	30,35	4.0	4.6
B_6	56	75	200	100	56	40	6.0	D_6	56	75	200	100	56	40	35,40	6.0	6.8
B_7	75	85	250	140	63	45	16.0	D_7	75	85	250	140	63	45	40,45	16.0	18.0
B_8	85	110	315	180	80	50	25.0	D_8	85	110	315	180	80	50	45,50	25.0	28.0
B_9	110	130	400	212	90	56	52.0	D_9	110	130	400	212	90	55	50,55	52.0	57.0
B_{10}	130	150	500	280	100	60	74.0	D_{10}	130	150	500	280	100	60	55	74.0	—

IS: 2693–1964

Table 13.2 *(b) Dimensions of Flexible Couplings, Bush and Disc Types (Fig. 13.6(a), (b) and (c))*

	BUSH						DISC				
Coupling No.	Bolt Recess	PCD of Bolts	No. of Bolt Holes	Bolt Dia	Bush Dia	Nominal Gap Between Coupling Halves	Coupling No.	Bolt Recess	PCD of Bolts	*No. of Bolt Holes	Bolt Dia
	H Min	D_2		d		c	H Min		D_2		d
(1)	(2)	(3)	(4)	(5)	(6)	(7)	(8)	(9)	(10)	(11)	(12)
B_1	10	53	3	8	20	2	D_1	10	53	6	8
B_2	12	63	3	10	22	2	D_2	12	63	6	10
B_3	12	73	3	10	22	2	D_3	12	73	6	10
B_4	15	90	4	12	25	4	D_4	15	90	8	12
B_5	15	120	4	12	25	4	D_5	15	120	8	12
B_6	15	150	4	12	30	4	D_6	15	150	8	12
B_7	22	190	6	16	40	5	D_7	22	190	12	16
B_8	22	250	6	16	40	5	D_8	22	250	12	16
B_9	28	315	8	18	45	6	D_9	28	315	16	18
B_{10}	28	400	8	18	45	6	D_{10}	28	400	16	18

All dimensions in millimeters

*Half the number of pinholes in each coupling half shall be clearance holes.

IS: 2693–1964

Table 13.2 *(c) Dimension of Bush Type Flexible Couplings for Power Transmission (Fig. 13.6(d))*

Coupling No.	Load Rating per 100 rev/min kW	Bore Diameter D		D_3	D_1	L	b	c
		Min.	Max.					
FB 1	0.368	15	22	80	40	32	18	2
FB 2	0.441	18	25	90	44	35	25	3
FB 3	0.736	20	30	100	50	40	25	3
FB 4	1.18	25	35	112	62	45	25	3
FB 5	1.84	28	40	125	65	50	28	3
FB 6	2.94	32	45	140	76	55	28	3
FB 7	4.63	35	50	160	85	60	38	3
FB 8	7.36	42	60	180	102	70	38	3
FB 9	10.3	50	70	200	120	80	38	4
FB 10	14.7	57	80	225	134	90	42	4
FB 12	20.6	64	90	250	154	100	45	4
FB 13	38.2	78	110	315	180	125	55	4
FB 14	58.8	85	120	355	200	140	68	5
FB 15	80.9	92	130	400	218	160	80	5
FB 16	110	100	140	450	240	180	80	5
FB 17	235	114	160	560	300	220	122	5
FB 18	331	128	180	630	340	240	122	5
FB 19	456	135	190	710	370	260	145	6
FB 20	618	170	240	800	405	290	245	6
FB 21	883	185	260	900	440	320	165	6
FB 22	1250	200	290	1000	490	350	165	6

All dimensions in millimetres.

IS: 2693–1980

Table 13.3 *Service Factors for use in Equation 13.5*

Type Driven Machine	Service Factors for Prime-Movers					
	Electric Motor Steam or Water Turbine	High Speed Steam or Gas Engine	Petrol Engine		Oil Engine	
			4 or more cyl.	less than 4 cyl.	6 or more cyl.	4 cycle or less
Alternators and generators (excluding welding generators), induced draught fans, printing machinery, rotary pumps compressors and exhausters, conveyors	1.5	2.0	2.5	3.0	3.5	5.0
Woodworking machinery, machine tools (cutting) excluding planing machines, calenders, mixers, elevators	2.0	2.5	3.0	3.5	4.0	5.5
Forced draught fans, high speed reciprocating compressors, high speed crushers and pulverisers, machine tools (forming)	2.5	3.0	3.5	4.0	4.5	6.0
Rotary screens, rod mills, tube, cable and wire machinery, vacuum pumps	3.0	3.5	4.0	4.5	5.0	6.5
Low speed reciprocating compressors haulage gears, metal planning machines brick and tile machinery, rubber macninery, tube mills generators (welding)	3.5	4.0	4.5	5.0	5.5	7.0

IS: 2693–1964

Table 13.4 *Friction Materials For Clutches**

Contact Surfaces		Friction co-efficient		Max. temperature °C	Max pressure*** MN/m²	Relative cost	Comment
Wearing	Opposing	Wet	Dry				
Cast bronze	Cast iron or steel	0.05	..	150	0.55 – 0.83	Low	Subject to seizing
Cast iron	Cast iron	0.05	0.15 – 0.2	315	0.98 – 1.18	Very low	Good at low speed
Cast iron	Steel	0.06	..	260	0.83 – 1.37	Very low	Fair at low speeds
Hard steel	Hard steel	0.05	..	260	0.69	Moderate	Subject to galling
Hard steel	Hard steel, chromium plated	0.03	..	260	1.37	High	Durable combination
Hard-drawn phosphor bronze	Hard steel, chromium plated	0.03	..	260	0.98	High	Good wearing qualities
Power metal**	Cast iron or steel	0.05 – 0.1	0.1 – 0.4	540	0.98	High	Good wearing qualities
Power metal**	Hard steel chromium plated	0.05 – 0.1	0.1 – 0.3	540	2.06	Very High	High energy absorption
Wood	Cast iron or steel	0.16	0.2 – 0.35	150	0.39 – 0.59	Lowest	Unsuitable at high speed
Leather	Cast iron or steel	0.12 – 0.15	0.3 – 0.5	90	0.07 – 0.29	Very low	Subject to glazing
Cork	Cast iron or steel	0.15 – 0.25	0.3 – 0.5	90	0.06 – 0.09	Very low	Cork-insert type preferred
Felt	Cast iron or steel	0.18	0.22	90	0.03 – 0.07	Low	Resinent engagement
Vulcanized fiber or paper	Cast iron or steel	..	0.3 – 0.5	90	0.07 – 0.09	Very low	Low speeds, light duty
Woven asbestos**	Cast iron or steel	0.1 – 0.2	0.3 – 0.6	175 – 260	0.34 – 0.69	Low	Prolonged slip service ratings given
Woven asbestos	Cast iron or steel	0.1 – 0.2	..	260	0.69 – 1.37	Low	This rating for short infrequent engagement
Woven asbestos	Hard steel, Chromium plated	0.1	..	..	1.37	Moderate	Used in Napier Sabre engine
Molded asbestos**	Cast iron or steel	0.08 – 0.12	0.2 – 0.5	260	0.34 – 0.98	Very low	Wide field of applications
Impregnated asbestos	Cast iron or steel	0.12	0.32	260 – 400	0.98	Moderate	For demanding applications
Carbon graphite	Steel	0.05 – 0.1	0.25	370 – 540	2.06	High	For critical requirements

*Conservative values should be used to allow for possible glazing of cloth surfaces in service and for adverse operating conditions

**For specific material within this group the coefficient usually is maintained within plus or minus 5 percent

***To obtain the values in Metric Units (kgf/mm²), divide the given values by 9.8067

Table 13.5 *Service Factors for Clutches*

Type of Service	Factor Not including Starting factor
Driving machine:	
Electric motor, steady load	1.0
Fluctuating load	1.5
Gas engine, single cylinder	1.5
Multiple cylinder	1.0
Diesel engine, high speed	1.5
Large, slow speed	2.0
Driven machine:	
Generator, steady load	1.0
Fluctuating load	1.5
Blower	1.0
Compressor, depending on the number of cylinders ..	2.0 – 2.5
Pumps, centrifugal	1.0
Single acting	2.0
Double acting	1.5
Line shaft	1.5
Woodworking machinery	1.75
Hoists, elevators, cranes, shovels	2.0
Hammer mills, ball mills, crushers	2.0
Brick machinery	3.0
Rock crushers	3.0

Table 13.6 *(a) Size of wheels of Brakes*

Diameter, mm	160 200 250	320 400 500	630 800
Width, mm	50 65 80	100 125 160	200 250
Radial clearance, mm	1 to 1.5	1.5 to 2.0	2.0 to 2.5

Table 13.6 (b) Comparison of Hoist Brakes

Brake Characteristics		Block Brakes		Band Brakes		Axial Brakes	
		Double Block	V-ground Sheave	Simple	Both Directions of Rotations	Cone	Multidisk
Force ratio $\dfrac{F}{F_t}$	..	$\dfrac{b}{fa}$	$\dfrac{b\sin\alpha}{fa}$	$\dfrac{b}{a(c^{f\theta}-1)}$	$\dfrac{b(e^{f\theta}+1)}{a(e^{f\theta}-1)}$	$\dfrac{b\sin\alpha}{fa}$	$\dfrac{b}{nfa}$
Average numerical value	..	0.667	0.282	0.0323	0.165	0.161	0.097
Relative value	..	20.6	8.7	1.0	5.1	5.0	3.00
Travel at lever end	..	$\dfrac{ha}{b}$	$\dfrac{ha}{b\sin\alpha}$	$\dfrac{ha\theta}{2\pi b}$	$\dfrac{ha\theta}{4\pi b}$	$\dfrac{ha}{b\sin\alpha}$	$\dfrac{ih'a}{b}$
Average travel, mm	..	3.13	7.40	29.43	14.71	12.92	2.19
Maximum capacity, kW (MHP)	..	150 (200)	20 (25)	220 (300)	75 (100)	35 (50)	90 (120)

Table 13.7 Working Pressures for Brake Blocks

Rubbing velocity, m/s	Pressure, MN/m² (kgf/mm²)		
	Wood blocks	Asbestos Fabric	Asbestos Blocks
1	0.549 (0.056)	0.687 (0.070)	1.103 (0.1125)
2	0.451 (0.046)	0.549 (0.050)	1.035 (0.1055)
3	0.343 (0.035)	0.412 (0.042)	0.896 (0.0914)
4	0.245 (0.025)	0.275 (0.028)	0.687 (0.0700)
5	0.173 (0.018)	0.206 (0.021)	0.483 (0.0492)
6	0.173 (0.018)	0.206 (0.021)	0.275 (0.0280)

Table 13.8 *Design Value for Brake Facings*

Facing Material		Design Co-efficient of Friction, f	Permissible Unit Pressure p, MN/m^2 (kgf/mm^2)	
			1 m/s	10 m/s
Cast iron on cast iron:				
Dry	..	0.20	..	..
Oily	..	0.07	..	..
Wood on cast iron	..	0.25 – 0.30	0.549 – 0.687 (0.056 – 0.070)	0.137 – 0.173 (0.014 – 0.0176)
Leather on cast iron:				
Dry	..	0.40 – 0.50	0.0549 – 0.103 (0.0056 – 0.0105)	..
Oily	..	0.15	..	..
Asbestos fabric on metal:				
Dry	..	0.35 – 0.40	0.621 – 0.687 (0.0633 – 0.070)	0.173 – 0.206 (0.0176 – 0.021)
Oily	..	0.25	..	..
Molded asbestos on metal, dry		0.30 – 0.35	1.035 – 1.206 (0.1055 – 0.1230)	0.206 – 0.275 (0.021 – 0.028)

Table 13.9 *Radiating Factors for Brakes*

Temperature difference degree centigrade	Radiating factor K
50	2.95×10^{-5} (0.30×10^{-5})
100	3.68×10^{-5} (0.375×10^{-5})
150	4.08×10^{-5} (0.416×10^{-5})
200	4.42×10^{-5} (0.451×10^{-5})

Table 13.10 *Values of $e^{f\theta}$*

Proportion of Contact to Whole Circumference, $\dfrac{\theta}{2\pi}$	Steel Band on Cast iron $f = 0.18$	Leather Belt on			
		Wood		Cast Iron	
		Slightly Greasy; $f = 0.47$	Very Greasy; $f = 0.12$	Slightly Greasy; $f = 0.28$	Damp; $f = 0.38$
0.1	1.12	1.34	1.08	1.19	1.27
0.2	1.25	1.81	1.16	1.42	1.61
0.3	1.40	2.43	1.25	1.69	2.05
0.4	1.57	3.26	1.35	2.02	2.60
0.425	1.62	3.51	1.38	2.11	2.76
0.45	1.66	3.78	1.40	2.21	2.93
0.475	1.71	4.07	1.43	2.31	3.11
0.500	1.76	4.38	1.46	2.41	3.30
0.525	1.81	4.71	1.49	2.52	3.50
0.6	1.97	5.88	1.57	2.81	4.19
0.7	2.21	7.90	1.66	3.43	5.32
0.8	2.47	10.60	1.83	4.09	6.75
0.9	2.77	14.30	1.97	4.87	8.57
1.0	3.10	19.20	2.12	5.81	10.90

Table 13.11 *Friction Coefficients and Allowable Pressures*

Materials in Contact	Friction Coefficient			Allowable Pressure MN/m^2
	Dry	Greasy	Lubricated	
Cast iron on cast iron	0.2–0.15	0.10–0.06	0.10–0.05	1.0–1.75
Bronze on case iron	...	0.10–0.05	0.10–0.05	0.55–0.85
Steel on cast iron	0.30–0.20	0.12–0.07	0.10–0.06	0.80–1.40
Wood on cast iron	0.25–0.20	0.12–0.08	...	0.40–0.62
Fiber on metal	...	0.20-0.10	...	0.10–0.20
Cork on metal	0.35	0.30–0.25	0.25–0.22	0.05–0.10
Leather on metal	0.5–0.3	0.20–0.15	0.15–0.12	0.07–0.20
Wire asbestos on metal	0.5–0.35	0.30–0.25	0.25–0.20	0.28–0.55
Asbestos blocks on metal	0.48–0.40	0.30–0.25	...	0.28–1.10
Asbestos on metal, short action	...	...	0.25–0.20	1.40–2.10
Metal on cast iron, short action	...	...	0.10–0.05	1.40–2.10

14

Flexible Machine Elements

Symbols	Description and Units
A	net area of wire in rope, mm^2
b	width of belt, mm (Table 14.1)
B	width of pulley face, mm
C	centre distance between pulleys, mm
d, D	diameters of smaller and larger pulleys respectively, mm
F	effort, N (kgf)
F_t	net belt pull, N (kgf)
g	acceleration due to gravity, m/s^2
t	thickness of belt, mm
T_1, T_2	tensions of belt on tight and slack sides respectively, N (kgf)
T_c	centrifugal force on the belt, N (kgf)
v	velocity of belt, m/s
μ	coefficient of friction between belt and pulley (Table 14.2)
σ_1, σ_2	unit tensions of belt on tight and slack sides respectively, MN/m^2 (kgf/mm^2)
σ_c	cantrifugal coefficient for leather belts, MN/m^2 (kgf/mm^2)
σ_d	allowable stress or design stress, MN/m^2 (kgf/mm^2)
θ	arc of contact

Particular	Equation	Eqn. No.
Flat Belts		
(i) angle of contact in the open belt drive:		
(a) on smaller pulley, rad (Fig. 14.1(a))	$\theta_s = \pi - 2\sin^{-1}\dfrac{D-d}{2C} \approx \pi - \dfrac{D-d}{C}$	14.1(a)
(b) on larger pulley, rad (Fig. 14.1(a))	$\theta_L = \pi + 2\sin^{-1}\dfrac{D-d}{2C} \approx \pi + \dfrac{D-d}{C}$	14.1(b)
(ii) angle of contact in the Crossed belt drive, rad (Fig. 14.1(b))		
	$\theta = \theta_s = \theta_L = \pi + 2\sin^{-1}\dfrac{D+d}{2C} \approx \pi + \dfrac{D+d}{C}$	14.2(a)

289

Particular	Equation	Eqn. No.

Length of open belts

$$L = \sqrt{4C^2 - (D-d)^2} + \tfrac{1}{2}(D\theta_L + d\theta_s) \approx 2C + \frac{\pi}{2}(D+d) + \frac{(D-d)^2}{4C} \qquad \text{14.2(b)}$$

Length of Crossed belts

$$L = \sqrt{4C^2 - (D+d)^2} + \frac{\theta}{2}(D+d) \approx \left[\frac{\pi}{2} + \frac{D+d}{2C}\right](D+d) + \sqrt{4C^2 - (D+d)^2} \qquad \text{14.2(c)}$$

An empirical formula to select the centre distance from the condition of longevity of the belt

$$C \approx (0.07 \text{ to } 0.10)v \quad \text{or} \quad C \geq (1.5 \text{ to } 2.0)(D+d) \qquad \text{14.2(d)}$$

At low velocities (neglecting the centrifugal force on the belt) the relation between the belt tensions. (Fig. 14.2)	$T_1/T_2 = e^{\mu\theta}$	14.3(a)
	$\sigma_1/\sigma_2 = e^{\mu\theta}$	14.3(b)
At high velocities the relation between the belt tensions (Fig. 14.2)	$\dfrac{T_1 - T_c}{T_2 - T_c} = e^{\mu\theta}$	14.3(c)
	$\dfrac{\sigma_1 - \sigma_c}{\sigma_2 - \sigma_c} = e^{\mu\theta}$	14.3(d)

$$\text{where } \mu = 0.54 - \frac{0.712}{2.542 + v}, \text{ coefficient of friction (Barth's formula)}$$

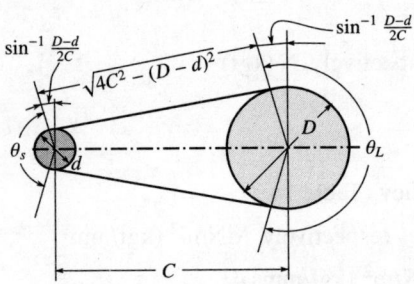

Fig. 14.1(a): *Open belt drive*

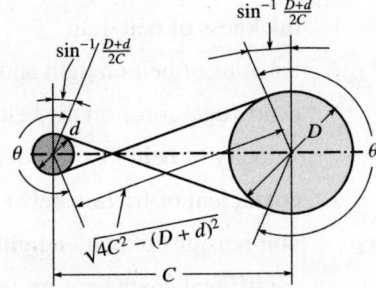

Fig. 14.1(b): *Closed belt drive*

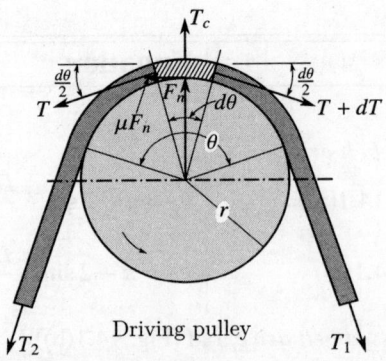

Fig. 14.2: *Forces on element of belt*

Particular	Equation	Eqn. No.
The centrifugal force on the belt, N (kgf)	$T_c = \dfrac{w'v^2}{g} = \dfrac{wbtv^2}{10^6 \times g}$	14.3(e)
Stress in the belt due to centrifugal force T_c MN/m² (kgf/mm²)	$\sigma_c = \dfrac{wv^2}{10^6 \times g}$	14.3(f)

The effective pull, N (kgf)

$$F_t = (T_1 - T_2) = (T_1 - T_c)\left[\frac{e^{\mu\theta}-1}{e^{\mu\theta}}\right] = bt(\sigma_d - \sigma_c)\left[\frac{e^{\mu\theta}-1}{e^{\mu\theta}}\right] = bt\left[\sigma_d - \frac{wv^2}{10^6 g}\right]\left[\frac{e^{\mu\theta}-1}{e^{\mu\theta}}\right] \qquad 14.4$$

where σ_d = 2.06 MN/m² (0.21 kgf/mm²), design stress in the leather belt with long life

v is the velocity of the belt, m/s

w' = (wbt)/10^6, weight of belt, N/m (kg/m) length of belt

w = weight density of belt material, N/m³ (kg/m³)

g is the acceleration due to gravity, 9.81 m/s²

Power transmitted, kW (SI Units)

$$P = \frac{(T_1 - T_2)v}{1000} = \frac{bt\,v}{1000}\left[\sigma_d - \frac{wv^2}{10^6 g}\right]\left[\frac{e^{\mu\theta}-1}{e^{\mu\theta}}\right] \qquad 14.5(a)$$

Power transmitted, MHP (Metric Units)

$$P = \frac{(T_1 - T_2)v}{75} = \frac{bt\,v}{75}\left[\sigma_d - \frac{wv^2}{10^6 g}\right]\left[\frac{e^{\mu\theta}-1}{e^{\mu\theta}}\right] \qquad 14.5(b)$$

Power transmitted per square mm of belt:

(a) at high velocities, kW/mm² (SI units)	$P/mm^2 = \dfrac{v}{1000}(\sigma_d - \sigma_c)\left[\dfrac{e^{\mu\theta}-1}{e^{\mu\theta}}\right]$	14.6(a)
at high velocities, MHP/mm² (Metric units)	$P/mm^2 = \dfrac{v}{75}(\sigma_d - \sigma_c)\left[\dfrac{e^{\mu\theta-1}}{e^{\mu\theta}}\right]$	14.6(b)
(b) at low velocities, kW/mm² (SI units)	$P/mm^2 = \dfrac{v\sigma_d}{1000}\left[\dfrac{e^{\mu\theta}-1}{e^{\mu\theta}}\right]$	14.6(c)
at low velocities, MHP/mm² (Metric units)	$P/mm^2 = \dfrac{v\sigma_d}{75}\left[\dfrac{e^{\mu\theta}-1}{e^{\mu\theta}}\right]$	14.6(d)

Forces in flat belts:

The relation between the stress 'σ' and elongation, e	$\sigma = C_1^2 e^2$	14.7

where σ is the stress in the belt, MN/m²(kgf/mm²); e is the elongation, mm/mm

C_1 = 70 (22.35) constant for leather belts

The relation between the initial tension and power tensions	$\sqrt{T_1} + \sqrt{T_2} = 2\sqrt{T_o}$	14.8

where T_o is the initial tension, N (kgf)

Particular	**Equation**	**Eqn. No.**

Cast iron pulley design: (Fig. 14.3 and Table 14.13)

Saverin's empirical formula to determine the diameter of the smaller pulley* (Table 14.13(b))

$$d = D_{\min} = (525 - 630) \sqrt[3]{\frac{P(kW)}{\omega_{\max}}} = (525 - 630) \sqrt[3]{\frac{P(kW)}{2\pi n_{\max}}} \qquad \text{14.9(a)}$$

The diameter of the driven pulley (Table 14.13(b))	$D = (1 - \epsilon)di$	14.9(b)

where $\epsilon = 0.01$ to 0.03, coefficient of creep; i = velocity ratio

The face width of pulley (Barth's formula) (Table 14.13(c))	$B = 1\dfrac{3}{16}b + 10$ mm for heavy duty belts	14.9(c)
	$= 1\dfrac{3}{32}b + 5$ mm for light duty belts	14.9(d)

Number of arms: (Table 14.13(f))

$i = 4$ for $D = 200$ mm to 450 mm $i = 6$ for $D > 450$ mm.

For pulleys upto $D = 200$ mm, use webs

The thickness of elliptical arm a, near the boss (mm)	$a = 2.94 \sqrt[3]{BD/4i}$ for single belt	14.9(e)
	$= 2.94 \sqrt[3]{BD/2i}$ for double belt	14.9(f)
Thickness of arm a_1, near rim	Taper 4 mm per 100 mm	14.9(g)
Radius of the cross section of arms	$r = \dfrac{3}{4}a$	14.9(h)

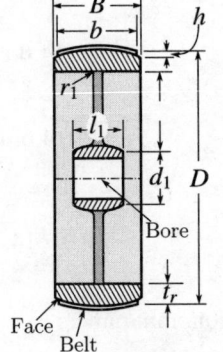 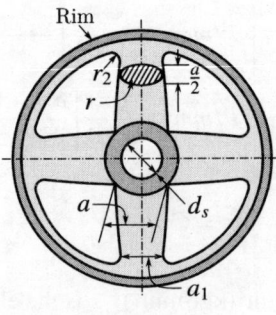

B is the width of pulley, mm
b is the width of belt, mm
D is the diameter of pully, mm
d_1 is the hub diameter, mm
d_s is the shaft diameter, mm
t_r is the thickness of rim, mm
l_1 is the hub length
h is the crown height

Fig. 14.3: *Cast iron pulley*

---

*$d = D_{\min}$ only in a step-down drive
$D_{\min} = D$ for a step-up drive. Instead of selecting the diameter of the pulley, the belt velocity v may be specified and then d determined.

Particular	Equation	Eqn. No.
The crown height (Table 14.13(d) and (e))	$h = 0.003D$	14.9(i)
The relation between the shaft diameter and hub diameter, d_1		
	$\dfrac{d_1 - d_s}{2} = 0.412 \sqrt[3]{BD} + 6$ mm for single belt	14.9(j)
	$= 0.529 \sqrt[3]{BD} + 6$ mm for double belt	14.9(k)
The thickness of the rim, mm	$t_r = \dfrac{D}{200} + 3$ mm for single belt	14.9(l)
	$= \dfrac{D}{200} + 6$ mm for double belt	14.9(m)
The hub length	$l_1 \geq (2/3)B$ or $l_1 \leq B$ or $l_1 \geq 1.5d_s$	14.9(n)
Another equation to determine the thickness of the arm, a (Assuming that only one-half the total number of arms carry the load), mm	$a = 2.73 \sqrt[3]{(F_t D / i\sigma_d)}$	14.9(o)

where σ_d is the allowable stress, MN/m^2 (kgf/mm^2)

Mild Steel Pulleys: (Fig. 14.4) (Table 14.13)

Number of arms in pulleys (refer Table 14.13)		
Length of boss or hub	$l_1 = \frac{1}{2}B$	14.10(a)

$l_1 = 100$ mm minimum in case of pulleys with 19 mm diameter spokes

$l_1 = 140$ mm minimum for pulleys with 22 mm diameter spokes

Short–Centre Drives: **(Fig. 14.5)**

Pivoted motor drive or Rockwood drive: **(Fig. 14.5)**

The relation between the weight of the motor and the tensions in the belt (Fig. 14.5)	$W = \dfrac{T_1 a + T_2 e}{m}$	14.11(a)

where W = weight of the motor, N (kgf); $\quad e = f \cos\theta_2 + m \sin\theta_2 + r_1$

$a = f \cos\theta_1 - m \sin\theta_1 - r_1; \qquad \theta_1 = \phi - \gamma; \quad \theta_2 = \phi + \gamma$

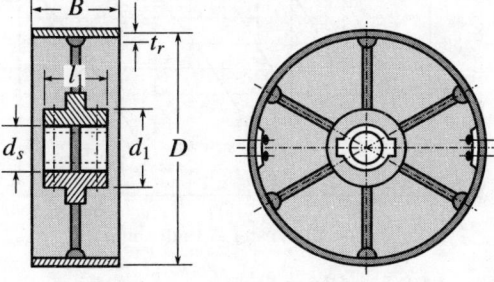

t_r is the thickness of rim, mm

$t_r = 0.252 \sqrt{D} + 1.6$mm for light duty

$t_r = 0.3775 \sqrt{D} + 3.2$mm for heavy duty pully

B is the width of pully, mm

l_1 is the length of hub, mm

Fig. 14.4: *Mild Steel pulley*

Particular	Equation	Eqn. No.
The value of T_1	$T_1 = \dfrac{mW + eF_t}{a + e}$	14.11(b)
The value of T_2	$T_2 = \dfrac{mW - aF_t}{a + e}$	14.11(c)
The required pivot arm length for motor of weight W	$m = \dfrac{F_t\left(a\frac{T_1}{T_2} + e\right)}{W\left(\frac{T_1}{T_2} - 1\right)}$	14.11(d)
	where $F_t = T_1 - T_2$, required net pull, N(kgf)	

V-Belts (Fig. 14.6) (Table 14.14 to 14.24)

At high velocities the relation between the belt tensions in the case of V-belts	$\dfrac{T_1 - T_c}{T_2 - T_c} = e^{\mu_1 \theta}$	14.12

where $\mu_1 = \mu / \sin(\alpha/2)$, apparent coefficient of friction

α is the groove angle of the pulley, deg (Table 14.16) (Fig. 14.6(b))

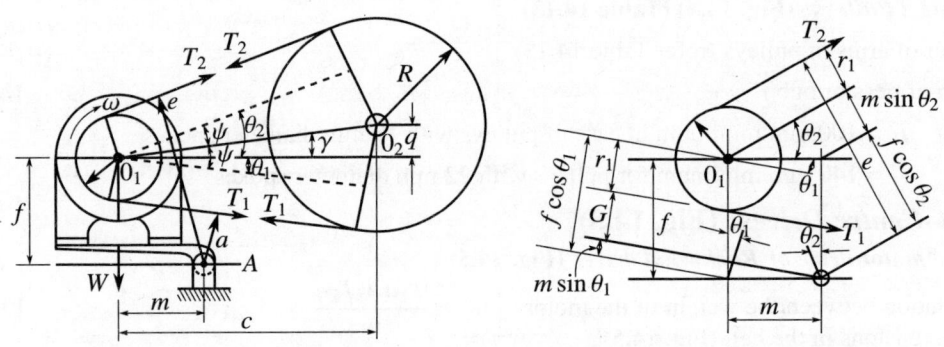

Fig. 14.5: *Pivoted motor drive*

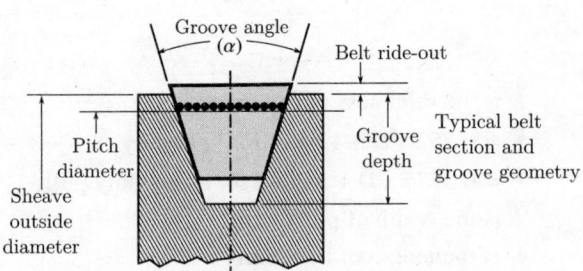

Fig. 14.6(a): *Cross-section of V-belt and sheave groove*

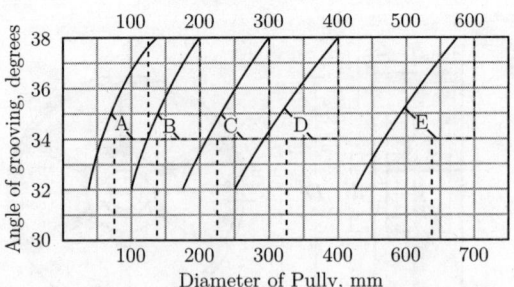

Fig. 14.6(b): *Chart for determination of groove angle*

Particular	Equation	Eqn. No.

Formulae for Transmitting Capacities: (Table 14.18)

The maximum power in kilowatt which the V-belts of Sections A, B, C, D and E can transmit shall be calculated from the following formulae:

Belt Cross-section Symbol	Formula	Maximum value of d_e in the formula, mm	
A	$kW = \left(0.61v^{-0.09} - \dfrac{26.68}{d_e} - 1.04 \times 10^{-4}v^2\right) \times 0.7355v$	125	14.13(a)
B	$kW = \left(1.08v^{-0.09} - \dfrac{69.68}{d_e} - 1.78 \times 10^{-4}v^2\right) \times 0.7355v$	175	14.13(b)
C	$kW = \left(2.01v^{-0.09} - \dfrac{194.8}{d_e} - 3.18 \times 10^{-4}v^2\right) \times 0.7355v$	300	14.13(c)
D	$kW = \left(4.29v^{-0.09} - \dfrac{690}{d_e} - 6.48 \times 10^{-4}v^2\right) \times 0.7355v$	425	14.13(d)
E	$kW = \left(6.22v^{-0.09} - \dfrac{1294}{d_e} - 9.59 \times 10^{-4}v^2\right) \times 0.7355v$	700	14.13(e)

where kW = maximum power in kilo-watts at 180° arc of contact for a belt of average length

v = belt speed, m/s; $d_e = d \times K_d$, equivalent pitch diameter;

K_d is the small diameter factor (Table 14.15); d is the pitch diameter of the smaller pulley (Table 14.22)

The number of belts required $\qquad \left| \quad n' = \dfrac{PK_s}{(kW)K_L K_a} \right. \qquad$ 14.14

where P is the drive power in kW

K_s is the correction factor according to service (Table 14.19)

K_L is the correction factor for length (Table 14.20)

K_a is the correction factor for arc of contact (Table 14.21)

(kW) is the ratings of the V-belt (Table 14.18) (Eqn. 14.13)

The centre distance $\qquad \left| \quad C = A + \sqrt{(A^2 - B)} \right. \qquad$ 14.15(a)

$\qquad$ where $A = \dfrac{L}{4} - \dfrac{\pi(D+d)}{8}$; $\quad B = \left[\dfrac{D-d}{8}\right]^2$

Pitch length of belt $\qquad \left| \quad L = 2C + 1.57(D + d) + \dfrac{(D-d)^2}{4C} \right. \qquad$ 14.15(b)

In the absence of tables from manufacturers, to determine the power ratings of Vee belts SI – Units $\qquad \left| \quad P(kW) = \dfrac{n'av}{1000}\left[\sigma_d - \dfrac{wv^2}{10^6 g}\right]\left[\dfrac{e^{\mu_1\theta} - 1}{e^{\mu_1\theta}}\right] \right. \qquad$ 14.16(a)

Particular	Equation	Eqn. No.
Metric Units	$P(MHP) = \dfrac{n'av}{75}\left[\sigma_d \dfrac{wv^2}{10^6 g}\right]\left[\dfrac{e^{\mu_1\theta}}{e^{\mu_1\theta}}\right]$	14.16(b)

where a = area of cross section of the belt, mm^2; σ_d = 2.26 MN/m^2 (kgf/mm^2), working stress,

w = weight density of belt material

= 10.89×10^3 N/m^3 (kg/m^3); n' = number of belts

Strength of Manila rope:

The ultimate load, N (kgf)	$P_u = k_1 d^2$	14.17(a)

where d is the diameter of the rope, mm; k_1 = 48.30 (4.925), constant in SI (Metric) Units

For continuous driving the maximum tension on the tight side, N (kgf)	$T_1 = k_2 d^2 = F_t + \dfrac{F_t}{2} + T_c$	14.17(b)
According to C.W. Hunt, the effective tension which transmits power is given by	$F_t = \dfrac{2}{3}(T_1 - T_c)$	14.17(c)
The power transmitted (SI Units)	$P(kW) = \dfrac{2}{3}\dfrac{(T_1 - T_c)v}{1000}$	14.17(d)
(Metric Units)	$P(MHP) = \dfrac{2}{3}\dfrac{(T_1 - T_c)v}{75}$	14.17(c)

where v = velocity, m/s g = 9.81 m/s^2, acceleration due to gravity,

$T_c = \dfrac{w'v^2}{g}$ k_2 = constant = 1.373 (0.14) in SI (Metric) Units

w' = weight of rope, N/metre (kg/metre) length of rope

Hoisting Tackle:

The relation between the effort F and the resistance Q in the case of single sheave pulley (Fig. 14.7)	$F = \left[\dfrac{D + \mu d + 2e}{D - \mu d - 2e'}\right]Q = C_h Q$	14.18(a)

where $C_h = \left[\dfrac{D + \mu d + 2e}{D - \mu d - 2e^1}\right]$, a constant depends on the size of rope, size of sheave and pin

and on coefficient of friction

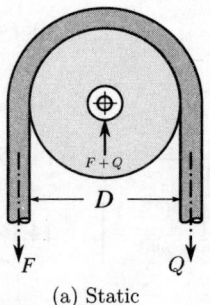

(a) Static

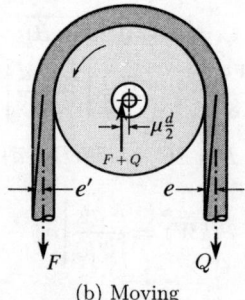

(b) Moving

D is the diameter of sheave

d is the diameter of pin

μ is the coefficient of friction

C_h = constant (Table 14.23)

= 1.15, for manila rope

= 1.07, for wire rope

= 1.10, for dry chain

= 1.04, for greased chain

Fig. 14.7: *Rope passing over sheave*

Particular	Equation	Eqn. No.
The effort F, on the rope in a hoist (Fig. 14.8)		
(a) For raising the load	$F = \dfrac{C_h^n(C_h - 1)}{(C_h^n - 1)} Q$	14.18(b)
(b) For lowering the load	$F = \dfrac{(C_h - 1)}{C_h(C_h^n - 1)} Q$	14.18(c)
Efficiency of the hoist	$\eta = \dfrac{(C_h^n - 1)}{n C_h^n(C_h - 1)}$	14.18(d)

where n is the number of times a rope passes over the sheave

Particular	Equation	Eqn. No.
Differential Chain Block: (Fig. 14.9)		
The effort required for raising the load without friction (Fig. 14.9)	$F_o = \dfrac{Q}{2}(1 - n_1')$ where $n_1' = d/D = r/R$	14.19(a)
The effort required for raising the load with friction	$F = \left[\dfrac{C_h^2 - n_1'}{1 + C_h}\right] Q$	14.19(b)
The efficiency	$\eta = \left[\dfrac{1 - n_1'}{2}\right]\left[\dfrac{1 + C_h}{C_h^2 - n_1'}\right]$	14.19(c)
The effort for lowering the load with friction	$F = \dfrac{Q}{C_h}\left[\dfrac{1 - n_1' C_h^2}{1 + C_h}\right]$	14.19(d)
The efficiency	$\eta = \dfrac{2}{C_h}\left[\dfrac{1 - n_1' C_h^2}{(1 - n_1')(1 + C_h)}\right]$	14.19(e)

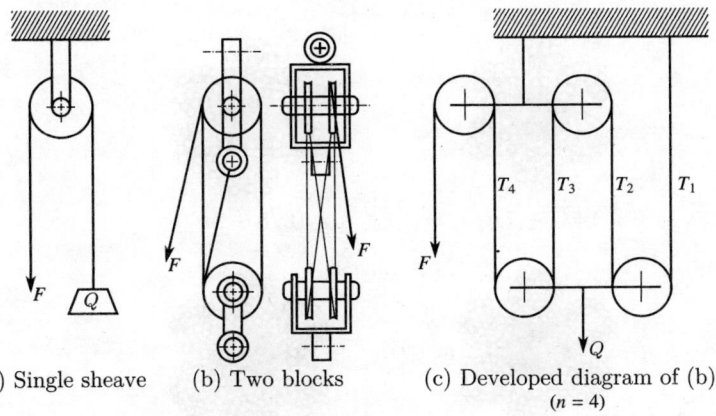

(a) Single sheave   (b) Two blocks   (c) Developed diagram of (b)
(n = 4)

Fig. 14.8: *Hoisting tackle*

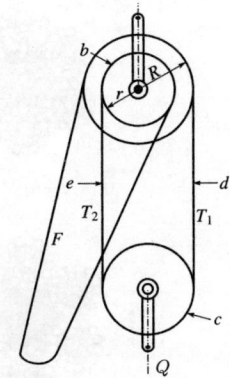

Fig. 14.9: *Differential chain block*

Particular	Equation	Eqn.	No.

Wire Rope: (Fig. 14.10 & Table 14.25 to 14.33)

In the case of wire rope the bending stress is directly proportional to the diameter of the wire (d_w) and inversely proportional to the diameter of the sheave (D)	$\sigma_b = K\dfrac{d_w}{D}$	14.20(a)
The bending load	$F_b = \sigma_b A = KA\dfrac{d_w}{D}$	14.20(b)
The relation between ultimate load, bending and service load in wire rope	$\dfrac{F_u}{(FS)} > F_b + F_s$	14.20(c)

where F_u is the ultimate strength of rope, N (kgf) A = net area of wire in rope, (Table 14.32)

F_s is the service load on rope, N (kgf) d_w = diameter of wire in rope, (Table 14.32)

F_b is the bending load, N (kgf) D = pitch diameter of sheave, (Table 14.32)

K = constant of proportionality FS = factor of Safety (Table 14.33)

   $= 82.8 \times 10^3 MN/m^2 (8.44) \times 10^3$ (kgf/mm²)

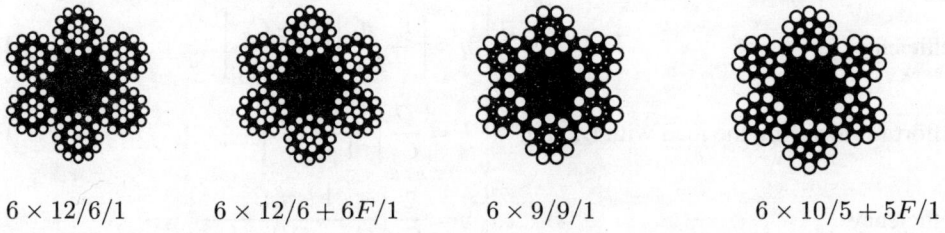

$6 \times 12/6/1$	$6 \times 12/6 + 6F/1$	$6 \times 9/9/1$	$6 \times 10/5 + 5F/1$

Fig. 14.10(a): *Construction of group* 6×19 *wire rope*

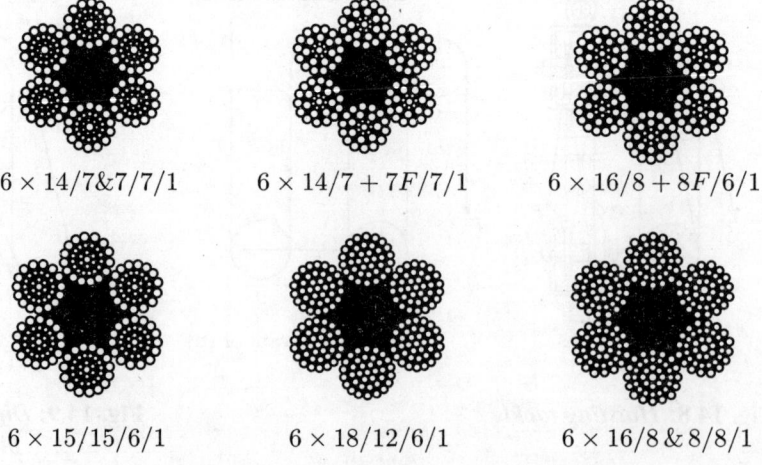

$6 \times 14/7\&7/7/1$	$6 \times 14/7 + 7F/7/1$	$6 \times 16/8 + 8F/6/1$
$6 \times 15/15/6/1$	$6 \times 18/12/6/1$	$6 \times 16/8 \& 8/8/1$

Fig. 14.10(b): *Construction of group* 6×37 *wire rope*

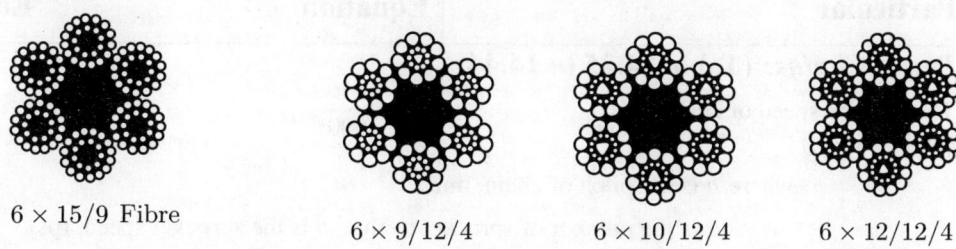

$6 \times 15/9$ Fibre

Fig. 14.10(c): 6×24 *fibre core*

$6 \times 9/12/4$ $6 \times 10/12/4$ $6 \times 12/12/4$

Fig. 14.10(d): *Compound flattened strand*

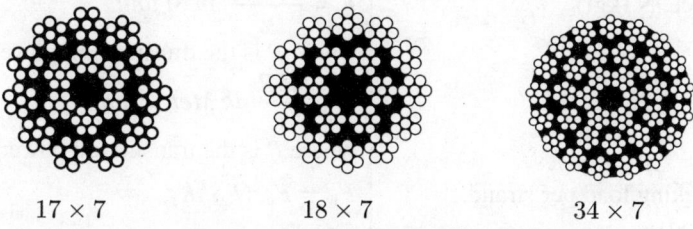

17×7 18×7 34×7

Fig. 14.10(e): *Multi Strand non-rotating ropes*

Fig. 14.10: Construction of wire ropes

Particular	Equation	Eqn. No.
Hoisting and Power Chains:		
Hoisting chain:		
Working load for the ordinary common coil chain, N (kgf)	$F_w = 93.75d^2$ *in SI units*	14.21(a)
	$= 9.56d^2$ *in Metric units*	14.21(b)
The safe working load for coil chain when the chain is subjected to shock, N (kgf)	$F_w = 50.35d^2$ *in SI units*	14.21(c)
	$= 5.134d^2$ *in Metric units*	14.21(d)
The safe working load for stud chain when the chain is subjected to shock, N (kgf)	$F_w = 60.41d^2$ *in SI units*	14.21(e)
	$= 6.16d^2$ *in Metric units*	14.21(f)
The sheave diameter	$D = 20d$ to $30d$	14.21(g)

where *d* is the diameter of rod from which the chain is made, mm

Particular	Equation	Eqn. No.
***Power Chains:* (Table 14.35 to 14.44)**		
The average speed of chain, m/s (Fig. 14.11(a))	$v = \dfrac{pzn}{1000}$	14.22(a)

where p is the pitch of chain, mm

z is the number of sprocket teeth; n is the sprocket speed, rps

The empirical formula to determine pitch, mm	$p \le 10\left[\dfrac{60.67}{n_1}\right]^{2/3}$	14.22(b)

where n_1 is the speed of smaller sprocket, rev/s

The tangential force, N (kgf)	$F = \dfrac{1000P}{v}$ *in SI units*	14.22(c)

where P is the transmitting power, kW

$$F = \frac{75P}{v} \quad \textit{in Metric units} \qquad 14.22(d)$$

where P is the transmitted power, *MHP*

The allowable working load per strand, N/strand (kgf/strand)	$F_w = F_u/(FS)K_s$	14.22(e)

where F_u = ultimate strength of the chain, N/strand (kgf/strand);

K_s = Service factor depending on the nature of the load, efficiency of lubrication and the position of the chain (Table 14.35)

FS = Factor of safety (Table 14.37)

According to AGMA the formula for the allowable working load per strand (neglecting the centrifugal force)	$F_w = \dfrac{98.07A}{v + 3.05}$ *in SI units* (N/Strand)	14.22(f)
	$= \dfrac{10A}{v + 3.05}$ *in Metric units* (kgf/strand)	14.22(g)

where A is the projected bearing area of the pin bushing joint, mm^2

v is the speed of the chain, m/s

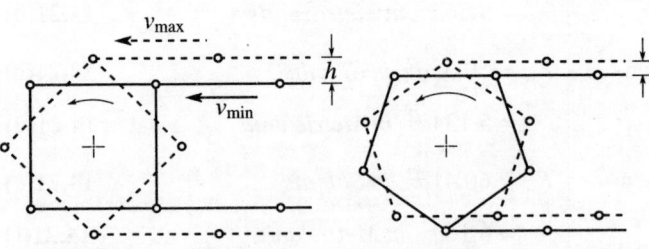

(i) Variation in chain velocity for a uniformly rotating sprocket with four teeth

(ii) Rise and fall of chain on sprocket with five teeth

Fig. 14.11(a): *Action of chain engaging sprocket*

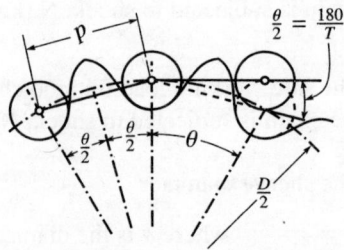

Fig. 14.11(b): *Action of chain engaging sprocket teeth*

Particular	Equation	Eqn. No.
The minimum number of strands in a chain (if $F > F_w$)	$j = \dfrac{F}{F_w}$	14.22(h)
The optimum centre distance between sprockets in pitches	$C_p = (30 \text{ to } 50)$ where $C = p\, C_p$	14.22(i)
Minimum centre distance	$C\min = K_1 C_1$	14.22(j)

where $C_1 = \dfrac{D_{01} + D_{02}}{2}$

D_{01} is the tip diameter of smaller sprocket; D_{02} is the tip diameter of larger sprocket

K_1 = a constant (Table 14.36(b))

The chain length in pitches:

$$L_p = 2C_p \cos\alpha + \tfrac{1}{2}(z_1 + z_2) + \alpha\frac{(z_2 - z_1)}{180} \quad \text{(exact)} \tag{14.22(k)}$$

$$= 2C_p + 0.5(z_1 + z_2) + \frac{0.026(z_2 - z_1)^2}{C_p} \quad \text{(approx.)} \tag{14.22(l)}$$

where C_p is the centre distance in pitches

z_2, z_1 are the number of teeth on larger and smaller sprockets respectively

D_1, D_2 are the pitch diameters of smaller and larger sprockets respectively

α = angle between tangent to the sprocket pitch circle and the centre line

$= \sin^{-1}\left[\dfrac{D_2 - D_1}{2C}\right]$

The chain length	$L = pL_p$	14.22(m)
The pitch diameter of a sprocket (Fig. 14.11(b))	$D = \dfrac{p}{\sin(180/z)}$	14.22(n)

To check the actual factor of safety:

Actual factor of safety	$FS = \dfrac{F_u}{F + F_c + F_s}$	14.22(o)

where F_u is the breaking load of chain, N (kgf); F is the tangential force, N (kgf)

v is the chain velocity, m/s; $F_c = \dfrac{w^1 v^2}{g}$, centrifugal tension, N (kgf)

w' = weight per metre length of chain, N (kgf)

$g = 9.81$ m/s^2, acceleration due to gravitational pull

$F_2 = k_2 w' C_1$, tension due to sagging of chain, N (kgf)

K_2 = coefficient for sag, (Table 14.38); C_1 = centre distance, m

Particular	Equation	Eqn. No.
Precision Roller Chains (Dimensions and Tolerances): (Fig. 14.12) (Table 14.39)		
The minimum value of tooth gap	Minimum $SR_1 = 0.505 D_r$	
Minimum $SA_1 = 140° - \dfrac{90°}{z}$;	Minimum $FR_1 = 0.12 D_r(z+2)$	14.23(a)
The maximum value of tooth gap	$SR_2 = (0.505 D_r + 0.069 \sqrt[3]{D_r}) mm$	
$SA_2 = 120° - \dfrac{90°}{z}$;	$FR_2 = 0.008 D_r(z^2 + 180)$	14.23(b)
The maximum top diameter	$TD_{max} = PCD + 0.625 p - D_r$	14.23(c)
The minimum top diameter	$TD_{min} = PCD + p\left(0.5 - \dfrac{0.4}{z}\right) - D_r$	14.23(d)

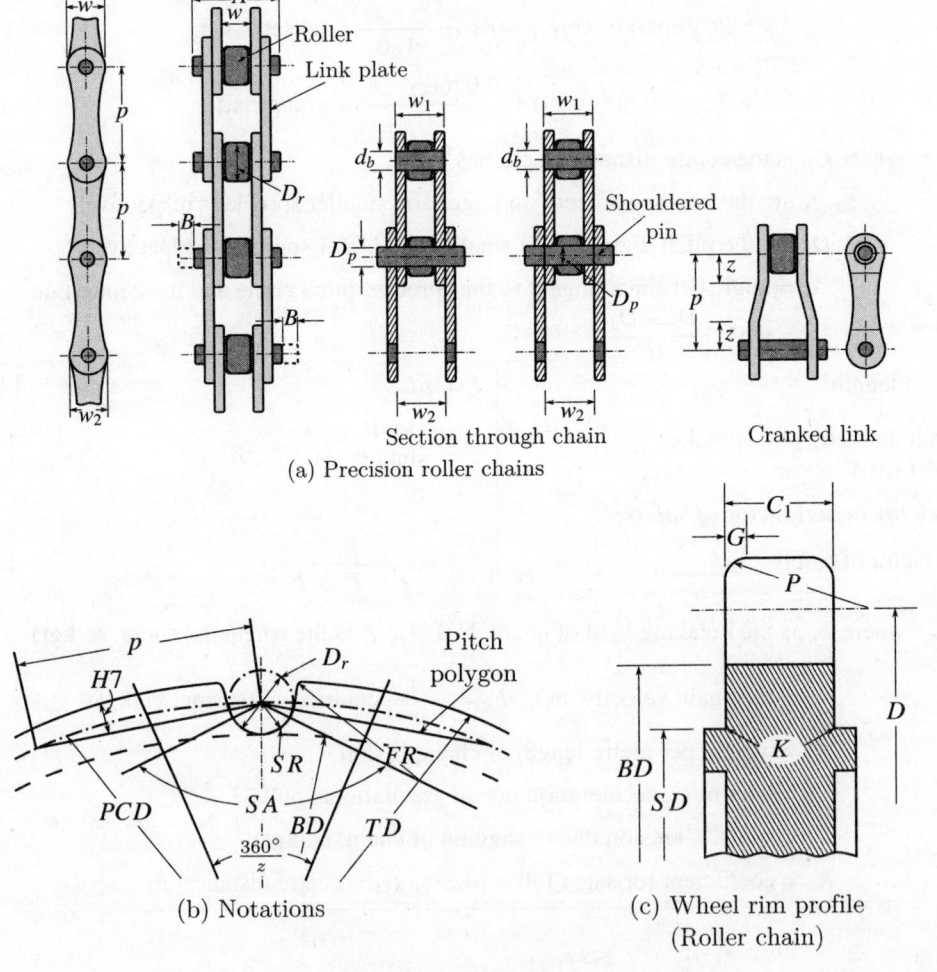

(a) Precision roller chains

(b) Notations

(c) Wheel rim profile (Roller chain)

Fig. 14.12: Roller chains

Particular	Equation	Eqn. No.
Precision Bush Chains: (Dimensions and Tolerances) **(Fig. 14.13) (Table 14.40)**		

| The minimum value of tooth gap | $SR_1 = 0.505D_b$ | |

$$SA_1 = 140° - \frac{90°}{z}; \quad FR_1 = 0.12\,D_b(z+2) \qquad 14.24(a)$$

| The maximum value of tooth gap | $SR_2 = (0.505D_b + 0.069\sqrt[3]{D_b})mm$ | 14.24(b) |

$$SA_2 = 120° - \frac{90°}{z} \qquad 14.24(c)$$

$$FR_2 = 0.008D_b(z^2 + 180) \qquad 14.24(d)$$

$$\text{where } D_b = \text{Bush diameter in mm}$$

| The maximum top diameter | $TD_{max} = PCD + 1.25p - D_b$ | 14.24(e) |
| The minimum top diameter | $TD_{min} = PCD + p\left(1 - \dfrac{1.6}{z}\right) - D_b$ | 14.24(f) |

Wheel Rim Profiles: (Fig. 14.13(c))

The value of the tooth width C_1:

(a) for simple chain wheels	$C_1 = 0.93W$	14.25(a)
(b) for duplex and triplex chain wheels	$C_1 = 0.91W$	14.25(b)
(c) for quadruplex chain wheels and above	$C_1 = 0.88W$	14.25(c)

$$\text{where } W = \text{Minimum width between inner plates}$$

$$C_2 \text{ and } C_3 = \text{Width over teeth}$$

| The tooth side relief | $G = 0.1p \text{ to } 0.15p$ | 14.25(d) |

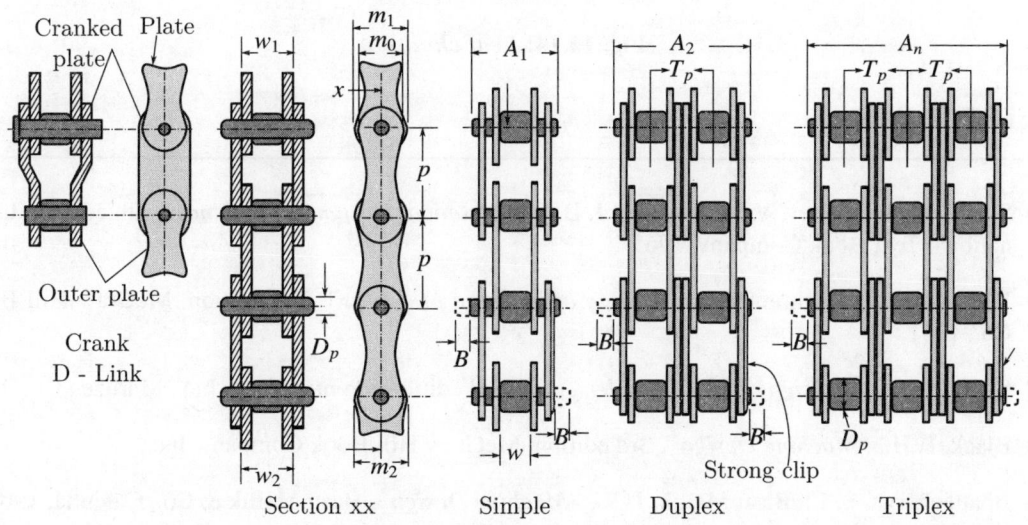

Fig. 14.13(a): *Precission bush chain*

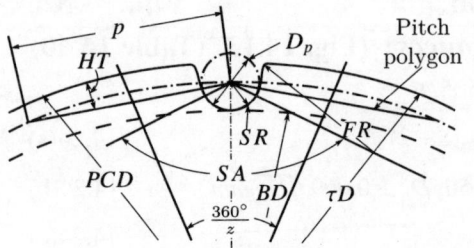

Fig. 14.13(b): *Notations (Bush chain)*

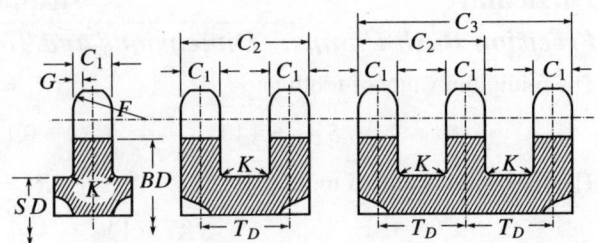

Fig. 14.13(c): *Wheel rim profile (Bush chain)*

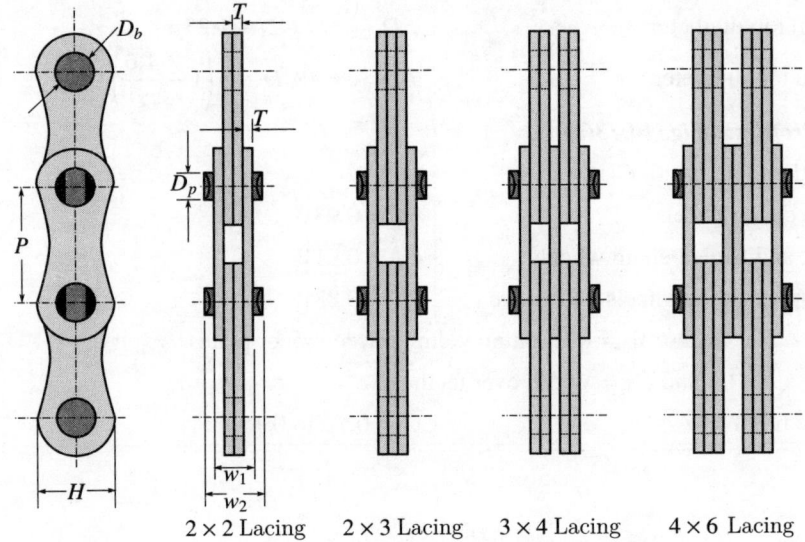

2 × 2 Lacing   2 × 3 Lacing   3 × 4 Lacing   4 × 6 Lacing

Fig. 14.14: *Leaf chains*

References

[1] Siegel, M. J., Maleev, V. L., Hartman J. B., *"Mechanical Design of Machines"*, 4th edition, International Text Book Company, 1965.

[2] Vallance, A., Doughtie, V. L., *"Design of Machine Members"*, 3rd Edition, McGraw Hill Book Co., 1951.

[3] Spotts, M. E., *"Design of Machine Elements"*, 3rd edition, Prentice Hall, Inc., Maruzen Co., Ltd.

[4] Black, P. H., *"Machine Design"*, 3rd edition, McGraw Hill Book Company, Inc.,

[5] Bhattacharya, S. C., Basu Mallik, J. R., *"Machine Design"*, Basu Mallik & Co., Calcutta, 1966.

Table 14.1 *Leather Belt Data*

Grading of belting	Thickness, mm				Increment of width mm
	Single to 200mm	Double to 300mm	Triple to 600mm	quadruple	
Light	3	6	—	—	12 to 24 by 3
					24 to 102 by 6
					102 to 198 by 12
Medium	4	8	12.5	17.5	200 to 800 by 25
					800 to 1400 by 50
Heavy	5	10	15	20	1500 to 2100 by 100

Table 14.2 *(a) Coefficients of Friction for Belts and Pulley Materials*

Belt Material	Pulley Material					
	Iron-steel	Wood	Paper	Wet Iron	Greasy Iron	Oily Iron
Oak-tanned leather	0.25	0.30	0.35	0.20	0.15	0.12
Mineral-tanned leather	0.40	0.45	0.50	0.35	0.25	0.20
Canvas stitched	0.20	0.23	0.25	0.15	0.12	0.10
Balata	0.32	0.35	0.40	0.20	—	—
Cotton woven	0.22	0.25	0.28	0.15	0.12	0.10
Camel-hair	0.35	0.40	0.45	0.25	0.20	0.15
Rubber-friction	0.30	0.32	0.35	0.18	—	—
Rubber-covered	0.32	0.35	0.38	0.15	—	—
Rubber on fabric	0.35	0.38	0.40	0.20	—	—

Table 14.2 *(b) Coefficients of Friction of Leather Belts on Iron Pulleys*

v(m/s)	μ	v(m/s)	μ	v(m/s)	μ	v(m/s)	μ	v(m/s)	μ
0.00	0.260	2.00	0.384	4.50	0.440	9.00	0.479	20.00	0.508
0.25	0.285	2.50	0.400	5.00	0.446	10.00	0.482	22.50	0.512
0.50	0.307	3.00	0.413	6.00	0.458	12.50	0.490	25.00	0.514
1.00	0.340	3.50	0.423	7.00	0.466	15.00	0.499	27.50	0.516
1.50	0.365	4.00	0.432	8.00	0.473	17.50	0.505	30.00	0.518

Table 14.3 Values of Exponential $e^{\mu\theta}$

μ_θ	$e^{\mu\theta}$	μ_θ	$e^{\mu\theta}$	μ_θ	$e^{\mu\theta}$	μ_θ	$e^{\mu\theta}$	μ_θ	$e^{\mu\theta}$	μ_θ	$e^{\mu\theta}$	μ_θ	$e^{\mu\theta}$
0.30	1.350	0.45	1.568	0.60	1.822	0.72	2.117	0.90	2.460	1.05	2.858	1.20	3.320
0.31	1.363	0.46	1.584	0.61	1.840	0.76	2.138	0.91	2.484	1.06	2.886	1.21	3.354
0.32	1.377	0.47	1.600	0.62	1.859	0.77	2.160	0.92	2.509	1.07	2.915	1.22	3.387
0.33	1.391	0.48	1.616	0.63	1.878	0.78	2.181	0.93	2.535	1.08	2.945	1.23	3.421
0.34	1.405	0.49	1.632	0.64	1.896	0.79	2.203	0.94	2.560	1.09	2.974	1.24	3.456
0.35	1.419	0.50	1.649	0.65	1.916	0.80	2.226	0.95	2.586	1.10	3.004	1.25	3.490
0.36	1.433	0.51	1.665	0.66	1.933	0.81	2.248	0.96	2.612	1.11	3.034	1.26	3.525
0.37	1.448	0.52	1.682	0.67	1.954	0.82	2.270	0.97	2.638	1.12	3.065	1.27	3.561
0.38	1.462	0.53	1.699	0.68	1.974	0.83	2.293	0.98	2.664	1.13	3.096	1.28	3.597
0.39	1.477	0.54	1.716	0.69	1.994	0.84	2.316	0.99	2.691	1.14	3.127	1.29	3.633
0.40	1.492	0.55	1.733	0.70	2.014	0.85	2.340	1.00	2.718	1.15	3.158	1.30	3.699
0.41	1.507	0.56	1.751	0.71	2.034	0.86	2.363	1.01	2.746	1.16	3.190	1.31	3.706
0.42	1.522	0.57	1.768	0.72	2.054	0.87	2.387	1.02	2.773	1.17	3.222	1.32	3.743
0.43	1.537	0.58	1.786	0.73	2.075	0.88	2.411	1.03	2.801	1.18	3.254	1.33	3.781
0.44	1.553	0.59	1.804	0.74	2.096	0.89	2.435	1.04	2.829	1.19	3.287	1.34	3.819

Table 14.4 *Allowable Tension in N (kgf) per mm Width of Belt*

Material in belt	Ply or Number of Thicknesses of Material											
	1	2	3	4	5	6	7	8	9	10	11	12
Leather, Light	—	16.67 (1.70)	—	—	—	—	—	—	—	—	—	—
Leather, Medium	14.71 (1.50)	24.52 (2.50)	—	—	—	—	—	—	—	—	—	—
Leather, Heavy	17.65 (1.8)	28.44 (2.9)	35.30 (3.6)	—	—	—	—	—	—	—	—	—
Canvas (Stitched)	—	—	—	6.86 (0.7)	8.83 (0.9)	10.79 (1.1)	—	11.77 (1.2)	—	13.73 (1.4)	—	15.69 (1.6)
Rubber	—	—	7.85 (0.8)	10.79 (1.1)	12.75 (1.3)	15.69 (1.6)	18.63 (1.9)	22.56 (2.3)	25.50 (2.6)	28.44 (2.9)	30.40 (3.1)	33.34 (3.4)
Balata	—	—	4.90 (0.5)	6.86 (0.7)	8.83 (0.9)	10.79 (1.1)	11.77 (1.2)	13.73 (1.4)	25.50 (2.6)	28.44 (2.9)	30.40 (3.1)	33.34 (3.4)

Table 14.5 *Relative Strength of Belt Joints*

Type of joint	Relative strength of joint to an equal section of solid leather, Efficiency
Cemented, endless, cemented at factory	90 to 100
Cemented, endless, cemented in shop	80 to 90
Laced, wire, by machine	75 to 85
by hand	70 to 80
rawhide, small holes	60 to 70
large holes	50 to 60
Hinged, wire hooks	40
metal hooks	35 to 40

Table 14.6 *Rating in kW per mm of width-Oak-Tanned Leather Belts*

Belt speed, m/s	Single ply			Double ply		Triple ply	
	4.35	5.16	7.14	7.94	9.13	11.91	13.5
3	0.0324	0.0353	0.0441	0.0530	0.0647	0.0736	0.0824
4	0.0412	0.0500	0.0588	0.0706	0.0780	0.0971	0.1059
5	0.0530	0.0618	0.0765	0.0912	0.1059	0.1206	0.1324
6	0.0618	0.0736	0.0912	0.1089	0.1265	0.1442	0.1589
7	0.0736	0.0853	0.1030	0.1265	0.1442	0.1677	0.1854
8	0.0824	0.0971	0.1177	0.1442	0.1648	0.1912	0.2089
9	0.0941	0.1089	0.1353	0.1589	0.1824	0.2148	0.2354
10	0.1030	0.1206	0.1412	0.1765	0.2030	0.2383	0.2618
12	0.1236	0.1442	0.1736	0.2074	0.2412	0.2795	0.3052
14	0.1442	0.1648	0.2000	0.2412	0.2795	0.3236	0.3545
16	0.1589	0.1854	0.2236	0.2707	0.3111	0.3604	0.3972
18	0.1736	0.2045	0.2242	0.2942	0.3436	0.3935	0.4340
20	0.1883	0.2177	0.2648	0.3200	0.3700	0.4266	0.4707
22	0.2045	0.2324	0.2824	0.3435	0.3935	0.4523	0.4965
24	0.2118	0.2442	0.2964	0.3604	0.4141	0.4751	0.5222
26	0.2207	0.2530	0.3089	0.3751	0.4289	0.4928	0.5443
28	0.3000	0.2589	0.3170	0.3847	0.4413	0.5075	0.5590
30	0.3030	0.2618	0.3200	0.3876	0.4465	0.5163	0.5663

Table 14.7 Correction Factor for Centre Distance and small Pulley Diameter

Small pulley diameter, mm	Center distance, m															
	Upto 1.2		1.2 to 1.8		1.8 to 2.4		2.4 to 3.0		3.0 to 3.6		3.6 to 4.6		4.6 to 6.0		6.0 and up	
	Tight side		Tight side		Tight side		Tight side		Tight side		Tight side		Tight side		Tight side	
	Above	below	Above	below	Above	below	Above	below	Above	below	Above	below	Above	below	Above	below
75	0.45	0.45	0.46	0.47	0.47	0.48	0.47	0.49	0.48	0.50	0.49	0.52	0.48	0.54	0.48	0.55
100	0.53	0.53	0.54	0.55	0.55	0.57	0.56	0.59	0.57	0.61	0.58	0.63	0.59	0.65	0.59	0.65
125	0.59	0.59	0.60	0.62	0.62	0.64	0.63	0.66	0.63	0.68	0.65	0.70	0.66	0.72	0.66	0.74
150	0.62	0.62	0.63	0.65	0.65	0.68	0.66	0.70	0.67	0.72	0.68	0.74	0.69	0.76	0.70	0.78
200	0.66	0.66	0.67	0.69	0.69	0.72	0.70	0.74	0.71	0.76	0.72	0.78	0.73	0.80	0.74	0.82
250	0.68	0.68	0.70	0.71	0.71	0.74	0.73	0.77	0.73	0.79	0.75	0.81	0.76	0.83	0.77	0.85
300	0.70	0.70	0.72	0.74	0.73	0.77	0.75	0.79	0.76	0.81	0.77	0.83	0.78	0.86	0.79	0.88
375	0.73	0.73	0.74	0.76	0.76	0.79	0.77	0.82	0.78	0.84	0.80	0.86	0.81	0.89	0.82	0.91
450	0.75	0.75	0.76	0.78	0.78	0.81	0.79	0.84	0.80	0.86	0.82	0.89	0.83	0.91	0.84	0.93
600	0.77	0.77	0.79	0.81	0.81	0.84	0.82	0.87	0.83	0.89	0.85	0.92	0.86	0.94	0.87	0.96
750	0.79	0.79	0.81	0.82	0.82	0.86	0.84	0.89	0.85	0.91	0.87	0.94	0.88	0.96	0.89	0.98
900	0.80	0.80	0.82	0.84	0.83	0.87	0.85	0.90	0.86	0.92	0.88	0.95	0.89	0.98	0.90	1.00

Table 14.8 *Service Correction Factors*

Select the one appropriate factor from each of the five divisions in Table 14.8

(1)	Atmospheric Condition	Clean, scheduled maintenance on large drives	..	1.2
		Normal	.. .. ..	1.0
		Oily, wet or dusty	.. .. ..	0.7
(2)	Angle of Center line	Horizontal to 60 degrees from horizontal	..	1.0
		60 to 75	.. .. ..	0.9
		75 to 90	.. .. ..	0.8
(3)	Pulley Material	Fibre on motor and small pulleys	.. .. ..	1.2
		Cast iron or steel	.. .. ..	1.0
(4)	Service	Temporary or infrequent	.. .. ..	1.2
		Normal	.. .. ..	1.0
		Important or continuous	.. .. ..	0.8

(5)		All electric motor drives, motor pulley diameters (mm)	
		75 to 90	0.5
		100 to 115	0.55
		125 to 140	0.58
		150 to 250	0.60
	Peak loads	280 to 330	0.63
		355 to 430	0.65
		455 to 580	0.68
		600 to 760	0.70

Light, steady load, such as steam engines, steam turbines, diesel engines, and multi-cylinder gasoline engines	1.0
Jerkey loads, reciprocating machines such as normal-starting-torque squirrel-cage motors, shunt-wound d-c motors, and single-cylinder engines	0.8
Shock and reversing loads: full-voltage start such as squirrelcage and synchronous motors	0.6

Table 14.9 *(a) Specification for Friction Surface Rubber Transmission Belting (IS: 1370–1965)*

Nominal belt widths of friction surface Rubber Transmission belting (mm)
25, 32, 40, 50, 63, 71, 80, 90, 100, 112, 125, 140, 160
180, 200, 224, 250, 280, 315, 355, 400, 450, 500.

Table 14.9 *(b) Thickness of friction surface rubber transmission belting*

Ply construction	Nominal belt thickness Hard type fabric	Tolerance
	(mm)	(mm)
3 ply	3.9	± 0.5
4 ply	5.1	± 0.7
5 ply	6.4	± 0.8
6 ply	7.7	± 0.9
7 ply	9.1	± 1.0
8 ply	10.4	± 1.1

Table 14.10 *Tensile strength of Fabric in finished belting*

Ply construction	Weight of fabric per square meter	Tensile strength	
		Warp	Weft
	$N/m^2(Kg/m^2)$	N/mm(Kg/mm) of width	N/mm (Kg/mm) of width
Soft	8.00 (0.815)	61.30 (6.25)	29.42 (3.00)
Hard	8.83 (0.900)	61.30 (6.25)	35.30 (3.60)
Soft	9.12 (0.930)	69.62 (7.10)	32.36 (3.30)
Hard	9.56 (0.975)	69.62 (7.10)	44.12 (4.50)

Table 14.11 *The maximum ratings in kW (MHP) per mm width of belting at 180°*
arc of contact

Type of Fabric	Weight of Fabric. N/m²	Pulley Diameter	Belt Speed m/s	Rating per mm Width per ply
	(Kg/m²)	mm		kW (MHP)
Soft	8.00 (0.815)	250	5	0.012 (0.0163)
	9.12 (0.930)	250	5	0.015 (0.020)
Hard	8.83 (0.900)	250	5	0.012 (0.0163)
	9.56 (0.975)	250	5	0.015 (0.020)

Table 14.12 *Minimum pulley diameters for given belt speeds and belt plies in mm*

No. of Plies	Maximum Belt Speed, m/s				
	10	15	20	25	30
2	50	63	80	90	112
3	90	100	112	140	180
4	140	160	180	200	250
5	200	224	250	315	355
6	250	315	355	400	450
7	355	400	450	500	560
8	450	500	560	630	710
9	560	630	710	800	900
10	630	710	800	900	1000

Table 14.13 *(a) Specification for Cast Iron and Mild Steel Flat Pulleys*
(IS: 1691–1968) Maximum rim speed

Type of pulley	Maximum Rim Speed m/s
a) Cast iron pulleys:	
1) Solid, with flat or crown face	25
2) Split, with flat or crown face	17
b) Mild steel pulleys, solid or split, with flat or crown face and	
mild steel spokes	25

Table 14.13 (b) Nominal diameters of Cast iron and mild steel pulleys, mm

40, 45, 50, 56, 63, 71, 80, 90, 100, 112, 125, 140, 160, 180, 200, 224, 250, 280, 315, 355, 400, 450, 500, 560, 630, 710, 800, 900, 1000, 1120, 1250, 1400, 1600, 1800, 2000.

Table 14.13 (c) Width of Flat cast iron and mild steel pulleys, mm

20, 25, 32, 40, 50, 53, 71, 80, 90, 100, 112, 125, 140, 160, 180, 200, 224, 250, 280, 315, 355, 400, 450, 500, 560, 630.

Table 14.13 (d) Crown of Cast iron and Mild steel pulleys of diameters from 40 to 355 mm inclusive

Nominal diameter D (mm)	40 to 112	125 and 140	160 and 180	200 and 224	250 and 280	315 and 355
Crown (h) mm	0.3	0.4	0.5	0.6	0.8	1.0

Table 14.13 (e) Crown of Cast iron and Mild Steel pulleys of Diameters from 400 to 2000 mm

Nominal Diameter D mm	Crown h (in mm) of Pulleys of Width (in mm)						
	125 and smaller	140 and 160	180 and 200	224 and 250	280 and 315	355	400 and Larger
400 to 450	1	1.2	1.2	1.2	1.2	1.2	1.2
500 to 560	1	1.5	1.5	1.5	1.5	1.5	1.5
630	1	1.5	2	2	2	2	2
710	1	1.5	2	2	2	2	2
800	1	1.5	2	2.5	2.5	2.5	2.5
900	1	1.5	2	2.5	2.5	2.5	2.5
1000	1	1.5	2	2.5	3	3	3
1120	1.2	1.5	2	2.5	3	3	3.5
1250	1.2	1.5	2	2.5	3	3.5	4
1400	1.5	2	2.5	3	3.5	4	4
1600	1.5	2	2.5	3	2.5	4	5
1800	2	2.5	3	3.5	4	5	5
2000	2	2.5	3	3.5	4	5	6

Table 14.13 (f) Number of Arms in Pulleys

Diameter, mm	Details of Spokes	Diameter, mm	Details of Spokes	Diameter, mm	Details of Spokes
280 to 500	6 Spokes of 19 mm dia	1120	12 Spokes 22 mm dia	1600	18 Spokes 22 mm dia
560 to 710	8 Spokes 19 mm dia	1250	14 Spokes 22 mm dia	1800	18 Spokes 22 mm dia
800 to 1000	10 Spokes 22 mm dia	1400	16 Spokes 22 mm dia	2000	22 Spokes 22 mm dia

Table 14.14 Classification of V-Belts

V-belt Symbol	A	B	C	D	E
Nominal top width, b(mm)	13	17	22	32	38
Nominal thickness, (mm)	8	11	14	19	23
Maximum recommended velocity, m/s	25	25	25	30	30
Recommended power ranges kW	0.4 - 4.0	1.5 - 15	10 - 70	35 - 150	70 - 260
(Mhp)	(0.5 - 50)	(2 - 20)	(15 - 100)	(50 - 200)	(100 - 350)
Max. no. of strands	6	9	12	14	20

Table 14.15 Small Diameter Factor, K_d

Speed Ratio Range	K_d	Speed Ratio Range	K_d	Speed Ratio Range	K_d
1.000 to 1.019	1.00	1.110 to 1.142	1.05	1.341 to 1.429	1.10
1.020 to 1.032	1.01	1.143 to 1.178	1.06	1.430 to 1.562	1.11
1.033 to 1.055	1.02	1.179 to 1.222	1.07	1.563 to 1.814	1.12
1.056 to 1.081	1.03	1.233 to 1.274	1.08	1.815 to 2.948	1.13
1.082 to 1.109	1.04	1.275 to 1.340	1.09	2.949 and over	1.14

Table 14.16 Minimum Pitch Diameters in Relation to Groove Angles

Groove Section	Minimum pitch diameters, mm		
	When $\alpha = 38°$	When $\alpha = 36°$	When $\alpha = 34°$
A	125	—	75
B	200	—	125
C	300	300	—
D	500	355	—
E	630	500	—

Table 14.17 *Nominal inside length, Nominal pitch length and Permissible length variations for standard sizes of V-belts*

All dimensions in mm

	Nominal pitch length, cross-sections					Pitch length Variation	
Nominal inside length	A	B	C	D	E	Pitch length limits	Maximum Variation in Length within a matched set
(1)	(2)	(3)	(4)	(5)	(6)	(7)	(8)
610	645	—	—	—	—	+11.4	
660	696	—	—	—	—	− 6.4	
711	747	—	—	—	—		
787	828	—	—	—	—		
830	848	—	—	—	—	+12.5	
889	925	932	—	—	—	−5.7	
914	950	—	—	—	—		2.5
965	1001	1008	—	—	—		
991	1026	—	—	—	—		
1016	1051	1059	—	—	—	+14.0	
1067	1102	1110	—	—	—	−8.9	
1092	1128	—	—	—	—		
1168	1204	1212	—	—	—		
1219	1255	1262	—	—	—		
1295	1331	1339	1351	—	—		
1372	—	1415	—	—	—		
1397	1433	1440	—	—	—	+16.0	
1422	1458	1466	—	—	—	−9.0	
1473	1509	—	—	—	—		
1524	1560	1567	1580	—	—		5.0
1600	1636	—	—	—	—		
1626	1661	—	—	—	—	+17.8	
1651	1687	1694	—	—	—	−12.5	
1727	1763	1770	1783	—	—		
1778	1814	1824	—	—	—		
1905	1941	1948	1961	—	—	+17.8 −12.5	

(1)	(2)	(3)	(4)	(5)	(6)	(7)	(8)
1981	2017	2024	—	—	—		
2032	2068	—	—	—	—		
2057	2093	2101	2113	—	—	+30.0	7.5
2159	2195	2202	2215	—	—	−16.0	
2286	2322	2329	2342	—	—		
2438	2474	—	2494	—	—		
2464	—	2507	—	—	—		
2540	—	2583	—	—	—	+34.0	
2667	2703	2710	2723	—	—	−18.0	
2845	2880	2888	2901	—	—		
3048	3084	3091	3104	3127	—		
3150	—	—	3205	—	—		10
3251	3287	3294	3307	3330	—	+38.0	
3404	—	—	3459	—	—	−21.0	
3658	3693	3701	3713	3736	—		
4013	—	4056	4069	4092	—	+43.0 −24.0	
4115	—	4158	4171	4194	—	+43.0	
4394	—	4437	4450	4473	—	−24.0	
4572	—	4615	4628	4651	—		
4953	—	4996	5009	5032	—	+49.0	12.5
5334	—	5377	5390	5413	5426	−28.0	
6045	—	—	6101	6124	6137		
6807	—	—	6863	6886	6899	+56.0 −32.0	
7569	—	—	7625	7648	7661	+56.0 −32.0	15
8331	—	—	8387	8410	8423	+65.0	
9093	—	—	9143	9172	9168	−37.0	
9855	—	—	—	9934	9947	+65.0 −37.0	
10617	—	—	—	10696	10709	+76.0	17.5
12141	—	—	—	12220	12233	−43.0	
13665	—	—	—	13744	13757	+89.0	
15189	—	—	—	15268	15281	−50.0	
16713	—	—	—	16792	16805	+105.0 −59.0	

IS: 2494–1964

Table 14.18 *(a) Ratings For V-Belts in Kilo watt*

Cross-section A

Belt Speed (m/s)	Equivalent pitch diameter d_e in mm					
	80	**90**	**100**	**110**	**120**	**125** and over
0.5	0.13	0.13	0.14	0.14	0.15	0.15
1	0.22	0.24	0.25	0.27	0.28	0.29
2	0.37	0.40	0.43	0.46	0.49	0.51
3	0.51	0.58	0.64	0.68	0.72	0.74
4	0.58	0.74	0.81	0.88	0.93	0.96
5	0.74	0.85	0.95	1.04	0.13	1.18
6	0.81	0.94	1.05	1.15	1.25	1.32
7	0.88	1.08	1.25	1.39	1.50	1.54
8	0.96	1.17	1.35	1.50	1.62	1.69
9	1.03	1.32	1.54	1.69	1.77	1.84
10	1.10	1.40	1.62	1.77	1.91	1.99
11	1.18	1.47	1.69	1.91	2.06	2.13
12	1.25	1.54	1.84	3.06	2.21	2.28
13	1.32	1.62	1.91	2.13	2.35	2.43
14	1.32	1.69	1.99	2.28	2.50	2.50
15	1.32	1.77	2.06	2.35	2.57	2.65
16	1.40	1.84	2.13	2.43	2.65	2.79
17	1.40	1.84	2.21	2.50	2.79	2.87
18	1.40	1.84	2.28	2.57	2.87	2.94
19	1.40	1.84	2.28	2.65	2.94	3.02
20	1.32	1.91	2.35	2.72	3.02	3.09
21	1.32	1.91	2.35	2.72	3.02	3.16
22	1.25	1.91	2.35	2.72	3.09	3.24
23	1.25	1.84	2.35	2.79	3.09	3.24
24	1.18	1.84	2.35	2.79	3.16	3.31
25	1.10	1.77	2.28	2.79	3.16	3.31
26	1.03	1.69	2.28	2.72	3.16	3.31
27	0.88	1.62	2.20	2.72	3.09	3.31
28	0.81	1.54	2.13	2.65	3.09	3.24
29	0.66	1.47	2.06	2.57	3.02	3.24
30	0.51	1.32	1.99	2.50	2.94	3.16

1kW=1.35966 hp(metric)   IS: 2494–1964

Table 14.18 *(b)* *Ratings for V-Belts in Kilowatt*

Cross-section B

Belt Speed (m/s)	Equivalent Pitch diameter d_e in mm.					
	130	140	150	160	170	180 and over
0.5	0.22	0.22	0.22	0.22	0.22	0.29
1	0.37	0.44	0.44	0.44	0.51	0.51
2	0.66	0.74	0.81	0.81	0.88	0.88
3	0.96	1.03	1.10	1.17	1.25	1.39
4	1.18	1.32	1.40	1.47	1.50	1.62
5	1.47	1.54	1.69	1.84	1.91	1.99
6	1.62	1.84	1.99	2.06	2.21	2.28
7	1.91	2.13	2.21	2.35	2.50	2.65
8	2.06	2.28	2.43	2.65	2.79	2.94
9	2.21	2.43	2.65	2.87	3.02	3.16
10	2.35	2.65	2.87	3.09	3.31	3.46
11	2.50	2.79	3.09	3.31	3.53	3.75
12	2.65	3.02	3.31	3.53	3.75	3.97
13	2.79	3.16	3.46	3.75	3.97	4.19
14	2.87	3.16	3.60	3.90	4.19	4.56
15	2.94	3.38	3.75	4.05	4.34	4.63
16	3.02	3.46	3.90	4.19	4.49	4.78
17	3.09	3.60	3.97	4.34	4.71	4.92
18	3.16	3.60	4.03	4.49	4.78	5.07
19	3.16	3.68	4.19	4.56	4.92	5.22
20	3.16	3.75	4.19	4.63	5.00	5.44
21	3.16	3.75	4.27	4.71	5.07	5.44
22	3.16	3.75	4.27	4.78	5.15	5.52
23	3.09	3.75	4.27	4.78	5.22	5.59
24	3.02	3.68	4.27	4.78	5.22	5.66
25	2.94	3.60	4.19	4.78	5.22	5.66
26	2.79	3.53	4.19	4.71	5.22	5.66
27	2.65	3.46	4.12	4.63	5.15	5.66
28	2.50	3.31	3.97	4.56	5.15	5.59
29	2.43	3.16	3.82	4.49	5.00	5.52
30	2.13	2.94	3.68	4.34	4.92	5.44

1kW=1.35966 hp(metric)   IS: 2494–1964

Table 14.18 *(c) Ratings for V-Belts in Kilowatt*

Cross-section C

Belt Speed (m/s)	Equivalent pitch diameter d_e in mm.						
	180	200	220	240	260	280	300 and over
0.5	0.37	0.44	0.44	0.51	0.51	0.51	0.51
1	0.64	0.73	0.81	0.88	0.88	0.96	0.96
2	1.15	1.32	1.47	1.50	1.69	1.77	1.84
3	1.62	1.84	2.06	2.21	2.35	2.50	2.57
4	2.06	2.35	2.57	2.79	3.02	3.16	3.31
5	2.35	2.79	3.09	3.38	3.60	3.75	3.97
6	2.72	3.16	3.60	3.90	4.19	4.41	4.63
7	3.02	3.60	4.05	4.40	4.71	5.00	5.22
8	3.31	3.97	4.49	4.84	5.22	5.59	5.81
9	3.60	4.27	4.85	5.37	5.81	6.10	6.40
10	3.82	4.56	5.22	5.81	6.25	6.62	6.99
11	4.04	4.92	5.59	6.18	6.69	7.13	7.58
12	4.19	5.15	5.96	6.62	7.13	7.72	8.00
13	4.34	5.44	6.25	6.96	7.58	8.16	8.46
14	4.49	5.59	6.55	7.28	7.94	8.53	8.97
15	4.63	5.81	6.77	7.58	8.31	8.90	9.41
16	4.71	5.96	7.06	7.87	8.61	9.27	9.78
17	4.78	6.10	7.21	8.09	8.90	9.56	10.15
18	4.78	6.25	7.35	8.38	9.19	9.93	10.51
19	4.78	6.33	7.58	8.53	9.41	10.15	10.81
20	4.78	6.33	7.65	8.68	9.63	10.44	11.11
21	4.71	6.33	7.72	8.83	9.86	10.66	11.33
22	4.56	6.33	7.80	8.90	10.00	10.81	11.62
23	4.34	6.25	7.80	8.97	10.08	11.03	11.77
24	4.19	6.18	7.72	9.05	10.15	11.11	11.91
25	4.05	6.03	7.72	9.05	10.15	11.18	11.99
26	3.82	5.88	7.58	8.97	10.15	11.18	12.06
27	3.60	5.66	7.43	8.90	10.15	11.18	12.13
28	3.24	5.44	7.35	8.75	10.08	11.18	12.13
29	2.79	5.15	7.06	8.06	9.93	11.03	12.06
30	2.43	4.78	6.77	8.38	9.71	10.80	11.99

1kW=1.35966 hp(metric)   IS: 2494–1964

Table 14.18 *(d)* *Ratings for V-Belts in Kilowatt*

Cross-section D

Belt Speed (m/s)	Equivalent Pitch Diameter d_e in mm							
	300	320	340	360	380	400	420	430 and over
0.5	0.81	0.88	0.96	0.96	1.03	1.03	1.10	1.10
1	1.47	1.54	1.69	1.77	1.84	1.91	1.91	1.99
2	2.50	2.79	2.94	3.09	3.24	3.38	3.53	3.53
3	3.46	3.75	4.04	4.34	4.56	4.71	4.92	5.00
4	4.34	4.78	5.15	5.44	5.74	6.03	6.25	6.40
5	5.07	5.66	6.10	6.55	6.91	8.21	7.58	7.65
6	5.81	6.55	7.06	7.51	7.94	8.38	8.75	8.90
7	6.47	7.28	7.94	8.46	8.97	9.41	9.86	10.08
8	7.13	7.94	8.68	9.34	10.00	10.52	10.96	11.25
9	7.65	8.68	9.49	10.22	10.96	11.47	12.06	12.28
10	8.23	9.34	10.22	11.03	11.84	12.43	13.02	13.31
11	8.68	9.86	10.88	11.84	12.58	13.39	14.05	14.34
12	9.12	10.37	11.47	12.50	13.39	14.19	14.93	15.30
13	9.49	10.88	12.06	13.16	14.05	15.00	15.74	16.11
14	9.79	11.25	12.58	13.75	14.56	15.74	16.55	16.99
15	10.00	11.62	13.09	14.34	15.44	16.40	17.28	17.72
16	10.30	11.91	13.46	14.78	15.96	16.99	18.02	18.46
17	10.44	12.21	13.83	15.22	16.55	17.58	18.61	19.05
18	10.51	12.43	14.12	15.59	16.99	18.09	19.20	19.71
19	10.51	12.50	14.27	15.89	17.36	18.53	19.86	20.23
20	10.51	12.58	14.49	16.11	17.65	18.98	20.15	20.74
21	10.37	13.31	14.56	16.40	17.87	19.27	20.52	21.11
22	10.22	12.58	14.56	16.47	18.02	19.49	20.81	21.48
23	9.93	12.43	14.56	16.40	18.17	19.71	21.11	21.70
24	9.63	12.21	14.34	16.40	18.24	19.78	21.26	21.99
25	9.19	11.91	14.27	16.25	18.17	19.78	21.33	22.06
26	8.68	11.47	13.97	16.11	17.87	19.78	21.33	21.99
27	8.16	11.03	13.53	15.81	17.80	19.56	21.26	21.99
28	7.51	10.51	13.09	15.44	17.43	19.34	21.11	21.84
29	6.77	9.86	12.58	15.00	17.14	19.12	20.89	21.62
30	5.96	9.12	11.91	14.42	16.70	18.68	20.52	21.33

1kW=1.35966 hp(metric)   IS: 2494–1964

Table 14.18 *(e) Ratings for V-Belts in Kilowatt*

Cross-section E

Belt Speed (m/s)	Equivalent Pitch Diameter d_e in mm					
	450	500	550	600	650	700 and over
0.5	1.40	1.47	1.54	1.62	1.69	1.77
1	2.43	2.65	2.87	2.94	3.09	3.24
2	4.34	4.78	5.15	5.44	5.66	5.88
3	6.03	6.69	7.21	7.65	8.02	8.38
4	7.58	8.46	9.19	9.78	10.22	10.74
5	9.05	10.15	11.03	11.77	12.36	13.02
6	10.44	11.69	12.80	13.68	14.49	15.07
7	11.77	13.32	14.49	15.51	16.40	17.14
8	13.02	14.78	16.11	17.28	18.31	19.05
9	14.12	16.11	17.72	18.98	20.15	21.11
10	15.22	17.43	19.12	20.59	21.85	22.95
11	16.25	18.61	20.59	22.20	23.61	24.71
12	17.21	19.78	21.92	23.68	25.15	26.40
13	18.02	20.81	23.17	25.08	26.69	28.02
14	18.84	21.85	24.35	26.40	28.10	29.57
15	19.56	22.80	25.45	27.65	29.49	31.04
16	20.15	23.61	26.60	28.83	30.82	32.44
17	20.74	24.42	27.36	29.86	31.99	33.76
18	21.18	25.08	28.24	30.89	33.10	35.01
19	21.55	25.60	28.97	31.77	34.13	36.72
20	21.77	26.11	29.71	32.58	35.08	37.22
21	21.99	26.48	30.23	33.17	35.97	38.17
22	22.06	26.77	30.74	33.90	36.70	38.98
23	21.99	27.07	31.04	34.42	37.29	39.72
24	21.92	27.07	31.33	34.79	37.88	40.38
25	21.71	26.99	31.48	35.08	38.25	40.89
26	21.25	26.92	31.48	35.30	38.54	41.26
27	20.74	26.62	31.41	35.38	38.69	41.56
28	20.15	25.89	31.18	35.30	38.83	41.78
29	19.49	25.74	30.89	35.08	38.76	41.78
30	18.61	25.08	30.45	34.79	38.54	41.70

Note:-1. Belt speed is calculated using the pitch diameter and revolutions per second of one of the pulleys on the drive.

Note:-2. If belt speeds are over 25 metres per second, the pulleys may require special construction or special material. They may also require dynamic balancing. Such applications should be referred to the manufacturer.

1kW=1.35966 hp(metric)   IS: 2494–1964

Table 14.19 Correction Factors for Industrial Service, K_s

Severity of Service	Type of Driven Machines	Type of Driving Units					
		Type - M			Type - N		
		Upto 10 h	Over 10 h to 16 h	Over 16 h and continuous service	Upto 10 h	Over 10 h to 16 h	Over 16 h and continuous service
Light-duty	Agitators for liquids, blowers and exhausters, centrifugal pumps and compressors, fans upto 7.5kW (10 hp), and light-duty conveyors	1.0	1.1	1.2	1.1	1.2	1.3
Medium duty	Belt conveyors for sand, grain etc; dough mixers; fans over 7.5 kW (10hp); generators; line shafts; laundry machinery; machine tools; punches, presses and shears; printing machinery; positive displacement rotary pumps; and revolving and vibrating screens.	1.1	1.2	1.3	1.2	1.3	1.4
Heavy duty	Brick machinery, bucket elevators, exciters, piston compressors, conveyors (drag-pan-screw), hammer mills, paper mill beaters, piston pumps, positive displacement blowers, pulverizers, sawmill and wood-working machinery and textile machinery	1.3	1.4	1.5	1.5	1.6	1.8
Extra-heavy duty	Crushers (gyratory-jaw-roll), mills (ball-rod-tube), hoists, and rubber (calenders-extruders-mills)	1.3	1.4	1.5	1.5	1.6	1.8

Note 1–The table gives only a few examples of particularly representative machines.

Note 2–If am idler pulley is used, the following values must be added to the service factor:

Idler pulley on the slack side { inside : 0, outside : 0.1 }   Idler pulley on the tight side { inside : 0.1, outside : 0.2 }

Note 3, Type-A AC Motors; Normal Torque, Squirrel Cage, Synchronous and Split Phase DC Motors; Shunt Wound, Multiple Cylinder Internal Combustion Engines Over 10 rev/s

Note 4, Type-B AC Motors; Hign Torque, High Slip Repulsion-Induction, Single Phase Series Wound and Slip Ring DC Motors; Series Wound and Compound Wound, Single Cylinder Internal Combustion Engines. Multiple Cylinder Internal Combustion Engines Under 10 rev/s, Line Shafts, Clutches, Brakes, Direct on LIne Starting

IS: 2499–1964

Table 14.20 *Correction Factors for Belt Length* K_L

Nominal Inside length mm	Belt-Cross-Section symbols				
	A	B	C	D	E
(1)	(2)	(3)	(4)	(5)	(6)
610	0.80	—	—	—	—
660	0.81	—	—	—	—
711	0.82	—	—	—	—
787	0.84	—	—	—	—
813	0.85	—	—	—	—
889	0.87	0.81	—	—	—
914	0.87	—	—	—	—
965	0.88	0.83	—	—	—
991	0.88	—	—	—	—
1016	0.89	0.84	—	—	—
1067	0.90	0.85	—	—	—
1092	0.90	—	—	—	—
1168	0.92	0.87	—	—	—
1219	0.93	0.88	—	—	—
1295	0.94	0.89	0.80	—	—
1372	—	0.90	—	—	—
1397	0.96	0.90	—	—	—
1422	0.96	0.90	—	—	—
1473	0.97	—	—	—	—
1524	0.98	0.92	0.82	—	—
1600	0.99	—	—	—	—
1626	0.99	—	—	—	—
1651	1.00	0.94	—	—	—
1727	1.00	0.95	0.85	—	—
1778	1.01	0.95	—	—	—
1905	1.02	0.97	0.87	—	—
1981	1.03	0.98	—	—	—
2032	1.04	—	—	—	—

(1)	(2)	(3)	(4)	(5)	(6)
2057	1.04	0.98	0.89	—	—
2159	1.05	0.99	0.90	—	—
2286	1.06	1.00	0.91	—	—
2438	1.08	—	0.92	—	—
2464	—	1.02	—	—	—
2540	—	1.03	—	—	—
2667	1.10	1.04	0.94	—	—
2845	1.11	1.05	0.95	—	—
3048	1.13	1.07	0.97	0.86	—
3150	—	—	0.97	—	—
3251	1.14	1.08	0.98	0.87	—
3404	—	—	0.99	—	—
3658	—	1.11	1.00	0.90	—
4013	—	1.13	1.02	0.92	—
4115	—	1.14	1.03	0.92	—
4394	—	1.15	1.04	0.93	—
4572	—	1.16	1.05	0.94	—
4953	—	1.18	1.07	0.96	—
5334	—	1.19	1.08	0.96	0.94
6045	—	—	1.11	1.00	0.96
6807	—	—	1.14	1.03	0.99
7569	—	—	1.16	1.05	1.01
8331	—	—	1.19	1.07	1.03
9093	—	—	1.21	1.09	1.05
9855	—	—	1.23	1.11	1.07
10617	—	—	1.24	1.12	1.09
12141	—	—	—	1.16	1.12
13665	—	—	—	1.18	1.14
15189	—	—	—	1.20	1.17
16713	—	—	—	1.23	1.19

IS: 2494–1964

Table 14.21 *Correction Factors for Arc of Contact, K_a*

Arc of Contact on smaller pulley (in deg)	Correction Factor (proportion of 180° rating)	
	V-V	**V-Flat**
180	1.00	0.75
177	0.99	0.76
174	0.99	0.76
171	0.98	0.77
169	0.97	0.78
166	0.97	0.79
163	0.96	0.79
160	0.95	0.80
157	0.94	0.81
154	0.93	0.81
151	0.93	0.82
148	0.92	0.83
145	0.91	0.83
142	0.90	0.84
139	0.89	0.85
136	0.88	0.85
133	0.87	0.86
130	0.86	0.86
127	0.85	0.85
123	0.83	0.83
120	0.82	0.82
117	0.81	0.81
113	0.80	0.80
110	0.78	0.78
106	0.77	0.77
103	0.75	0.75
99	0.73	0.73
95	0.72	0.72
91	0.70	0.70
87	0.68	0.68
83	0.65	0.65

Note: 1–Arcs of contact below 120° should not be used unless full drive details are first submitted to the V-drive manufacturer concerned for confirmation.

Note: 2–It should be noted that the advantage of using V-Flat drive diminishes increasingly for arcs of contact greater than 133°, and the use of such drives is usually not found to be practical for arcs of contact greater than 151°.

IS: 2494–1964

Table 14.22 *Recommended Standard Pulley Pitch Diameters*

Series of pitch diameters			Degree of Preference for Pitch Diameters According to the Groove Section*				
Nominal Value	Pitch Diameter Limits		A	B	C	D	E
	Min.	Max.					
(1)	(2)	(3)	(4)	(5)	(6)	(7)	(8)
mm	mm	mm					
75	75	76.3	3	—	—	—	—
80	80	81.3	3	—	—	—	—
85	85	86.4	3	—	—	—	—
90	90	91.4	1	—	—	—	—
95	95	96.5	2	—	—	—	—
100	100	101.6	1	—	—	—	—
106	106	107.7	2	—	—	—	—
112	112	113.8	1	—	—	—	—
118	118	119.9	2	—	—	—	—
125	125	127.0	1	2	—	—	—
132	132	134.1	2	2	—	—	—
140	140	142.2	1	1	—	—	—
150	150	152.4	2	2	—	—	—
160	160	162.6	1	1	—	—	—
170	170	172.7	3	2	—	—	—
180	180	182.9	1	1	—	—	—
190	190	193.0	3	3	—	—	—
200	200	203.2	1	1	1	—	—
212	212	215.4	—	—	2	—	—
224	224	227.6	2	2	1	—	—
236	236	239.8	—	—	2	—	—
250	250	254.0	1	1	1	—	—
265	265	269.5	—	—	2	—	—
280	280	284.5	2	2	1	—	—
300	300	304.8	2	2	2	—	—
315	315	320.0	1	1	1	—	—
355	355	360.7	2	2	2	1	—
375	375	381.0	—	2	2	2	—
400	400	406.4	1	1	1	1	—
425	425	431.8	—	—	—	2	—

(1)	(2)	(3)	(4)	(5)	(6)	(7)	(8)
450	450	457.2	2	2	2	1	—
475	475	482.6	—	—	—	2	—
500	500	508.0	1	1	1	1	1
530	530	538.5	—	3	3	3	2
560	560	569.0	2	2	2	2	1
600	600	609.6	—	2	2	2	2
630	630	640.0	1	1	1	1	1
670	670	680.7	—	—	—	—	2
710	710	721.4	2	2	2	2	1
750	750	762.0	—	2	2	2	3
800	800	812.8	3	1	1	1	1
900	900	914.4	—	2	2	2	2
1000	1000	1016.0	—1	1	1	1	
1060	1060	1077.0	—	—	—	2	—
1120	1120	1137.9	—	3	2	2	2
1250	1250	1270.0	—	—	1	1	1
1400	1400	1422.4	—	—	2	2	2
1500	1500	1524.0	—	—	—	2	2
1600	1600	1625.6	—	—	1	1	1
1800	1800	1828.8	—	—	—	2	2
1900	1900	1930.4	—	—	—	—	2
2000	2000	2032.0	—	—	—	1	1
2240	2240	2275.8	—	—	—	—	2
2500	2500	2540.0	—	—	—	—	1

*For each groove section the pitch diameters marked 1 are recommended, marked 2 are second preference and marked 3 are not recommended.

IS: 3142–1965

Table 14.23 *Values of C*

			C
Manila rope	...	...	1.15
Wire rope	...	...	1.07
Dry Chain	...	...	1.10
Greased chain	...	...	1.04

Table 14.24 *Dimensions for Standard V-Grooved Pulleys*

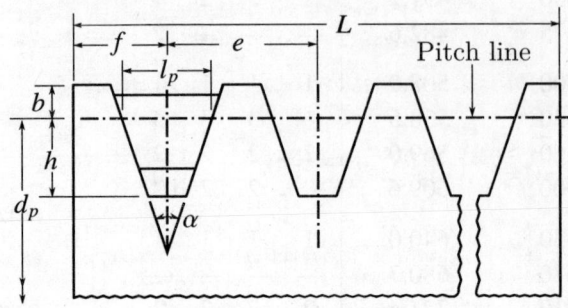

$M_{ax}L = (n' - 1)e + 2f$, where n' is the number of grooves

Groove Section	Pitch width mm 1_p	Minimum Height of Groove above pitch line b, mm	Minimum depth of Groove below pitch line h, mm	Centre to Centre Distance of Grooves, e, mm	Edge of pulley to first groove centre, f, mm
A	11	3.3	8.7	15 ± 0.3	10^{+2}_{-1}
B	14	4.2	10.8	19 ± 0.4	12.5^{+2}_{-1}
C	19	5.7	14.3	25.5 ± 0.5	17^{+2}_{-1}
D	27	8.1	19.9	37 ± 0.6	24^{+3}_{-1}
E	32	9.6	23.4	44.5 ± 0.7	29^{+4}_{-1}

IS: 3142–1965

Table 14.25 *Specification for Steel Wire Ropes for General Engineering Purposes*

Construction	Diameter of rope, mm	Approximate weight N/m (Kg/m)	Nominal Breaking Strength of Rope	
			Tensile Strength of wire 1569 to 1716 MN/m² (160 to 175 kgf/mm²)	Tensile Strength of wire 1716 to 1863 MN/m² (175 to 190 kgf/mm²)
(1)	(2)	(3)	(4)	(5)
			kN(tonne)	kN(tonne)
(a) Group 6 × 19	8	2.354 (0.24)	—	36.28 (3.7)
(Fig. 14.10(a))	10	4.315 (0.44)	64.72 (6.6)	70.61 (7.2)
6 × 12/6/1;	12	5.296 (0.54)	84.34 (8.6)	92.18 (9.4)
	14	7.453 (0.76)	106.89 (10.9)	116.70 (11.9)
6 × 12/6 + 6F/1	16	9.218 (0.94)	131.41 (13.4)	144.16 (14.7)

(1)	(2)	(3)	(4)	(5)
6 × 9/9/1	18	12.258 (1.25)	189.27 (19.3)	206.92 (21.1)
	20	14.416 (1.47)	221.63 (22.6)	241.24 (24.6)
	22	18.044 (1.84)	254.00 (25.9)	278.51 (28.4)
	24	20.888 (2.13)	294.20 (30.0)	232.62 (33.0)
Group 6 × 19	25	23.634 (2.41)	333.43 (34.0)	368.73 (37.6)
(Fig. 14.10(a))	29	29.910 (3.05)	423.65 (43.2)	462.87 (47.2)
	32	36.873 (3.76)	522.69 (53.3)	572.21 (58.4)
	35	44.620 (4.55)	632.53 (64.5)	692.35 (70.6)
	38	53.250 (5.43)	752.17 (76.7)	826.70 (84.3)
	41	62.468 (6.37)	886.52 (90.4)	971.84 (99.1)
	44	72.373 (7.38)	1026.76 (104.7)	1125.80 (114.8)
	48	83.160 (8.48)	1175.82 (119.9)	1298.40 (132.4)
	51	94.536 (9.64)	1345.47 (137.2)	1474.92 (150.4)
	54	106.794 (10.89)	1514.15 (154.4)	1664.19 (169.7)
(*b*) Group 6 × 37	10	4.413 (0.45)	60.80 (6.2)	66.69 (6.8)
6 × 14/7 and 7/7/1;	12	5.884 (0.60)	79.43 (8.1)	87.28 (8.9)
6 × 14/7 + 7*F*/7/1;	14	7.257 (0.74)	101.01 (10.3)	110.82 (11.3)
6 × 16/8 + 8*F*/6/1;	16	9.022 (0.92)	124.55 (12.7)	136.32 (13.9)
6 × 15/15/6/1;	18	12.945 (1.32)	179.46 (18.3)	196.13 (20.0)
6 × 18/12/6/1;	20	15.495 (1.58)	209.86 (21.4)	230.46 (23.5)
6 × 16/8 and 8/8/1	22	17.750 (1.81)	241.24 (24.6)	263.80 (26.9)
	24	20.594 (2.10)	278.51 (28.4)	304.01 (31.0)
(Fig. 14.10(b))	25	23.242 (2.37)	318.71 (32.5)	349.12 (35.6)
	29	29.322 (2.99)	398.15 (40.6)	438.36 (44.7)
	32	36.187 (3.69)	493.27 (50.3)	543.29 (55.4)
	35	52.171 (5.32)	711.96 (72.6)	782.57 (79.8)
	41	61.292 (6.25)	836.51 (85.3)	916.92 (93.5)
	44	71.000 (7.24)	971.94 (99.1)	1065.98 (108.7)
	48	81.591 (8.32)	1116.00 (113.8)	1225.83 (125.0)
	51	92.771 (9.46)	1266.04 (129.1)	1394.51 (142.2)
	54	104.735 (10.68)	1434.71 (146.3)	1573.97 (160.5)
	57	117.484 (11.98)	1604.37 (163.6)	1763.24 (179.8)
	64	145.040 (14.79)	1982.91 (202.2)	2172.17 (221.5)
	70	175.343 (17.88)	2401.65 (244.9)	2630.14 (268.2)

(1)	(2)	(3)		(4)		(5)	
(*c*) Group 6 × 24	8	2.059	(0.21)	29.42	(3.0)	32.36	(3.3)
Fibre Core	10	3.825	(0.39)	53.94	(5.5)	59.82	(6.1)
6 × 15/9/Fibre	12	5.296	(0.54)	74.33	(7.6)	81.40	(8.3)
	14	6.571	(0.67)	92.18	(9.4)	102.00	(10.4)
	16	7.845	(0.80)	112.78	(11.5)	123.56	(12.6)
(Fig. 14.10(c))	18	11.670	(1.19)	164.75	(16.8)	181.42	(18.5)
	20	13.827	(1.41)	196.13	(20.0)	214.77	(21.9)
	22	16.083	(1.64)	228.50	(23.3)	249.09	(25.4)
	24	18.240	(1.86)	258.90	(26.4)	278.09	(28.4)
	25	20.398	(2.08)	289.30	(29.5)	313.81	(32.0)
	29	26.282	(2.68)	368.73	(37.6)	406.00	(41.1)
	32	31.774	(3.24)	448.16	(45.7)	493.28	(50.3)
	35	38.834	(3.96)	548.19	(55.9)	603.19	(61.5)
	38	46.680	(4.76)	662.93	(77.7)	836.51	(85.3)
	44	63.057	(6.43)	891.42	(90.9)	976.74	(99.6)
	48	72.962	(7.44)	1025.78	(104.6)	1125.80	(114.8)
	51	81.984	(8.36)	1166.01	(118.9)	1274.87	(130.0)
	54	93.359	(9.52)	1315.07	(134.1)	1405.29	(147.3)
(*d*) Compound	14	8.336	(0.85)	112.78	(11.5)	121.60	(12.4)
Flattened strand,	16	10.200	(1.04)	143.18	(14.6)	155.93	(15.9)
Group II F	18	13.729	(1.40)	208.88	(21.3)	224.57	(22.9)
6 × 9/12/4,	20	16.279	(1.66)	246.15	(25.1)	263.80	(26.9)
6 × 10/12/4,	22	20.104	(2.05)	284.39	(29.0)	308.91	(31.5)
6 × 12/12/4,	24	23.242	(2.37)	323.62	(33.0)	349.12	(35.6)
	25	26.282	(2.68)	363.83	(37.1)	393.25	(40.1)
(Fig. 14.10(d))	29	33.245	(3.39)	462.87	(47.2)	498.18	(50.8)
	32	41.188	(4.20)	572.71	(58.4)	622.72	(63.5)
	35	49.622	(5.06)	682.54	(69.6)	737.46	(75.2)
	38	59.036	(6.02)	816.89	(83.3)	886.52	(90.4)
	41	69.137	(7.05)	966.94	(98.6)	1036.56	(105.7)
	44	81.003	(8.26)	116.00	(113.8)	1216.06	(124.0)
	48	92.673	(9.45)	1275.85	(130.1)	1374.89	(140.2)
	51	105.029	(10.71)	1454.33	(148.3)	1574.00	(160.5)

Table 14.26 *(a) Specification for Steel Wire Ropes for General Engineering Purposes*

Construction	Diameter of rope, mm	Approximate weight N/m (Kg/m)	Nominal Breaking Strength of Rope, kN (tonne) Tensile Strength of wire 1716 to 1863 MN/m² (175 to 190 kgf/mm²)
(a) Multi-strand	8	2.452 (0.25)	35.30 (3.6)
non-rotating	10	4.119 (0.42)	68.65 (7.0)
Ropes, 17 × 7	12	5.590 (0.57)	87.28 (8.9)
and 18 × 7	14	7.845 (0.80)	113.76 (11.6)
(Fig. 14.10(e))	16	9.611 (0.98)	142.20 (14.5)
	18	12.945 (1.32)	210.04 (20.5)
	20	15.200 (1.55)	237.32 (24.2)
	22	18.927 (1.93)	268.70 (27.4)
	24	21.861 (2.23)	313.81 (32.0)
	25	24.811 (2.53)	358.92 (36.6)
	29	31.381 (3.20)	443.26 (45.2)
	32	38.834 (3.96)	548.19 (55.9)
	35	46.778 (4.77)	672.74 (68.6)
	38	55.898 (5.70)	802.18 (81.8)
(b) Multi-strand	16	10.200 (1.04)	134.35 (13.7)
non-rotating	18	13.435 (1.37)	193.19 (19.7)
ropes, 34 × 7	20	15.985 (1.63)	225.55 (23.0)
	22	19.809 (2.02)	263.80 (26.9)
(Fig. 14.10(e))	24	22.751 (2.32)	299.10 (30.5)
	25	25.989 (2.65)	344.21 (35.1)
	29	32.852 (3.35)	433.45 (44.2)
	32	40.600 (4.14)	538.39 (54.9)
	35	49.033 (5.00)	647.24 (66.0)
	38	58.350 (5.95)	771.78 (78.7)
	44	79.532 (8.11)	1025.78 (104.6)
	51	103.852 (10.59)	1334.69 (136.1)

IS: 2266–1963

Table 14.27 *Specification for Steel Wire Suspension Ropes for Lifts and Hoists*

Construction	Diameter of rope, mm	Approximate weight N/m (Kg/m)	Nominal Breaking Strength KN (tonne)	
			Tensile Strength of wire 1079 to 1226 MN/m^2 (110 to 125 kgf/mm^2)	Tensile Strength of wire 1226 to 1373 MN/m^2 (125 to 140 kgf/mm^2)
(1)	(2)	(3)	(4)	(5)
		kN(tonne)		
(a) 6 × 19 Group	6	1.471 (0.15)	14.710 (1.5)	16.670 (1.7)
6 × 12/6/1;	8	2.452 (0.25)	22.555 (2.3)	26.478 (2.7)
6 × 19(12/6/1)	10	3.922 (0.40)	39.227 (4.0)	44.130 (4.5)
6 × 12/6 + 6F/1	12	5.394 (0.55)	53.937 (5.5)	58.840 (6.0)
6 × 19(9/9/1)	14	7.355 (0.75)	75.511 (7.7)	86.299 (8.8)
	16	9.316 (0.95)	94.144 (9.6)	107.873 (11.0)
	18	12.258 (1.25)	124.544 (12.7)	139.254 (14.2)
	20	14.220 (1.45)	147.010 (15.0)	166.713 (17.0)
	22	18.142 (1.85)	184.365 (18.8)	207.901 (21.2)
	25	22.065 (2.95)	225.553 (23.0)	254.973 (26.0)
(b) 8 × 19 Group	8	1.961 (0.20)	21.575 (2.2)	24.517 (2.5)
8 × 19 Filler wire,	10	3.423 (0.35)	37.265 (3.8)	42.169 (4.3)
i.e. 8 × 12/6 + 6F/1	12	4.903 (0.50)	49.033 (5.0)	53.937 (5.5)
8 × 19(9/9/1) Seale	14	6.865 (0.70)	68.647 (7.0)	79.434 (8.1)
	16	8.336 (0.85)	88.260 (9.0)	98.067 (10.0)
	18	10.787 (1.10)	112.777 (11.5)	132.390 (13.5)
	20	13.239 (1.35)	137.223 (14.0)	152.003 (15.5)
	22	16.671 (1.70)	184.423 (18.5)	205.940 (21.0)
	25	19.613 (2.00)	201.036 (20.5)	235.360 (24.0)

IS: 2365–1963

Table 14.28 *Specification for Small Wire Ropes*

Construction	Nominal diameter, mm	Approximate weight N/m (kg/m)	Nominal Breaking load, kN (tonne)
6 × 7(6/1),	2	0.1471 (0.015)	2.550 (0.26)
fibre core	3	0.3236 (0.033)	5.884 (0.60)
	4	0.5590 (0.057)	10.395 (1.06)
	5	0.8728 (0.089)	16.270 (1.66)
	6	1.2553 (0.128)	23.536 (2.40)
	7	1.6966 (0.173)	31.970 (3.26)
6 × 12 (12/fibre)	3	0.2354 (0.024)	3.727 (0.38)
fibre core	4	0.4119 (0.042)	6.570 (0.67)
	5	0.6374 (0.065)	10.297 (1.05)
	6	0.9218 (0.094)	14.906 (1.52)
	7	1.2553 (0.128)	16.377 (2.07)
6 × 19 (12/6/1)	3	0.3138 (0.032)	4.903 (0.50)
fibre core	4	0.5394 (0.055)	8.728 (0.89)
	5	0.8434 (0.086)	13.533 (1.38)
	6	1.2062 (0.123)	19.613 (2.00)
	7	1.6475 (0.168)	26.576 (2.71)
6 × 24 (15/9/fibre)	4	0.5296 (0.054)	8.630 (0.88)
fibre core	5	0.8336 (0.085)	13.337 (1.36)
	6	1.1964 (0.122)	19.319 (1.97)
	7	1.6181 (0.165)	26.282 (2.62)

IS: 3459–1966

Table 14.29 *Specification for Round Strand Galvanized Steel Wire Ropes for Shipping Purposes*

Construction	Nominal (diameter), mm	Approximate weight N/m (kg/m)		Minimum Breaking Strength of Wire Rope Tensile Strength of wire 1373 to 1569 MN/m^2 (140 to 160 kgf/mm^2) kN (tonne)	
(1)	(2)	(3)		(4)	
6 × 7 Fibre	8	2.158	(0.22)	30.89	(3.15)
core ropes	9	2.746	(0.28)	38.74	(3.95)
	10	3.334	(0.34)	47.07	(4.80)
	11	4.021	(0.41)	56.88	(5.80)
	12	5.100	(0.52)	72.57	(7.40)
	14	6.767	(0.69)	96.11	(9.80)
	16	8.728	(0.89)	123.56	(12.60)
	18	10.885	(1.11)	153.96	(15.70)
	20	13.925	(1.42)	198.09	(20.20)
	22	16.573	(1.69)	236.34	(24.10)
	24	19.515	(1.99)	278.51	(28.40)
	26	22.751	(2.32)	232.62	(33.00)
	28	27.006	(2.76)	385.40	(39.30)
	32	34.716	(3.54)	494.26	(50.40)
	36	44.522	(4.54)	634.49	(64.70)
	40	54.329	(5.54)	773.75	(78.90)
6 × 19 Fibre	8	1.961	(0.20)	27.95	(2.85)
core ropes	9	2.844	(0.29)	30.21	(4.10)
	10	3.432	(0.35)	47.07	(4.80)
	11	3.923	(0.40)	53.94	(5.50)
	12	5.100	(0.52)	71.10	(7.25)
	14	6.472	(0.66)	90.22	(9.20)
	16	8.826	(0.90)	122.58	(12.50)
	18	10.591	(1.08)	147.10	(15.00)

(1)	(2)	(3)	(4)
6 × 14 Fibre	20	13.533 (1.38)	188.29 (19.20)
core ropes	22	15.691 (1.60)	218.69 (22.30)
	24	19.221 (1.96)	267.72 (27.30)
	26	23.144 (2.36)	321.66 (32.80)
	28	25.988 (2.65)	360.88 (36.80)
	32	33.735 (3.44)	468.76 (47.80)
	36	42.365 (4.32)	588.40 (60.00)
	40	54.133 (5.52)	753.15 (76.80)
	44	65.116 (6.64)	905.15 (92.30)
	48	77.963 (7.95)	1084.62 (110.60)
	52	90.025 (9.18)	1251.33 (127.60)
	56	104.049 (10.61)	1446.48 (147.50)
7 × 7 Wire	10	3.726 (0.38)	51.98 (5.30)
Core ropes	11	4.413 (0.45)	62.76 (6.40)
	12	5.688 (0.58)	80.41 (8.20)
	14	7.511 (0.77)	106.89 (10.90)
	16	9.709 (0.99)	137.29 (14.00)
	18	12.062 (1.23)	171.62 (17.50)
	20	15.495 (1.58)	219.67 (22.40)
	22	18.535 (1.89)	262.82 (26.80)
	24	21.869 (2.23)	308.91 (31.50)
	26	25.399 (2.59)	359.90 (36.70)
	28	30.205 (3.08)	427.57 (43.60)
	32	38.736 (3.95)	549.17 (56.00)
	36	49.720 (5.07)	704.12 (71.80)

IS: 2581–1968

Table 14.30 *Specification for Flat Hoisting Wire Ropes used in Mines*

Construction	Nominal size $b \times s$ mm	Nominal wire diameter, mm	Cross section of Strands, mm^2	Minimum Weight, N/m (kg/m)	Breaking strength of rope having Wires of Tensile strength of 1569 MN/m^2 (160 kgf/mm^2) kN(tonne)
$6 \times 4 \times 7$	52×10	1.20	190	18.633 (1.9)	298.12 (30.4)
	56×11	1.30	223	21.575 (2.2)	349.12 (35.6)
	60×12	1.40	259	25.497 (2.6)	406.00 (41.4)
	65×14	1.50	297	29.420 (3.0)	465.82 (47.5)
	70×15	1.60	338	33.343 (3.4)	529.56 (54.0)
	74×16	1.70	381	37.265 (3.8)	597.23 (60.9)
	78×17	1.80	427	42.169 (4.3)	669.79 (68.3)
	82×18	1.90	477	47.062 (4.8)	747.27 (76.2)
	87×19	2.00	528	51.975 (5.3)	827.68 (84.4)
	91×20	2.10	581	56.879 (5.8)	911.04 (92.9)
	95×21	2.20	638	62.763 (6.4)	1000.28 (102.0)
$8 \times 4 \times 7$	70×10	1.20	253	24.517 (2.5)	396.19 (40.4)
	75×11	1.30	298	29.420 (3.0)	466.80 (47.6)
	80×12	1.40	345	34.323 (3.5)	541.33 (55.2)
	86×14	1.50	396	39.227 (4.0)	620.76 (63.3)
	92×15	1.60	450	44.130 (4.5)	706.08 (72.0)
	98×16	1.70	508	50.014 (5.1)	796.30 (81.2)
	104×17	1.80	569	55.898 (5.7)	892.41 (91.0)
	110×18	1.90	636	62.763 (6.4)	997.34 (101.7)
	116×19	2.00	703	68.649 (7.0)	1102.27 (112.4)
	122×20	2.10	775	76.492 (7.8)	1216.03 (124.0)
	128×21	2.20	851	83.357 (8.5)	1334.69 (136.1)

IS: 4202–1969

Table 14.31 *Ratio of Drum and Sheave Diameter to Rope Diameter*

Purpose	Construction	Minimum Ratio*		
Mining Installations	All	100		
		Class 1	Class 2 and 3	Class 4
Cranes and allied hoisting equipment	6 × 37 8 × 19 Filler wire	15	17	22
	8 × 19 8 × 19 Warrington 8 × 19 Seale 34 × 7 Non-rotating	17	18	24
	6 × 24	18	19	25
	6 × 19 Filler Wire	18	20	23
	6 × 19 6 × 19 Warrington 17 × 7 Non-rotating 18 × 7 Non-rotating	19	23	27
	6 × 19 Seale	24	28	35

*The ratio of the diameters specified are valid for rope speeds up to 50m/min. For speeds above 50 m/min. The drum or sheave dia. should be increased prorata by 8 percent for each additional 50 m/min. of rope speed where practicable.

IS: 3973–1967

Table 14.32 *Approximate Wire Rope and Sheave Data*

Rope Construction	Weight N/m (kg/m)	Wire dia (d_w) (mm)	Area, mm^2	Recommended sheave dia	
				Average	Minimum
6 × 7	0.0333d^2 (0.0034d^2)	0.106d	0.38d^2	75d	42d
6 × 19	0.0363d^2 (0.0037d^2)	0.063d	0.38d^2	45d	30d
6 × 37	0.0343d^2 (0.0035d^2)	0.045d	0.38d^2	27d	18d
8 × 19	0.0339d^2 (0.00346d^2)	0.050d	0.38d^2	31d	21d

Table 14.33 *Factors of Safety for Wire Ropes*

Rope Application	Factors of Safety		
Mining ropes	10 or other figure laid down by the satutory authority		
Mine Shafts: Depths (metres)			
To 150	8		
300 to 600	7		
600 to 900	6		
Over 900	5		
Haulage rope	5		
Small electric and air hoists	7		
Hot ladle cranes	8		
Slings	8		
	Class 1	Class 2 & 3	Class 4
Fixed guys, Unreeved rope bridles of jib cranes or ancillary appliances, such as lifting beams,. Ropes which are straight between terminal fittings	3.5	4.0	4.5
Hoisting, luffing and reeved bridle systems of inherently flexible cranes (for example, mobile, crawler tower, guy derrick, stiff leg derrick) where jibs are supported by ropes or where equivalent shock absorbing devices are incorporated in jib supports	4.0	4.5	5.5
Cranes and hoists in general hoist blocks	4.5	5.0	6.0

IS: 3973–1967

Table 14.34 *Strength of Hoisting chains in terms of the bars from which they are made*

Type of chain		% of bar
Coil chain	..	120
Standard close link chain	..	138
Stud chain	..	165

Table 14.35 *Service Factor for Chains,* K_s

Operating Conditions	Intermittent few hours per day	Normal 8 to 10 h per day	Continuous 24 hours per day
Easy starting, smooth, steady load	0.60 – 1.00	0.90 – 1.50	1.20 – 2.00
Light to medium shock or Vibrating load	0.90 – 1.40	1.20 – 1.90	1.50 – 2.40
Medium to heavy shock or Vibrating load	1.20 – 1.80	1.50 – 2.30	1.80 – 2.80

Table 14.36 *(a) Number of Teeth on Smaller Sprocket*

Transmission ratio, $i = \dfrac{z_2}{z_1}$	1-2	2-3	3-4	4-5	5-7
No. of teeth on smaller sprocket	30-27	27-25	25-23	23-21	21-17

Table 14.36 *(b) Minimum Centre Distance Coefficient, K_1*

Transmission Ratio	K_1
3	C min = 30 to 50 mm
3 to 4	1.2
4 to 5	1.3
5 to 6	1.4
6 to 7	1.5

Table 14.37 *Factor of Safety*

Chains	Speed of Smaller Sprocket, rev/min								
	50	200	400	600	800	1000	1200	1600	2000
Bush-roller chain									
p = 12-15 mm	7.0	7.8	8.55	9.35	10.2	11.0	11.7	13.2	14.8
p = 20-25 mm	7.0	8.2	9.35	10.30	11.7	12.9	14.0	16.3	—
p = 30-35 mm	7.0	8.55	10.20	13.20	14.8	16.3	19.5	—	—
Silent Chain									
p = 12.7-15.87 mm	20	22.2	24.4	28.7	29.0	31.0	33.4	37.8	42.0
p = 19.05-25.4 mm	20	23.4	26.7	30.0	33.4	36.8	40.0	46.5	53.5

Table 14.38 *Coefficient for Sag K_2*

Coefficient for sag	Position of chain drive			
	Horizontal	Upto 40°	More than 40°	Vertical
K_2	6	4	2	1

Table 14.39 (a) Chain Dimensions, Measuring loads and Breaking loads of Base chains

All dimensions in millimeters.

ISO Chain Number	Pitch p	Roller Diameter d_1 Max	Width Between Inner Plates b_1 Min	Bearing Pin Body Diameter d_2 Max	Chain Path Depth h_1 Min	Inner Plate Depth h_2 Max	Outer Intermediate Plate Depth h_3 Max	Cranked Link Dimensions* l_1 Min	l_2 Min	c	Transverse Pitch p_t	Width Over inner Link b_2 Max	Width Between Outer Plates b_3 Min	Width Over Bearing Pins Simple b_4 Max	Duplex b_5 Max	Triplex b_6 Max	Additional Width for Joint Fastener** b_7 Max	Measuring Load, kg Simple	Duplex	Triplex	Breaking Load, kg Simplex Min	Duplex Min	Triplex Min
05B	8.00	5.00	3.00	2.31	7.37	7.11	7.11	3.71	3.71	0.08	5.64	4.77	4.90	8.6	14.3	19.9	3.1	5	10	15	460	800	1140
06B	9.525	6.35	5.72	3.28	8.52	8.26	8.26	4.32	4.32	0.08	10.24	8.53	8.66	13.5	23.8	34.0	3.3	8	15	22	910	1730	2540
08B	12.70	8.51	7.75	4.45	12.07	11.81	10.92	5.66	6.12	0.08	13.92	11.30	11.43	17.0	31.0	44.9	3.9	13	26	39	1820	3180	4540
10B	15.875	10.16	9.65	5.08	14.99	14.73	13.72	7.11	7.62	0.10	16.59	13.28	13.41	19.6	36.2	52.8	4.1	20	40	60	2270	4540	6810
12B	19.05	12.07	11.63	5.72	16.39	16.13	16.13	8.33	8.33	0.10	19.46	15.62	15.75	22.7	42.2	61.7	4.6	29	57	86	2950	5900	8850
16B	25.40	15.88	17.02	8.28	21.34	21.08	21.08	11.15	11.15	0.13	31.88	25.45	25.58	36.1	68.0	99.9	5.4	51	102	152	4310	8620	12930
20B	31.75	19.05	19.56	10.19	26.68	26.42	26.42	13.89	13.89	0.15	36.45	29.01	29.14	43.2	79.7	116.1	6.1	79	159	238	6580	13160	19740
24B	38.10	25.40	25.40	14.63	33.73	33.40	33.40	17.55	17.55	0.18	48.36	37.92	38.05	53.4	101.8	150.2	6.6	113	227	340	9980	19960	29940
28B	44.45	27.94	30.99	15.90	37.46	37.08	37.08	19.51	19.51	0.20	59.56	46.58	46.71	65.1	124.7	184.3	7.4	154	308	463	13160	26320	39480
32B	50.80	29.21	30.99	17.81	42.72	42.29	42.29	22.20	22.50	0.20	58.55	45.57	45.70	67.4	126.0	184.5	7.9	204	408	612	17240	34480	51720
40B	63.50	39.37	38.10	22.89	53.49	52.96	52.96	27.76	27.76	0.20	72.29	55.75	55.88	82.6	154.9	227.2	10.2	318	635	953	26770	53540	80310
48B	76.20	48.26	45.72	29.24	64.52	63.88	63.88	33.45	33.45	0.20	91.21	70.56	70.69	99.1	190.4	281.6	10.5	454	907	1361	40830	81650	122470
56B	88.90	53.98	53.34	34.32	78.64	77.85	77.85	40.61	40.61	0.20	106.60	81.33	81.46	114.6	221.2	—	11.7	621	1243	—	55340	110680	—
64B	101.60	63.50	60.96	39.40	91.08	90.17	90.17	47.07	47.07	0.20	119.89	92.02	92.15	130.9	250.8	—	13.0	812	1624	—	72580	145150	—
72B	114.30	72.39	68.58	44.48	104.67	103.63	103.63	53.37	53.37	0.20	136.27	103.81	103.94	147.4	283.7	—	14.3	1030	2059	—	91630	183260	—

IS: 2403–1975

Note– Regarding chains 08B and 10B, narrow versions of the simple chain having widths between inner plates of 5.21 mm *Min* and 6.48 mm *Min*, may be used for motorcycle applications.

*Cranked links are not recommended for use on chains which are intended for onerous applications.

**The actual dimensions will depend on the type of fastener used but they should not exceed the dimensions in this column, details of which should be obtained by the purchaser from the manufacturer.

Flexible Machine Elements

Table 14.39 (b) Chain Dimensions, Measuring Loads and Breaking Loads of Precision Roller Chains (Fig. 14.12)

All dimensions in millimeters.

Chain Number	Pitch, p	Roller Dia, D_r Max.	Width Between Inner Plates, W Min.	Bearing Pin Body Dia, D_p Max.	Bush Bore, d_b Min.	Chain Path Depth, H_c Min.	Plate Depth, H Max.	Cranked Link Dimension, X Min.	Width Over Inner Link, W_1 Max.	Width Between Outer Plates, W_2 Min.	Width Over Bearing Pin, A Max.	Additional Width For Joint* Fastener, B Max.	Measuring Load	Breaking Load Minimum
(1)	(2)	(3)	(4)	(5)	(6)	(7)	(8)	(9)	(10)	(11)	(12)	(13)	(14)	(15)
													N(kgf)	kN (tonne)
208A	25.40	7.92	7.95	3.96	4.01	12.33	12.07	6.9	11.18	11.31	17.8	3.9	127.50 (13)	13.83 (1.40)
208B	25.40	8.51	7.75	4.45	4.50	12.17	11.81	6.9	11.30	11.43	17.0	3.9	127.50 (13)	17.85 (1.82)
210A	31.75	10.16	9.53	5.08	5.13	15.35	15.09	8.4	13.84	13.97	21.8	4.1	196.13 (20)	21.77 (2.22)
210B	31.75	10.16	9.65	5.08	5.13	14.99	14.73	8.4	13.28	13.41	19.6	4.1	196.13 (20)	22.66 (2.27)
212A	38.10	11.91	12.70	5.94	5.99	18.34	18.08	9.9	17.75	17.88	26.9	4.6	284.39 (29)	31.19 (3.18)
212B	38.10	12.07	11.68	5.72	5.77	16.39	16.13	9.9	15.62	15.75	22.7	4.6	284.39 (29)	28.94 (2.95)
216A	50.80	15.88	15.88	7.92	7.97	24.39	24.13	13.0	22.61	22.74	33.5	5.4	500.14 (51)	55.60 (5.67)
216B	50.80	15.88	17.02	8.28	8.33	21.34	21.08	13.0	25.45	25.58	36.1	5.4	500.14 (51)	42.27 (4.31)
220A	63.50	19.05	19.05	9.53	9.58	30.48	30.18	16.0	27.46	27.59	41.1	6.1	747.73 (79)	86.79 (8.85)
220B	63.50	19.05	19.56	10.19	10.24	26.68	26.42	16.0	29.01	29.14	43.2	6.1	747.73 (79)	64.53 (6.58)
224A	76.20	22.23	25.40	11.10	11.15	36.55	36.20	19.1	35.46	35.59	50.8	6.6	1108.15 (113)	124.55 (12.70)
224B	76.20	25.40	25.40	14.63	14.68	33.73	33.40	19.1	37.92	38.05	53.4	6.6	1108.15 (113)	98.87 (9.98)
228B	88.90	27.94	30.99	15.90	15.95	37.46	37.08	21.3	46.58	46.71	65.1	7.4	1510.22 (154)	129.06 (13.16)
232B	101.60	29.21	30.99	17.81	17.86	42.72	42.29	24.4	45.57	45.70	67.4	7.9	2000.56 (204)	169.07 (17.24)

Note 1–The chain path depth H_c is the minimum depth of channel through which the assembled chain will pass.

Note 2–The overall width of chain with joint fastener is:

A+B for riveted pin end and fastener on one side,

A+1.6B for headed pin end and fastener on one side, and

A+2B for fasteners on both sides.

*The actual dimensions will depend on the type of fastener used but they should not exceed the dimensions in this column and should be obtained by the purchaser from the manufacturer.

IS: 3542–1966

Table 14.40 Chain Dimensions, Measuring Loads and Breaking Loads of Precision Bush Chains (Fig. 14.13(a))

All dimensions in mm

Chain Number	Pitch, D_p	Bush Dia B_r Max.	Width Between Inner Plates, W Min.	Bearing Pin Body Dia D_p Max.	Bush Bore d_b Min.	Chain Path Depth H_c Min.	Inner Plate Depth H_i Max.	Outer or Intermediate Plate Depth H_o Max.	Cranked Link Dimensions* X Min.	r Min.	C	Transverse Pitch T_p	Width Over Inner Link W_1 Max.	Width Between Outer Plates W_2 Min.
0.4C	6.35	3.30	3.18	2.29	2.34	6.27	6.02	5.21	2.64	3.06	0.08	6.40	4.80	4.93
0.6C	9.525	5.08	4.77	3.59	3.63	6.30	9.05	7.80	3.96	4.60	0.08	10.13	7.47	7.60

Width Over Bearing Pins			Additional Width for Joint Fasteners B	Measuring Load			Breaking Load		
Simple A_1 Max.	Duplex A_2 Max.	Triplex A_3 Max.	Max.	Simple N(kgf)	Duplex N(kgf)	Triplex N(kgf)	Simple Min. N(kgf)	Duplex Min. N(kgf)	Triplex Min. N(kgf)
9.1	15.5	21.8	2.5	49.03 (5)	98.07 (10)	147.10 (15)	3432.32 (350)	6864.66 (700)	10296.98 (1050)
13.2	23.4	33.5	3.3	68.65 (7)	137.29 (14)	205.94 (21)	7747.25 (790)	15494.51 (1580)	23241.76 (2370)

Note 1–Dimension C represents the clearance between the cranked link plates and the straight plates available during articulation.

Note 2–The chain path depth H_c is the minimum depth of channel through which the assembled chain passes.

Note 3–Width over bearing pins for chains wider than triples = $A_1 + T_p$ (number of stranos in chain–1).

*Cranked links are not recommended for use on chains which are intended for onerous applications.

IS: 3560–1966

Table 14.41 *Pitch Circle Diameter*

The following table gives correct pitch circle diameters for wheels to suit a chain of unit pitch (for example, 1mm). The pitch circle diameters for wheels to suit a chain of any other pitch are directly proportional to the pitch of the chain:

Number of Teeth z	Pitch Circle Diameter	Number of Teeth z	Pitch Circle Diameter	Number of Teeth z	Pitch Circle Diameter
(1)	(2)	(1)	(2)	(1)	(2)
5	1.701 3	21	6.709 5	37	11.791 6
$5\frac{1}{2}$	1.849 6	$21\frac{1}{2}$	6.868 1	$37\frac{1}{2}$	11.950 6
6	2.000 0	22	7.026 6	38	12.109 5
$6\frac{1}{2}$	2.151 9	$22\frac{1}{2}$	7.185 3	$38\frac{1}{2}$	12.268 5
7	2.304 8	23	7.343 9	39	12.427 5
$7\frac{1}{2}$	2.458 6	$23\frac{1}{2}$	7.502 6	$39\frac{1}{2}$	12.586 5
8	2.613 1	24	7.661 3	40	12.745 5
$8\frac{1}{2}$	2.768 2	$24\frac{1}{2}$	7.820.0	$40\frac{1}{2}$	12.904 5
9	2.923 8	25	7.978 7	41	13.063 5
$9\frac{1}{2}$	3.079 8	$25\frac{1}{2}$	8.137 5	$41\frac{1}{2}$	13.222 5
10	3.236 1	26	8.296 2	42	13.381 5
$10\frac{1}{2}$	3.392 7	$26\frac{1}{2}$	8.455 0	$42\frac{1}{2}$	13.540 5
11	3.549 4	27	8.613 8	43	13.699 5
$11\frac{1}{2}$	3.706 5	$27\frac{1}{2}$	8.772 6	$43\frac{1}{2}$	13.858 5
12	3.863 7	28	8.931 4	44	14.017 6
$12\frac{1}{2}$	4.021 1	$28\frac{1}{2}$	9.090 2	$44\frac{1}{2}$	14.176 5
13	4.178 6	29	9.249 1	45	14.335 6
$13\frac{1}{2}$	4.336 2	$29\frac{1}{2}$	9.408 0	$45\frac{1}{2}$	14.494 6
14	4.494 0	30	9.566 8	46	14.658 7
$14\frac{1}{2}$	4.651 8	$30\frac{1}{2}$	9.725 6	$46\frac{1}{2}$	14.812 7
15	4.809 7	31	9.884 4	47	14.971 7
$15\frac{1}{2}$	4.967 7	$31\frac{1}{2}$	10.043 4	$47\frac{1}{2}$	15.130 8

Table 14.41 *Pitch Circle Diameter (Contd...)*

(1)	(2)	(1)	(2)	(1)	(2)
16	5.125 8	32	10.202 3	48	15.289 8
$16\frac{1}{2}$	5.284 0	$32\frac{1}{2}$	10.361 2	$48\frac{1}{2}$	15.448 8
17	5.442 2	33	10.520 1	49	15.607 9
$17\frac{1}{2}$	5.600 5	$33\frac{1}{2}$	10.679 0	$49\frac{1}{2}$	15.766 9
18	5.758 8	34	10.838 0	50	15.926 0
$18\frac{1}{2}$	5.917 1	$34\frac{1}{2}$	10.996 9	$50\frac{1}{2}$	16.085 0
19	6.075 5	35	11.155 8	51	16.244 1
$19\frac{1}{2}$	6.234 0	$35\frac{1}{2}$	11.314 8	$51\frac{1}{2}$	16.403 1
20	6.392 5	36	11.473 7	52	16.562 2
$20\frac{1}{2}$	6.550 9	$36\frac{1}{2}$	11.632 7	$52\frac{1}{2}$	16.721 2
53	16.880 3	61	19.425 5	69	21.971 0
$53\frac{1}{2}$	17.039 3	$61\frac{1}{2}$	19.584 7	$69\frac{1}{2}$	22.130 3
54	17.198 4	62	19.743 7	70	22.289 2
$54\frac{1}{2}$	17.357 5	$62\frac{1}{2}$	19.902 9	$70\frac{1}{2}$	22.448 5
55	17.516 6	63	20.061 9	71	22.607 4
$55\frac{1}{2}$	17.675 6	$63\frac{1}{2}$	20.221 0	$71\frac{1}{2}$	22.766 7
56	17.834 7	64	20.280 0	72	22.925 6
$56\frac{1}{2}$	17.993 8	$64\frac{1}{2}$	20.539 3	$72\frac{1}{2}$	23.084 9
57	18.152 9	65	20.698 2	73	23.243 8
$57\frac{1}{2}$	18.311 9	$65\frac{1}{2}$	20.857 5	$73\frac{1}{2}$	23.403 1
58	18.471 0	66	21.016 4	74	23.562 0
$58\frac{1}{2}$	18.630 1	$66\frac{1}{2}$	21.175 7	$74\frac{1}{2}$	23.721 3
59	18.789 2	67	21.334 6	75	23.860 2
$59\frac{1}{2}$	18.948 2	$67\frac{1}{2}$	21.493 9		
60	19.107 3	68	21.652 8		
$60\frac{1}{2}$	19.266 5	$68\frac{1}{2}$	21.812 1		

IS: 3542–1966

Table 14.42 *Pitch circle diameters*

Number of Teeth	Pitch Circle Diameter	Number of Teeth	Pitch Circle Diameter	Number of Teeth	Pitch Circle Diameter
(1)	(2)	(1)	(2)	(1)	(2)
76	24.198 5	85	27.062 5	94	29.926 7
77	24.516 7	86	27.380 7	95	30.244 9
78	24.834 9	87	27.699 0	96	30.563 2
79	25.153 1	88	28.017 2	97	30.881 5
80	25.471 3	89	28.335 5	98	31.199 7
81	25.789 6	90	28.653 7	99	31.518.0
82	26.107 8	91	28.971 9	100	31.836 2
83	26.426 6	92	29.290 2	101	32.154 5
84	26.744 3	93	29.608 4	102	32.472 7
103	32.791 0	119	37.883 3	135	42.975 7
104	33.109 3	120	38.201 6	136	43.294 0
105	33.427 6	121	38.519 8	137	43.612 3
106	33.745 8	122	38.838 1	138	43.930 6
107	34.064 0	123	39.156 4	139	44.248 8
108	34.382 3	124	38.474 6	140	44.567 1
109	34.700 6	125	39.792 9	141	44.885 4
110	35.018 8	126	40.111 2	142	45.203 7
111	35.337 1	127	40.429 5	143	45.522 0
112	35.655 4	128	40.747 8	144	45.840 3
113	35.973 7	129	41.066 0	145	46.158 5
114	36.291 9	130	41.384 3	146	46.476 8
115	36.610 2	131	41.702 6	147	46.795 1
116	36.928 5	132	42.020 9	148	47.113 4
117	37.246 7	133	42.339 1	149	47.431 7
118	37.565 0	134	42.657 4	150	47.750 0

IS: 3560–1966

Table 14.43 Leaf Chain Dimensions, Measuring Loads and Breaking Loads (Fig. 14.14)

All dimensions in mm

Chain Number	Pitch, p mm	inch	Lacing	Chain Width W_1	Width Over Breaking Pins W_2	Pin Body Diameter D_p	Articulating Plates Bore Diameter D_b	Plate Depth H	Plate Thickness T	Measuring load	Breaking Load Min.
						Maximum	Minimum	Maximum	Maximum	N (kgf)	kN (tonne)
(1)	(2)	(3)	(4)	(5)	(6)	(7)	(8)	(9)	(10)	(11)	(12)
0822	12.70	(0.500)	2 × 2	6.45	8.69	4.45	4.48	11.81	1.57	187.31 (19.1)	18.73 (1.91)
0823	12.70	(0.500)	2 × 3	8.08	10.31	4.45	4.48	11.81	1.57	187.31 (19.1)	18.73 (1.91)
0834	12.70	(0.500)	3 × 4	11.30	13.54	4.45	4.48	11.81	1.57	280.47 (28.6)	28.05 (2.86)
0846	12.70	(0.500)	4 × 6	16.13	18.36	4.45	4.48	11.81	1.57	373.63 (38.1)	37.36 (3.81)
1022	15.88	(0.625)	2 × 2	7.26	9.80	5.08	5.10	14.73	1.78	249.09 (25.4)	24.91 (2.54)
1023	15.88	(0.625)	2 × 3	9.09	11.63	5.08	5.10	14.73	1.78	249.09 (25.4)	24.91 (2.54)
1034	15.88	(0.625)	3 × 4	12.73	15.27	5.08	5.10	14.73	1.78	391.29 (39.9)	39.13 (3.99)
1046	15.88	(0.625)	4 × 6	18.16	20.70	5.08	5.10	14.73	1.78	498.18 (50.8)	49.82 (5.08)
1222	19.05	(0.750)	2 × 2	12.50	15.90	6.78	6.80	16.13	3.07	445.22 (45.4)	44.52 (4.54)
1223	19.05	(0.750)	2 × 3	15.62	19.02	6.78	6.80	16.13	3.07	445.22 (45.4)	44.52 (4.54)
1234	19.05	(0.750)	3 × 4	21.87	25.27	6.78	6.80	16.13	3.07	666.85 (68.0)	66.69 (6.80)
1246	19.05	(0.750)	4 × 6	31.24	34.65	6.78	6.80	16.13	3.07	889.46 (90.7)	88.95 (9.07)

Table 14.43 *Leaf Chain Dimensions, Measuring Loads and Breaking Loads (Fig. 14.14) (Contd...)*

(1)	(2)	(3)	(4)	(5)	(6)	(7)	(8)	(9)	(10)	(11)	(12)
1623	25.40 (1.000)		2 × 3	21.34	25.48	8.28	8.30	21.08	4.22	622.72 (63.5)	62.27 (6.35)
1634	25.40 (1.000)		3 × 4	29.87	34.01	8.28	8.30	21.08	4.22	1022.83 (104.3)	102.28 (10.43)
1646	25.40 (1.000)		4 × 6	42.67	46.81	8.28	8.30	21.08	4.22	1245.44 (127.0)	124.54 (12.70)
2023	31.75 (1.250)		2 × 3	23.24	28.35	10.19	10.22	26.42	4.60	978.70 (99.8)	97.87 (9.98)
2034	31.75 (1.250)		3 × 4	32.54	37.64	10.19	10.22	26.42	4.60	1512.19 (154.2)	151.22 (15.42)
2046	31.75 (1.250)		4 × 6	46.48	51.59	10.19	10.22	26.42	4.60	1957.41 (199.6)	195.74 (19.96)
2423	38.10 (1.500)		2 × 3	30.73	38.05	14.63	14.66	33.40	6.10	1601.43 (163.3)	160.14 (16.33)
2434	38.10 (1.500)		3 × 4	43.03	50.34	14.63	14.66	33.40	6.10	2401.65 (244.9)	240.17 (24.49)
2446	38.10 (1.500)		4 × 6	61.47	68.78	14.63	14.66	33.40	610	3202.85 (326.6)	320.29 (32.66)
2823	44.45 (1.750)		2 × 3	35.94	43.89	15.90	15.92	37.08	7.14	2134.91 (217.7)	213.49 (21.77)
2834	44.45 (1.750)		3 × 4	50.32	58.27	15.90	15.92	37.08	7.14	3202.85 (326.6)	320.29 (32.66)
2846	44.45 (1.750)		4 × 6	71.88	79.83	15.90	15.92	37.08	7.14	4270.80 (435.5)	427.08 (43.55)
3223	50.80 (2.000)		2 × 3	40.51	49.43	17.81	17.84	42.29	8.05	2757.63 (281.2)	275.76 (28.12)
3234	50.80 (2.000)		3 × 4	56.72	65.63	17.81	17.84	42.29	8.05	4136.45 (421.8)	413.65 (42.18)
3246	50.80 (2.000)		4 × 6	81.03	89.94	17.81	17.84	42.29	8.05	5516.24 (562.5)	551.62 (56.25)

IS: 1072–1967

Table 14.44 *Dimensions for Leaf Chain Sheaves*

All dimensions in mm

Chain Number (1)	Distance Between Flanges L Minimum (2)	Sheave Diameter SD Minimum (3)	Flange Diameter FD Minimum (4)
0822	9.12	63.50	88.90
0823	10.80	63.50	88.90
0834	14.20	63.50	88.90
0846	19.28	63.50	88.90
1022	10.29	79.38	104.78
1023	12.22	79.38	104.78
1034	16.03	79.38	104.78
1046	21.74	79.38	104.78
1222	16.69	95.25	120.65
1223	19.96	95.25	120.65
1234	26.54	95.25	120.65
1246	36.37	95.25	120.65
1623	26.75	127.00	152.40
1634	35.71	127.00	152.40
1646	49.15	127.00	152.40
2023	29.77	158.75	184.15
2034	39.52	158.75	184.15
2046	54.18	158.75	184.15
2423	39.95	190.50	215.90
2334	52.86	190.50	215.90
2446	72.21	190.50	215.90
2823	46.08	222.25	247.65
2834	61.19	222.25	247.65
2846	83.82	222.25	247.64
3223	51.89	254.00	279.40
3234	68.92	254.00	279.40
3246	94.44	254.00	279.40

IS: 1072–196

15

Journal Bearings

Symbols	Description and Units
c	radial clearance, mm
C	bearing characteristic number
d	journal diameter, mm
e	eccentricity, mm
f	coefficient of friction
h	oil film thickness, mm
h_o	minimum film thickness, mm
H_D	heat dissipated, J/s (kgf m/s)
H_g	heat generated, J/s (kgf m/s)
l	length of bearing, mm
n	speed of the journal, rev/s
N	speed of the journal, rev/min
p	bearing pressure on projected area, MN/m^2 (kgf/mm^2)
S	Sommerfeld number without side leakage, s/min
S_o	sommerfeld number with side leakage, s/min
t_A	ambient temperature, °C
t_o	temperature of the oil film in the bearing, °C
t_R	temperature rise of the bearing wall, °C
v	velocity, m/s
W	load, N (Kgf)
Z	absolute or dynamic viscosity of oil, Ns/m^2 or pascal-seconds, P_{as} ($kgf\ s/m^2$)
Z_k	kinematic viscosity of oil, m^2/s
ϵ	eccentricity ratio
ρ	specific gravity
ρ_{15}	specific gravity of the oil at 15°C

Particular	Equation	Eqn. No.
Viscosity: Newton's law of viscous flow states that the shearing stress in the fluid is proportional to the rate of change of velocity (Fig. 15.1)	$$\tau = \frac{F}{A} = Z\frac{dv}{dy}$$	15.1(a)
If the rate of shear is constant then the shearing stress, MN/m^2 (kgf/mm²)	$$\tau = \left(Z\frac{v}{h}\right) \times 10^{-3}$$	15.1(b)

where $\dfrac{dv}{dy}$ = rate of change of velocity with distance and may be called the rate of shear or the velocity gradient

Z is the absolute or dynamic viscosity of oil, Ns/m^2 (P_{a-s})

v = velocity, m/s; h = thickness of lubricant, mm

The kinematic viscosity based upon seconds saybolt (S') or Saybolt Universal Viscosity (SUV) in seconds		

$$\text{(i) in centistoke (cm}^2/\text{s)} \quad Z'_k = \left\{0.22S' - \frac{180}{S'}\right\} \qquad \text{15.1(c)}$$

$$\text{(ii) in m}^2/\text{s} \qquad Z_k = \left\{0.22S' - \frac{180}{S'}\right\} \times 10^{-6} \qquad \text{15.1(d)}$$

where S' is the number of seconds saybolt, sec

The absolute or dynamic viscosity of oil in SI units (Ns/m^2) or pascal-seconds (P_{a-s}),	$$Z = \rho Z_k = \rho\left\{0.22S' - \frac{180}{S'}\right\} \times 10^{-6}$$	15.1(e)
Specific gravity of oil at any temperature, $t°C$	$\rho_t = \rho_{15} - 0.00063(t° - 15)$ or	15.1(f)
	$\quad = \rho_{15} - 0.000657(t°)$	

where ρ_{15} is the specific gravity of oil at 15°C (Table 15.1)

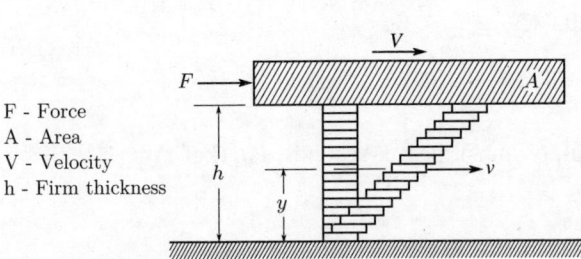

F - Force
A - Area
V - Velocity
h - Firm thickness

Fig. 15.1: *Load on moving plate (Newton's viscous effect)*

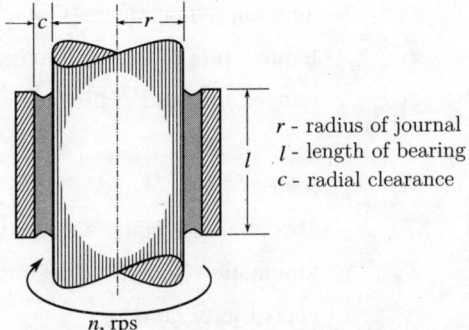

r - radius of journal
l - length of bearing
c - radial clearance

Fig. 15.2(a): *Loaded journal in bearing*

Particular	Equation	Eqn. No.
The kinematic viscosity in centistokes from Redwood units		
(a) For Redwood No. 1	$Z'_k = 0.260R - \dfrac{179}{R}$ when $34 < R < 100$	15.2(a)
	$Z'_k = 0.247R - \dfrac{50}{R}$ when $R > 100$	15.2(b)
(b) For Redwood Admiralty	$Z'_k = 2.7R - \dfrac{2000}{R}$	15.2(c)
	where R is the number of seconds Redwood	

The kinematic viscosity in centistokes from Engler number

$$Z'_k = 0.147E - \frac{347}{E} \quad \text{where } E \text{ is the Engler number} \qquad \text{15.2(d)}$$

In the case of a vertical shaft rotating in a guide bearing (Fig. 15.2) (considering the clearance uniform)

(a) The shearing stress in the lubricant (Fig. 15.2), MN/m^2(Kgf/mm^2)

$$\tau = Z\frac{v}{c} = (2\pi rZn \times 10^{-6})/c \qquad \text{15.3(a)}$$

(b) The viscous of shearing force on the shaft, N(kgf)

$$F_s = \tau \times \text{Area} = \tau \times 2\pi rl = (4\pi^2 r^2 lZn \times 10^{-6})/c \qquad \text{15.3(b)}$$

(c) The shearing torque, N mm (Kgf mm)

$$T = F_s \times r = (4\pi^2 r^3 lZn \times 10^{-6})/c \qquad \text{15.3(c)}$$

The frictional torque, N mm (Kgf mm)	$T_f = fWr = (f)(2rlp)(r) = 2r^2 flp$	15.3(d)

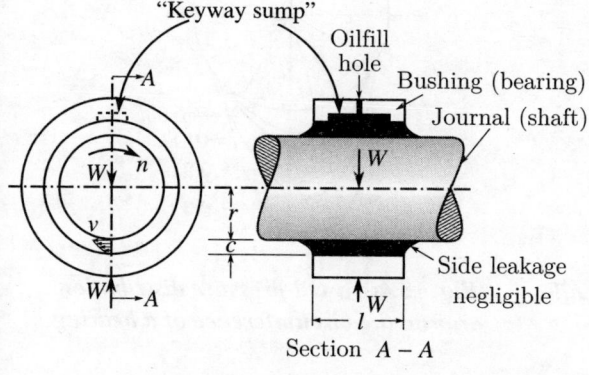

r is the radius of the journal, mm

l is the length of the bearing, mm

c is the radial clearance, mm

W is the force or load on bearing, N(kgf)

f is the coefficient of friction, mm

$p = \dfrac{W}{2rl}$, average pressure, MN/m^2 (kgf/mm^2)

Fig. 15.2(b): *Loaded journal in bearing*

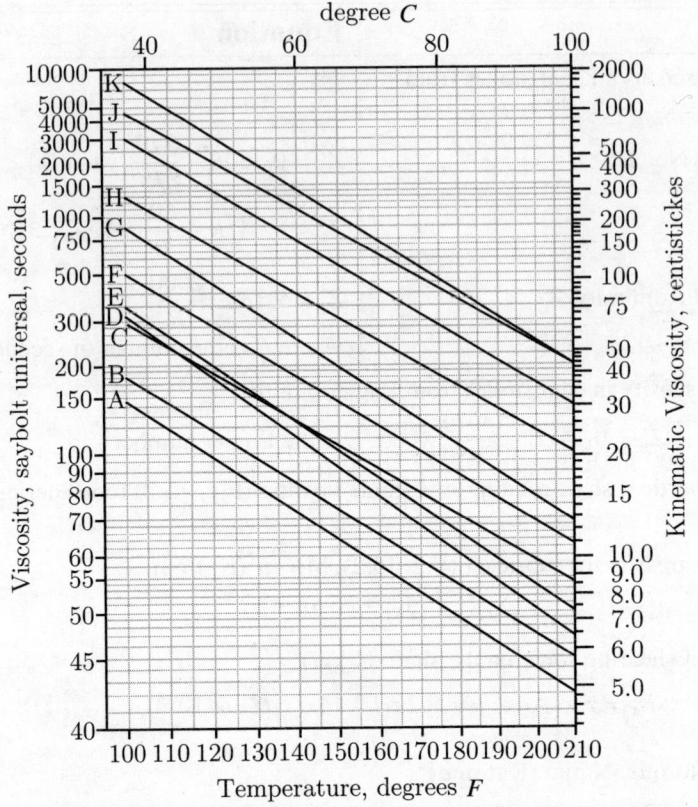

Fig. 15.3: *Viscosity-temperature chart (Table 15.1)*

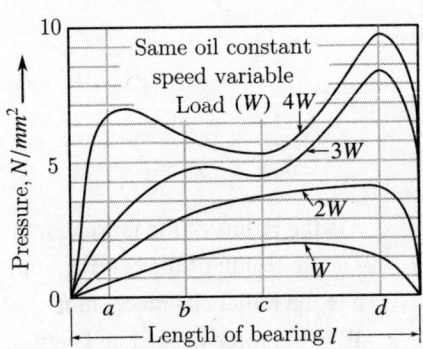

Fig. 15.4(a): *Longitudinal distribution of oil pressure*

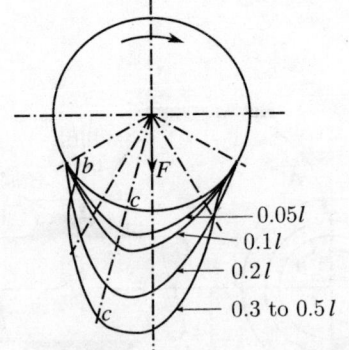

Fig. 15.4(b): *Oil-pressure distribution around the circumference of a bearing*

1 poise (P) = 10^{-1} Ns/m^2 (1.02×10^{-2} kgf s/m^2)   1 stoke (St) = 10^{-4} m^2/s

1 centipoise (cP) = 10^{-3} Ns/m^2 (1.02×10^{-4} kgf s/m^2)   1 centistoke (cSt) = 10^{-6} m^2/s

Particular	Equation	Eqn. No.
Petroff's relation to determine the coefficient of friction for lightly loaded bearing	$f = (2\pi^2 \times 10^{-6})\left(\dfrac{Zn}{p}\right)\left(\dfrac{r}{c}\right)$	15.4(a)

where the minimum value of Zn/p is called bearing modulus or bearing characteristic (Fig. 15.5(a))

| The empirical equation developed by Mc Kcc, S.A., and Mc Kcc, T.R., that is used for estimating values of coefficient of friction for well lubricated bearings | $f = K_a\left(\dfrac{Zn}{p}\right)\left(\dfrac{r}{c}\right) \times 10^{-10} + (\Delta f)$ | 15.4(b) |

where $K_a = 541.33\,\beta$, where β is the circumferential length of the bearing in deg

$= 0.195 \times 10^6$ for a full bearing i.e., $\beta = 360°$

$(\Delta f) = 0.002$ for bearing having $l/d = 0.75$ to 2.8 (Fig. 15.5(b))

| When the bearings are partially lubricated, the coefficient of friction according to Louis Illmer | $f = \dfrac{C_1 C_2}{269.44}\sqrt[4]{p_a/v}$ SI Units | 15.4(c) |
| | $= \dfrac{C_1 C_2}{152.26}\sqrt[4]{p_a/v}$ Metric units | 15.4(d) |

average p_a is the pressure on projected area, but must never be assumed to be less than

one-half of the maximum pressure imposed during a complete

revolution, MN/m^2 (kgf/mm^2)

v = rubbing velocity of the journal, m/s

C_1 = constant (Table 15.4); C_2 = constant (Table 15.5)

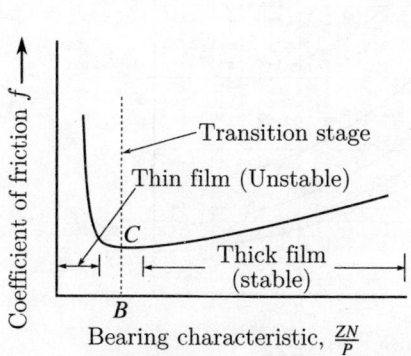

Fig. 15.5(a): *Variation of the coefficient of friction with Bearing*

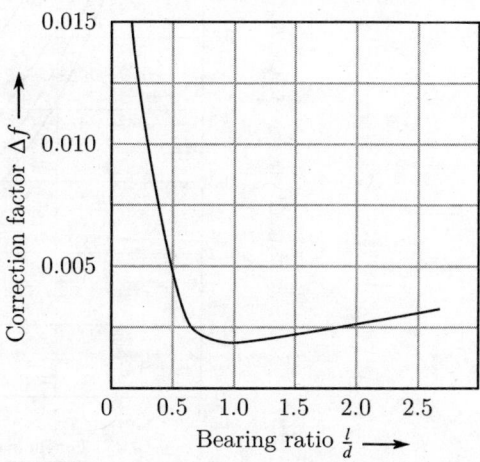

Fig. 15.5(b): *Correction factor for Eq. 15.4(b)*

Particular	Equation	Eqn. No.
Bearing Pressure:		
General electric company's formula for bearing pressure in the design of motor and generator bearing	$p = 0.622 \sqrt[3]{v}$ SI Units $= 0.0634 \sqrt{v}$ Metric units	15.5(a)
The safe operating bearing pressure due to Tatarinoff, MN/m² (kgf/mm²)	$p = \dfrac{13.30}{10^6} Zn \left(\dfrac{d}{c}\right)^2 \left(\dfrac{l}{d+l}\right)$	15.5(b)
Moore equation for unit pressure	$p = 0.726 \sqrt{v}$ SI units $= 0.074 \sqrt{v}$ Metric units	15.5(c)
The Sommerfeld number (s/min)		
(a) without side leakage	$S = \left(\dfrac{r}{c}\right)^2 \left(\dfrac{ZN}{p}\right) \times 10^{-6}$	15.6(a)
(b) with side leakage	$S_o = \left(\dfrac{r}{c}\right)^2 \left(\dfrac{ZN}{p}\right) K_w \times 10^{-6}$	15.6(b)

where K_w is the load correction factor for side leakage (Fig. 15.6)

N is the speed, rev/min; p = bearing pressure, MN/m² (kgf/mm²)

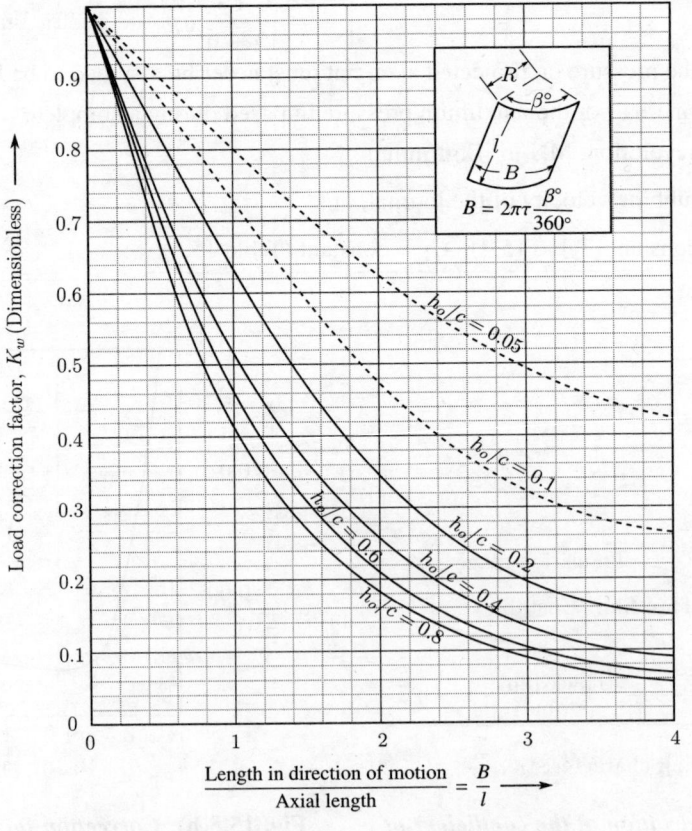

Fig. 15.6: *Load correction factor for side flow*

Particular	Equation	Eqn. No.
Unit load or average pressure	$p = \dfrac{W}{2rl}$	15.6(c)
Friction variable (Fig. 15.7)*	$(FV) = \dfrac{r}{c}f$	15.6(d)
Coefficient of friction (a) without side leakage	$f = (FV)\dfrac{c}{r}$	15.6(e)
(b) with side leakage	$f = (FV)\dfrac{cK_F}{rK_w}$	15.6(f)
where K_F is the friction correction factor (Fig. 15.8)		
The friction torque, N mm (kgf mm)	$T = fWr$	15.6(g)
Power loss, kW	$P = \left(\dfrac{2\pi}{10^6}\right)Tn$ SI Units	15.6(h)
Power loss, (mhp)	$P = \left(\dfrac{2\pi}{75 \times 10^3}\right)Tn$ Metric Units	15.6(i)

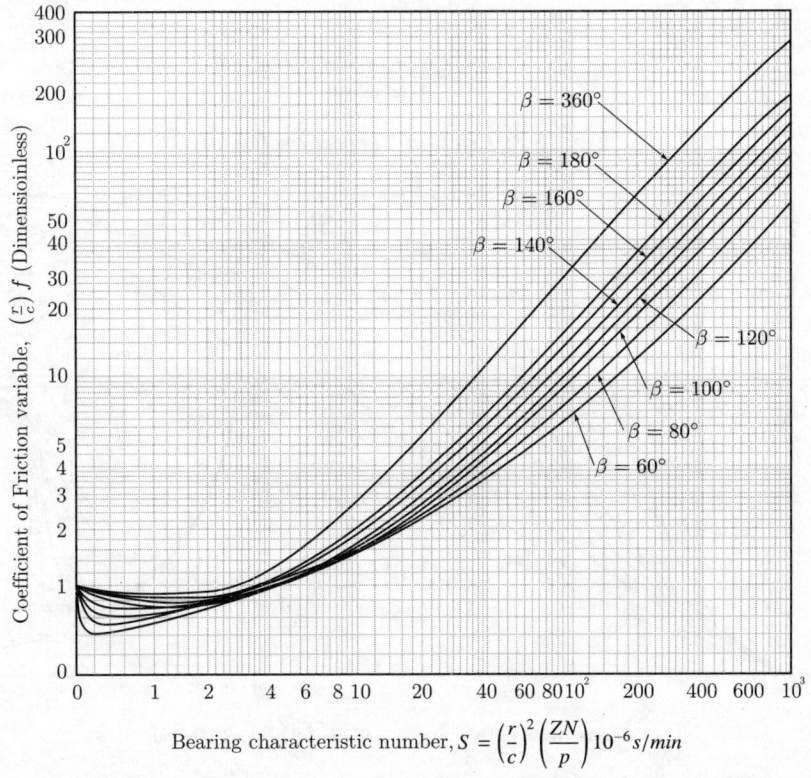

Fig. 15.7: *Chart for determining the coefficient of friction, based on no side flow*

*with side leakage use S_o

Particular	Equation	Eqn. No.
Power loss or heat generated, J/s (kgf m/s)	$H_g = fWv$ where $v = \dfrac{\pi dn}{1000}$, rubbing velocity, m/s	15.6(j)
(a) The minimum film thickness variable (Fig. 15.9)[†]	$(MFT) = h_o/c$	15.7(a)
(b) The smallest oil film thickness (h_o) when the journal is rotating	$h_o = c - e = c\left(1 - \dfrac{e}{c}\right)$	15.7(b)

where e is the eccentricity (distance between the center of the journal and the
centre of the bearing), mm
c is the radial clearance, mm

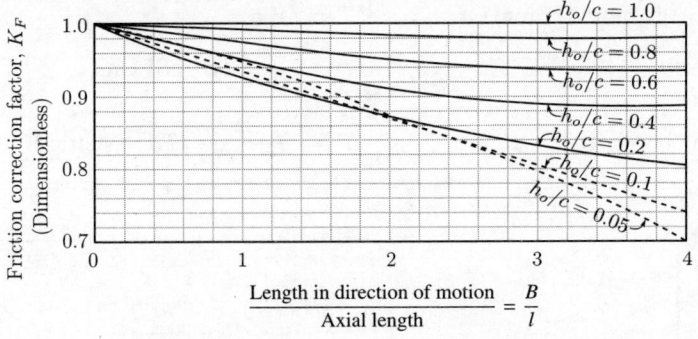

Fig. 15.8: *Friction Correction Factor*

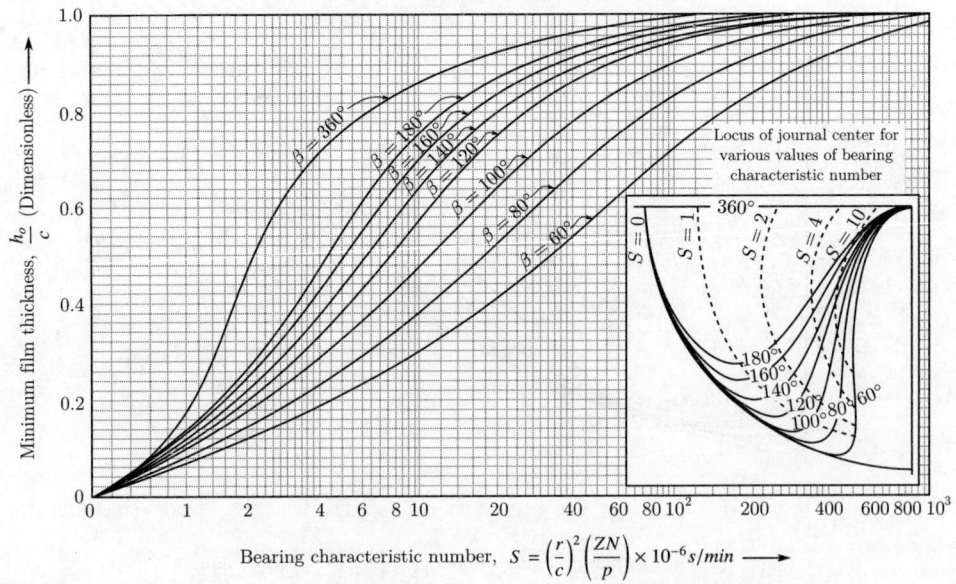

Fig. 15.9: *Minimum film thickness variable (with no side flow)*

[†]with side leakage use S_o

Particular	Equation	Eqn. No.
The eccentricity ratio[‡]	$\epsilon = \dfrac{e^{‡}}{c} = \cos\phi = 1 - \dfrac{h_o}{c}$	15.7(b)
The relation between the eccentricity ratio and a constant K for different values of β (refer Fig. 15.10 and Fig. 15.12) where the constant K is given by (for C_L refer Fig.15.11)	$K = 5884\dfrac{Zn}{p}\left(\dfrac{r}{c}\right)^2$	15.7(c)
In general the safe thickness for a bearing in good condition ($v_m \geqq 1m/s$)	$h_{\min} = 0.018 v_m^{0.4}\left(\dfrac{A}{10^6}\right)^{0.2}$	15.7(d)

where v_m is the peripheral or rubbing velocity of the journal, m/s

$A = ld$, projected area of the bearing, mm^2

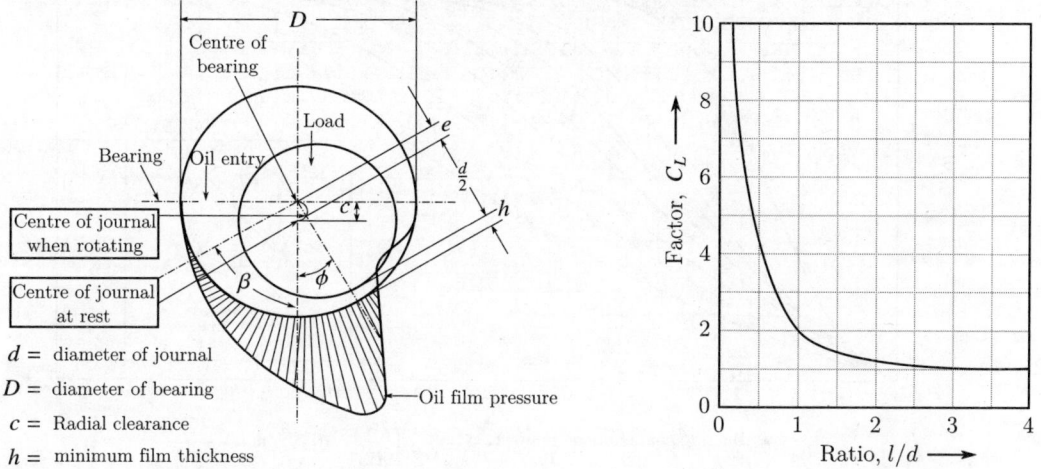

Fig. 15.10: *Operating conditions of a loaded journal*   Fig. 15.11: *Factor C_L*

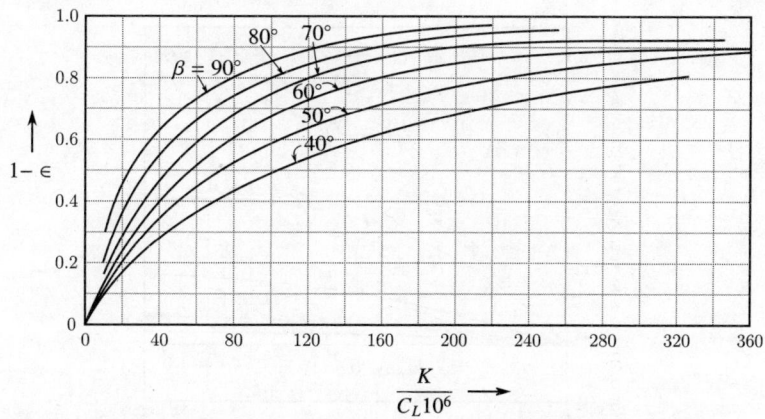

Fig. 15.12: *Variation of journal eccentricity coefficient with K/C_L*

[‡]The magnitude of e is a function of the pressure (p) on the projected bearing area, the relative clearance (c/r), the oil viscosity (Z), the speed of the journal (n) and the angle β.

Particular	Equation	Eqn. No.
Flow:		
The flow variable (Fig. 15.13)	$(FVL) = \dfrac{Q}{rcNl}$	15.8(a)
(a) flow without side leakage, mm³/min	$Q = (FLV)rcNl$	15.8(b)
(b) flow with side leakage, mm³/min	$Q = (FLV)rcNlK_Q$	15.8(c)

where N is the spped, rpm; K_Q is the flow correction factor (Fig. 15.14)

Note: If a central groove is used, then l is one-half the length of the bearing; in this case, the total flow should be found for two half bearings

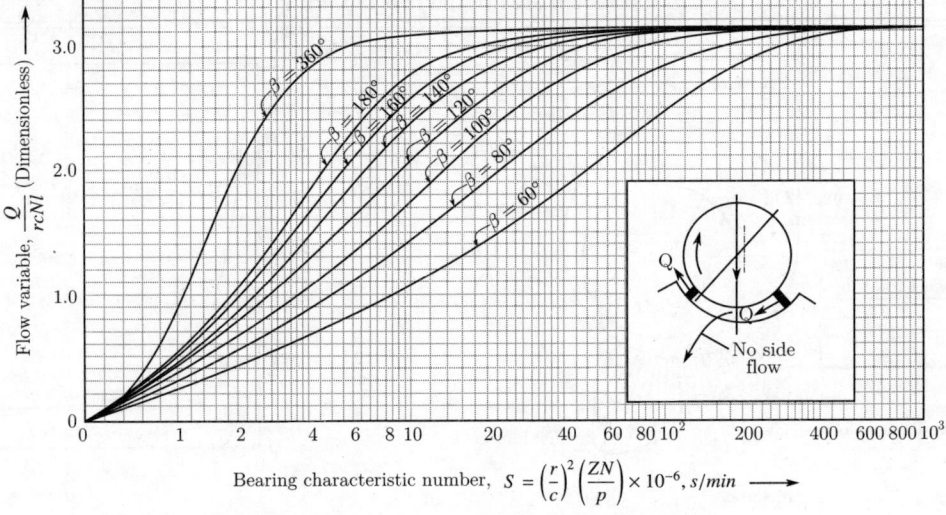

Bearing characteristic number, $S = \left(\dfrac{r}{c}\right)^2\left(\dfrac{ZN}{p}\right) \times 10^{-6}, s/min$ ⟶

Fig. 15.13: *Oil flow variable (without side flow)*

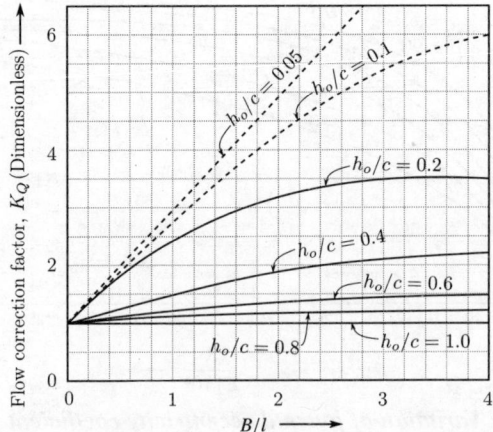

B/l ⟶

Fig. 15.14: *Flow correction factor with side flow*

Particular	Equation	Eqn. No.
Temperature rise, °C	$(\Delta T) = \dfrac{402 \times 10^3 H_g}{Q}$ (SI units)	15.9(a)
	$(\Delta T) = \dfrac{3.95 \times 10^6 H_g}{Q}$ Metric units	15.9(b)

where H_g is the heat generated (Egn. 15.6(j)); Q is the flow of oil, mm^3/min

The average temperature of the oil at which the viscosity is to be determined	$T_{av} = T_1 + \dfrac{(\Delta T)}{2}$ where T_1 is the inlet temp of the oil, °C	15.9(c)

Pressure-fed Bearings: (Full annular groove)

Oil Flow:

The average velocity, m/s	$v_{av} = \left(\dfrac{0.1 \times 10^6}{6}\right)\left(\dfrac{p_s c^2}{Zl}\right)$	15.10(a)

where p_s is the supply pressure, MN/m^2 (kgf/mm^2)

The quantity of oil flow from the end of supply pressure of the bearing, mm^3/s	$Q' = 1000 A v_{av} = 1000(2\pi rc)v_{av}$	15.10(b)
	$Q' = \left(\dfrac{3}{0.1 \times 10^9}\right)\dfrac{\pi p_s c^3 r}{Zl}$	15.10(c)

where A is the area of the clearance space, mm^2

The quantity of oil flow from both ends of the bearing after applying the eccentricity correction factor, mm^3/s	$Q' = k_2 \left(\dfrac{3}{0.1 \times 10^9}\right)\dfrac{\pi p_s c^3 r}{Zl}$	15.10(d)

where $k_2 = \left(1 + \left(\dfrac{3}{2}\right)\dfrac{e}{c}\right)$, eccentricity correction factor (due to Dennison)

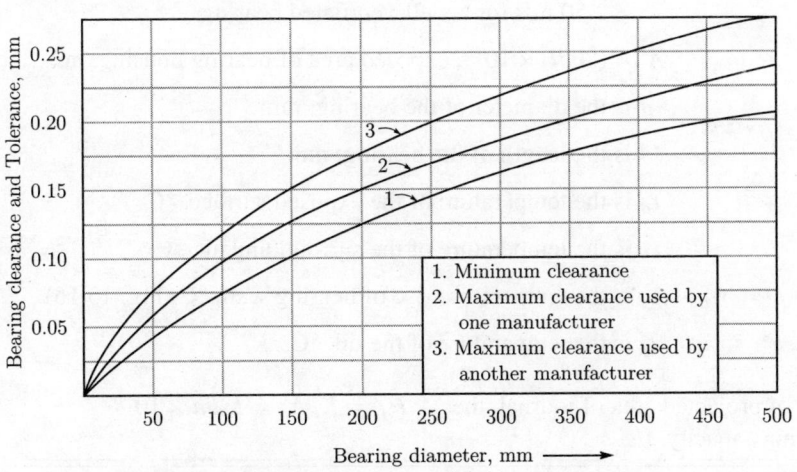

1. Minimum clearance
2. Maximum clearance used by one manufacturer
3. Maximum clearance used by another manufacturer

Fig. 15.15: *Clearances used in babbitted bearings*

Particular	Equation	Eqn. No.
In the case of pressure-fed bearings to determine the coefficient of friction from Petroff's law by applying an eccentricity correction factor	$f = k_1(2\pi^2 \times 10^{-6})\left(\dfrac{Z_n}{p}\right)\dfrac{r}{c}$ where $k_1 = 1/\left(\sqrt{1 - \left(\dfrac{e}{c}\right)^2}\right)$, eccentricity correction factor (due to Dennison)	15.10(e)
Temperature rise, °C	$(\Delta T) = \dfrac{80\pi^2}{10^{18}}\left(\dfrac{k_1}{k_2}\right)\left(\dfrac{nrl}{c^2}\right)^2 \dfrac{Z^2}{p_s}$	15.10(f)

Heat Dissipation of Bearings:

Heat generated in the bearing J/s (kgf m/s)	$H_g = fWv$	15.11(a)

where f is the coefficient of friction; W is the bearing load, N; $v = \pi dn/1000$ rubbing velocity, m/s

General expression for the heat dissipating capacity of a bearing, J/s (kgf m/s)	$H_D = K_h A'(t_B - t_A)$	15.11(b)

where $K_h = Mv^{0.89}$, the film coefficient, J/sm^2 °C

$= 11.4$ J/sm^2 °C for still air

$= 15.3$ J/sm^2 °C for average design conditions

$= 33.5$ J/sm^2 °C for air moving at 2.5 m/s

$M = 14.82$, a constant for the selected units of K_h

$v =$ the air velocity, m/s

≈ 0.75 m/s for normal conditions without ventilation

≈ 2.50 m/s for a well-ventilated bearing

$A' = (20dl) \times 10^{-6}$, exposed area of bearing housing, m^2

d is the diameter of the bearing, mm

l is the length of the bearing, mm

t_B is the temperature of the exposed surface, °C

t_A is the temperature of the surrounding air, °C

$(t_B - t_A)$ is the temperature rise of bearing wall, °C (Fig. 15.16)

t_0 is the temperature of the oil, °C

On the basis of projected area of journal, the heat dissipating capacity, J/s	$H_D = K_P A_p = K_P l d \times 10^{-6}$	15.11(c)

Particular	Equation	Eqn.	No.

where $K_P = \dfrac{(t_B - t_A + 18)^2}{k_p}$, coefficient depends on temperature rise, J/sm² (Fig. 15.17)

$k_p = 0.273$ sm² °C/J, for bearing of heavy construction well ventilated

$\quad = 0.484$, (sm² °C/J), for bearing of light or medium construction in still air

$(t_B - t_A) = \dfrac{1}{2}(t_0 - t_A)$, t_o is the operating temperature, °C

$A_p = (ld) \times 10^{-6}$, projected area of journal, m²

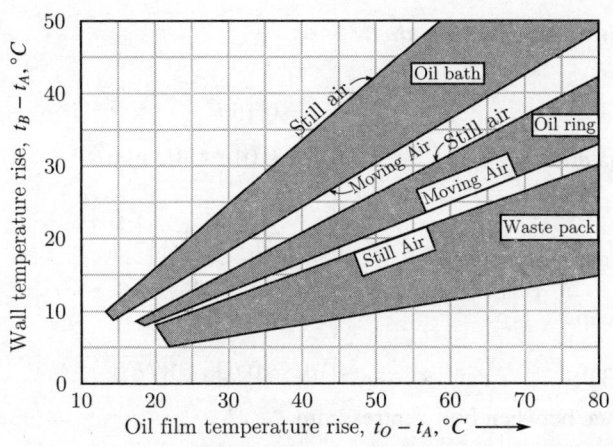

Fig. 15.16: *Relation between oil-film temperature and bearing-wall temperature*

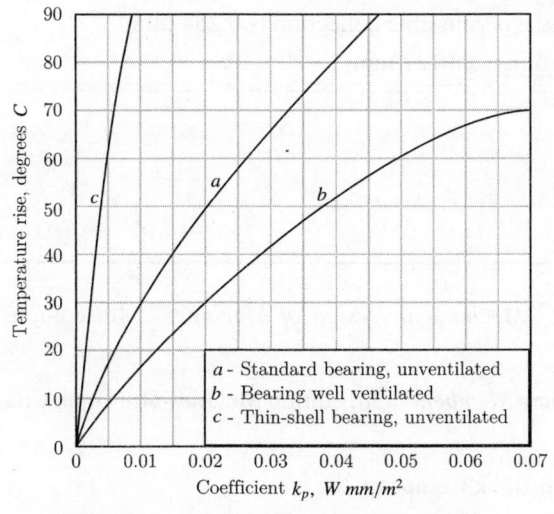

Fig. 15.17: *Heat dissipation by bearings*

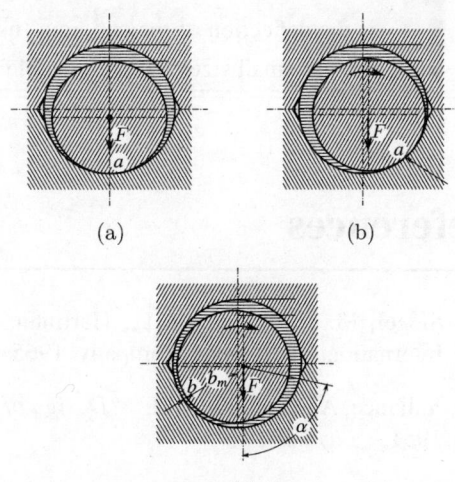

Fig. 15.18: *Oil film at various phases of rotation of a journal*

Particular	Equation	Eqn. No.
Bearing Shells:		
The thickness of small brass and bronze shells	$t = 0.08d + 2.5$ mm	15.12
The thickness of medium size bearings (about 75 mm):		
(a) made up of cast iron	$t = 0.2d$	15.13(a)
(b) made of babbitt material	$t = 0.02d + 3.2 mm$	15.13(b)
The thickness of engine main bearing shells (for 225 mm and up):		
(a) made of cast steel	$t = 0.15d$	15.14(a)
(b) made of babbitt material	$t = 0.01d + 3.2$ mm	15.14(b)
Bearing Caps:		
The bearing cap thickness, mm	$h_b = \left(\dfrac{3}{2} \times \dfrac{Wa}{l\sigma_b}\right)^{\frac{1}{2}}$	15.15
The deflection of the cap	$y = Wa^3/4EIh_b^3$	15.16
The thickness of the cap	$h_b = 0.63a\sqrt[3]{W/EIy}$	15.17

where a is the distance between bolt centres, mm;

σ_b = allowable bending stress, MN/m^2 (kgf/mm^2)

l is the length of bearings, mm; E is modulus of elasticity, MN/m^2 (kgf/mm^2)

y is the deflection of the cap, mm (usually the permissible deflection is 0.254 mm, in small sizes the permissible deflection is 0.0127 mm)

References

[1] Siegel, M. J., Maleev, V. L., Hartman, J. B., *"Mechanical Design of Machines"*, 4th edition, International Text Book Company, 1965

[2] Vallance, A., Doughtie, V. L., *"Design of Machine Members"*, 3rd edition McGraw Hill Book Co., 1951.

[3] Shigley, J. E., *"Machine Design"*, McGraw Hill Book Company, Inc.

[4] Bhattacharya, S. C., Basu Mallik, J. R., *"Machine Design"*, Basu Mallik & Co., Calcutta, 1966.

Table 15.1 *Specific Gravity of Oils at 15°C (Fig. 15.3)*

No.	Oil Characteristic	ρ_{15}
A	Turbine oil, ring-oiled bearing	0.8877
B	Turbine oil, ring-oiled bearing, SAE 10	0.8894
C	All-year automobile oil, SAE 20	0.9036
D	Ring-oiled bearing oil, high-speed machinery	0.9346
E	Automobile oil, SAE 20	0.9254
F	Automobile oil, SAE 30	0.9263
G	Automobile oil, SAE 40, medium-speed machinery	0.9275
H	Airplane oil 100, SAE 60	0.8927
I	Transmission oil, SAE 110, spur and bevel gears	0.9328
J	Gear oil, show-speed worm gears	0.9153
K	Transmission oil, SAE 160, slow-speed gears	0.9365

Table 15.2 *Recommended speed of some Machinery, rev./min*

Location of bearing	speed, rev/min	Location of bearings	speed, rev/min
Automobile crank shaft	900 to 14000	Stationary high speed main	360
Aeronautic engine crank shaft	1800 to 2000	-do- crank pin	360
Stationary gas-engine main	250 to 800	-do- cross head	360
-do- crank pin	250 to 800	Locomotive drive wheel	250
-do- cross head	250 to 800	-do- crank pin	250
Diesel engine main	60 to 160	-do- cross head	250
-do- crank pin	60 to 160	Marine steam turbine	2000
Marine steam engine main	180	Stationary steam turbine	2000
-do- main crank pin	180	De Laval 5 kW steam turbine	30000
Stationary slow speed main	40 to 80	Railway car axle	300
-do- -do- crank pin	40 to 80	Generator and motor	150 to 500
-do- -do- cross head	40 to 80	Rolling mill main	60
Cotton mill spindle	8000 to 12000	Gyroscope	800 to 1500

Table 15.3 *Journal Bearing Materials and Applications*

Material	Material	Material
1. Babbitt or white metal alloys (tin base)	Very expensive	Used for general purpose resistance to corrosive effects of acids. I.C. engine bearings.
2. Lead-base white metals	Low cost, lower strength and susceptibility to corrosion, high coefficient of friction	General machinery purpose. Used at moderately high temperatures. Lead ranging from 0.981 MN/m^2 (0.10 kgf/mm^2) to 2.158 MN/m^2 (0.22 kgf/mm^2) at 1 m/s
3. Plastic bronze	Alloy of copper and lead, resistance to seizure, conformability and embed-ability. Less corrodible metals. Low coefficient of friction	Used in automobiles, locomotive and rolling mills where there are heavy loads, Max. load carrying capacity is approx. 10.297 MN/m^2 (1.05 kgf/mm^2) at 15 m/s
4. Phosphor bronze	Good mechanical and anti friction properties	All machines. The permissible load is 68.65 MN/m^2 (7.0 kgf/mm^2). Max. rubbing speed 5 m/s
5. Gun metal	Chill casting gives a finer structure and is preferable to sand casting	Light loads
6. Brass	Low cost than Babbitt material	At high pressures
7. Aluminium	Good corrosion fatigue resistance and thermal conductivity low embadability, high thermal expansion	Suitable for heavy loads upto about 24 MN/m^2 (2.45 kgf/mm^2) peak load and 13.73 MN/m^2 (1.40 kgf/mm^2) continuous load at moderate speeds of 4 to 6 m/s
8. Cast Iron	Low friction, must have good lubrication	Cam shaft, light transmission. Max. speed 0.65 m/s. Max. load 3.43 MN/m^2 (0.35 kgf/mm^2)
9. Cadmium base bearing metals	Allow much higher operating temperatures than are safe with babbitt	Used for severe service in internal combustion engines
10. Porous bearings	Oil impregnated bearings	Medium duty applications in small size bearings. Where supply of lubricant is difficult, inadequate or infrequent. Rubbing speed from 0.4 to 7.5 m/s with light load
11. Wood bearing (Lignum vitae, rock maple or oak)	Low cost, self lubricating	Conveyors
12. Rubber	Low coefficient of rubbing friction	Hydraulic turbines, centrifugal and deep well pumps and washers

Table 15.4 *Values of the Circumstance Constant C_1 in Eqn. 15.4(c) & (d)*

Lubrication	Workmanship	Attendance	Location	Constant C_1
Oil bath or flooded	High-grade	First class	Clean and protected	1
Oil, free drop (constant feed)	Good	Fairly good	Favourable (ordinary conditions)	2
Oil cup or grease (intermittent feed)	Fair	Poor	Exposed to dirt, grit or other unfavourable conditions	4

Table 15.5 *Values of the Constant C_2 in Eqn. 15.4(c) & (d)*

Type of Bearing	Constant C_2
1. Rotating journals, such as rigid bearings and crank pins ..	1
2. Oscillating journals, such as rigid wrist pins and pintle block ..	1
3. Rotating bearings lacking ample rigidity, such as eccentrics and the like ..	2
4. Rotating flat surfaces lubricated from the centre to the circumference, such as annular step or pivot bearings ..	2
5. Sliding flat surfaces wiping over the guide ends, such as reciprocating corsshead shoes. Use 2 for relatively long guides and 3 for short guides ..	2-3
6. Sliding or wiping surfaces lubricated from the periphery or outer wiping edge. Marine thrust bearings, and worm gears ..	3-4
7. Long power-screw nuts and similar wipping parts over which it is difficult to effect a uniform distribution of lubricant or load ..	4.6

Table 15.6 *Values of C for Various Combinations of Journal and Bearings*

Shaft	Bearing	Bearing modulus	
		(Zn/p)	ZN/p
Hardened and ground steel	Babbitt	48.36×10^{-3}	2.902
Machined, soft steel	Babbitt	60.51×10^{-3}	3.631
Hardened and ground steel	Plastic bronze	72.58×10^{-3}	4.355
Machined, soft steel	Plastic bronze	84.65×10^{-3}	5.079
Hardened and ground steel	Rigid bronze	96.71×10^{-3}	5.803
Machined, soft steel	Rigid bronze	120.85×10^{-3}	7.251

Table 15.7 *Design Data for Bearings*

Machinery (1)	Bearing (2)	Maximum p** MN/m² (3)	Suitable Z** Ns/m² (4)	Minimum (ZN/p)* (5)	$\dfrac{c}{r}$ (6)	$\dfrac{l}{d}$ (7)
1. Automobile and aircraft engines	Main Crank pin Wrist pin	5.5-12.0 10.0-24.0 16.0-34.5	0.007-0.008	2.18 1.45 1.16	— — —	0.8-1.8 0.7-1.4 1.5-2.2
2. Gas and oil engines, four stroke	Main Crank pin wrist pin	4.8-8.2 9.6-12.4 12.4-15.2	0.020-0.065	2.90 1.45 0.73	0.001 < 0.001 < 0.001	0.6-2.0 0.6-1.5 1.5-2.0
3. Gas and oil engines, two stroke	Main Crank pin Wrist pin	3.4-5.5 6.9-10.3 8.2-12.4	0.020-0.065	3.63 1.74 1.45	0.001 < 0.001 < 0.001	0.6-2.0 0.6-1.5 1.5-2.0
4. Marine Steam engines	Main Crank pin Wrist pin	3.4 4.1 10.3	0.030 0.040 0.030	2.90 2.18 1.45	< 0.001 < 0.001 < 0.001	0.7-1.5 0.7-1.2 1.2-1.7
5. Stationary slow-speed steam engines	Main Crank pin Wrist pin	2.8 10.3 12.4	0.060 0.080 0.060	2.90 0.87 0.73	< 0.001 < 0.001 < 0.001	1.0-2.0 0.9-1.3 1.2-1.5
7. Reciprocating pump and compressors	Main Crank pin Wrist pin	1.8 4.1 6.9	0.030-0.080	4.36 2.90 1.45	0.001 < 0.001 < 0.001	1.0-2.2 0.9-1.7 1.5-2.0
8. Steam locomotives	Driving axle Crank pin Wrist pin	3.7 13.7 27.5	0.100 0.040 0.030	4.36 0.73 0.73	0.001 < 0.001 < 0.001	1.6-1.8 0.7-1.1 0.8-1.3
9. Railway cars	Axle	3.0	0.100	7.25	0.001	1.8-2.0
10. Steam turbines	Main	0.7-1.9	0.002-0.016	14.50	0.001	1.0-2.0
11. Gyroscope	Rotor	5.9	0.030	7.98	0.0013	—
12. Transmission shafting	Light, fixed self-aligning Heavy	0.2 1.0 1.0	0.025-0.060	145.00 4.36 4.36	0.001 0.001 0.001	2.0-3.0 2.5-4.0 2.0-3.0
13. Cotton mill	Spindle	0.007	0.002	1450.00	0.005	—
14. Machine tools	Main	2.1	0.040	5.80	0.001	1.0-4.0
15. Punching and shearing Machines	Main Crank pin	27.5 55.0	0.100 0.100	— —	0.001 0.001	1.0-2.0 1.0-2.0
16. Rolling mills	Main	20.6	0.050	1.45	0.0015	1.1-1.5
17. Generators, motors, centrifugal pumps	Rotor	0.7-1.4	0.025	29.01	0.0013	1.0-2.0

*N = speed, rev/min

**The values of p and Z in metric units can be obtained by dividing the given values with 9.80665.

Table 15.8 *Bearing Clearances in Industrial Applications*

Type of Service, Material, and Finish of Journal and Bearing	Running Clearance c, in mm $\times 10^{-3}$ for Shaft Diameter d mm				
	d = 12	d = 25	d = 50	d = 90	d = 140
Precision spindle, hardened and ground steel, lapped-in bronze bearing, rubbing speed under 2.5 m/s, pressure $p < 3.5$ N/mm	3.5-9.5	9.5-19.0	19.0-31.5	31.5-44.0	44.0-62.5
Precision spindle, hardened and ground steel, lapped-in bronze bearing, rubbing speed over 2.5 m/s, pressure $p > 3.5$ N/m	6.5-12.5	12.5-25.0	25.0-37.5	37.5-56.5	56.5-81.5
Electric motors and generators, ground journals in broached or reamed bronze bearings or reamed babbit bearings	6.5-19.0	12.5-25.0	19.0-42.5	25.0-50.0	32.5-75.0
General machinery, continuous rotating or oscillating motion, turned or cold-rolled steel journals in bored and reamed bronze bearings or poured and reamed babbit bearings.	25.0-50.0	31.5-56.5	37.5-62.5	50.0-87.5	62.5-100.0
Rougn machinery, turned or cold-rolled steel journals in poured babbit bearings	37.5-75.0	62.5-100.0	100-150	150-200	200-250

Table 15.9 *(a) Allowable Bearing, Pressure, Reciprocating Motion*

Type of Bearing	Type of Machinery	Pressure p N/mm^2
Crosshead	Steam engine, stationary	2.5-4.2
	Steam engine, marine	4.0-7.0
	Steam engine, locomotive	5.0-6.0
	Gas and oil engines, stationary	3.0-5.0
	Compressors and pumps	4.5-6.0
Trunk piston	Gas and oil engines, stationary	1.5-2.0
	Automotive and aircraft engines	1.5-2.0

Table 15.9 *(b) Allowable Bearing Pressures for Semifluid Lubrication*

Journal Material	Bearing Material	Allowable Pressure p N/mm^2
Hardened tool steel	Lumen of phosphor bronze	17.5
Hardened alloy steel	Hardened steel	14.5
SAE 1050 steel	Hard babbitt	10.3
Hardened alloy steel	Bronze	9.3
Cast iron	Cast iron	7.5
Alloy steel	Bronze	6.0
SAE 1040 Steel	Babbit, soft	5.0
Mild steel, smooth finish	Bronze	4.0
Mild steel, ordinary finish	Bronze	3.0
Cast iron	Bronze	3.0
Mild steel	Cast iron	2.5
Mild steel	Lignum vitae, water-lubricated	2.5

Table 15.10 *Permissible Bearing Pressure on Journal Bearings*

Type of bearing		Permissible bearing pressure on projected area, MN/m^2 (kgf/mm^2)
Diesel engines:	Main bearing	5.49 –10.30 (0.56–1.05)
	Crank pin	6.87 –13.73 (0.70–1.40)
	Wrist pin	12.36 –13.73 (1.26–1.40)
Electric motor bearings:		0.69 – 1.37 (0.07–0.14)
Marine Diesel Engines:	Main bearings	3.43 – 4.12 (0.35–0.42)
	Crank pin	6.87 – 9.61 (0.70–0.98)
Steam turbines and reduction gears		0.69 – 1.47 (0.07–0.1)
Automotive engines:	Main bearings	3.43 – 4.12 (0.35–0.42)
	Crank pin	10.30 –13.73 (1.05–1.40)
Air compressors:	Main bearings	0.79 – 1.57 (0.08–0.16)
	Crank pin	1.57 – 2.55 (0.16–0.26)
Air craft-engine:	Crank pin	4.81 –13.73 (0.49–1.40)
Centrifugal pumps:		0.59 – 0.69 (0.06–0.07)
Steam engine:	Main bearings	0.98 – 3.53 (0.10–0.36)
	Cross head pin	6.87–12.26 (0.70–1.25)
	Crank pin	5.39 –10.30 (0.55–1.05)
Marine Steam engine:	Main bearings	1.96 – 3.43 (0.20–0.35)
	Crank pin	2.94 – 3.92 (0.30–0.40)
Miscellaneous bearings:		0.49 – 0.98 (0.05–0.10)

Table 15.11 *Values of the Sommerfeld Variable for Various h_o/c and L/d Ratios*

L^*/d \\ h_o/c	1	0.2	0.1	0.067	0.05	0.04	0.033	0.0286	0.025
0.1	0	43.5	8.76	4.32	2.50	1.79	1.37	1.10	0.962
0.2	0	18.9	4.39	2.20	1.32	0.970	0.775	0.649	0.581
0.3	0	11.6	2.96	1.52	0.952	0.714	0.585	0.503	0.452
0.4	0	8.27	2.22	1.18	0.770	0.595	0.495	0.438	0.396
0.5	0	6.21	1.81	1.00	0.680	0.537	0.452	0.406	0.369
0.6	0	5.12	1.60	0.909	0.640	0.510	0.436	0.390	0.357
0.8	0	3.98	1.40	0.833	0.599	0.483	0.416	0.377	0.346
1.0	0	3.41	1.29	0.787	0.568	0.467	0.403	0.366	0.338
1.2	0	3.12	1.21	0.752	0.549	0.450	0.394	0.357	0.330
1.5	0	2.86	1.12	0.715	0.526	0.435	0.380	0.347	0.321
2.0	0	2.53	1.06	0.681	0.505	0.420	0.370	0.339	0.314
∞	0	2.07	0.922	0.611	0.411	0.394	0.352	0.322	0.301

*L = effective bearing length. Fer a central annular groove

$$^*L = \frac{l - w}{2} = \frac{\text{bearing length} - \text{groove width}}{2}$$

Table 15.12 *Product of Pressure and Velocity*

Type of Bearing	Pressure × velocity	
	(MN/m^2) (m/s)	(kgf/mm^2) (m/s)
Axles, locomotive ..	4.20	(0.428)
Railway car ..	4.20	(0.428)
Crank pins, aircraft ..	87.60	(8.933)
Crank pins, Gas engine ..	14.00	(1.428)
Crank pins, Steam, H.S. ..	14.00	(1.428)
Crankshaft and Main bearings: Aircraft ..	70.10	(7.143)
-do- Diesel ..	35.00	(3.572)
Generators, motors ..	1.75	(0.178)
Line shafts ..	0.88	(0.089)
Reducing gears ..	3.50	(3.572)
Machine tools ..	0.35	(0.036)
Steam turbines ..	35.00	(3.572)
Mill shafting, with self-aligning cast iron bearing, grease or imperfect oil lubrication maximum value	0.43	(0.043)
Mill shafting, self-aligning, ring-oiled babbit bearings, maximum ..	0.85	(0.086)
Self-aligning ring-oiled bearings, continuous load in one direction ..	1.40	(0.143)
Crankshaft journals with bronze bearings ..	0.78	(0.080)
Crankshaft bearings with babbitted bearings, maximum ..	2.06	(0.210)
For excellent radiating conditions ..	4.67	(0.476)

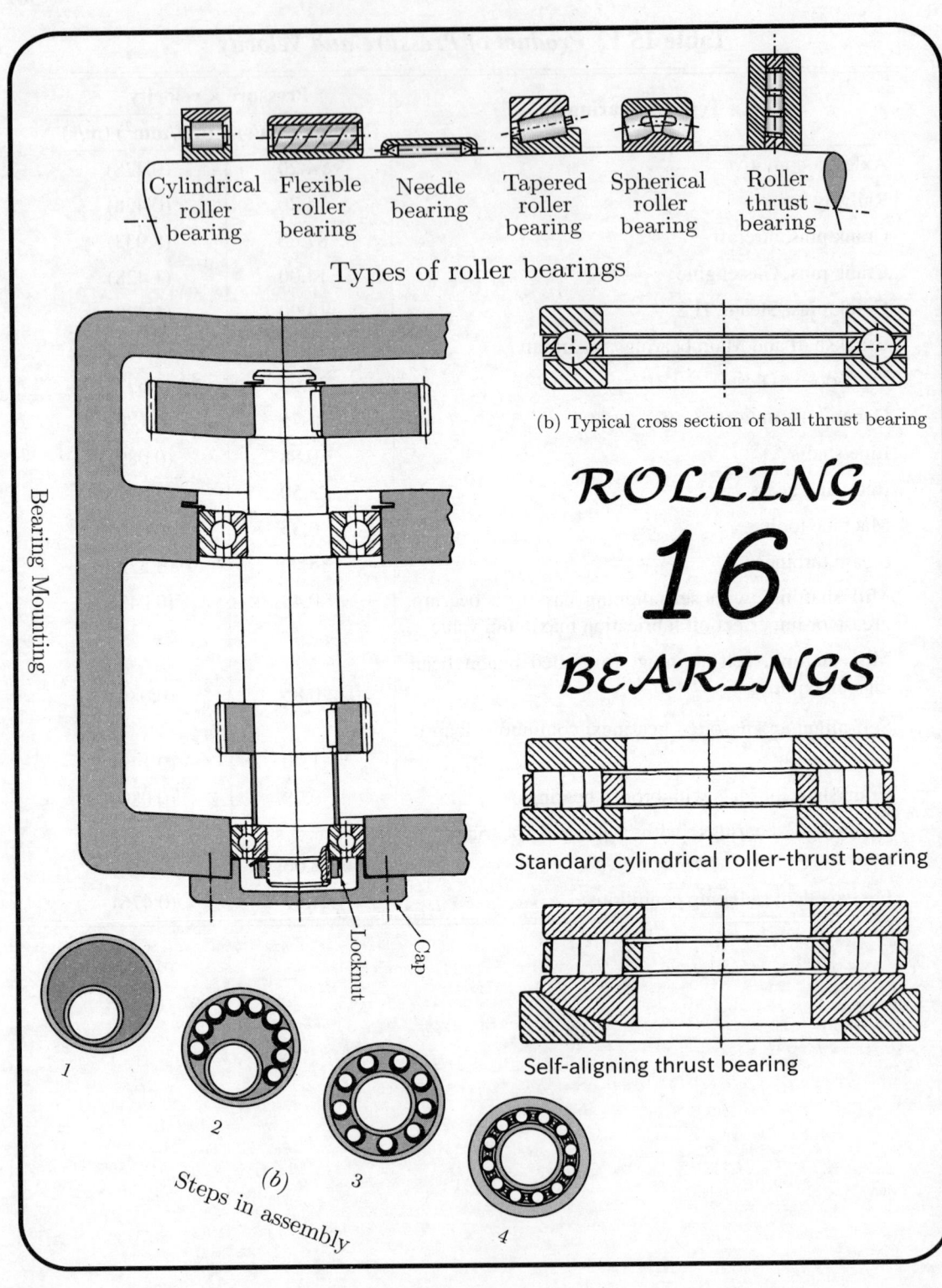

Types of roller bearings

Cylindrical roller bearing   Flexible roller bearing   Needle bearing   Tapered roller bearing   Spherical roller bearing   Roller thrust bearing

(b) Typical cross section of ball thrust bearing

ROLLING
16
BEARINGS

Standard cylindrical roller-thrust bearing

Self-aligning thrust bearing

Bearing Mounting

Locknut

Cap

1

2

3

4

(b)

Steps in assembly

16

Rolling Bearings

Symbols	Description and Units
C	specific capacity or the basic load rating of the bearing, N (kgf)
C_o	the basic static load rating, N (kgf)
D	ball diameter, mm
F	effective belt pull, N (kgf)
F_1, F_2	the constant loads during N_1, N_2.–revolution respectively, N (kgg)
F_a	thrust load, N (kgf)
F_c	radial load, N (kgf)
F_m	the constant mean load, N (kgf)
i	number of rows of balls in any one bearing
L_N	the life of the bearing in millions of revolutions
L_h	the life of the bearing in hours
z	number of balls per row

Particular	Equation	Eqn. No.
The tooth load in a gear	$F_{ef} = f_k f_d F$	16.1

where F is the thoretical tooth load, N(kgf)

  f_k = a factor for the additional forces created in the gearing itself

    = 1.05 to 1.10 for precision gears (errors in pitch and-form less than 0.025 mm)

    = 1.10 to 1.30 for commercial gears (errors in pitch and form 0.025 to 0.125 mm)

  f_d = a factor for additional force emanating from the mechanisms coupled to the gearing

    = 1.0 to 1.2 for shock free rotary machines e.g. electric machines and turbo-compressors

    = 1.2 to 1.5 for reciprocating engines, according to the degree of balance

    = 1.5 to 3.0 for machinery subjected to heavy shock loading, such as rolling mills

| The shaft load in a belt drive, N (kgf) | $F_s = F \times f$ | 16.2 |

where f = a factor, the value of which depends upon the kind of belt used and its initial tension

    = 2.0 to 2.5 for Vee-belts

    = 2.5 to 3.0 for single leather belts, with jockey pulleys

    = 4.0 to 5.0 for single leather belts, balata belts, rubber belts

  F = Effective belt pull, N (kgf)

Particular	**Equation**	**Eqn. No.**

Dynamic load ratings of rolling bearings:

(a) Radial ball bearings:

The relation between load and life

$$\frac{F_1}{F_2} = \sqrt[3]{L_2/L_1} \text{ or } F_1 \sqrt[3]{L_1} = F_2 \sqrt[3]{L_2}$$ 16.3

The rating life in millions of revolutions:

(a) for ball bearings

$$L_n = (C/P)^3$$ 16.4(a)

(b) for roller bearings

$$L_n = (C/P)^{\frac{10}{3}}$$ 16.4(b)

where (C/P) is the loading ratio (Table 16.1)

The basic load rating or specific capacity C in N(kgf) for radial and angular contact ball bearings, (except filling slot bearing)

$$C = f_c(i \cos \alpha)^{0.7} z^{2/3} D^{1.8} \text{ for } D < 25.4 \text{ mm}$$ 16.5(a)

$$C = f_c(i \cos \alpha)^{0.7} z^{2/3}(3.647)D^{1/4} \text{ for } D > 25.4\text{mm}$$ 16.5(b)

where f_c is the factor which depends on the geometry of the bearing components, the accuracy to which the various bearing parts are made and the material (Table 16.2)

The equivalent load P for a radial and angular contact ball bearing (except filling slot bearing) under combined constant radial (F_r) and constant thrust (F_a) loads

$$P = XVF_r + YF_a$$ 16.6

where X = radial factor (Table 16.3); V = rotation factor (Table 16.3);

Y = thrust factor (Table 16.3)

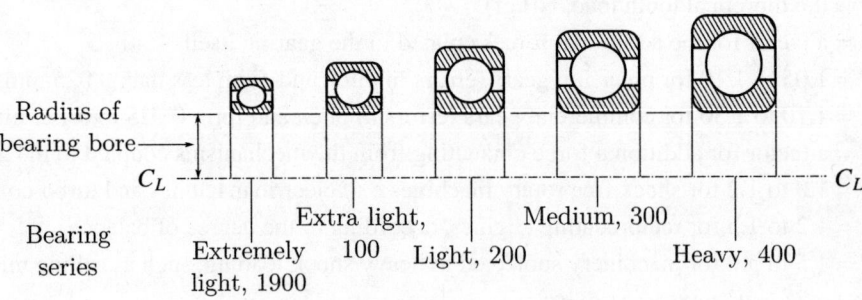

Radius of bearing bore

C_L ———————————————————————————————— C_L

Bearing series

Extremely light, 1900

Extra light, 100

Light, 200

Medium, 300

Heavy, 400

Fig. 16.1: *Relative Sizes of Bearing Series*

Particular	Equation	Eqn. No.
(b) Radial Roller bearings:		
The basic load rating C in N (kgf) for radial roller bearing	$C = f_c(il_{ef} \cos \alpha)^{7/9} z^{3/4} D^{29/27}$	16.7(a)

where f_c = a factor which depends on the units use the exact geometrical shape of the load carrying surface of the rollers and ring the accuracy to which the various bearing parts are made and the material. For roller bearings of good quality hardened roller bearing steel, the values of f_c are obtained from Table 16.4

l_{ef} = effective length of contact between one roller and that ring where the contact is the shortest (overall roller length minus roller chamfers or minus grinding undercuts), mm

Particular	Equation	Eqn. No.
The equivalent load P for a radial roller bearings	$P = XVF_r + YF_a$	16.7(b)
	X, V and Y, refer Table 16.5	

(c) Taper roller bearings:

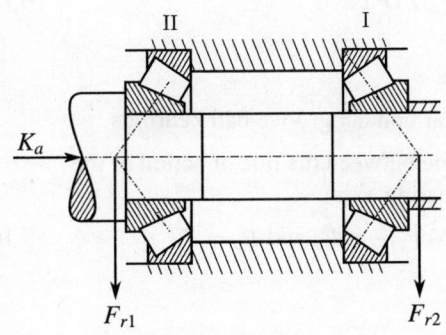
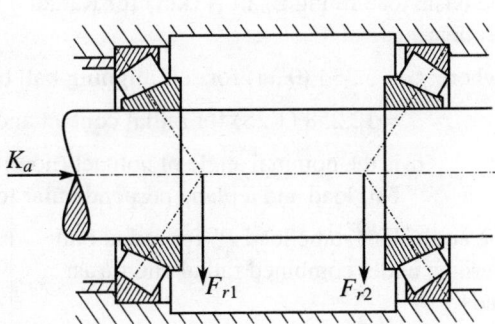

	Conditions	Thrust loads	
1)	$\dfrac{F_{r1}}{Y_1} \geq \dfrac{F_{r2}}{Y_2}$ $K_a \geq AO$	$F_{a1} = \dfrac{0.5F_{r1}}{Y_1}$	16.8(a)
2)	$\dfrac{F_{r1}}{Y_1} < \dfrac{F_{r2}}{Y_2}$ $K_a \leq 0.5\left(\dfrac{F_{r2}}{Y_2} - \dfrac{F_{r1}}{Y_1}\right)$	$F_{a2} = F_{a1} + K_a$	16.8(b)
3)	$\dfrac{F_{r1}}{Y_1} < \dfrac{F_{r2}}{Y_2}$ $K_a \leq 0.5\left(\dfrac{F_{r2}}{Y_2} - \dfrac{F_{r1}}{Y_1}\right)$	$F_{a1} = F_{a2} - K_a$ $F_{a2} = \dfrac{0.5F_{r2}}{Y_2}$	16.8(c) 16.8(d)

Particular	Equation	Eqn. No.
Fluctuating bearing load:		
An approximate value of the constant mean load	$F_m = \left(\dfrac{F_1^3 N_1 + F_2^3 N_2 + F_3^3 N_3 + - - -}{N} \right)^{\frac{1}{3}}$	16.9(a)

where F_1 is the constant load during N_1 revolutions

F_2 is the constant load during N_2 revolutions, etc.

$N = N_1 + N_2 + N_3 + - - -$

= the total no. of revolutions during which the loads $F_1, F_2, F_3, - - -$ act

| If the bearing speed and the direction of loading are constant, and the load fluctuates more or less linearly over a certain period, the constant mean load for this period is obtained from the formula | $F_m = \dfrac{2F_{max} + F_{min}}{3}$

where F_{max} is the maximum load, N

F_{min} is the minimum load, N | 16.9(b) |

Static load rating of Rolling bearings:

| The basic load rating C_o in N (kgf) for Radial ball bearings | $C_o = f_o i Z D^2 \cos \alpha$ | 16.10(a) |

where $f_o = 3.334$ (0.34) for self aligning ball bearings

= 12.258 (1.25) for radial contact and angular contact groove ball bearings

α is the nominal angle of contact (nominal angle between the line of action of the ball load and a plane perpendicular to the bearing axis)

| The equivalent static load P_o for radial ball bearings under combined radial and thrust loads | $P_o = X_o F_r + Y_o F_a$ and $P_o = F_r$ | 16.10(b) |

where X_o, Y_o are radial and thrust factors respectively, (Table 16.6)

| The basic static load rating C_o for radial roller bearings | $C_o = f_o i Z l_{ef} D \cos \alpha$ | 16.10(c) |

where $f_o = 21.572$ (2.20), factor for different kinds of bearings

| The basic static load C_{oa} in $N(kgf)$ for thrust ball bearings | $C_{oa} = f_{oa} Z D^2 \sin \alpha$ | 16.10(d) |

where $f_{oa} = 49.033$ (5.0), factor for thrust ball bearings

| The static equivalent load P_{oa} for thrust ball bearings with constant angle $\alpha \neq 90°$ under combined radial and thrust loads | $P_{oa} = F_a + 2.3 F_r \tan \alpha$ | 16.10(e) |

| The basic static load rating C_{oa} in N(kgf) for thrust roller bearings | $C_{oa} = f_{oa} Z l_{ef} D \sin \alpha$ | 16.10(f) |

where $f_{oa} = 98.067$ (10.0), factor for thrust roller bearings

Particular	Equation	Eqn. No.
The static equivalent load P_{oa} for thrust roller bearings with contact angle $\alpha \neq 90°$ under combined radial and thrust loads	$P_{oa} = F_a + 2.3F_r \tan\alpha$	16.10(g)
The static equivalent load P_o for radial roller bearings and combined radial and thrust loads	$P_o = X_o F_r + Y_o F_a$ and $P_o = F_r$	16.10(h)

where X_o = a radial factor (Table 16.6); Y_o = a thrust factor (Table 16.6)

The relationship between the life in millions of revolutions and the life in working hours	$L_N = \dfrac{60NL_h}{1000000} = 0.03\,N,$	16.11(a)

when $L_h = 500$ hrs, life of bearing in hours

N is the speed in revolutions per minute

The load rating C_n at the speed of rotation N	$C_n = \dfrac{C}{\sqrt[3]{0.03N}} = f_n C$	16.11(b)

where f_n is a coefficient from the monogram (Fig. 16.1)

Life Factors:

The specific capacity	$C = f_N P$	16.12(a)

where $f_N = \sqrt[3]{L_N}$, a life factor (Fig. 16.2)

P is the Equivalent load, N (kgf)

L_N is the life offering in millions of revolutions

If the speed of rotation is constant, the load rating	$C_n = f_h P$	16.12(b)

where $f_h = \sqrt[3]{(N_h/500)}$ is the life factor for the life figured in hrs. (from Fig. 16.2)

References

[1] "S. K. F. Ball and Roller Bearings". Catalogue No. 2401. E. AB Svenska Kullagerfabriken, 1962.

[2] Arvid Palmgreen, *"Ball and Roller Bearing Engg."*, S. H. Burbank & Co. Inc., Philadelphia, 1945.

[3] Vallance, A., Doughtie, V. L., *"Design of Machine Members"*, 3rd edition. McGraw Hill Book Company, 1951.

[4] Indian Standard – Methods of evaluating static load ratings of rolling bearing. [IS: 3823 (Part I to IV) – 1966.]

[5] Indian Standard – Methods of evaluating dynamic load rating of rolling Bearings. [IS: 3824 (Part I and II)–1966]

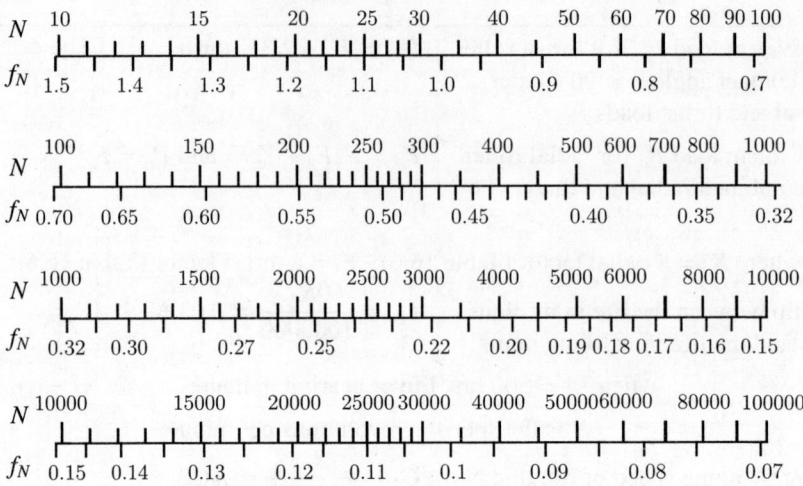

Fig. 16.2: *Speed and speed factor f_N*

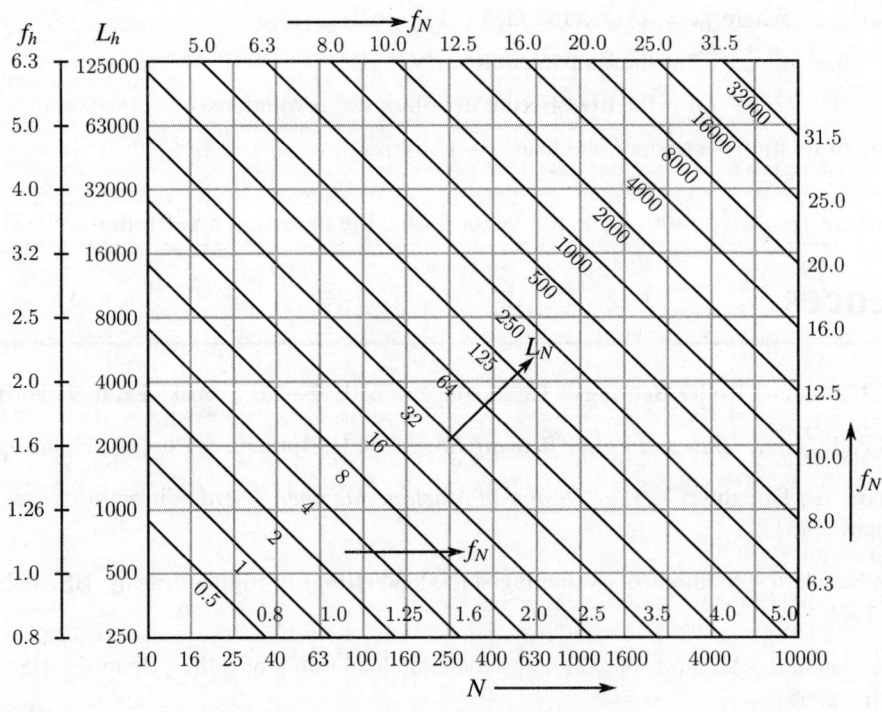

Fig. 16.3: *Speed and life factors*

Table 16.1 *Loading ratio C/P for different lives expressed in millions of revolutions*

(a) BALL BEARINGS

Life in millions of revolutions L_n (1)	$\dfrac{C}{P}$ (2)	Life in millions of revolutions L_n (1)	$\dfrac{C}{P}$ (2)	Life in millions of revolutions L_n (1)	$\dfrac{C}{P}$ (2)	Life in millions of revolutions L_n (1)	$\dfrac{C}{P}$ (2)
0.5	0.793	80	4.31	600	8.43	3200	14.7
0.75	0.909	90	4.48	650	8.66	3400	15.0
1	1	100	4.64	700	8.88	3600	15.3
1.5	1.14	120	4.93	750	9.09	3800	15.6
2	1.26	140	5.19	800	9.28	4000	15.9
3	1.44	160	5.43	850	9.47	4500	16.5
4	1.59	180	5.65	900	9.65	5000	17.1
5	1.71	200	5.85	950	9.83	5500	17.7
6	1.82	220	5.04	1000	10.0	6000	18.2
8	2	240	6.21	1100	10.3	6500	18.7
10	2.15	260	6.38	1200	10.6	7000	19.1
12	2.29	280	6.54	1300	10.9	7500	19.6
14	2.41	300	6.69	1400	11.2	8000	20.0
16	2.52	320	6.84	1500	11.4	8500	20.4
18	2.62	340	6.98	1600	11.7	9000	20.8
20	2.71	360	7.11	1700	11.9	9500	21.2
25	2.92	380	7.24	1800	12.2	10000	21.5
30	3.11	400	7.37	1900	12.4	12000	22.9
35	3.27	420	7.49	2000	12.6	14000	24.1
40	3.42	440	7.61	2200	13.0	16000	25.2
45	3.56	460	7.72	2400	13.4	18000	26.2
50	3.68	480	7.83	2600	13.8	20000	27.1
60	3.91	500	7.94	2800	14.1	25000	29.2
70	4.12	550	8.19	3000	14.4	30000	31.1

Table 6.1 *Loading ratio C/P for different lives in (L_n)* *(Contd...)*

(b) ROLLER BEARINGS							
(1)	**(2)**	**(1)**	**(2)**	**(1)**	**(2)**	**(1)**	**(2)**
0.5	0.812	80	3.72	600	6.81	3200	11.3
0.75	0.917	90	3.85	650	6.98	3400	11.5
1	1	100	3.98	700	7.14	3600	11.7
1.5	1.13	120	4.20	750	7.29	3800	11.9
2	1.24	140	4.40	800	7.43	4000	12.0
3	1.39	160	4.58	850	7.56	4500	12.5
4	1.52	180	4.75	900	7.70	5000	12.9
5	1.62	200	4.90	950	7.82	5500	13.2
6	1.71	220	5.04	1000	7.94	6000	13.6
8	1.87	240	5.18	1100	8.17	6500	13.9
10	2.00	260	5.30	1200	8.39	7000	14.2
12	2.11	280	5.42	1300	8.59	7500	14.5
14	2.21	300	5.54	1400	8.79	8000	14.8
16	2.30	320	5.64	1500	8.97	8500	15.1
18	2.38	340	5.75	1600	9.15	9000	15.4
20	2.46	360	5.85	1700	9.31	9500	15.6
25	2.63	380	5.94	1800	9.48	10000	15.8
30	2.77	400	6.03	1900	9.63	12000	16.7
35	2.91	420	6.12	2000	9.78	14000	17.5
40	3.02	440	6.21	2200	10.1	16000	18.2
45	3.13	460	6.29	2400	10.3	18000	18.9
50	3.23	480	6.37	2600	10.6	20000	19.5
60	3.42	500	6.45	2800	10.8	25000	20.9
70	3.58	550	6.64	3000	11.0	30000	22.0

Table 16.2 *Value of Factors f_c*

$\dfrac{D \cos \alpha}{d_m^*}$	For Single Row Radial Contact, Groove Ball Bearings, Single and Double Row Angular Contact, Groove Ball Bearings	For Double Row Radial Contact Groove Ball Bearings	For Self Aligning Ball Bearings	For Single Row Radial Contact Separatable Ball Bearings
0.05	46.68 (4.76)	44.23 (4.51)	17.26 (1.76)	16.18 (1.65)
0.06	49.03 (5.00)	46.48 (4.74)	18.63 (1.90)	17.36 (1.77)
0.07	51.09 (5.21)	48.45 (4.94)	19.91 (2.03)	18.54 (1.89)
0.08	52.86 (5.39)	50.11 (5.11)	21.08 (2.15)	19.52 (1.99)
0.09	54.33 (5.54)	51.39 (5.24)	22.26 (2.27)	20.59 (2.10)
0.10	55.51 (5.66)	52.66 (5.37)	23.34 (2.38)	21.48 (2.19)
0.12	57.47 (5.86)	54.43 (6.55)	25.60 (2.61)	23.44 (2.39)
0.14	58.84 (6.00)	55.70 (5.68)	27.66 (2.82)	25.30 (2.58)
0.16	59.62 (6.08)	56.49 (5.76)	29.71 (3.03)	27.07 (2.76)
0.18	59.92 (6.11)	56.78 (5.79)	31.68 (3.23)	28.83 (2.94)
0.20	59.92 (6.11)	56.78 (5.79)	33.54 (3.42)	30.50 (3.11)
0.22	59.62 (6.08)	56.49 (5.76)	35.21 (3.59)	32.07 (3.27)
0.24	58.93 (6.01)	55.90 (5.70)	36.78 (3.75)	33.64 (3.43)
0.26	58.15 (5.93)	55.11 (5.62)	38.25 (3.90)	35.11 (3.58)
0.28	57.17 (5.83)	54.13 (5.52)	39.42 (4.02)	36.48 (3.72)
0.30	56.00 (5.71)	53.05 (5.41)	40.31 (4.11)	37.85 (3.86)
0.32	54.72 (5.58)	51.98 (5.30)	40.90 (4.18)	38.93 (3.97)
0.34	53.25 (5.43)	50.50 (5.15)	41.19 (4.20)	39.82 (4.06)
0.36	51.68 (5.27)	49.03 (5.00)	41.29 (4.21)	40.40 (4.12)
0.38	50.04 (5.10)	47.46 (4.84)	40.99 (4.18)	40.70 (4.15)
0.40	48.25 (4.92)	45.80 (4.67)	40.40 (4.12)	40.89 (4.17)

$^*d_m$ is the pitch diameter of the ball set in mm

Note 1–For values of $\dfrac{D \cos \alpha}{d_m}$ other than those given in this table, f_e is obtained by linear interpolation.

Table 16.2 *Values of factor f_c (Contd...)*

Note 2–When calculating the basic load rating for a unit consisting of two similar single row radial contact ball bearings in a duplex mounting, the unit shall be considered as one double row radial contact ball bearing.

The values of f_c as given in this table shall apply to bearings whose raceways have a cross-sectional radius not larger than the following:

In radial contact and angular contact groove ball bearing inner rings	52 percent of the ball diameter
In radial contact and angular contact groove ball bearing outer rings	53 percent of the ball diameter
In self-aligning ball bearing inner rings	53 percent of the ball diameter

The basic load rating is not necessarily increased by the use of smaller groove radii but is reduced by the use of larger radii than those given above.

Note 3–When calculating the basic load rating for a unit consisting of two similar single row angular contact ball bearings in a duplex mounting, 'face to face' or 'back to back', the unit shall be considered as one double row angular contact ball bearing.

Note 4–When calculating the basic load rating for a unit consisting of two similar single row angular contact ball bearings mounted 'in tandem', properly manufactured and mounted for equal load distribution, the rating of the unit is the number of bearings to the 0.7 power times the load rating of a single row ball bearing. If for some technical reason the unit may be treated as a number of individually inter changeable single row bearings, this shall not apply.

IS: 3824 (part I)–1966.

Table 16.3 *Value of Factors V, X and Y*

Bearing Type	$\dfrac{iF_a}{C_o^*}$, $\dfrac{F_a}{ZD^2}$	$\dfrac{F_a}{ZD^2}$	$\dfrac{F_a}{C_o^*}$	$\dfrac{F_a}{iZD^2}$	V — Rotating	V — Stationary	X Single Row** when $\dfrac{F_a}{VF_r} \le e$	X Double Row @ when $\dfrac{Fa}{VF_r} \le e$	X Double Row @ when $\dfrac{F_a}{VF_r} > e$	Y Single Row when $\dfrac{F_a}{VF_r} > e$	Y Double Row @ when $\dfrac{F_a}{VF_r} \le e$	Y Double Row @ when $\dfrac{F_a}{VF_r} > e$	e†
(1)	(2)	(3)	(4)	(5)	(6)	(7)	(8)	(9)	(10)	(11)	(12)	(13)	(14)
Non-filling slot assembly, radial contact, groove ball bearings//	—	—	0.014	0.018	1.0	1.2*//	0.56	1.0	0.56	2.30	0.0	2.30	0.19
			0.028	0.035						1.99		1.99	0.22
			0.056	0.070						1.71		1.71	0.26
			0.084	0.110						1.55		1.55	0.28
			0.110	0.140						1.45		1.45	0.30
			0.170	0.210						1.31		1.31	0.34
			0.280	0.350						1.15		1.15	0.38
			0.420	0.530						1.04		1.04	0.42
			0.560	0.700						1.00		1.00	0.44
Angular contact groove ball bearings// $\alpha = 5^o$	0.014	0.018	—	—	1.0	1.2*//	For this type, use X, Y and e values applicable to single row, non-filling slot assembly, radial contact, groove ball bearings	1.0	0.78	For this type, use the X, Y & e values applicable to single row, non-filling slot assembly, radial contact, groove ball bearings	2.78	3.74	0.23
	0.028	0.035									2.40	3.23	0.26
	0.056	0.070									2.07	2.78	0.30
	0.085	0.110									1.87	2.52	0.34
	0.110	0.140									1.75	2.36	0.36
	0.170	0.210									1.58	2.13	0.40
	0.280	0.350									1.39	1.87	0.45
	0.420	0.530									1.26	1.69	0.50
	0.560	0.700									1.21	1.63	0.52

Table 16.3   Value of Factors V, X and Y (Contd...)

(1)	(2)	(3)	(4)	(5)	(6)	(7)	(8)	(9)	(10)	(11)	(12)	(13)	(14)
Angular contact groove ball bearings//													
α = 10°	0.014	0.018	—	—	1.0	1.2°//	0.46	1.0	0.75	1.88	2.18	3.06	0.29
	0.029	0.035								1.71	1.98	2.78	0.32
	0.057	0.070								1.52	1.76	2.47	0.36
	0.086	0.110								1.41	1.63	2.29	0.38
	0.110	0.140								1.34	1.55	2.18	0.40
	0.170	0.210								1.23	1.42	2.00	0.44
	0.290	0.350								1.10	1.27	1.79	0.49
	0.430	0.530								1.01	1.17	1.64	0.54
	0.570	0.700								1.00	1.16	1.63	0.54
α = 150°	0.015	0.018	—	—	1.0	1.2°//	0.44	1.0	0.72	1.47	1.65	2.39	0.38
	0.029	0.035								1.40	1.57	2.28	0.40
	0.058	0.070								1.30	1.46	2.11	0.43
	0.087	0.110								1.23	1.38	2.00	0.46
	0.120	0.140								1.19	1.34	1.93	0.47
	0.170	0.210								1.12	1.26	1.82	0.50
	0.290	0.350								1.02	1.14	1.66	0.55
	0.440	0.530								1.00	1.12	1.63	0.56
	0.580	0.700								1.00	1.12	1.63	0.56
α = 20°					1.0	1.2*//	0.43	1.0	0.70	1.00	1.09	1.63	0.57
α = 25°					1.0	1.2	0.41	1.0	0.67	0.87	0.92	1.41	0.68
α = 30°					1.0	1.2	0.39	1.0	0.63	0.76	0.78	1.24	0.80
α = 35°					1.0	1.2	0.37	1.0	0.60	0.66	0.66	1.07	0.95
α = 40°					1.0	1.2	0.35	1.0	0.57	0.57	0.55	0.93	1.14
Self aligning ball bearing			—	—	1.0	1.0	0.40	1.0	0.65	0.4 cot α	0.42 cot α	0.65 cot α	1.5 cot α
Single row radial contact separable ball bearings (magnetic bearings)	—	—	—	—	1.0	1.0	0.5	—	—	2.5	—	—	0.2

(Contd...)

Table 16.3 *Value of Factors V, X and Y (Contd...)*

*C_2 is the static basic load rating.

[†]Values of X, Y and e for a load or a contact angle, other than those shown in this table, are obtained by linear interpolation.

** For Single row bearings, when $\frac{F_a}{VF_r} \leq e$, use X = 1 and Y = 0

(a) when calculating the equivalent load for a unit consisting of two similar single row-angular contact ball bearings in a duplex mounting, 'face to face' or 'back to back', the units shall be considered as one double row angular contact ball bearing.

(b) when calculating the equivalent load for a unit consisting of two or more single row radial or angular contact ball bearings mounted 'in tandem', the X and Y values for single row ball bearings shall be used

@ Double row bearings are presumed to be symmetrical

*// Because experimental data are incomplete, no correct value of factor V for radial and angular contact groove ball bearings with inner ring stationary in relation to the load can be stated. The values shown in this table are, however, well on the safe side.

// Permissible maximum value of $\frac{F_a}{C_o}$ depends on the bearing design.

Table 16.4 Value of Factor f_c

$\dfrac{D\cos\alpha}{d_m^*}$	0.01	0.02	0.03	0.04	0.05	0.06	0.07	0.08	0.09	0.10	1.12	0.14	0.16	0.18	0.20	0.22	0.24	0.26	0.28	0.30
f_c	45.70	53.45	58.45	62.27	65.02	66.78	69.43	71.69	72.77	73.84	76.10	77.18	77.67	78.26	77.67	78.26	77.18	76.10	74.92	73.84
	(4.66)	(5.45)	(5.96)	(6.35)	(6.63)	(6.91)	(7.08)	(7.31)	(7.42)	(7.53)	(7.76)	(7.87)	(7.92)	(7.98)	(7.92)	(7.87)	(7.76)	(7.64)	(7.53)	

d_m^* = pitch diameter of the roller set in mm

IS: 3824 (Part II)–1966

Table 16.5 Value of Factors V, X and Y for radial roller bearings

Bearing Type	V		X				Y				e
	If, in Relation to the load, the inner Ring is		For Single-Row Roller Bearings		For Double-Row Roller Bearings*		For Single-Row Roller Bearings		For Double-Row Roller Bearings*		For single and Double-row Roller Bearings†
	Rotating	Stationary†	when $\dfrac{F_a}{VF_r} \le e$	when $\dfrac{F_a}{VF_r} > e$	when $\dfrac{F_a}{VF_r} \le e$	when $\dfrac{F_a}{VF_r} > e$	when $\dfrac{F_a}{VF_r} \le e$	when $\dfrac{F_a}{VF_r} > e$	when $\dfrac{F_a}{VF_r} \le e$	when $\dfrac{F_a}{VF_r} > e$	
Self-aligning roller bearings and tapered roller bearings $\alpha \neq 0°$	1.0	1.2	1.0	0.4	1.0	0.67	0.0	0.4 cot α	0.45 cot α	0.67 cot α	1.5 tan α

* Double-row bearings are presumed to be symmetrical

† Because experimental data are incomplete, no correct value of factor V for roller bearings with inner ring stationary in relation to the load can be stated. The value V = 1.2 is, however, well on the safe side.

‡ For $\alpha = 0°$, $F_a = 0$ and $X = 1$

IS: 3824 (Part II)–1966

Table 16.6 *Values of Factors X_o and Y_o*

Bearing Type		Single Row* Bearings		Double Row† Bearings	
		X_o	Y_o	X_o	Y_o
Radial contact groove ball bearings*‡		0.6	0.5	0.6	0.5
Angular contact groove ball bearings//	$\alpha = 20°$	0.5	0.42	1.0	0.84
	$\alpha = 25°$	0.5	0.38	1.0	0.76
	$\alpha = 30°$	0.5	0.33	1.0	0.66
	$\alpha = 35°$	0.5	0.29	1.0	0.58
	$\alpha = 40°$	0.5	0.26	1.0	0.52
Self-aligning ball bearings		0.5	$0.22 \cot \alpha$	1.0	$0.44 \cot \alpha$
Self-aligning and tapered roller bearings	$\alpha \neq 0°$	0.5	$0.22 \cot \alpha$	1.0	$0.44 \cot \alpha$

*P_o is always $\geq F_r$.

†Double row bearings are presumed to be symmetrical.

‡Permissible maximum value of F_o/C_o depends on the bearing design (groove depth and internal clearance).

//For two similar single row-angular contact ball bearings, mounted 'face-to-face' or 'back-to-back' use the values of X_o and Y_o which apply to a double row angular contact ball bearings. For two or more similar single row-angular contact ball bearings, mounted 'in tandem', use the values of X_o and Y_o which apply to a single row angular contact ball bearing.

IS: 3823 (Part I)–1966

Table 16.7 *Bearing Life*

Class of machine	Life in working hours L_h
Instruments and apparatus that are used only seldom:	
Demonstration apparatus; mechanisms for operating sliding doors	500
Machines used for short period or intermittently and whose breakdown would not have serious consequences:	
Handtools; lifting tackle on workshops; hand-operated machines generally; agricultural machines; cranes in erecting shops; domestic machines	4000–8000
Machines working intermittently and whose breakdown would have serious consequences:	
Auxiliary machinery in power stations; conveyor plant for flow production; lifts; cranes for piece goods; machine tools used infrequently	8000–12000
Machines for use-8 hours per day and not always fully utilised:	
Stationary electric motors; general-purpose gear units	12000-20000
Machines for use 8 hours per day and fully utilised:	
Machines for the engineering industry generally; cranes for bulk goods; ventilating fans; countershafts	20000–30000
Machines for continuous use 24 hours per day:	
Sperarators; compressors; pumps; mine hoists; stationary electric machines; machines in continuous operations on board naval vessels	40000–60000
Machines required to work with a high degree of reliability 24 hours per day	
Pulp and papermaking machinery; public power plants; mine pumps; water works; machines in continuous operation on board merchant ships	100000–200000

Table 16.8 *Reduction in Carrying Capacity with Temperature*

Bearing temperature $°C$	125	150	175	200	225	250
Decrease in carrying capacity	5%	10%	15%	25%	35%	40%

Table 16.9 *(a) Deep Groove Ball Bearings (Series 62)*

ISI No.	Bearing of basic design No. (SKF)	d	D	B	r	Basic capacity,* N		Max. permissible speed rev/min
						Static C_o	Dynamic C	
		mm	mm	mm	mm			
(1)	(2)	(3)	(4)	(5)	(6)	(7)	(8)	(9)
10BC02	6200	10	30	9	1.0	2160	3925	20000
12BC02	01	12	32	10	1.0	2940	5250	20000
15BC02	02	15	35	11	1.0	3430	5980	16000
17BC02	6203	17	40	12	1.0	4315	7355	16000
20BC02	04	20	47	14	1.5	6375	9805	16000
25BC02	05	25	52	15	1.5	6965	10690	13000
30BC02	6206	30	62	16	1.5	9805	14710	13000
35BC02	07	35	72	17	2.0	13535	19615	10000
40BC02	08	40	80	18	2.0	15495	22165	10000
45BC02	6209	45	85	19	2.0	17750	24910	8000
50BC02	10	50	90	20	2.0	20595	27070	8000
55BC02	11	55	100	21	2.5	25300	33340	8000
60BC02	6212	60	110	22	2.5	31580	40210	6000
65BC02	13	65	120	23	2.5	35715	42905	6000
70BC02	14	70	125	24	2.5	38440	47070	5000
75BC02	6215	75	130	25	2.5	41385	50600	5000
80BC02	16	80	140	26	3.0	44130	55505	5000
85BC02	17	85	150	28	3.0	53450	63745	4000
90BC02	6218	90	160	30	3.0	60800	74040	4000
95BC02	19	95	170	32	3.5	71100	82870	4000
100BC02	20	100	180	34	3.5	79925	97145	3000
105BC02	6221	105	190	36	3.5	90710	101500	3000
110BC02	22	110	200	38	3.5	101010	108850	3000
120BC02	24	120	215	40	3.5	101010	110815	3000
	6226	130	230	40	4.0	112780	120130	2500
	28	140	250	42	4.0	127680	126510	2500
	30	150	270	45	4.0	139745	135330	2500
	32	160	290	48	4.0	151020	140235	2000
	6234	170	310	52	5.0	184365	159850	2000
	36	180	320	52	5.0	200060	169165	1600
	38	190	340	55	5.0	235360	196130	1600
	40	200	360	55	5.0	259880	205940	1600

SKF Page 88

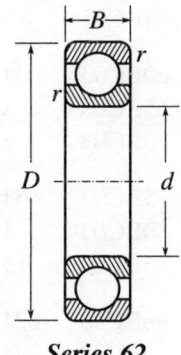

Series 62

*Basic capacity in Metric units, i.e. kgf can be obtained by dividing the values given in columns 7 & 8 with 9.80665.

Table 16.9 *(b) Deep Groove Ball Bearings (Series 63) (Contd.)*

(1)	(2)	(3)	(4)	(5)	(6)	(7)*	(8)*	(9)
10BC03	6300	10	35	11	1.0	3570	6080	16000
12BC03	01	12	37	12	1.5	4220	7550	16000
15BC03	02	15	42	13	1.5	5100	8580	16000
17BC03	6303	17	47	14	1.5	6080	10300	13000
20BC03	04	20	52	15	2.0	7550	12260	13000
25BC03	05	25	62	17	2.0	10150	15985	10000
30BC03	6306	30	72	19	2.0	14220	20990	10000
35BC03	07	35	80	21	2.5	16970	25300	8000
40BC03	08	40	90	23	2.5	20990	31380	8000
45BC03	6309	45	100	25	2.5	29225	40700	8000
50BC03	10	50	110	27	3.0	34720	47070	6000
55BC03	11	55	120	29	3.0	41190	53940	6000
60BC03	6312	60	130	31	3.5	47070	62270	5000
65BC03	13	65	140	33	3.5	53450	71100	5000
70BC03	14	70	150	35	3.5	60800	79925	5000
75BC03	6315	75	160	37	3.5	71100	89280	4000
80BC03	16	80	170	39	3.5	78450	94140	4000
85BC03	17	85	180	51	4.0	85810	101500	4000
90BC03	6318	90	190	43	4.0	96110	107870	3000
95BC03	19	95	200	45	4.0	107870	117680	3000
100BC03	20	100	215	47	4.0	129450	135330	3000
105BC03	6321	105	225	49	4.0	140240	140235	2500
110BC03	22	110	240	50	4.0	160730	152980	2500
120BC03	24	120	260	55	4.0	162790	157890	2500
	6326	130	280	58	5.0	191230	173580	2500
	28	140	300	62	5.0	215750	196130	2000
	30	150	320	65	5.0	249090	210840	2000

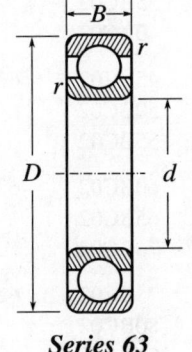

Series 63

SKF Page 90

*Basic capacity in Metric units i.e., kgf can be obtained by dividing the values given in columns 7 & 8 with 9.80665.

Table 16.10 *(a) Self-Aligning Ball Bearings*

Bearing with cylindrical bore No. (SKF)	Bearing with taper bore No.(SKF)	d mm	D mm	B mm	r mm	Basic capacity,* N		Max. permissible speed rev/min
						Static C_o	Dynamic C	
(1)	(2)	(3)	(4)	(5)	(6)	(7)	(8)	(9)
2200		10	30	14	1.0	1670	5540	20000
01		12	32	14	1.0	1960	5640	20000
02		15	35	14	1.0	2110	5740	16000
2203		17	40	16	1.0	2745	7500	16000
04	2204 K	20	47	18	1.5	3825	9610	16000
05	05 K	25	52	18	1.5	4120	9610	13000
2206	2206 K	30	62	20	1.5	5390	11770	13000
07	07 K	35	72	23	2.0	7845	16180	10000
08	08 K	40	80	23	2.0	8825	16920	10000
2209	2209 K	45	85	23	2.0	9810	17410	8000
10	10 K	50	90	23	2.0	10490	17410	8000
11	11 K	55	100	25	2.5	12455	20200	8000
2212	2212 K	60	110	28	2.5	15300	25810	6000
13	13 K	65	120	31	2.5	19610	33340	6000
14	–	70	125	31	2.5	21080	34080	5000
2215	2215 K	75	130	31	2.5	21575	34080	5000
16	16 K	80	140	33	3.0	24520	37850	5000
17	17 K	85	150	36	3.0	29030	44620	4000
2218	2218 K	90	160	40	3.0	35550	53450	4000
19	19 K	95	170	43	3.5	42170	63740	4000
20	20 K	100	180	46	3.5	49030	76000	3000
2221	—	105	190	50	3.5	53940	82870	3000
22	2222 K	110	200	53	3.5	62270	96600	3000

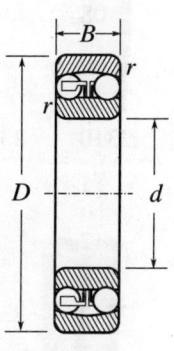

22 Series

Table 16.10 *(b) Self-Aligning Ball Bearings (Contd.)*

(1)	(2)	(3)	(4)	(5)	(6)	(7)*	(8)*	(9)
2301		12	37	17	1.5	2940	8925	16000
02		15	42	18	1.5	3285	9070	13000
03		17	47	19	1.5	4070	10790	13000
2304	2304 K	20	52	21	2.0	5345	13730	10000
05	05 K	25	62	24	2.0	7600	18490	10000
06	06 K	30	72	27	2.0	9810	24030	8000
2307	2307 K	35	80	31	2.5	12945	29810	8000
08	08 K	40	90	33	2.5	15450	34720	6000
09	09 K	45	100	36	2.5	19220	40940	6000
2310	2310 K	50	110	40	3.0	23630	50750	5000
11	11 K	55	120	43	3.0	28050	56390	5000
12	12 K	60	130	46	3.5	32750	66693	4000
2313	2313 K	65	140	48	3.5	38490	73550	4000
14	—	70	150	51	3.5	43640	82375	4000
15	15 K	75	160	55	3.5	50750	92670	3000
16	16 K	80	170	58	3.5	56390	102970	3000
2317	2317 K	85	180	60	4.0	59580	106890	2500
18	18 K	90	190	64	4.0	68160	115720	2500

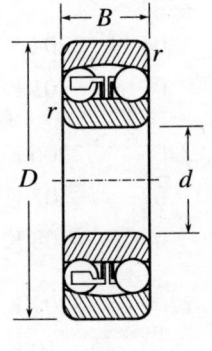

23 Series

SKF Page 106

*Basic capacity in Metric units, i.e. kgf can be obtained by dividing the values given in columns 7 & 8 with 9.80665.

Table 16.11 *(a) Single Row Angular Contact Ball Bearings (Series 72B)*

ISI No.	Bearing No. (SKF)	d mm	D mm	B mm	r mm	r_1 mm	a mm	Basic capacity,* N Static C_o	Dynamic C	Max. permissible speed rev/min
(1)	(2)	(3)	(4)	(5)	(6)	(7)	(8)	(9)	(10)	(11)
15BA02	7202 B	15	35	11	1.0	0.5	16	3680	6080	13000
17BA02	03 B	17	40	12	1.0	0.8	18	4460	7700	13000
20BA02	04 B	20	47	14	1.5	0.8	21	6370	10150	10000
25BA02	7205 B	25	52	15	1.5	0.8	24	7700	11280	10000
30BA02	06 B	30	62	16	1.5	0.8	27	10790	15400	10000
35BA02	07 B	35	72	17	2.0	1.0	31	14710	20590	8000
40BA02	7208 B	40	80	18	2.0	1.0	34	18490	24520	8000
45BA02	09 B	45	85	19	2.0	1.0	37	21180	27655	6000
50BA02	10 B	50	90	20	2.0	1.0	39	23140	28440	6000
55BA02	7211 B	55	100	21	2.5	1.2	43	29175	36285	6000
60BA02	12B	60	110	22	2.5	1.2	47	36285	42900	5000
65BA02	13B	65	120	23	2.5	1.2	50	42410	49030	5000
70BA02	7214 B	70	125	24	2.5	1.2	53	44620	52470	5000
75BA02	15 B	75	130	25	2.5	1.2	56	49030	54430	4000
80BA02	16 B	80	140	26	3.0	1.5	59	55650	60800	4000
85BA02	7217 B	85	150	28	3.0	1.5	64	63740	69630	4000
90BA02	18 B	90	160	30	3.0	1.5	67	75760	81400	4000
95BA02	19 B	95	170	32	3.5	2.0	71	85810	92670	3000
100BA02	7220 B	100	180	34	3.5	2.0	76	90710	98070	3000
105BA02	21 B	105	190	36	3.5	2.0	80	101500	106890	2500
110BA02	22 B	110	220	38	3.5	2.0	84	112780	117680	2500

Series 72B

SKF Page 112

Table 16.11 *(b) Single Row Angular Contact Ball Bearings (Series 73B)*

(1)	(2)	(3)	(4)	(5)	(6)	(7)	(8)	(9)	(10)	(11)
17BA03	7303 B	17	47	14	1.5	0.8	21	7110	11283	10000
20BA03	04 B	20	52	15	2.0	1.0	23	8140	13580	10000
25BA03	05 B	25	62	17	2.0	1.0	27	12260	18930	10000
30BA03	7306 B	30	72	19	2.0	1.0	31	15840	24025	8000
35BA03	07 B	35	80	21	2.5	1.2	35	20005	28050	8000
40BA03	08 B	40	90	23	2.5	1.2	39	24910	34715	6000
45BA03	7309 B	45	100	25	2.5	1.2	43	33340	44620	6000
50BA03	10 B	50	110	27	3.0	1.5	47	40210	51485	6000
55BA03	11 B	55	120	29	3.0	1.5	52	46580	59820	5000
60BA03	7312 B	60	130	31	3.5	2.0	55	53450	69630	5000
65BA03	13 B	65	140	33	3.5	2.0	60	61290	78450	5000
70BA03	14 B	70	150	35	3.5	2.0	64	72570	87280	4000
75BA03	7315 B	75	160	37	3.5	2.0	68	80415	96600	4000
80BA03	16 B	80	170	39	3.5	2.0	72	89240	102970	4000
85BA03	17 B	85	180	41	4.0	2.0	76	98070	111550	3000
90BA03	7318 B	90	190	43	4.0	2.0	80	111500	120130	3000
95BA03	19 B	95	200	45	4.0	2.0	84	122580	129250	2500
100BA03	20 B	100	215	47	4.0	2.0	90	149060	144650	2500
105BA03	7321 B	105	225	49	4.0	2.0	94	160090	153230	2500
110BA03	22 B	110	240	50	4.0	2.0	99	188780	168920	2500

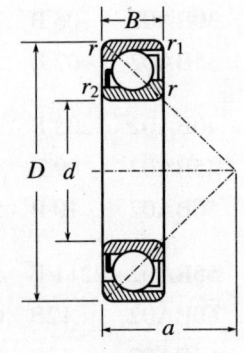

Series 73B

SKF Page 113

*Basic capacity in Metric units i.e kgf can be obtained by dividing the values given in columns 9 & 10 with 9.80665.

Table 16.12 *Double Row Angular Contact Ball Bearings (Series 33A)*

Bearing No. (SKF)	d mm	D mm	B mm	mm	Basic capacity,* N		Max. permissible speed, rev/min
					Static C_o	Dynamic C	
(1)	(2)	(3)	(4)	(5)	(6)	(7)	(8)
3302 A	15	42	19.0	1.5	9070	13730	10000
03 A	17	47	22.2	1.5	12650	18930	8000
04 A	20	42	22.2	2.0	13730	18930	8000
3305 A	25	62	25.4	2.0	19615	26085	6000
06 A	30	72	30.2	2.0	27165	35300	6000
07 A	35	80	34.9	2.5	35600	43640	5000
3308 A	40	90	36.5	2.5	44620	53450	5000
09 A	45	110	39.7	2.5	54430	62270	4000
10 A	50	110	44.4	3.0	72570	80170	4000
3311 A	55	120	49.2	3.0	78450	85910	4000
12 A	60	130	54.0	3.5	94630	98070	3000
13 A	65	140	58.7	3.5	108950	115720	3000
3314 A	70	150	63.5	3.5	126510	135820	3000
15 A	75	160	68.3	3.5	138080	140235	2500
16 A	80	170	86.3	3.5	153965	157890	2500
3317 A	85	180	73.0	4.0	173580	173580	2500
18 A	90	190	73.0	4.0	205940	200150	2500

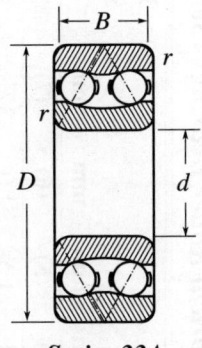

Series 33A

SKF Page 119

*Basic capacity in Metric units i.e. kgf can be obtained by dividing the values given in columns 6 & 7 with 9.80665

Table 16.13 (a) Cylindrical Roller Bearings (Series NU22)

| Bearing No. (SKF) | d mm | D mm | B mm | r mm | r_1 mm | F mm | Basic capacity, N* | | Max. permissible speed, rev/min |
| | | | | | | | Static C_o | Dynamic C | |
(1)	(2)	(3)	(4)	(5)	(6)	(7)	(8)	(9)	(10)
NU 2205	25	52	18	1.5	1.0	32	11030	15790	13000
2206	30	62	20	1.5	1.0	38.5	16970	23140	13000
2207	35	72	23	2.0	1.0	43.8	27655	35600	10000
NU 2208	40	80	23	2.0	2.0	50	32750	40700	10000
2209	45	85	23	2.0	2.0	55	35600	43640	8000
2210	50	90	23	2.0	2.0	60.4	38540	45500	8000
NU 2211	55	100	25	2.5	2.0	66.5	45500	52560	8000
2212	60	110	28	2.5	2.5	73.5	59820	69630	6000
2213	65	120	31	2.5	2.5	79.6	74040	81640	6000
NU 2214	70	125	31	2.5	2.5	84.5	78450	85910	5000
2215	75	130	31	2.5	2.5	88.5	84730	96350	5000
2216	80	140	33	3.0	3.0	95.3	98070	109340	5000
NU 2217	85	150	36	3.0	3.0	101.8	117680	127000	4000
2218	90	160	40	3.0	3.0	107	135820	140235	4000
2219	95	170	43	3.5	3.5	113.5	160340	173580	4000
NU 2220	100	180	46	3.5	3.5	120	184855	196130	3000
2222	110	200	53	3.5	3.5	132.5	226435	254170	3000
2224	120	215	58	3.5	3.5	143.5	271645	280470	3000
NU 2226	130	230	64	4.0	4.0	156	306700	296650	2500
2228	140	250	68	4.0	4.0	169	378540	362850	2500
2230	150	270	73	4.0	4.0	182	436400	423650	2500

Series NU 22

SKF Page 146

Table 16.13 (b) Cylindrical Roller Bearings (Contd.)

(1)	(2)	(3)	(4)	(5)	(6)	(7)	(8)	(9)	(10)
Series NU 23									
NU 2305	25	62	24	2.0	2.0	35	21280	30205	10000
2306	30	72	27	2.0	2.0	42	26430	35305	10000
2307	35	80	31	2.5	2.0	46.2	30695	41780	8000
NU 2308	40	90	33	2.5	2.5	53.5	47270	58840	8000
2309	45	100	36	2.5	2.5	58.5	55700	74040	8000
2310	50	110	40	3.0	3.0	65	74040	90960	6000
NU 2311	55	120	43	3.0	3.0	70.5	82965	106890	6000
2312	60	130	46	3.5	3.5	77	103460	129250	5000
2313	65	140	48	3.5	3.5	83.5	120130	142690	5000
NU 2314	70	150	51	3.5	3.5	90	138270	155925	5000
2315	75	160	55	3.5	3.5	95.5	166710	200150	4000
2316	80	170	58	3.5	3.5	103	184855	213785	4000
NU 2317	85	180	60	4.0	4.0	108	196130	227415	3000
2318	90	190	64	4.0	4.0	115	222610	254000	3000
2319	95	200	67	4.0	4.0	121.5	260760	292140	3000
NU 2320	100	215	73	4.0	4.0	129.5	309890	341170	3000
2322	110	240	80	4.0	4.0	143	423650	455030	2500
2324	120	260	86	4.0	4.0	154	499160	557510	2500
NU 2326	130	280	93	5.0	5.0	167	637430	609970	2500
2328	140	300	102	5.0	5.0	180	726670	736480	2000
2330	150	320	108	5.0	5.0	193	815910	815910	2000

SKF Page 150

*Basic capacity in Metric units, i.e. kgf can be obtained by dividing the values given in columns 8 & 9 with 9.80665

Table 16.14 Taper Roller Bearings (Series 322)

Series 322

Bearing No. (SKF)	d mm	D mm	B mm	T mm	C mm	r mm	r_1 mm	a mm	Basic capacity, N* Static C_o	Dynamic C	Max. permissible speed, rev/min
(1)	(2)	(3)	(4)	(5)	(6)	(7)	(8)	(9)	(10)	(11)	(12)
32206	30	62	20	21.25	17	1.5	0.5	15	27165	31675	6000
07	35	72	23	24.25	19	2.0	0.8	18	36285	41430	6000
08	40	80	23	24.75	19	2.0	0.8	19	40210	45500	6000
32209	45	85	23	24.75	19	2.0	0.8	20	45500	49915	5000
10	50	90	23	24.75	19	2.0	0.8	21	47270	51580	5000
11	55	100	25	26.75	21	2.5	0.8	22	61050	65115	4000
32212	60	110	28	29.75	24	2.5	0.8	24	75710	78450	4000
13	65	120	31	32.75	27	2.5	0.8	26	90810	96105	4000
14	70	125	31	33.25	27	2.5	0.8	28	90810	96105	3000
32215	75	130	31	33.25	27	2.5	0.8	29	99930	101450	3000
16	80	140	33	35.25	28	3.0	1.0	30	113760	117680	3000
17	85	150	36	38.5	30	3.0	1.0	33	134840	135820	2500
32218	90	160	40	42.5	34	3.0	1.0	36	160730	158080	2500
19	95	170	43	45.5	37	3.5	1.2	38	180440	180440	2500
20	100	180	46	49	39	3.5	1.2	41	207705	202510	2500
32221	105	190	50	53	43	3.5	1.2	44	241240	236340	2000
22	110	200	53	56	46	3.5	1.2	46	271645	254000	2000
24	120	213	53	61.5	50	3.5	1.2	52	334410	298120	2000
32226	130	230	64	67.75	54	4.0	1.5	56	407960	369710	1600
28	140	250	68	71.75	58	4.0	1.5	60	481510	422670	1600
30	150	270	73	77	60	4.0	1.5	64	534460	480525	1600

SKF Page 159

*Basic capacity in Metric units, i.e. kgf can be obtained by dividing the values given in columns 10 & 11 with 9.80665

17

Fly-Wheel

Symbols	Description and Units
A	cross-sectional area of the rim, mm^2
B	width of rim, mm
d_h	hub diameter, mm
E	excess energy or the change in energy, J (kgf m)
i	number of arms
k	polar radius of gyration of the rim, m
L	length of hub, mm
n	mean speed, rev/s
T	transmitted torque, N mm (kgf mm)
t	thinkness of the rim, mm
U	kinetic energy, J (kgf m)
W	weight of the flywheel, N (kg)
W_r	weight of the rim, N (kg)
w	weight density of the material, N/m^3 (kg/m^3)
Z	section modulus, mm^3

Particular	Equation	Eqn. No.
The Kinetic energy (E_k) in the rim of a rotating wheel, J (kgf m)	$E_k = \dfrac{Wv^2}{2g}$	17.1(a)
where W is the fly-wheel rim weight, N(kg) v is the mean velocity of the rim, m/s $g = 9.81$ m/s^2, acceleration due to gravity		
When the velocity changes from v_1 to v_2, the energy released or absorbed during this change (Excess Energy or change in energy), J (kgf m)	$E = E_k - E_k = \dfrac{W(v_1^2 - v_2^2)}{2g} = \dfrac{W(v_1 - v_2)v}{g}$ $= \dfrac{WC_s v^2}{g} = \left(\dfrac{4\pi^2}{g}\right) WC_s k^2 n^2$	17.1(b)

Particular	Equation	Eqn. No.

The weight of fly-wheel rim*, N (kg)

$$W = \frac{2gE}{v_1^2 - v_2^2} = \frac{gE}{(v_1 - v_2)v} = \frac{gE}{C_s v^2} = \left(\frac{g}{4\pi^2}\right)\frac{E}{C_s k^2 n^2}$$ 17.1(c)

where $v = (v_1 + v_2)/2 = 2\pi k n$, mean velocity of rim, m/s

$k = (R_i + R_o)/2$, polar radius of gyration of the rim, m

$n = (n_1 + n_2)/2$, mean speed of the fly-wheel, rev/s

$C_s{}^\dagger = (v_1 - v_2)/v = (n_1 - n_2)/n$, coefficient of fluctuation of speed or rotation

v_1, v_2 are the maximum and minimum velocities respectively, m/s

| The fly-wheel effect or polar moment of inertia | $(Wk^2) = \left(\dfrac{g}{2\pi^2}\right)\dfrac{E}{n_1^2 - n_2^2} = \left(\dfrac{g}{4\pi^2}\right)\dfrac{E}{C_s n^2}$ | 17.1(d) |
| The relative speed variation or the coefficient of steadiness | $m = n/(n_1 - n_2)$ | 17.1(e) |

where n_1, n_2 are the maximum and minimum speeds respectively, rev/s

Engine Fly-wheels:

| The average energy delivered by the engine shaft per revolution, J | $E_a = \dfrac{1000P}{n}$ | 17.2(a) |
| The energy fluctuation or the change in energy, J | $E = C_e E_a = C_e \dfrac{1000P}{n}$ | 17.2(b) |

where P is the power of the engine, kw

C_e is the coefficient of fluctuation of energy (Table 17.2 and 17.3)

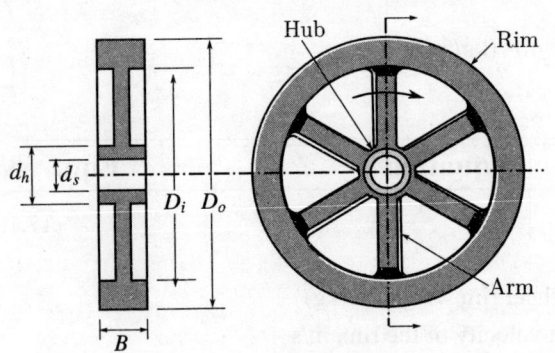

d_s - shaft diameter, mm

d_h - hub diameter, mm

D_i - Inner Diameter of rim, mm

D_o - Outer diameter of rim, mm

B - width of rim, mm

Fig. 17.1: *Flywheel*

Note : * The amount of energy in the arms and the hub is so small it is neglected

† The value of C_s or m depends on the nature of the service for which the machine is built; permissible variation between speed; method of connecting the driven machine to the driving motor.

Particular	Equation	Eqn. No.
The weight required in the fly-wheel rim, N (From Eqn. 17.1(b) and 17.2(b))	$$W = 1000\left(\frac{C_e}{C_s}\right)\frac{Pg}{nv^2} = \left(\frac{1000g}{4\pi^2}\right)\left(\frac{C_e}{C_s}\right)\frac{P}{n^3k^2}$$	17.2(c)
The velocity of the fly-wheel rim, m/s	$v = 2\pi kn$	17.2(d)

For Automobile Engines

$v = 25$ m/s for CI wheels of engines

under 75 kw (100 khp)

$= 30$ m/s for larger engines

$= 35$ m/s with special rim

design without blow holes in the rim

$= 50$ m/s for cast steel wheels

$v = 50$ m/s for CI fly-wheels

$= 75$ m/s for semisteel wheels

$= 100$ m/s for steel wheels

Rim Design:

| weight of rim, N (kg) | $$W = \frac{9}{10}W_F = \left(\frac{2\pi}{10^6}\right)ktBw = \left(\frac{2\pi}{10^6}\right)kAw$$ | 17.3 |

where w = weight density of the material,

$= 69600$ N/m^3 (7100 kg/m^3) for cast iron

$= 76500$ N/m^3 (7800 kg/m^3) for steel

W_F is the weight of flywheel, N(kg)

t is the thickness of rim, mm

B is the width of rim, mm

$t/B = 0.5$ to 1.25

The width of fly wheel when used as belt pulley	$B = b + (25$ to $50)$ mm	17.4(a)
	where b is the width of the belt, mm	
The hub diameter	$d_h = 2d_s$	17.4(b)
The length of hub	$L = 2d_s$, to $2.5d_s$	17.4(c)

Stresses in Fly-wheel Rim:
(a) Centrifugal stresses:
(i) Unstrained by the arms:

| The centrifugal force on one-half of the rim, N (kgf) | $$F_c = \left(\frac{2}{10^6}\right)\frac{Btwv^2}{g}$$ | 17.5(a) |
| The tensile stress at the rim section due to the centrifugal force, MN/m^2 (kgf/mm^2) | $$\sigma_t = \frac{wv^2}{10^6g}$$ | 17.5(b) |

Particular	Equation	Eqn. No.
(ii) Restrained by the arm: The bending stress	$\sigma_b = \dfrac{wv^2}{10^6 g} \times \dfrac{2000\pi^2 R}{ti^2}$	17.5(c)

where R is the mean radius, m; i is the number of arms

The resultant tensile stress	$\sigma_R = 0.75\sigma_t + 0.25\sigma_b$ ≤ 41.2 MN/m^2 (4.2 kgf/mm^2) for C.I.	17.5(d)

Stresses in arms:
Stress due to speed variation:

The bending stress due to the full torque at the time of starting or stopping, MN/m^2 (kgf/mm^2)	$\sigma_1 = \dfrac{T(D - d_S)}{iZD}$	17.6(a)

$\sigma_1 < 13.8$ MN/m^2 (1.40 kgf/mm^2) on account of uncertainties of the material and possible shrinkage stress

$= 6.9$ MN/m^2 (0.70 kgf/mm^2), under severe load conditions

When the flywheel is used as a belt pulley, the stress due to the net belt tension at the hub, MN/m^2 (kgf/mm^2)	$\sigma_2^* = \dfrac{(T_1 - T_2)(D - d_s)}{2iZ}$	17.6(b)
In case of thin rim wheel, the stress at the hub due to the net belt pull, MN/m^2 (kgf/mm^2)	$\sigma_2 = \dfrac{(T_1 - T_2)(D - d_s)}{iZ}$	17.6(c)

where D is the pulley diameter, mm
d_s is the shaft diameter, mm

The direct stress in the arm due to centrifugal force, MN/m^2 (kgf/mm^2)	$\sigma_3 = \dfrac{wv^2}{10^6 g}$	17.6(d)
The maximum tensile stress in the arms at the hub end	$\sigma_{\max} = \sigma_1 + \sigma_2 + \sigma_3$	17.6(e)

For cast iron $\sigma_{\max}$ should not exceed, 20.6 MN/m^2 (2.1 kgf/mm^2)

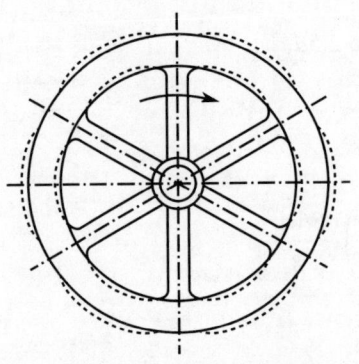

Fig. 17.2: *Strains in a flywheel*

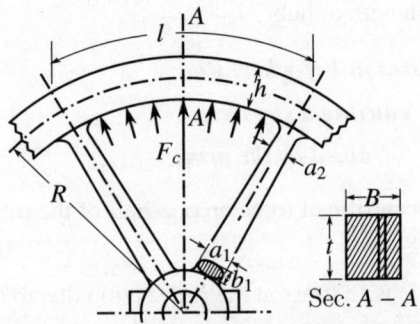

Fig. 17.3: *Bending of flywheel rim.*

Particular	Equation	Eqn. No.
The force necessary to stop the fly-wheel, N (kgf)	$F_r = \dfrac{Wa}{g}$	17.7(a)
	where W = weight of rim, N (kgf)	
	a = deceleration, m/s^2	
The bending moment at the centre of the hub	$M = F_r k$	17.7(b)
In case of elliptical section the major axis can be determined from the relation	$a_1 = \sqrt[3]{(64Z)/\pi}$	17.7(c)
	where $a_1 = 2b_1$, major axis of the arm, mm	
	b_1 = minor axis, mm	

*Experiments have shown that thin rim pulleys lacking rigidity do not distribute equally the loads to all arms. For this reason some designors think that half the no. of arms takes care of the total bending moment.

References

[1] Siegel, M. J., Maleev, V. L., Hartman, J. B., *"Mechanical Design of Machines"* 4th edition, International Text Book Company, 1965.

[2] Bhattacharya, S. C., Basu Mallik, J. R., *"Machine Design"*, Basu Mallik & Co., Calcutta, 1966.

Table 17.1 *Coefficient of Speed Fluctuation, (C_s) and coefficient of steadiness (m)*

Driven Machinery	Type of Drive	m	C_s
Hammers, crushers, punch presses	Belt	5	0.20
Comprssors, concrete mixers, excavators	Belt	7-10	0.14-0.10
Pumps, shears	Belt or flexible coupling	20-25	0.05-0.04
Metalworking and woodworking machinery	Belt	30	0.033
Flour, paper, and textile mills	Belt	40-50	0.025-0.020
Compressors, pumps, and similar machines	Gears	50	0.020
Spinning machinery, coarse to fine	Belt	50-65	0.020-0.015
D-C generators, single or parallel	Belt	35	0.029
D-C generators, single or parallel	Direct-coupled	70	0.014
A-C generators, single or parallel	Belt	60	0.017
A-C generators, single or parallel	Direct-coupled	100	0.010
Automobile (Idling)	Gears	5	0.20
Automobile (Normal speed)	Gears	10	0.10

Table 17.2 *Coefficient of Fluctuation of Energy for Steam Engine*

	Fluctuation of Energy C_e		
Cut off percentage	Single cylinder engine	Two cylinders with cranks 90° apart	Three cylinders with cranks 120° apart
10	0.35	0.088	0.040
20	0.33	0.082	0.037
40	0.31	0.078	0.034
60	0.29	0.072	0.032
80	0.28	0.070	0.031
100	0.27	0.068	0.030

Table 17.3 *Coefficient of Fluctuation of Energy C_e*
(For internal-combustion engines)

Type of engine	Number of cylinders	Angle between cranks	C_e	
			4-stroke cycle	2-stroke cycle
Single acting	1	360	2.35-2.40	0.95-1.00
twin	2	360	0.92-1.04	0.75-0.85
opposed	2	180	0.92-1.04	0.75-0.85
tandem	2	0	0.92-1.04	0.75-0.85
twin	2	180	1.50-1.60	0.20-0.25
opposed	2	360	1.50-1.60	0.20-0.25
vertical	3	120	0.60-0.75	0.15-0.18
vertical	4	180 and 90	0.15-0.20	0.075-0.10
vertical	6	180 and 60	0.10-0.12	0.016-0.02
Double acting	1	...	1.50-1.60	0.20-0.24
twin or tandem	2	...	0.18-0.20	0.18-0.20
twin-tandem	4	90	0.08-0.09	0.07-0.08

18

Cylinders and Pistons of Steam and Internal Combustion Engines

Symbols	Description and Units
F_p	the maximum load on the piston, N (kgf)
h	the depth of the piston ring, mm
i	number of studs or bolts
L	length of the piston, mm
L_c	length of cylinder, mm
l_1	length of the gudgeon pin bearing, mm
n	speed of the engine, rev/s
p	working pressure, MN/m² (kgf/mm²)
p_m	actual mean effective pressure, MN/m² (kgf/mm²)
t	thickness of the cylinder, mm
t_f	thickness of the cylinder flange, mm
t_1	thickness of the piston head, mm
t_r	the radial thickness of the piston ring, mm
v	mean speed of the piston, m/s (Table 18.1)
W_R	weight of the reciprocating parts, N (kg)
σ_t	allowable stress, MN/m² (kgf/mm²)

Particular	Equation	Eqn. No.
Steam Engine Cylinder:		
The diameter of a double acting eninge (steam engine)	$D = \left[\dfrac{1000(P)}{(\pi/4)p_m v} \right]^{\frac{1}{2}}$ SI units	18.1(a)
	$D = \left[\dfrac{75(P)}{(\pi/4)p_m v} \right]^{\frac{1}{2}}$ Metric units	18.1(b)

403

Particular	Equation	Eqn. No.
where P = indicative power, kw (Mhp); L_s = length of the storke, m $v = 2L_s n$ mean speed of the pistons, m/s; n = speed of the engine, rev/s p_m is mean effective pressure, MN/m² (kgf/mm²)		
An empirical rule to determine the thickness of ordinary grey C.I. cylinder without liner	$t = \dfrac{pD}{2\sigma_t} + 7.6$ mm	18.2(a)
where D = inside diameter of cylinder, mm σ_t = 10 to 40 MN/m² (1.02 to 4.08 kgf/mm²) for ordinary grey C.I.		
The thickness of the cylinder (Lame's equation) for brittle material, mm	$t = \dfrac{D_i}{2}\left[\left(\dfrac{\sigma_t + p_i}{\sigma_t - p_i}\right)^{\frac{1}{2}} - 1\right]$	18.2(b)
The thickness of the cylinder according to Grashof's equation, mm	$t = \dfrac{D_i}{2}\left[\left(\dfrac{3\sigma'_t + 2p_i}{3\sigma'_t - 4p_i}\right)^{\frac{1}{2}} - 1\right]$	18.2(c)
Clavarino's equation for the cylinder wall thickness, mm	$t = \dfrac{D_i}{2}\left[\left\{\dfrac{\sigma'_t + (1 - 2\mu)p_i}{\sigma'_t - (1 + \mu)p_i}\right\}^{\frac{1}{2}} - 1\right]$	18.2(d)

where D_i is the inside diameter of the cylinder, mm

σ'_t is the permissible working stress, MN/m² (kgf/mm²)

p_i is the pressure inside the cylinder, MN/m² (kgf/mm²)

μ is the poisson's ratio of lateral contraction

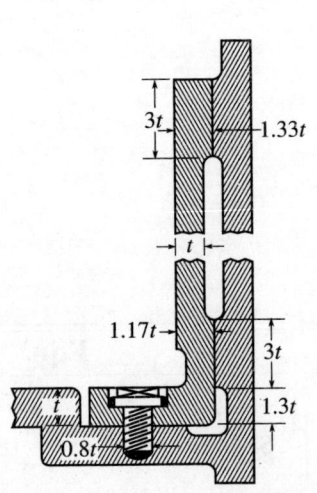

Fig. 18.1: *Cylinder with liner*

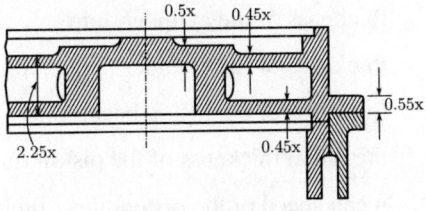

Fig. 18.2(a): *Cylinder cover*

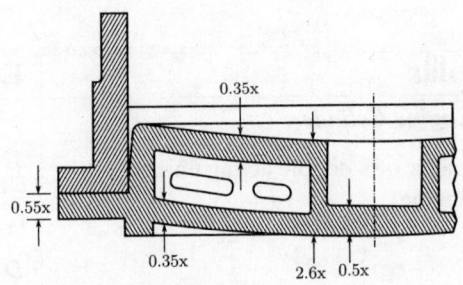

Fig. 18.2(b): *Cylinder cover*

Particular	Equation	Eqn. No.
The thickness of the cylinder flange	$t_f = 1.2t$ to $1.4t$	18.3(a)
Length of cylinder	L_c = stroke + width over piston rings	18.3(b)
The thickness of a flat cover plate firmly secured to the cylinder (Fig. 18.4)	$t = D\sqrt{p/6\sigma_t}$	18.3(c)

where p = pressure of steam, MN/m^2 (kgf/mm^2); σ_t = allowable stress on the cover plate,

$\sigma_t = 20.6$ MN/m^2 (2.10 kgf/mm^2) for C.I.; $\sigma_t = 55.0$ MN/m^2 (5.60 kgf/mm^2) for cast steel

| The root diameter of the stud | $d_r = D\sqrt{p/i\sigma_t}$ | 18.4(a) |

where i = number of studs used. It should be in multiples of 4

σ_t = working tensile stress in studs = $1.08d$, MN/m^2 ($0.11d$, kgf/mm^2)

$d \geq 20$ mm, major diameter of stud

| The maximum pitch of studs | $P_1 = 17\sqrt{t_f/P}$ | 18.4(b) |

Internal Combustion Engine Cylinder:

The diameter of a 4 stroke internal combustion engine, mm	$D = \left[\dfrac{1000 \times 4P}{(\pi/4)p_m v}\right]^{\frac{1}{2}}$ SI units(P in kw)	18.5(a)
	$D = \left[\dfrac{(75 \times 4P)}{(\pi/4)p_m v}\right]^{\frac{1}{2}}$ Metric units (P in Mhp)	18.5(b)
The thickness of the inner walls of automobile engine cylinder	$t = 0.045D + 1.5$ mm	18.6(a)
The Jacket wall thickness	$t_j = 0.032D + 1.5$ mm	18.6(b)
The water space, i.e. the distance between the outside of the cylinder and inside of the jacket:		
(a) For natural circulation cooling	$t_w = 8$ to 11 mm	18.6(c)
(b) For pump circulation	$t_w = 6$ to 8 mm	18.6(d)

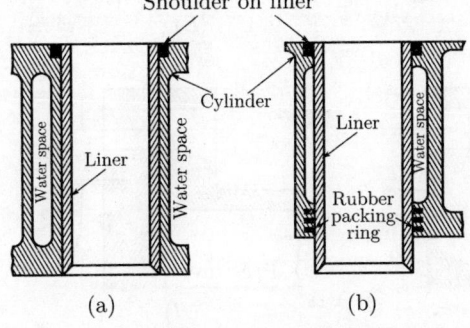

Fig. 18.3: *I.E. Engine cylinder linear*

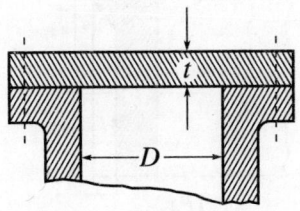

Fig. 18.4: *Cylinder cover*

Particular	Equation	Eqn. No.
Circular flat cylinder heads		
The minimum thickness of an unstayed flat head or cover plate, mm	$t_{min} = D_1 \left(\sqrt{\dfrac{kp}{\sigma_d}} \right)$	18.7(a)

where D_1 is the diameter of shortest span, mm (refer Fig. 18.5)

k is an empirical coefficient (Table 18.1)

p is the maximum inside pressure, MN/m^2 (kgf/mm^2)

σ_d is the allowable design stress, MN/m^2 (kgf/mm^2) (Table 18.2)

| The thickness of a plate uniformly loaded with a diameter of D_1 supported at the circumference, mm | $t = k_1 D_1 (\sqrt{p/\sigma_d})$ | 18.7(b) |

where k_1 is the coefficient (refer Table 18.3)

The maximum deflection of the cover plate $y = k_2 D_1^4 \dfrac{p}{Et^3}$

where k_2 is the coeffficient (refer Table 18.3)

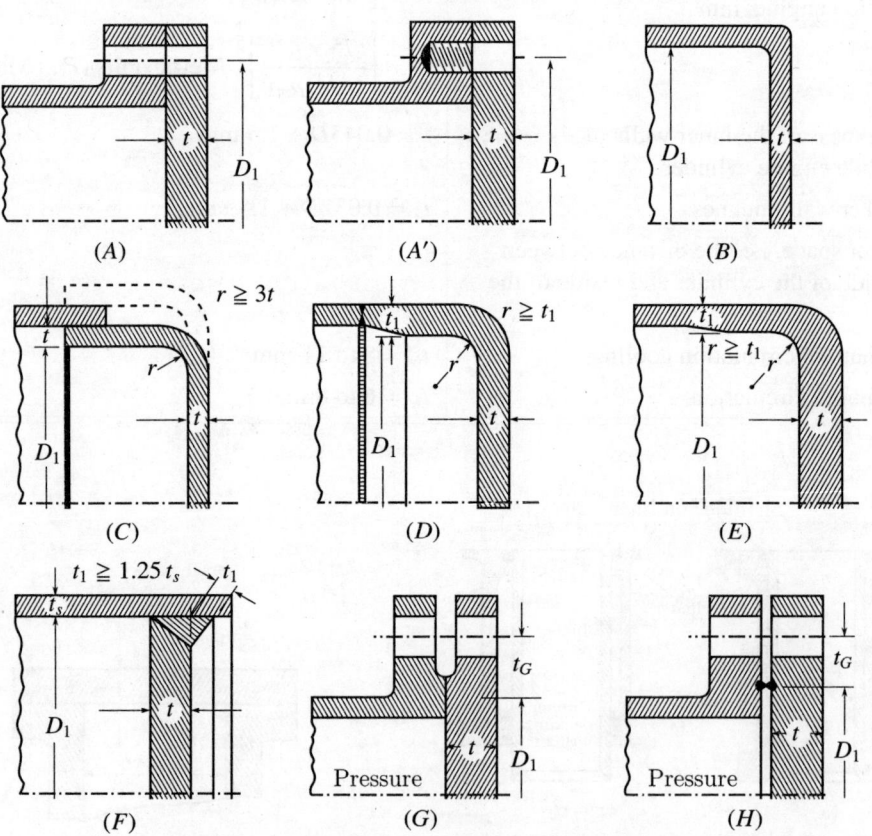

Fig. 18.5: *Types of cylinder heads and covers*

Particular	Equation	Eqn. No.
When a flat cast iron plate with a diameter D_1 and sujected to a load F distributed uniformly over an area $\frac{1}{4}\pi D^2$		
(a) Supported freely at the circumference		
(i) the thickness	$t = 1.2 \sqrt{\left(1 - \frac{0.67D}{D_1}\right)\frac{F}{\sigma_d}}$	18.7(c)
(ii) the deflection	$y = \left(\frac{0.12D_1^2 F}{Et^3}\right)$	18.7(d)
(b) Fixed rigidly around the circumference		
(i) the thickness	$t = 0.65 \sqrt{\frac{F}{\sigma_d} \log_e\left(\frac{D_1}{D}\right)}$	18.7(e)
(ii) the deflection	$y = \left(\frac{0.055D_1^2 F}{Et^3}\right)$	18.7(f)
The thickness of a flat cylinder head, mm	$t = 0.31D \sqrt{p/\sigma_d}$	18.7(g)

where p = maximum pressure inside the cylinder, MN/m^2 (kgf/mm^2)

$\quad\quad \sigma_d$ = allowable working stress; σ_d = 82.40 MN/m^2 (8.40 kgf/mm^2) low carbon cast steel

$\quad\quad\quad$ = 34.32 MN/m^2 (3.50 kgf/mm^2) for C.I.

$\quad\quad\quad$ = 42.00 MN/m^2 (4.28 kgf/mm^2) for Aluminum alloys

$\quad\quad\quad$ = 55.00 MN/m^2 (5.60 kgf/mm^2) for Nickel Cast Iron

Particular	Equation	Eqn. No.
The number of studs	$i = 0.015\,D + 4$	18.8
The flange thickness	$t_1 = 1.25d$ to $1.5d$; $t_1 > 1.10t$ to $1.25t$	18.9(a)
where d is the diameter of bolt, mm		
Length from the inside edge of cylinder to the centre of bolt, mm	$l = 1.25d$ to $1.50d$	18.9(b)
The depth (t_o) of tapped hole for studs inside the cylinder, mm		

	$t_0 = 1.25d$ in steel castings	
	$\quad = 1.50d$ to $1.75d$ in cast iron	18.9(c)
	$\quad = 1.75d$ to $2.00d$ in aluminium	
Cover plate diameter	D' = Flange diameter − (3 to 6) mm	18.9(d)

Particular	Equation	Eqn. No.

Bolts :

The pitch, distance between two bolts to insure a tight joint

$$p_c = 7d \text{ for low pressures from } 0.35 \text{ MN/m}^2 \qquad \text{18.9(d)}$$
$$= 3.5d \text{ for pressures from (1.2 to 1.4) MN/m}^2$$
$$\not< 3d$$

Note: The pitch gradually decreases with the increase in pressure

The number of bolts $\qquad i^* = 0.015D + 4 \qquad\qquad$ 18.9(e)

Steam Engine pistons:

(a) *Proportions of cast iron pistons*   18.10(a)

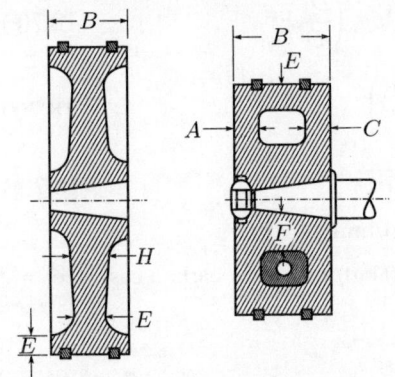

Fig. 18.6(a): *Cast iron pistons*

$$A = 0.4x$$
$$B = 1.5x \text{ to } 2.5x$$
$$C = 0.45x$$
$$D = 0.65x$$
$$E = 0.55x$$
$$F = 0.76x$$

(b) *Proportions of cast steel pistons*

$A = 0.48x$ for high pressure cylinder piston

$\quad = 0.54x$ for intermediate pressure cylinder piston

$\quad = 0.64x$ for low pressure cylinder piston

$C = 0.33x$ for high pressure cylinder piston

$\quad = 0.34x$ for intermediate pressure cylinder piston

$\quad = 0.38x$ for low-pressure cylinder piston

$B = 1.8x$ to $3.1x$, average $2.4x$

$E = 3.8x$ to $5.4x$, average $4.6x$

$F = 0.74x$

$H = 1.5x$ to $2.7x$, average $2.1x$

$\theta = 30°$

where $x = 0.1852D \sqrt{p}$ SI units

$\quad\quad = 0.58 D \sqrt{p}$ Metric units

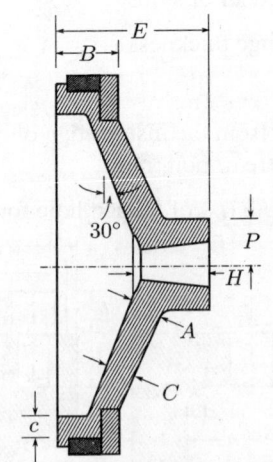

Fig. 18.6(b): *Cast steel piston*

---

*Note: The number of bolts must be multiples of 2 or 3 such as 4, 6, 8, 12 etc.

Particular	Equation	Eqn. No.
Diameter of piston Rod:		
The diameter of piston rod	$d = D\sqrt{p/\sigma_d}$	18.11

where p = unbalance pressure or difference between the steam inlet and

the exhaust pressure, MN/m^2 (kgf/mm^2)

σ_d = allowable stress in the piston rod, (in calculating σ_d, take the

factor of safety 10 for double acting engines and 8 for single acting

engines on the ultimate strength)

The inertia force of the reciprocating parts on the piston, N (kgf)	$F = 0.004032rn^2W_R\left(\cos\theta \pm \dfrac{\cos 2\theta}{n_1}\right)$	18.12

where r = crank radius, mm; W_R is the weight of reciprocating parts, N(kgf)

l = length of the connecting rod, mm; $n_1 = l/r$

θ = crank angle from the dead centre, positive sign is to be taken from inner

dead centre while the negative sign from outer dead centre

Trunk Pistons:		
The thickness of piston head (Table 18.4)	$t_1 = 0.43D\sqrt{p/\sigma_d}$	18.13(a)

where p is the fluid pressure, MN/m^2 (kgf/mm^2); D is the diameter of piston, mm

σ_d = allowable tensile stress,

= 38 MN/m^2 (3.90 kgf/mm^2) for good close grained cast iron or aluminium

alloys, with ultimate tensile strength of 137.0 MN/m^2 (14 kgf/mm^2)

= 55 MN/m^2 (5.6 kgf/mm^2) for Nickel Cast iron, semi-steel or special aluminium

alloy having ultimate tensile strength of 206 MN/m^2 (21 kgf/mm^2)

= 82.5 MN/m^2 (8.4 kgf/mm^2) for forged steel

An empirical formula to determine the thickness of the cast iron automobile engine piston head, mm	$t_1 = 0.032D + 1.5$mm	18.13(b)
The thickness of the Crown from the consideration of heat flow, mm	$t_1 = \dfrac{D^2 q}{1600K(T_c - T_e)}$	18.13(c)

Particular	Equation	Eqn. No.
where q = heat flow from gases, J/s m^2 (kgf m/s m^2), depends upon the piston material, mean effective pressure and stroke-bore ratio		
= 32000 to 128000 (3260 to 13050) for cast iron pistons in 4 stroke engines		
q = 64000 to 256000 (6525 to 26100) for aluminium pistons		
K = heat conductivity, J/sm^2°C/ mm (kgf m/s m^2°C/mm) length		
= 460 (46.91) for C.I.; K = 1600 (163.2) for Aluminium		
T_c = temperature at the centre, °C		
= 444°C for C.I. and 275°C for Aluminium		
T_e = temperature at the edge, °C		
$(T_c - T_e)$ = 222°C for cast iron and $(T_c - T_e)$ = 111° C for aluminium		
The maximum thickness of the piston barrel	$t_3 = 0.03D + b + 4.5$ mm	18.13(d)
where $b = t_r + 0.4$ mm, depth of ring grooves, mm		
t_r = radial width of piston ring, mm		
The wall thickness towards the open end of the piston, mm	$t_4 = 0.25t_3$ to $0.35t_3$	18.13(f)
The length of the piston*	$L = D$ to $1.5D$	18.14(a)
The stroke (Table 18.6)	$L_s = 1.3D$ to $1.4D$	18.14(b)

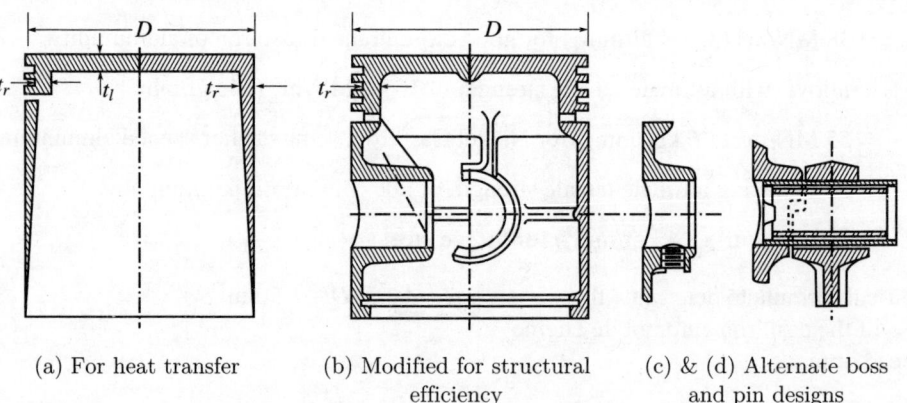

(a) For heat transfer   (b) Modified for structural   (c) & (d) Alternate boss
                                    efficiency   and pin designs

Fig. 18.6: *Trunk pistons*

*In aero engines the length of the piston may be as low as 0.75D, but in most medium and high speed engines it is about 1.5D. Lorry Diesel engines may have rather longer pistons, and in stationary and marine engines this may be as much as 2.5 D.

Particular	Equation	Eqn. No.
The diameter of the piston pin	$d = \dfrac{\pi D^2 p_{max}}{4 l_1 p_b}$	18.15(a)

where $l_1 = k_p d$, length of the gudgeon pin bearing, mm

k_p = 1.5 for petrol and gas engines and 2 for oil engines

p_b = bearing pressure

= 12.4 MN/m^2 (1.26 kgf/mm^2) for gas engines

= 15.0 MN/m^2 (1.54 kgf/mm^2) for oils engines

= 15.7 MN/m^2 (1.60 kgf/mm^2) for automotive engines

Another formula to determine the length of the gudgeon pin bearing	l_1 = 0.45D to 0.5D if it oscillates in the connecting rod	18.15(b)
	= 0.62D if it oscillates in the piston bosses	

To check the strength of the piston pin:

The bending stress	$\sigma_b = \dfrac{F_p D}{18 Z}$	18.16

where σ_b = bending stress

≤ 82.0 MN/m^2 (8.4 kgf/mm^2) for case hardened carbon steel

≤ 137.0 MN/m^2 (14.0 kgf/mm^2) for heat-treated alloy steel

F_p is the maximum load on the piston, N

Z is the section modulus, mm^3

Proportions of the Piston Rings:

The radial thickness of the cast iron snap ring	$t_r = D \sqrt{3 p_r / \sigma}$	18.17(a)

where σ = allowable stress for Cast iron

= 82.0 to 110 MN/m^2 (8.4 to 11.2 kgf/mm^2)

p_r = magnitude of radial pressure on the piston rings, MN/m^2 (kgf/mm^2) (Table 18.9)

The depth 'h' of the piston ring	$h = 0.7 t_r$ to t_r	18.17(b)
The minimum depth of the piston ring	$h = D/10i$	18.17(c)
	where i = number of piston rings	

The total depth of piston rings (according to Unwin)

$h_{total} = D/15 + 15.2$ mm for steam engines		18.17(d)

= $D/7 + 6$ mm for gas and oil engines; and $h_{total} = D/5.5$ for petrol engines

The distance from the top to the first groove	$t_g = t_1$ to $1.2 t_1$	18.18
The lands between the ring grooves	$t_{land} = h$ or slightly less than h	18.19

Table 18.1 *Coefficients for Determining Head Thickness (Fig 18.5)*

Type of Head in Fig. 18.5	Coefficient	Remarks
A or A'...	0.162	Plate rigidly riveted or bolted to the shell flange.
B...	0.162	Integral flat head; $D_1 \leqq 600$ mm; $t \geqq 0.05D_1$.
C...	0.30	Flanged plate attached by a lap joint; $r \geqq 3t$.
D or E...	0.25	Plate butt-welded or forged integral; $r \geqq 3t_f$.
F...	0.50	Plate fusion-welded with fillet weld; throat $t_1 \geqq 1.25t_s$.
G or H...	$0.30 + K$	Bolts tend to dish the plate; K is found by the relation $K = 1.4Wt_o/HD_1$, where W = total bolt load in N; H = total pressure on area bounded by the outside diameter of the gasket, in pounds; and h_0 and d are as shown in Fig. 18.5.

Table 18.2 *Design Stresses for Bolted Flanged Heads*

Maximum Temperature (Deg C)	Minimum of Specified Range of Tensile Strength of Flange Material at Room Temperature N/mm² (kgf/mm²)					Alloy Bolt Steel N/mm²
	310	345	380	415	485	
370	74(7.55)	82(8.36)	90(9.18)	115(11.73)	98(10.00)	
400	65(6.63)	72(7.34)	80(8.16)	87(8.87)	101(10.30)	87(8.87)
425	56(5.71)	62(6.32)	68(6.93)	75(7.65)	87(8.87)	75(7.65)
450	47(4.80)	52(5.30)	57(5.81)	62(6.32)	73(7.44)	62(6.32)
480	37(3.77)	42(4.28)	46(4.70)	50(5.10)	58(5.91)	50(5.10)
510	28(2.86)	32(3.26)	34(3.47)	37(3.77)	44(4.50)	37(3.77)

Table 18.3 *Coefficients in Formulas for Cover Plates*

Material of Cover Plate	Method of Holding Edges	Circular Plate		Rectangular Plate		Elliptical Plate
		k_1	k_2	k_3	k_4	k_5
Cast iron...	Supported, free	0.54	0.038	0.75	1.73	1.5
	Fixed	0.44	0.010	0.62	1.4; 1.6*	1.2
Mild steel...	Supported, free	0.42	...	0.60	1.38	1.2
	Fixed	0.35	...	0.49	1.12; 1.28	0.9

* With gasket.

Table 18.4 *Thickness of Piston Head*

Type of Engine	Piston Material	Four Stroke	Two Stroke
Compression-ignition oil engines	Cast iron	0.11D – 0.13D	0.16D – 0.18D
-do-	Aluminium	0.13D – 0.16D	0.17D – 0.20D
Spark ignition gas engines	Cast iron	0.12D – 0.14D	0.20D – 0.23D

Table 18.5 *Recommended Piston Speed*

Class of Engine	Speed of Piston in m/s
Ordinary direct-acting pumping engines	0.45 – 0.65
Ordinary horizontal engines	1.00 – 2.00
Horizontal compound and Triple-expansion engines	2.00 – 4.00
Ordinary marine engines	2.00 – 3.25
Locomotive engines (mail)	4.00 – 5.00
Internal combustion engine	3.25 – 18.00

Table 18.6 *Stroke-Bore Ratio*

Class of Engine	Ration, L_s/D
Ordinary horizontal mill engines	1.50 to 2.00
Vertical quick-running engines	1.25 to 1.60
Locomotive engines	1.20 to 1.55
Internal combustion engines	0.90 to 1.90
Air-cooled air-craft engines	1.00

Table 18.7 *Values of Inertia Factor* ($\cos\theta + \cos 2\theta/n_1$)

Crank Angle θ from Top Dead Centre	Ratio of connecting rod length to crank length, l/r					
	3.75	4.0	4.25	4.50	4.75	5.30
0	1.267	1.253	1.235	1.222	1.210	1.200
10	1.236	1.219	1.206	1.194	1.183	1.175
20	1.144	1.131	1.120	1.110	1.101	1.093
30	0.999	0.991	0.984	0.977	0.971	0.966
40	0.812	0.809	0.807	0.804	0.803	0.801
50	0.597	0.599	0.602	0.604	0.606	0.608
60	0.367	0.375	0.382	0.389	0.395	0.400
70	0.138	0.150	0.162	0.172	0.181	0.189
80	−0.077	−0.061	−0.047	−0.350	−0.024	−0.014
90	−0.267	−0.250	−0.235	−0.222	−0.210	−0.200
100	−0.425	−0.408	−0.395	−0.382	−0.372	−0.361
110	−0.546	−0.543	−0.522	−0.512	−0.512	−0.495
120	−0.633	−0.625	−0.618	−0.611	−0.605	−0.660
130	−0.689	−0.686	−0.684	−0.681	−0.679	−0.677
140	−0.723	−0.723	−0.725	−0.727	−0.729	−0.731
150	−0.733	−0.741	−0.748	−0.755	−0.761	−0.766
160	−0.733	−0.748	−0.760	−0.769	−0.779	−0.786
170	−0.733	−0.750	−0.764	−0.776	−0.787	−0.797
180	−0.733	−0.750	−0.765	−0.778	−0.790	−0.800

Table 18.8 *Weights of Reciprocating Parts*

Types of Engine	Weight W/A, MN/m^{2*} of Piston Area	
	Spark Ignition	**Compression Ignition**
Single Acting Engine		
Air-craft ..	$1.50 \times 10^{-3} - 2.75 \times 10^{-3}$	$2.06 \times 10^{-3} - 3.10 \times 10^{-3}$
Automobile ..	$2.06 \times 10^{-3} - 3.40 \times 10^{-3}$	–
Truck and tractor ..	$2.40 \times 10^{-3} - 5.15 \times 10^{-3}$	$2.40 \times 10^{-3} - 5.15 \times 10^{-3}$
Medium speed stationary ..	$10.30 \times 10^{-3} - 27.50 \times 10^{-3}$	$10.30 \times 10^{-3} - 30.90 \times 10^{-3}$

*Values in Metric units (kgf/mm^2 of piston area) can be obtained by dividing the given values with 9.8067

Table 18.9 *Magnitude of Radial Pressure of the Piston Rings on the Cylinder Barrel (according to Unwin)*

Type of engine	Steam Engines			Gas or Oil engines	Petrol engines
	H.p.	**I.P.**	**L.P.**		
p_r MN/m^2	0.02746	0.02060	0.01372	0.02402–0.03090	0.02746–0.03432
(kgf/mm^2)	(0.0028)	(0.0021)	(0.0014)	(0.00245–0.00315)	(0.0028–0.0035)

References

[1] Bhattacharya, S. C., Basu Mallik, J. R., *"Machine Design"*, Basu Mallik & Co., Calcutta, 1966.

[2] Vallance, A., Doughtle, V. L., *"Design of Machine Members"*, 3rd edition, McGraw Hill Book Company, 1951.

19

Connecting Rod

Particular	Equation	Eqn. No.
Assuring that the connecting rod has a uniform cross-section, the magnitude of the intertia force, N(kgf) (Fig. 19.1)	$F_i = \dfrac{Wv^2}{2gr} \sin\phi$	19.1(a)
The maximum inertia force, N(kgf)	$F_i = \dfrac{Wv^2}{2gr} = \left(\dfrac{2\pi^2}{g}\right) wAlrn^2 \times 10^{-12}$	19.1(b)
The maximum bending moment produced by the inertia force N-mm (kgf-mm)	$M = \dfrac{2F_i l}{9\sqrt{3}} = 0.2584 \times 10^{-12} wAl^2 rn^2$	19.1(c)
The maximum inertia bending stress or whipping stress, MN/m² (kgf/mm²)	$\sigma_b = \dfrac{M}{Z} = 0.2584 \times 10^{-12} wAl^2 rn^2 / Z$	19.1(d)

Where l is the length of the connecting rod, mm; r is the crank radius, mm

A is the area of cross-section, mm²; $v = \dfrac{2\pi rn}{1000}$, crank velocity, m/s

w is the weight of unit volume of rod, N/m³(kg/m³)

$g = 9.81$ m/s², acceleration due to gravity; n is the speed of crank, rev/s

$W = wAl \times 10^{-9}$ weight of the connection rod (without including ends), N(kgf)

Z is the section modulus of mean section of rod, mm³

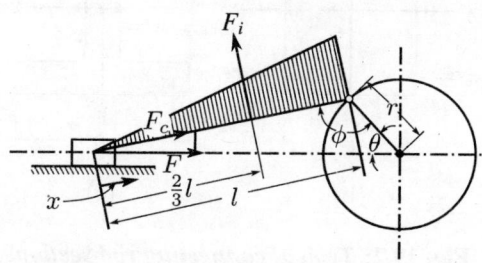

Fig. 19.1: *Forces acting on a connecting rod*

Note : The inertia force acts at a distance of $(2/3)l$ from the wrist pin.

Particular	Equation	Eqn.No.
The value of the crank angle, θ at which the bending moment is maximum for I.E. Engines (According to B.B. low), deg.	$\theta = 90 - \dfrac{3500}{(n_1 + 7.82)^2}$	19.2

When $n_1 = l/r$, ratio of length to radius

Treating the body of the connecting rod as a column with pin connected at both ends, the stress due to axial load (Rankine-Gordon formula), MN/m^2 (kgf/mm^2)	$\sigma_{cr} = \dfrac{F_c}{A} = \dfrac{\sigma_c}{1 + K(l/k)^2}$	19.3

where F_c is the crippling load, i.e. axial load on the rod due to steam or gas pressure

corrected for inertia effects of the piston and other reciprocating parts, N(kgf)

σ_c = allowable unit stress for designing MN/m^2 (kgf/m^2)

K = constant = 1/25000, for steel rod having both ends fixed

K = 4/25000 for steel rod, pin connected at both ends so that

the rod is free to bend in any plane

k = radius of gyration of cross-section about an axis

parallel to the point of the end joints (Fig. 19.2) (Table 1.3)

= $d/4$ for a circular section of diameter 'd'

= $0.289h$ for a rectangular section of depth 'h'

$= \left| \dfrac{bh^3 - b_1 h_1^3}{12(bh - b_1 h_1)} \right|^{\frac{1}{2}}$ for an I-section

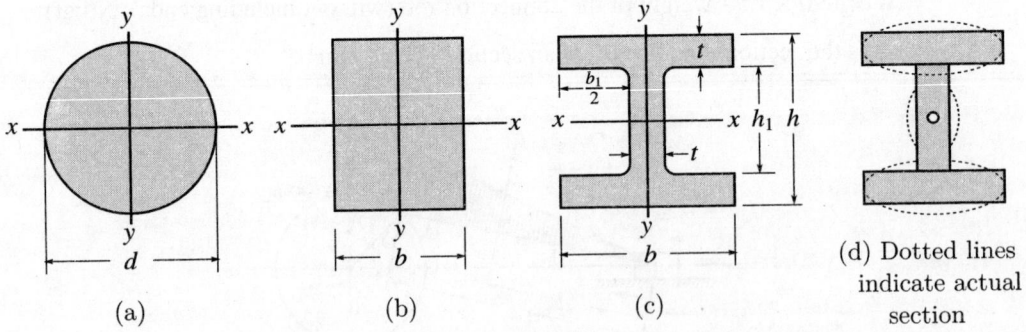

(d) Dotted lines indicate actual section

Fig. 19.2: *Typical connecting rod sections*

Particular	Equation	Eqn. No.
Reciprocating motion:		
The inertia force of the reciprocating parts	$F = \dfrac{1000 W_r v^2}{gr}\left(\cos\theta \pm \dfrac{\cos 2\theta}{n_1}\right)$	19.8(a)
	$= \dfrac{4\pi^2}{g} \times 10^{-3} rn^2 W_r\left(\cos\theta \pm \dfrac{\cos 2\theta}{n_1}\right)$	19.8(b)

where θ = crank angle from the dead centre (positive sign is to be taken
from inner dead centre while the negative sign from outer dead centre)

W_r = weight of the reciprocating parts, N (kgf)

$n_1 = l/r$; v is the crank velocity, m/s; r is the crank radius, mm; $g = 9.81$ m/s^2

The maximum value of inertia force F occurs when $0 = 0$ i.e. at the head-end dead centre	$F_{1\,\text{max}} = \dfrac{4\pi^2}{g} \times 10^{-3} rn^2 W_r\left(1 + \dfrac{1}{n_1}\right)$	19.9
At the crank-end dead centre when $\theta = 180°$, F attains the maximum negative value, acting in the opposite direction	$F_{2\,\text{max}} = \dfrac{4\pi^2}{g} \times 10^{-3} rn^2 W_r\left(1 - \dfrac{1}{n_1}\right)$	19.10
The ratio of l/r		

$l/r = 5$ to 7 for stationary steam engines; $l/r = 4$ to 5 for ordinary marine engines;

l/r 5.4 to 6 locomotive engines; $l/r = 3.2$ to 4 for I.C. engines

Cross-Section :		
In order to be equally resistant to buckling in either plane, the relation between the moment of inertias (Eulers Equation)	$I_{xx} = 4I_{yy}$	19.11
Small End and Big End :		
Length of bearing at small end	$l_1 = 0.45D$ to $0.5D$	19.12(a)
The ratio of length to diameter at small end (Refer Eqn. 18.15)	$l_1/d = 1.5$ to 2.0	19.12(b)
The diameter of crank pin (Refer Eqn. 3.13)	$dp_1 = 0.67D$ to $0.73D$	19.12(c)
The length of crank pin bearing (Refer Eqn. 3.14)	$l_p = 0.5 d_{p1}$ to $1.5 d_{p1}$	19.12(d)
Cap Thickness:		
The maximum bending moment, Nmm(kgf-mm)	$M = F_i l_3/6$	19.13(a)
The thickness of the cap, mm	$t_c = \sqrt{(6M/l_3\sigma_d)}$	19.13(b)

Particular	Equation	Eqn. No.

Where F_i is the inertia force due to reciprocating masses, MN/m^2(kgf/mm^2)

σ_d is the allowable stress in compression (use factor of safety

of 6 on yield stress), MN/m^2(kgf/mm^2)

l_3 = distance from centre to centre of bolts, mm

= bearing diameter d_{p1} + 2 (thickness of bearing shell + thickness of brearing)

+ bolt diameter d_b + allowance (3 mm to 10 mm)

Note : I-Section has been considered so that from Eulers equation $I_{xx} = 4I_{yy}$ for equal strength in both the planes (plane of motion and perpendicular plane) is satisfied. The dimensions width $B = 4t$ and Depth $H = 5t$ of I-Section give a value of $I_{xx} = 3.2I_{yy}$, where t is the thickness of the section.

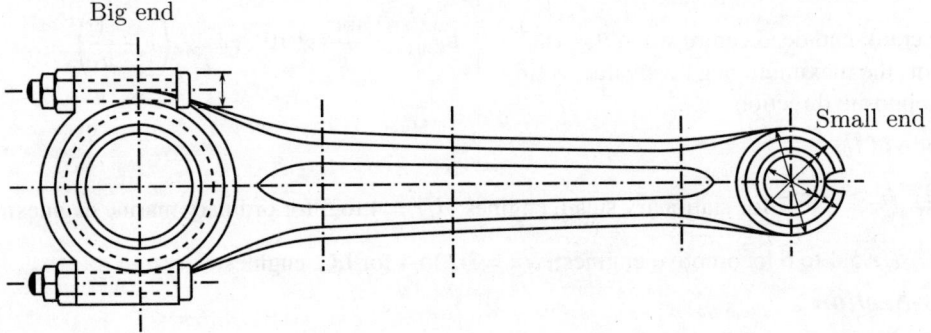

Fig. 19.3: *Forged connecting rod*

References

[1] Siegel, M. J., Maleev, V. L., Hartman, J. B., *"Mechanical Design of Machines"* 4th edition, International Text Book Company, 1965.

[2] Bhattacharya, S. C., Basu Mallik, J. E., "Machine Design", Basu Mallik & Co., Calcutta, 1966.

[3] Taylor, J. E., Wrigley, J. S., *"Engineering Design"*, Sir Isaac Pitman & Sons. Ltd., 1960.

[4] Vallance, A., Doughtie V. L., *"Design of Machine Members"*, 3rd Edition McGraw Hill Book Co., 1951.

[5] Low, D. A., *"A Pocket Book for Mechanical Engineers"*, Longmans, Green & Co. Ltd., London, 1955.

Table 19.1 *Strength of Some Varieties of Steel*

Material	Ultimate strength MN/m² (kgf/mm²)	Yield point MN/m² (kgf/mm²)	Elastic limit MN/m² (kgf/mm²)
Carbon steel (C-0.05% to 0.15%)	412 (42.0)	268 (27.3)	213 (21.7)
Carbon steel (C-0.15% to 0.25%)	460 (46.9)	295 (30.1)	240 (24.5)
Carbon steel (C-0.25% to 0.35%)	480 (49.0)	316 (32.2)	288 (29.4)
Carbon steel (C-0.35% to 0.45%)	585 (59.5)	378 (38.5)	343 (35.0)
Nickel steel (Ni-3.25% to 3.75%) (a) water quenched at 430°C	530 (53.9)	343 (35.0)	310 (31.5)
(b) water quenched at 700°C	960 (98.0)	755 (77.0)	— —

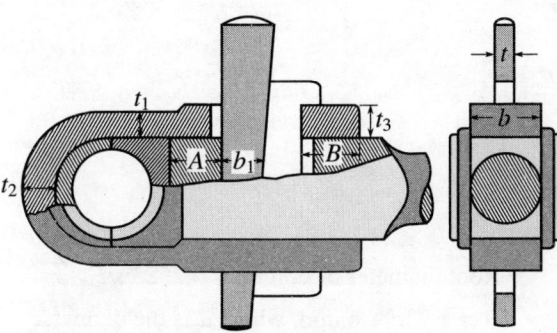

Fig. 19.4: *Common Strap End*

$t_1 = F_c/2b\sigma_d$; $t_2 = 1.2t_1$ to $1.5t_1$

$A = 2t_1$; $B = 2.5t_1$

$b_1 = 1.5d$; $t = 0.25b_1$

F_c = Maximum pull on the connecting rod, N (kgf)

σ_d = safe tensile stress for the material, MN/m² (kgf/mm²)

= 41.2 MN/m² (4.2 kgf/mm²) for wrought iron

= 48.0 MN/m² (4.9 kgf/mm²) for steel

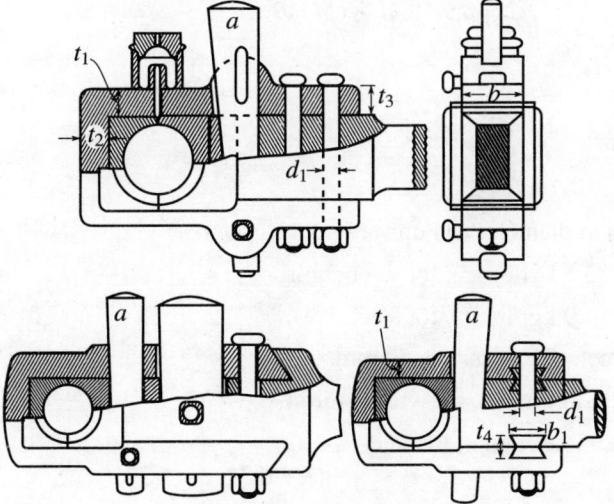

Fig. 19.5: *Fixed Strap end*

$$t_1 = \frac{F_c}{2b\sigma_d}$$
$t_2 = 1.2t_1$ to $1.5t_1$

$d_1 = 0.109 \sqrt{F_c}$ for wrought iron $\Big\}$ SI

= 0.096 $\sqrt{F_c}$ for steel units

$d_1 = 0.34 \sqrt{F_c}$ for wrought iron $\Big\}$ Metric

= 0.30 $\sqrt{F_c}$ for steel units

$d_1 = 0.7t_1$ $b_1 = 1.9t_1$ $t_4 = 1.3t_1$

Thickness of the cotter = $0.25b$

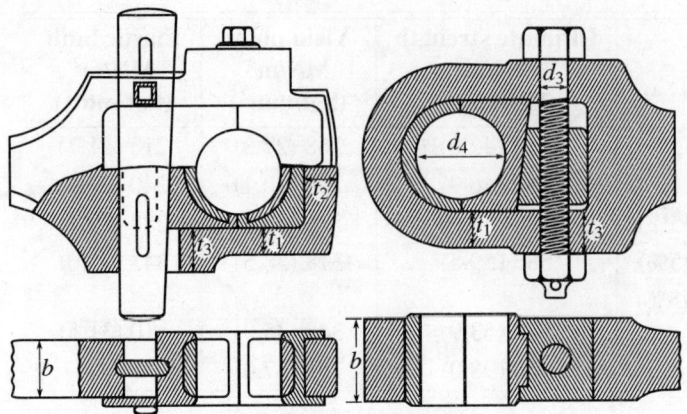

$$t_1 = \frac{F_c}{2b\sigma_d}$$
$$t_2 = t_3 = 1.2t \text{ to } 1.5t$$
$$d_2 = 0.2d_4 \text{ to } 0.3d_4$$

Fig. 19.6: *Solid or Box End*

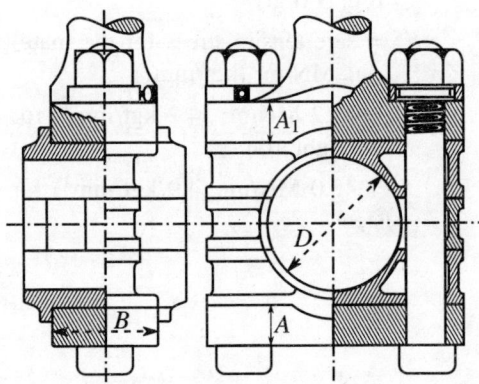

Root diameter of bolt $d_1 = 0.2525 \sqrt{F_c/\sigma_d}$

$B > 1.73d + 4$ mm, where d is the diameter
    of bolt over the screw thread

$A = 1.086d_1 \sqrt{D_1/B}$; $A_1 = A$ to $1.2A$

$C = 0.9d$ to $d \geq (1/2)B$

Fig. 19.7: *Marine type of connecting rod end*

For bolts 50 mm in diameter and upwards,
use $\sigma_d = 34.5$ MN/m^2 (3.5 kgf/mm^2), for wrought iron
$= 48.0$ MN/m^2 (4.9 kgf/mm^2), for steel
For smaller diameter i.e. less than 50 mm,
$\sigma \ngtr 20.6$ MN/m^2 (2.1 kgf/mm^2), for wrought iron
$\sigma \ngtr 29.0$ MN/m^2 (2.95 kgf/mm^2), for steel

20

Vibrations

Symbols:

Item	Rectilinear system		Rotational system	
	Symbol	Unit	Symbol	Unit
Time	t	s	t	s
Displacement	x	m	θ	rad
Velocity	$\dot{x}$	m/s	$\dot{\theta}$	rad/s
Acceleration	$\ddot{x}$	m/s^2	$\ddot{\theta}$	rad/s^2
Inertial mass	m	kg	J	Nms^2 (or) kg m^2
Spring constant	k	N/m (or) kg/s^2	k_t	Nm (or) kg m^2/s^2
Damping coefficient	c	Ns/m (or) kg/s	c_t	Nms (or) kg m^2/s
Angular natural frequency	ω_n	rad/s	ω_n	rad/s
Natural frequency	f_n	Hz	f_n	Hz

Particular	Equation	Eqn. No.

A) Undamped free Vibrations:

Rectilinear system	Rotational or Torsional system

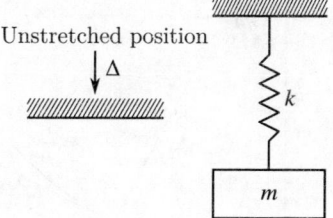

Fig. 20.1: *Spring mass system*

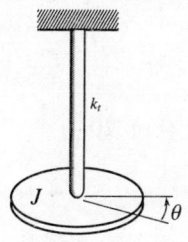

Fig. 20.2: *Torsional Pendulum*

Particular	Equation		Eqn. No.
	(i) Rectilinear	**(ii) Torsional**	
The differential equation of motion of the vibrating system	$m\ddot{x} + kx = 0$	$J\ddot{\theta} + k_t\theta = 0$	20.1
The natural period of vibration	$\tau = 2\pi\sqrt{\dfrac{m}{k}}$	$\tau = 2\pi\sqrt{\dfrac{J}{k_t}}$	20.2
	where $k = \dfrac{W}{\Delta}$	$k_t = \dfrac{\pi Gd^4}{32L}$	
The natural angular frequency of the system	$\omega_n = \sqrt{\dfrac{k}{m}} = \sqrt{\dfrac{g}{\Delta}}$	$\omega_n = \sqrt{\dfrac{k_t}{J}}$	20.3
The natural frequency	$f_n = \dfrac{1}{2\pi}\sqrt{\dfrac{k}{m}}$	$f_n = \dfrac{1}{2\pi}\sqrt{\dfrac{k_t}{J}}$	20.4
	$= \dfrac{1}{2\pi}\sqrt{\dfrac{g}{\Delta}}$		

Rayleigh's Method:

(a) *Spring mass system* (Fig. 20.3)

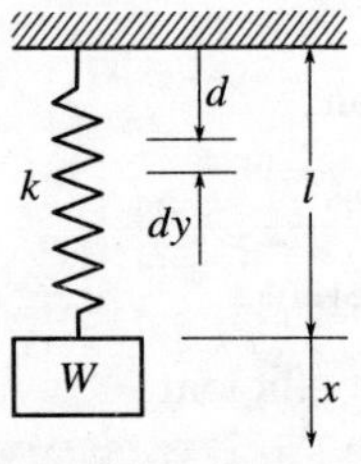

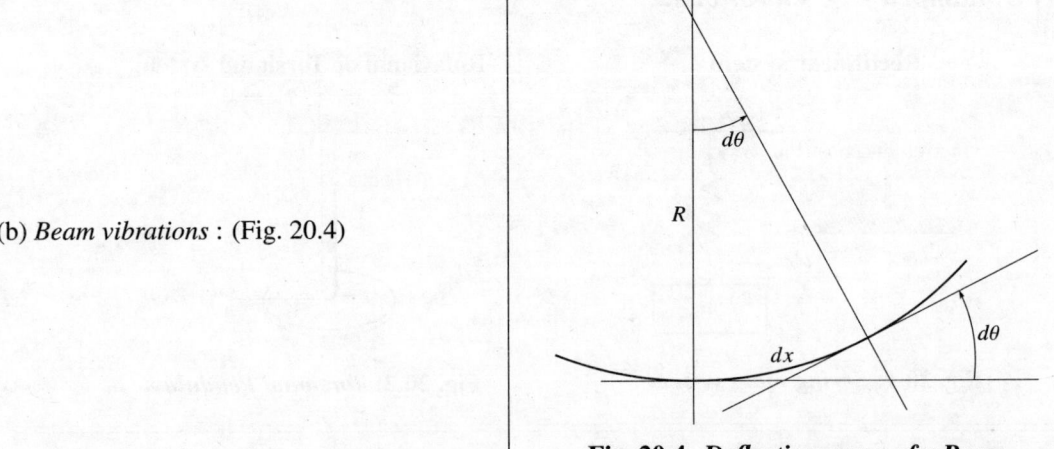

Fig. 20.3: *Spring mass system*

The natural frequency of the system
$$f_n = \frac{1}{2\pi}\sqrt{\frac{kg}{(W + \frac{1}{3}wl)}}$$
20.5

where l = length of the spring at static equilibrium

w = weight per unit length of the spring

(b) *Beam vibrations* : (Fig. 20.4)

Fig. 20.4: *Deflection curve of a Beam*

Particular	Equation	Eqn. No.
The fundamental frequency of the beam is determined from the equation	$$\omega^2 = \frac{\int EI\left(\frac{d^2y}{dx^2}\right)^2 dx}{\int y^2 dm}$$	20.6
Considering the tensile stress developed by the lateral deflection, the frequency equation	$$\omega^2 = \frac{\int EI\left(\frac{d^2y}{dx^2}\right)^2 dx + \int \frac{EA}{4}\left(\frac{dy}{dx}\right)^4 dx}{\int y^2 dm}$$	20.7

where m = mass per unit length along the beam

y = the amplitude of the assumed deflection curve

| If a beam is represented by a series of lumped weights $W_1, W_2, \ldots$, then the fundamental frequency equation is given by | $$\omega_1^2 = \frac{g(W_1 y_1 + W_2 y_2 + \ldots\ldots)}{(W_1 y_1^2 + W_2 y_2^2 + \ldots\ldots)}$$ $$= \frac{g \sum Wy}{\sum Wy^2}$$ | 20.8 |

Where $y_1, y_2\ldots$ are the static deflections of corresponding points due to the loads $W_1, W_2\ldots$ respectively

(B) Damped free Vibration:

(a) Viscous damping:

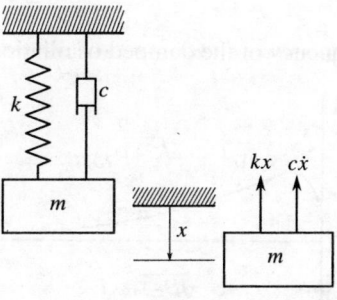

Fig. 20.5: *Free vibration with viscous damping*

The differential equation of motion (Fig. 20.5)	$m\ddot{x} + c\dot{x} + kx = 0$	20.9
The general solution for the damped free vibration	$x = Ae^{s_1 t} + Be^{s_2 t}$	20.10

where A and B are arbitrary constants whose values depend upon starting conditions,

s_1 and s_2 are constants determined by the equation,

$$s_{1,2} = -\frac{c}{2m} \pm \sqrt{\left(\frac{c}{2m}\right)^2 - \frac{k}{m}} = \left\{-\zeta \pm \sqrt{\zeta^2 - 1}\right\} \omega_n$$

where $\zeta = c/c_c$, damping ratio

c_c = critical damping = $2\sqrt{km} = 2m\omega_n$

Particular	Equation	Eqn. No.

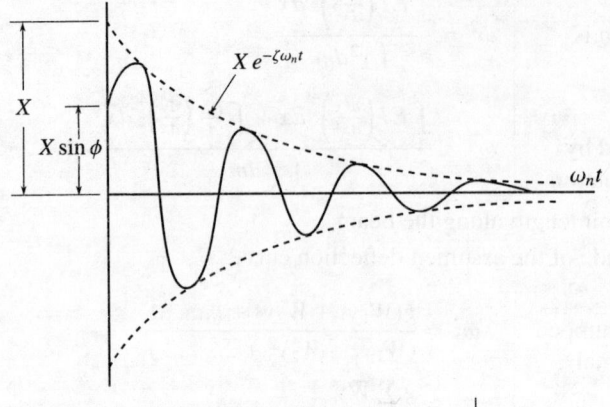

Fig. 20.6:

Damped oscillations: $\zeta < 1$

The equation for the general solution for under damping system ($\zeta < 1.0$) (Fig. 20.6)

$$x = e^{-\zeta \omega_n t}\left(Ae^{i\sqrt{1-\zeta^2}\omega_n t} + Be^{-i\sqrt{1-\zeta^2}\omega_n t}\right) = Xe^{-\zeta \omega_n t}\sin(\sqrt{1-\zeta^2}\omega_n t + \phi)$$ 20.11

The frequency of the damped oscillation

$$\omega_d = \sqrt{1-\zeta^2}\,\omega_n$$ 20.12

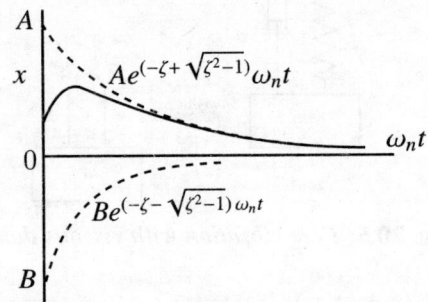

Fig. 20.7: *Aperiodic motion:*

$\zeta > 1.0$ with initial conditions x_o and v_o

The equation for the general solution for over damping system. ($\zeta > 1.0$) (Fig. 20.7)

$$x = Ae^{(-\zeta + \sqrt{\zeta^2-1})\omega_n t} + Be^{(-\zeta - \sqrt{\zeta^2-1})\omega_n t}$$ 20.13

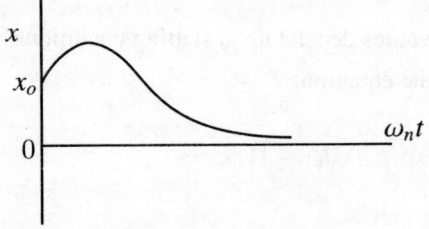

Fig. 20.8: *Critically damped motion:*

$\zeta = 1.0$ with initial conditions x_o and v_o

The equation for the general solution for critical damping ($\zeta = 1.0$) (Fig. 20.8)

$$x = (A + Bt)e^{-\omega_n t}$$ 20.14

Particular	Equation	Eqn. No.

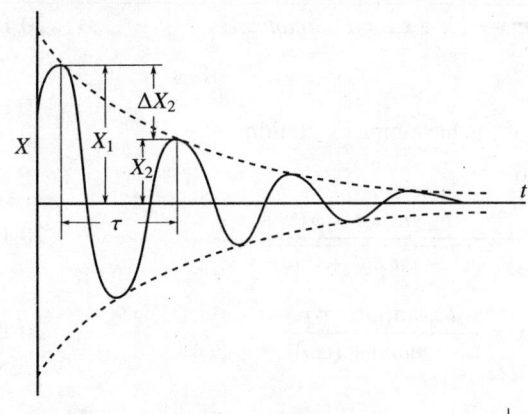

Fig. 20.9: *Rate of decay of oscillation is measured by the logarithmic decrement*

Logarithmic Decrement: (Fig. 20.9)

The logarithmic decrement

$$\delta = ln\ \frac{x_1}{x_2} = ln\ \frac{e^{-\zeta\omega_n t}}{e^{-\zeta\omega_n(t_1+\tau)}} = ln\ e^{\zeta\omega_n\tau} = \zeta\omega_n\tau = \frac{2\pi\zeta}{\sqrt{1-\zeta^2}} = \frac{1}{n}\ ln\ \frac{x_o}{x_n} = \frac{\Delta U}{U} \qquad 20.15$$

where $\tau = \dfrac{2\pi}{\omega_n\sqrt{1-\zeta^2}}$, period of damped oscillation

x_n = amplitude after n cycles have elapsed; U = vibrational energy

ΔU = energy dissipated per cycle; $U_i = \frac{1}{2}kx^2$

C) *Forced Vibration with Harmonic Excitation:*

(a) Steady state solution with viscous damping:

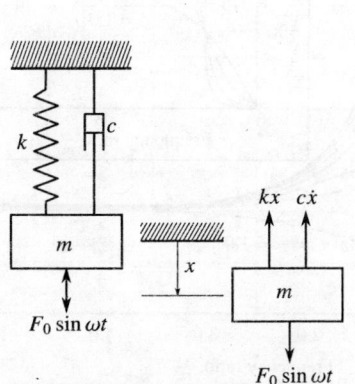

Fig. 20.10: *Forced vibration with viscous damping*

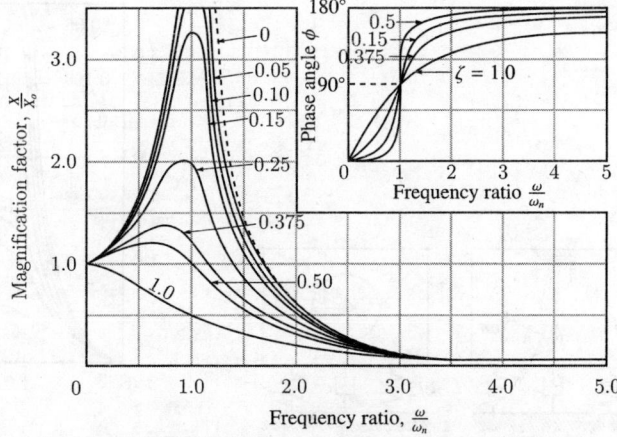

Fig. 20.11: *Plot of equations 20.19 and 20.20 for the vibration of a viscously damped system*

Vibrations

Particular	Equation	Eqn. No.
The differential equation of motion of the viscously damped spring-mass system (Fig. 20.10)	$m\ddot{x} + c\dot{x} + kx = F_o \sin\omega t$	20.16

where ω is the frequency of the harmonic excitation

The complete solution of the above equation 20.16

	$x = X_1 e^{-\zeta\omega_n t}\sin(\sqrt{1-\zeta^2}\,\omega_n t + \phi) + \dfrac{F_o\sin(\omega t - \phi)}{\sqrt{(k-m\omega^2)^2 + (c\omega)^2}}$	20.17
Steady state solution of equation 20.16	$x = \dfrac{F_o\sin(\omega t - \phi)}{(k-m\omega^2) + (c\omega)^2}$	20.18
Magnification factor (Fig. 20.11)	$\dfrac{X}{X_o} = \dfrac{1}{\sqrt{\left(1-\dfrac{m\omega^2}{k}\right)^2 + \left(\dfrac{c\omega}{k}\right)^2}} = \dfrac{1}{\sqrt{\left\{1-\left(\dfrac{\omega}{\omega_n}\right)^2\right\}^2 + \left\{2\zeta\left(\dfrac{\omega}{\omega_n}\right)\right\}^2}}$	20.19
Phase angle (Fig. 20.11)	$\tan\phi = \dfrac{\dfrac{c\omega}{k}}{1-\dfrac{m\omega^2}{k}} = \dfrac{2\zeta\left(\dfrac{\omega}{\omega_n}\right)}{1-\left(\dfrac{\omega}{\omega_n}\right)^2}$	20.20

where $X_o = \dfrac{F_o}{k}$ = zero frequency deflection of the spring-mass system under the action of a steady force F_o

(b) Reciprocating and Rotating unbalance

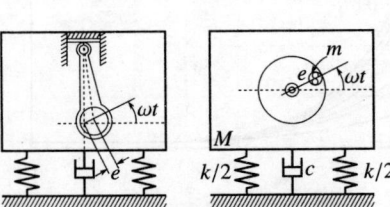

Fig. 20.12: *Periodic disturbing force resulting from a reciprocating or rotating unbalance*

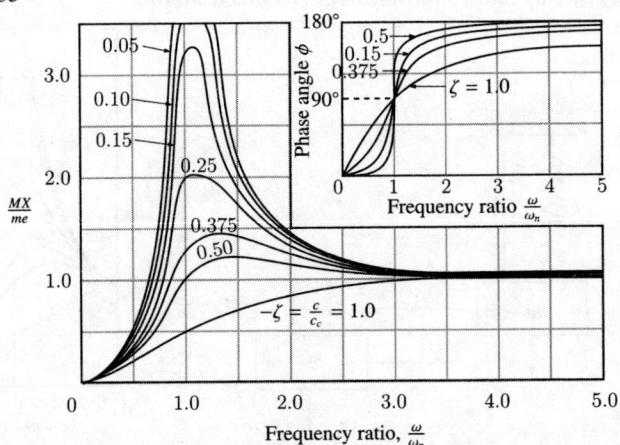

Fig. 20.13: *Plot of equations 20.22 and 20.23 for the forced vibration of a viscously damped system with a reciprocating or rotating unbalance*

Particular	Equation	Eqn. No.
The equation of motion of the system (Fig. 20.12)	$M\ddot{x} + c\dot{x} + kx = (me\omega^2)\sin\omega t$	20.21
The amplitude (Fig. 20.13) $$X = \frac{me\omega^2}{\sqrt{(k - M\omega^2)^2 + (c\omega)^2}} = \frac{\frac{m}{M}e\left(\frac{\omega}{\omega_n}\right)^2}{\sqrt{\left\{1 - \left(\frac{\omega}{\omega_n}\right)^2\right\}^2 + \left\{2\zeta\frac{\omega}{\omega_n}\right\}^2}}$$		20.22
The phase angle, (Fig. 20.13) $$\tan\phi = \frac{c\omega}{k - m\omega^2} = \frac{2\zeta\frac{\omega}{\omega_n}}{1 - \left(\frac{\omega}{\omega_n}\right)^2}$$		20.23

(c) Base Excitation

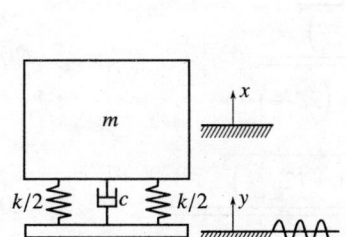

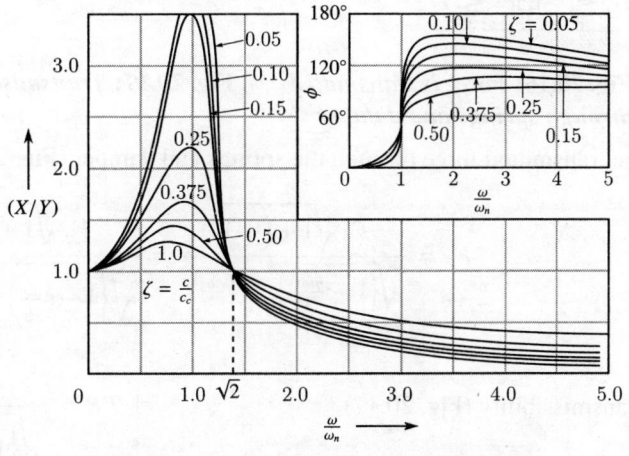

Fig. 20.14: *Base excitation of a spring mass system*

Fig. 20.15: *Plot of equations 20.25 and 20.26 for base excitation*

Particular	Equation	Eqn. No.
The differential equation of the system (Fig. 20.14)	$m\ddot{x} + c\dot{x} + kx = ky + cy$	20.24
The absolute value of the amplitude ratio (Fig. 20.15) $$\frac{X}{Y} = \sqrt{\frac{k^2 + (c\omega)^2}{(k - m\omega^2)^2 + (c\omega)^2}} = \frac{1 + \left(\frac{2\zeta\omega}{\omega_n}\right)^2}{\left\{1 - \left(\frac{\omega}{\omega_n}\right)^2\right\}^2 + \left(\frac{2\zeta\omega}{\omega_n}\right)^2}$$		20.25
The phase angle (Fig. 20.15) $$\tan\phi = \frac{mc\omega^3}{k^2\left\{1 - \left(\frac{\omega}{\omega_n}\right)^2\right\} + (c\omega)^2} = \frac{2\zeta\left(\frac{\omega}{\omega_n}\right)^3}{1 - \left(\frac{\omega}{\omega_n}\right)^2 + \left(\frac{2\zeta\omega}{\omega_n}\right)^2}$$		20.26

Particular	Equation	Eqn. No.

(d) Vibration isolation:

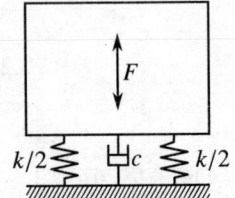

Fig. 20.17 graph showing curves labeled 0.05, 0.10, 0.15, 0.25, 0.375, 0.50, 1.0 with $\zeta = \frac{c}{c_c}$, axes Transmissibility TR (vertical) and $\frac{\omega}{\omega_n}$ (horizontal).

Fig. 20.16: *Force is transmitted through springs and damper*

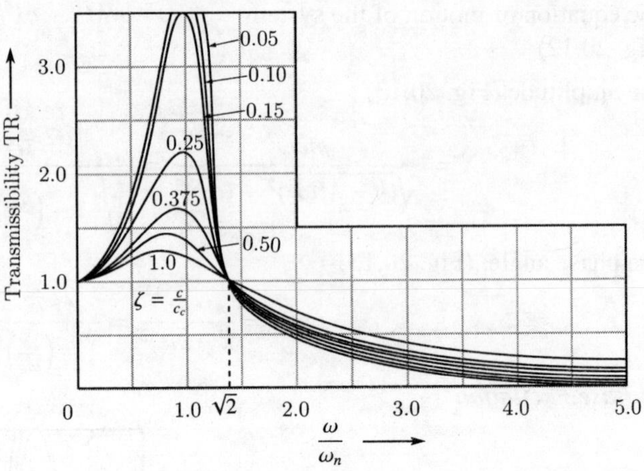

Fig. 20.17: *Transmissibility is less than 1.0 for frequency ratio $(\omega/\omega_n) > \sqrt{2}$*

The transmitted force through the springs and damper (Fig. 20.16)

$$F_T = \frac{F_o \sqrt{1 + \left(\frac{c\omega}{k}\right)^2}}{\sqrt{\left\{1 - \frac{m\omega^2}{k}\right\}^2 + \left(\frac{c\omega}{k}\right)^2}} = \frac{F_o \sqrt{1 + \left(2\zeta\frac{\omega}{\omega_n}\right)^2}}{\sqrt{\left\{1 - \left(\frac{\omega}{\omega_n}\right)^2\right\}^2 + \left(2\zeta\frac{\omega}{\omega_n}\right)^2}} \qquad 20.27$$

Transmissibility (Fig. 20.17)

$$TR = \frac{\sqrt{1 + \left(2\zeta\frac{\omega}{\omega_n}\right)^2}}{\sqrt{\left\{1 - \left(\frac{\omega}{\omega_n}\right)^2\right\}^2 + \left(2\zeta\frac{\omega}{\omega_n}\right)^2}} \qquad 20.28$$

When the damping is negligible the transmissibility

$$TR = \frac{1}{\left(\frac{\omega}{\omega_n}\right)^2 - 1} = \frac{1}{\frac{(2\pi f)^2 \Delta}{g} - 1} \qquad 20.29$$

where Δ = Static deflection of the system

(e) Whirling of Rotating Shafts:

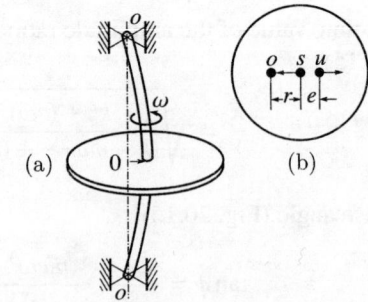

Fig. 20.18: *Whirling of shaft due to unbalance*

Particular	Equation	Eqn. No.
The dynamic deflection	$r = \dfrac{m^{\omega^2}e}{k - m\omega^2} = \dfrac{\left(\frac{\omega}{\omega_n}\right)^2 e}{1 - \left(\frac{\omega}{\omega_n}\right)^2}$	20.30

where $\omega_n = \sqrt{\dfrac{k}{m}}$, the natural frequency of lateral vibration of the shaft and disk at zero speed

The critical speed of the shaft	$\omega_c = \sqrt{\dfrac{k}{m}} = \sqrt{\dfrac{g}{\Delta}}$	20.31

Critical speed of a multi-rotor shaft system by Dunkerley equation

$$\frac{1}{\omega_c^2} = \frac{1}{\omega_s^2} + \frac{1}{\omega_1^2} + \frac{1}{\omega_2^2} + \ldots + \frac{1}{\omega_i^2} \ldots \qquad 20.32$$

where ω_s = critical speed of shaft only,
ω_1 = critical speed of shaft due to weight W_1 only
ω_2 = critical speed of shaft due to weight W_2 only
ω_i = critical speed of shaft due to weight W_i only

Torsional Vibrations:

(a) A two disk semi definite system (Fig. 20.19)

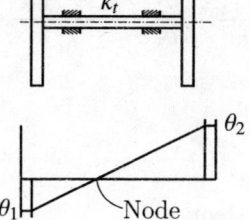

Fig. 20.19(a) : *Vibratory system*

Fig. 20.19(b) *Principal mode of vibration*

The equations of motion of the two rotors	$J_1 \ddot{\theta}_1 + K_t\theta_1 - k_t\theta_1 = 0$ $J_2 \ddot{\theta}_2 - k_t\theta_1 + k_t\theta_2 = 0$	20.33
The frequency equation	$\omega^2 \left\{ \omega^2 - \left(\dfrac{k_t}{J_1} + \dfrac{k_t}{J_2} \right) \right\} = 0$	20.34
The natural frequencies of the system	$\begin{cases} \omega_{n1} = 0 \\ \omega_{n2} = \sqrt{ k_t \left\{ \dfrac{J_1 + J_2}{J_1 J_2} \right\} } \end{cases}$	20.35
The amplitude ratio of the Principal modes	$\dfrac{\theta_1}{\theta_2} = \dfrac{k_t}{k_t - J_2\omega^2} = \dfrac{k_t - J_2\omega^2}{k_t}$	20.36

Particular	Equation	Eqn. No.

(b) A three disk semi definite system (Fig. 20.20)

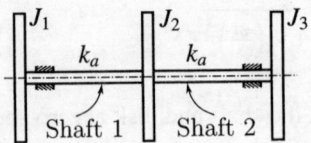

Fig. 20.20(a) : *Vibratory System*

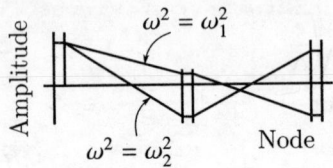

Fig. 20.20(b) : *Principal modes of vibration* $\omega_1^2 < \omega_2^2$

The equations of motion:

$$\begin{cases} J_1 \ddot{\theta}_1 + k_{t1}(\theta_1 - \theta_2) = 0 \\ J_2 \ddot{\theta}_2 + k_{t1}(\theta_1 - \theta_2) + k_{t2}(\theta_1 - \theta_3) = 0 \\ J_3 \ddot{\theta}_3 + k_{t2}(\theta_3 - \theta_2) = 0 \end{cases}$$ 20.37

The frequency equation for determining the natural frequencies of a three disk system

$$\omega^2 \left[\omega^2 - \left\{ k_{t1} \left(\frac{1}{J_1} + \frac{1}{J_2} \right) + k_{t2} \left(\frac{1}{J_2} + \frac{1}{J_3} \right) \right\} \omega^2 + k_{t1} k_{t2} \frac{J_1 + J_2 + J_3}{J_1 J_2 J_3} \right] = 0$$ 20.38

The amplitude ratios of the principal modes of vibration

$$\frac{\theta_1}{\theta_2} = \frac{k_{t1}}{k_{t1} - J_1 \omega^2}; \quad \frac{\theta_2}{\theta_3} = \frac{k_t^2 - J_3 \omega^2}{k_t^2}$$ 20.39

Geared systems: (Fig. 20.21)

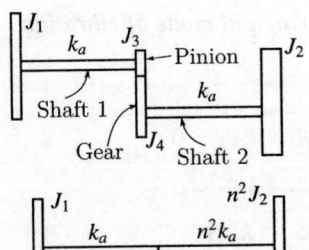

(a) Vibratory system

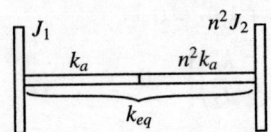

(b) Equivalent system, referring to shaft 1 and neglecting inertial effect of gears

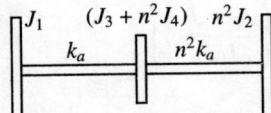

(c) Equivalent system, referring to shaft 1 and including internal effect of gears

Fig. 20.21 : *Geared Systems*

Particular	Equation	Eqn. No.
The equivalent inertia of J_2	$J_{2-eq} = n^2 J_2$	20.40
The equivalent spring constant of shaft 2	$K_{t2-eq} = n^2 k_{t2}$	20.41
Neglecting the inertial effect of the gears, the equivalent torsional spring constant	$k_{eq} = \dfrac{n^2 k_{t1} k_{t2}}{k_{t1} + n^2 k_{t2}}$	20.42
The natural frequencies	$\begin{cases} \omega_{n1} = 0 \\ \omega_{n2} = \sqrt{k_{eq}\left(\dfrac{J_1 + n^2 J_2}{n^2 J_1 J_2}\right)} \end{cases}$	20.43

where $n = \dfrac{Z_1}{Z_2}$, gear ratio

Z_1 = Number of teeth on the pinion

Z_2 = Number of teeth of the gear of shaft 2

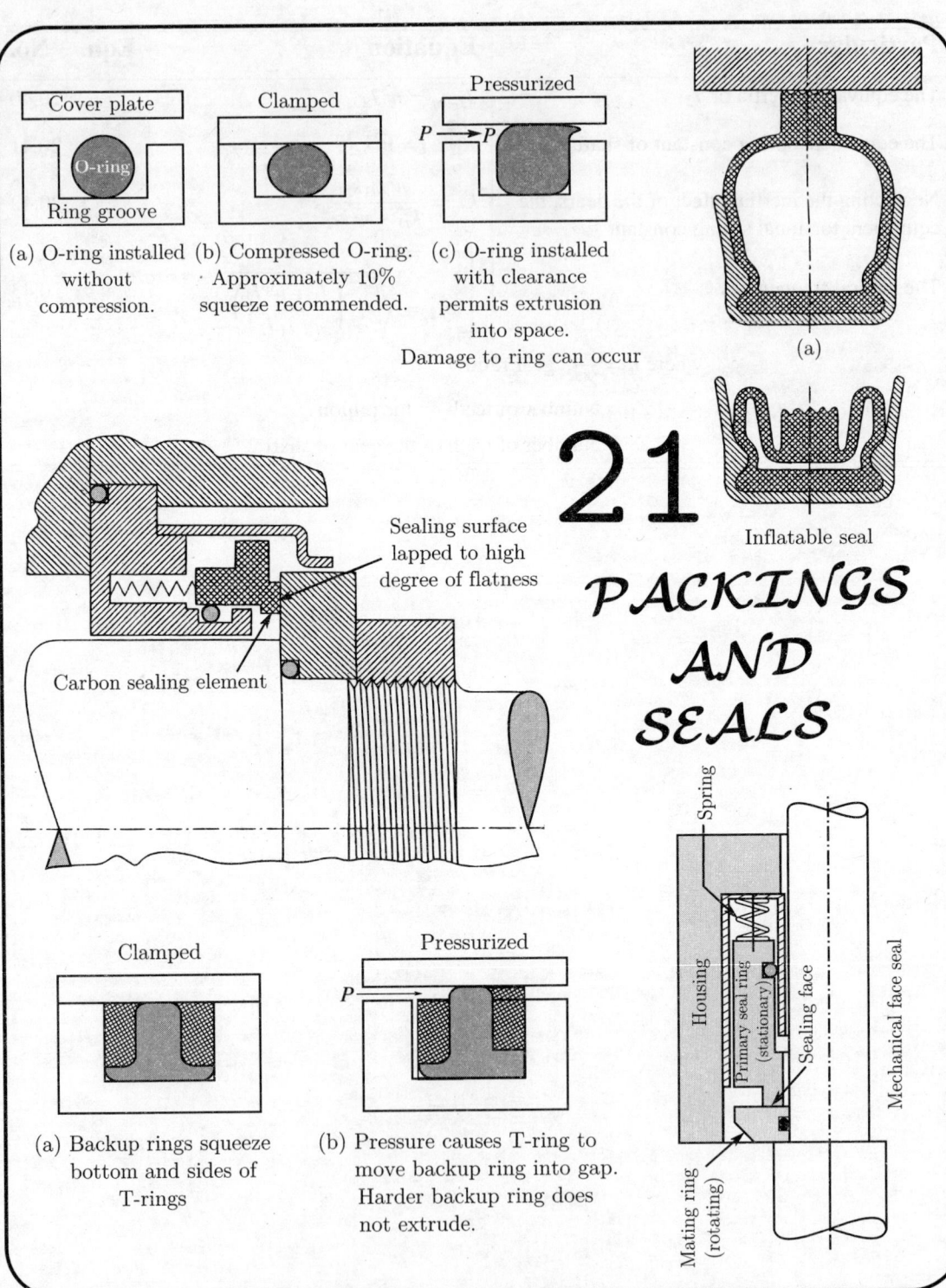

Cover plate

O-ring

Ring groove

(a) O-ring installed without compression.

Clamped

(b) Compressed O-ring. Approximately 10% squeeze recommended.

Pressurized

$P \longrightarrow P$

(c) O-ring installed with clearance permits extrusion into space. Damage to ring can occur

(a)

Inflatable seal

Sealing surface lapped to high degree of flatness

Carbon sealing element

21

PACKINGS AND SEALS

Clamped

(a) Backup rings squeeze bottom and sides of T-rings

Pressurized

P

(b) Pressure causes T-ring to move backup ring into gap. Harder backup ring does not extrude.

Spring

Housing

Primary seal ring (stationary)

Sealing face

Mating ring (rotating)

Mechanical face seal

Packings and Seals

Particular	Equation	Eqn. No.
Gaskets (Refer Fig. 21.1(a) and 21.1(b))		
Before the fluid pressure is acting, the force F_g in the bolt and on the gasket, N (kgf)	$F_g = A_g q$	21.1(a)
The force produced due to the internal fluid pressure only, N (kgf)	$F_i = A_i p$	21.1(b)
The force on the gasket required to prevent loss of pressure, N (kgf)	$F_l = A_g m p$	21.1(c)
where m is the gasket factor (Table 21.1) A_g is the effective area of the gasket, mm^2 A_i is the area subjected to internal pressure, mm^2 p is the fluid pressure, MN/m^2 (kgf/mm^2) q is the pressure on the gasket caused by tightening the bolts, MN/m^2 (kgf/mm^2)		
When the fluid pressure is acting, the bolt force F_b N(kgf)	$F_b = F_i + F_l = p(A_i + A_g m)$	21.1(d)
Equating F_g and F_b, the pressure on the gasket caused by tightening the bolts can be determined	$q = \dfrac{p(A_i + A_g m)}{A_g}$	21.1(e)
Thickness of gasket*		
$t_g = 0.25$ mm to 1.5 mm and not over 3 mm		21.2(a)
Thickness of asbestos gasket	$t_g = 0.75$ mm to 1.5 mm	21.2(b)
If the surfaces are finished, the thickness of copper gasket	$t_g \leq 0.4 mm$	21.2(c)

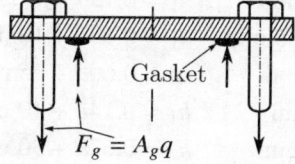
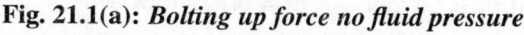

Fig. 21.1(a): *Bolting up force no fluid pressure*

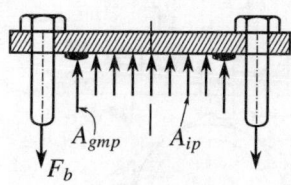

Fig. 21.1(b): *Forces when fluid pressure is acting*

---

*Ground joints without any gaskats are used for very high pressures.

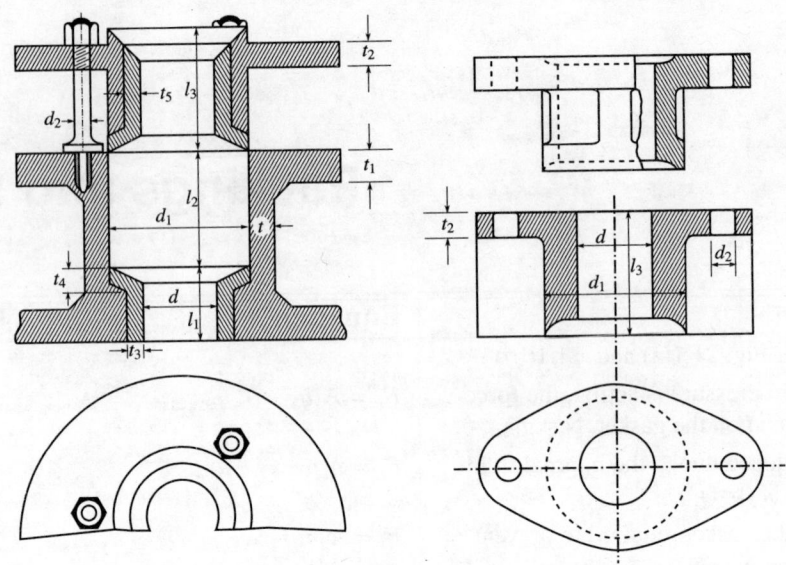

Fig. 21.2: *Stuffing Box*

Proportions:

d = diameter of rod, mm

$d_1 = 1.22d + 15$ mm

$l_1 = 0.4d + 25$ mm

$l_2 = d + 25$ mm to $1.3d + 25$ mm

$l_3 = 0.75l_2$

d_2 = diameter of bolts when two are used = $0.12d + 12.5$ mm

$t = 0.1d + 15$ mm

$t_1 = 1.4t - 0.14d + 21$ mm

$t_2 = t$

$t_3 = 0.04d + 5$ mm but not to exceed 12.5 mm

$t_4 = 0.1d + 3.3$ mm but not to exceed 25 mm

For i bolts, $d_1 = \dfrac{1.6}{\sqrt{i}}(0.12d + 12.5)$. when i is greater than two

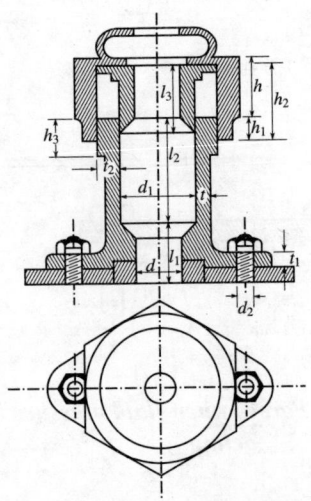

Proportions:

d = diameter of rod

$d_1 = 1.3d + 15$ mm

$d_2 = 0.15d + 12.5$ mm

$l_1 = 0.4d + 25$ mm

$l_2 = d + 37.5$ mm

$l_3 = 0.6d + 25$ mm

$t = 0.1d + 7.5$ mm

$t_1 = 0.15d + 12.5$ mm or

$t_1 = 0.13d + 10$ mm

$h = 0.60d + 25$ mm

$h_1 = 0.14d + 10$ mm

$h_2 = 0.67d + 30$ mm

$h_2 = 0.30d + 18$ mm

Fig. 21.3: *Brass stuffing box*

Particular	Equation	Eqn. No.
Packings: (a) Stuffing boxes (Refer Fig. 21.2 and Fig. 21.3)		
(b) Elastic packings		
The friction force, F_r exerted by a soft packing upon the reciprocating rod, N (kgf)	$F_r = kdp$	21.3(a)

where k = an empirical coefficient

= 0.2, when the nuts holding the gland are tightened only enough to prevent leakage

p = fluid pressure, MN/m^2 (kgf/mm^2) if p is less than 0.35 MN/m^2
(0.036 kgf/mm^2), use p = 0.35 MN/m^2 (0.036 kgf/mm^2)

The minor bolt diameter d_3 is found by equating the working strength of the bolts to the pressure p exerted by the fluid upon the gland and the frictional force F_r	$d_3 = \left[\dfrac{(d_1^2 - d^2)p + F_r}{i\sigma_d} \right]^{\frac{1}{2}}$	21.3(b)

where σ_d = 70 to 80 MN/m^2 (7.14 to 8.16 kgf/mm^2), allowable stress

(c) Self-sealing packings:

U – Collar

Particular	Equation	Eqn. No.
The approximate thickness of a U-shaped collar for great pressure (Based on the data of Houghton, Welch and Jenkins), mm	$h = 1.6d^{0.2}$	21.4(a)
The width of the collar, mm	$b = 4h$	21.4(b)
The depth of the collar, mm	$l = 1.2b$ to $1.8b$	21.4(c)
Maximum speed for leather collars[†]	$v_{max} = 1.00 m/s$	21.4(d)
Friction:		
The friction resistance, N (kgf)	$F_r = F_o + fAp$	21.5(a)

where F_o = friction force on the stuffing box when there is no fluid pressure, N (kgf)

f = coefficient of friction

= 0.01, for rubber and soft fabricated leather

= 0.15, for hard leather

Particular	Equation	Eqn. No.
Rotary motion friction:		
In the case of rotary motion, the tangential friction force	$F_r = kdp$	21.5(b)
For rotary motion the torsional resistance	$T = \dfrac{F_r d}{2} = \dfrac{kd^2 p}{2}$	21.5(c)

[†]*Note* : For high speeds use soft packing with a gland

Particular	Equation	Eqn. No.
Packingless seals: In the case of packingless seals, the leakage of the fluid past a rod (Fig. 21.6), mm³/s	$$Q_l = 260(100c)^3(p_1 - p_2)\frac{d}{lZ}$$	21.6

where Q_l is the discharge, mm³/s

c is the radial clearance between the rod and the bushing, mm

p_1, p_2 are the pressures on each end of the joint, MN/m² (kgf/mm²)

d is the rod diameter, mm; l is the length of the joint, mm

Z is the absolute viscosity of the fluid, cp (refer Table 21.3)

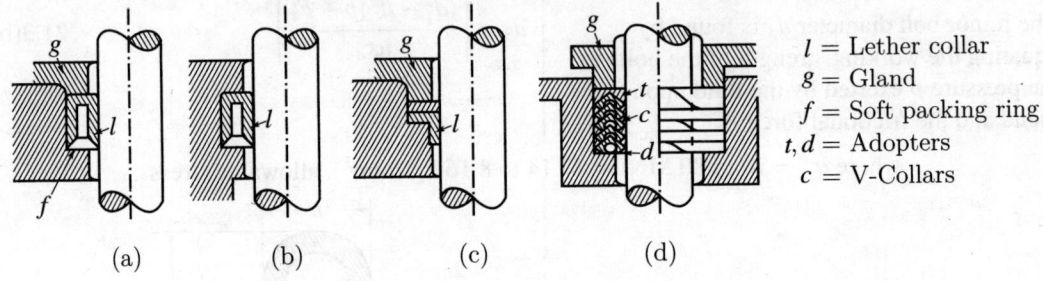

l = Lether collar
g = Gland
f = Soft packing ring
t, d = Adopters
c = V-Collars

(a)   (b)   (c)   (d)

Fig. 21.4: *Self-sealing packings*

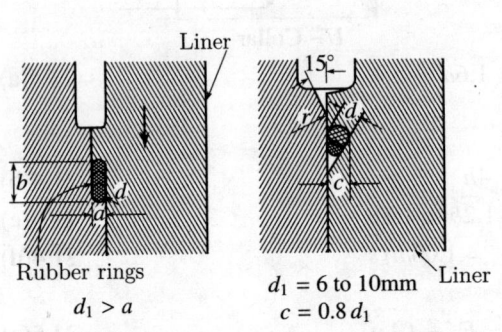

Fig. 21.5: *Joints with rubber packing ring*

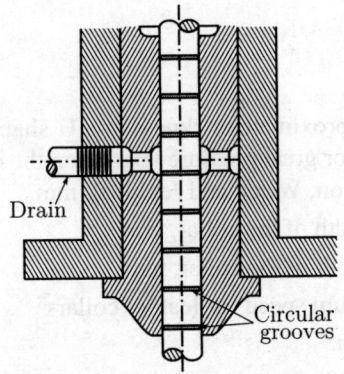

Fig. 21.6: *Labyrinth packing*

References

[1] Maleev, V. L., Hartman, J. B., *'Machine Design'*, 3rd edition, International Text Book Company, Pennsylvania, 1960.

[2] Spoots, M. F., *'Design of Machine Elements'*, 2nd edition, Prentice Hall, Inc., N. J., 1953.

[3] Low, D. A., *'A pocket book for Mechanical Engineers'*, New edition, Longmans, London, 1956.

Table 21.1

Gasket Factors *m* and Yield Values *y*		Gasket factor, m	Yield value, y	Refer to Table 21.2	
Gasket Material				Facing Limitation	Use Col.
Gum rubber sheet		0.50	0		
Hard rubber sheet		1.00	1.240	Use	
Cloth inserted soft rubber		0.75	0.345	1, 4, 6	
Cloth inserted hard rubber		1.25	2.760	only	
Vegetable fibre sheet (Hemp or Jute)		1.75	7.722		
Rubberized woven	3-Ply ..	2.25	15.170		
Wire inserted	2-Ply ..	2.50	19.858		
Asbestos	1-Ply ..	2.75	25.170		
Asbestos composition	3.2 mm thick ..	2.00	11.170	Use	
or	1.6 mm thick ..	2.75	25.170	1, 4, 6	
Compressed asbestos	0.8 mm thick ..	3.50	44.680	only	
Spiral-Wound Metal	Carbon steel	2.50	19.858		
Asbestos Filled	KA25 or type 316	3.00	31.030		
Serrated Steel, Asbestos Filled		2.75	25.170		
Corrugated Metal,	Soft Aluminum	2.50	19.858		
Asbestos Inserted	Soft copper or Brass	2.75	25.170		
or	Iron or soft steel	3.00	31.030		
Corrugated Metal	Monel or 4.6% Chrome	3.25	37.580		
Jacket, Asbestos Filled	11.13% Chrome, KA 25 or Type 316	3.50	44.680	Use 1	
	Soft Aluminum	2.75	25.170	only	
	Soft copper, or brass	3.00	31.030		
Corrugated Metal	Iron or soft steel	3.25	37.580		
	Monel or 4.6% Chrome	3.50	44.680		II
	11.13% Chrome, KA 25 or Type 316	3.75	52.402		
	Soft Aluminum	3.25	37580		
Flat Metal Jacket, Asbestos	Soft copper or Brass	3.50	44.680		
Filled	Iron or soft steel	3.75	52.402		
	Monel or 4.6% Chrome	4.00	60.814		
	11.13% Chrome, KA 25 or Type 316	4.25	69.780		
	Soft Aluminum	3.25	37.580		
Grooved Iron or Soft Steel	Soft Aluminum	3.25	44.680	Use	
Core, Metal Jacketed	Iron or soft steel	3.75	52.402	1, 4, 6	
	Monel or 4.6% Chrome	4.00	60.814	only	
	11.13% Chrome, KA 25 or Type 316	4.25	69.780		
	Soft Aluminum	4.00	60.814		
Solid Metal, 3.2 mm	Soft copper or Brass	4.75	89.635		
Thickness or More (For	Iron or soft steel	5.50	124.110		I
Thinner Gaskets see Note)	Monel or 4.6% Chrome	6.00	150.170		
	11.13% Chrome, KA 25 or Type 316	6.50	178.720		

Note:– For each 0.8 mm reduction in thickness below 3.2 mm increase m by 0.25, compute $y = 180(2m - 1)^2$.

Table 21.2 *Effective gasket width b*

Facing Sketch	Basic Gasket Yielding width bo	
	Col I	Col II
(1a)	$\dfrac{n}{2}$	$\dfrac{n}{2}$
(1b)	$\dfrac{w+t}{2}\left(\dfrac{w+n}{4}\,\max\right)$	$\dfrac{w+t}{2}\left(\dfrac{w+n}{4}\,\max\right)$
(2)	$\dfrac{w+n}{4}$	$\dfrac{w+3n}{8}$
(3)	$\dfrac{w}{2};\left(\dfrac{n}{4}\,\min\right)$	$\dfrac{w+n}{4};\left(\dfrac{3n}{8}\,\min\right)$
(4)	$\dfrac{3n}{8}$	$\dfrac{7n}{16}$
(5)		
(6)	$\dfrac{n}{4}$	$\dfrac{3n}{8}$
(7)		
(8)	$\dfrac{w}{8}$	

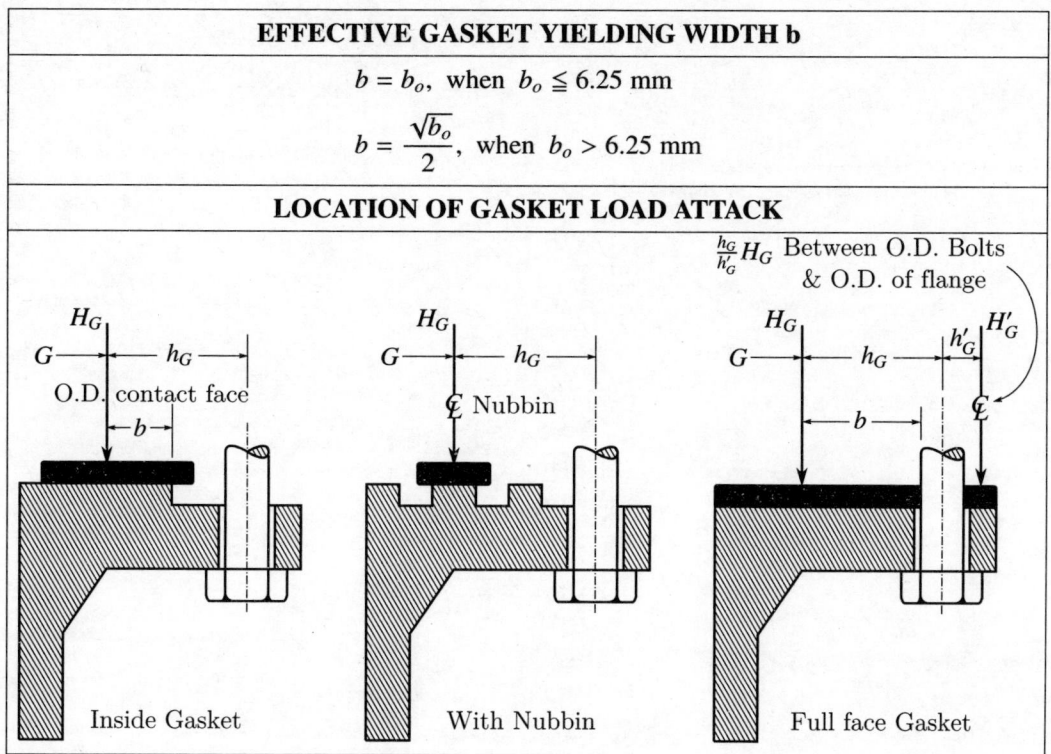

EFFECTIVE GASKET YIELDING WIDTH b

$b = b_o$, when $b_o \leqq 6.25$ mm

$b = \dfrac{\sqrt{b_o}}{2}$, when $b_o > 6.25$ mm

LOCATION OF GASKET LOAD ATTACK

$\dfrac{h_G}{h'_G} H_G$ Between O.D. Bolts & O.D. of flange

Inside Gasket   With Nubbin   Full face Gasket

Table 21.3 *Absolute viscosities of fluids (Z)**

Fluid	Temperature, °C	Absolute viscosity (cp)	Temperature, °C	Absolute viscosity (cp)
Steam	20	0.0097	260	0.018
Air	20	0.018	93.3	0.022
Water	0	1.790	37.8	0.690
Water	20	1.000	71.1	0.400
Gasoline	20	0.600	82.2	0.300
Kerosene	20	2.700	82.2	1.300
Fuel oil 30° Baume	20	5.000	82.2	1.600
Fuel oil, 24° Baume	20	40	82.2	4.000
Spindle oil	20	20-35	82.2	3-4
Machine oil	20	200-500	98.9	5.5-16.0
Castor oil	20	1000	43.3	200

*Viscosities at other temperatures may be determined by interpolation

22

Rotating Disks of Uniform Thickness

Particular	Equation	Eqn. No.
(a) *Thin Solid Disk*		

For a thin solid Disk of radius R_0, rotating with an angular velocity ω

(i) The circumferential or tangential stress at any radius r MN/m² (kgf/mm²)

$$\sigma_t = \frac{3+\mu}{8 \times 10^6}\rho\omega^2 R_0^2 - \frac{1+3\mu}{8 \times 10^6}\rho\omega^2 r^2 \qquad \text{22.1(a)}$$

$$= C_1 R_0^2 - C_2 r^2$$

where $C_1 = \dfrac{3+\mu}{8 \times 10^6}(\rho\omega^{2*})$ and $C_2 = \dfrac{1+3\mu}{8 \times 10^6}\rho\omega^2$

μ = Poisson's ratio; ρ = density of the material, kg/m³

R_0 = outer radius of the disk, m; r = radius, m

ω = angular velocity, rad/s

(ii) The radial stress at any radius r, MN/m² (kgf/mm²)

$$\sigma_r = \left(\frac{3+\mu}{8 \times 10^6}\right)\rho\omega^2 (R_0^2 - r^2) \qquad \text{22.1(b)}$$

$$= C_1 (R_0^2 - r^2)$$

(iii) The maximum tangential stress at the centre of the disk (i.e. at $r = 0$)

$$\sigma_{t\,max} = C_1 R_0^2 \qquad \text{22.1(c)}$$

(iv) The maximum radial stress at the centre of the disk ($r = 0$)

$$\sigma_{r\,max} = C_1 R_0^2 \qquad \text{22.1(d)}$$

(v) The radial outward displacement at $r = R_0$

$$Y_0 = \frac{(1-\mu)}{4 \times 10^9 E}\rho\omega^2 R_0^3 \qquad \text{22.1(e)}$$

where, E is the modulus of elasticity, MN/m² (kgf/mm²); Y = displacment, mm

$$Y_0 = 2\frac{1-\mu}{(3+\mu)E \times 10^3}C_1 R_0^3$$

*When using MKS units, substitute $(\rho\omega^2)/g$ in place of $\rho\omega^2$ in all the equations in this chapter.

Particular	**Equation**	**Eqn. No.**
(b) *Thin Circular Disk with a Hole:*		

For a thin circular disk of uniform thickness with a hole of radius R_i, rotating with an angular velocity ω

(i) The tangential stress at any radius r, MN/m^2, (kgf/mm^2)

$$\sigma_t = \left(\frac{3+\mu}{8 \times 10^6}\right)\rho\omega^2\left(R_0^2 + R_i^2 + \frac{R_i^2 R_0^2}{r^2} - \frac{1+3\mu}{3+\mu}r^2\right) = C_1\left(R_0^2 + R_i^2 + \frac{R_i^2 R_0^2}{r^2} - \frac{1+3\mu}{3+\mu}r^2\right) \qquad 22.2(a)$$

Particular	Equation	Eqn. No.
(ii) The radial stress at any radius r, MN/m^2 (kgf/mm^2)	$\sigma_r = C_1\left(R_0^2 + R_i^2 + \dfrac{R_i^2 R_0^2}{r^2} - r^2\right)$	22.2(b)
(iii) The maximum tangential stress at $r = R_i$	$\sigma_{t\,max} = 2C_1\left(R_0^2 + \dfrac{1-\mu}{3+\mu}R_i^2\right)$	22.2(c)
(iv) The maximum radial stress at $r = \sqrt{R_i R_0}$	$\sigma_{r\,max} = C_1(R_0 - R_i)^2$	22.2(d)
(v) The maximum tangential stress with a pinhole at the centre (i.e. $R_i \longrightarrow 0$)	$\sigma_{t\,max} = 2C_1 R_0^2$	22.2(e)
(vi) The maximum radial stress with a pinhole at the centre (i.e. $R_i \to 0$)	$\sigma_{r\,max} = C_1 R_0^2$	22.2(f)
(vii) The radial displacement at any radius, r	$Y_r = \dfrac{r}{10^3 \times E}(\sigma_t - \mu\sigma_r)$	22.2(g)
The radial displacement at $r = R_i$, mm	$Y_i = \dfrac{2C_1}{E \times 10^3}R_i\left(R_0^2 + \dfrac{1-\mu}{3+\mu}R_i^2\right)$ $= \dfrac{R_i \sigma_{t\,max}}{E \times 10^3}$	22.2(h)
The radial displacement at $r = R_0$, mm	$Y_0 = \dfrac{2C_1}{E \times 10^3}R_0\left(R_i^2 + \dfrac{1-\mu}{3+\mu}R_0^2\right)$	22.2(i)

Rotating Cylinders:

(a) *Hollow Cylinder:*

In the case of a uniformly rotating long hollow cylinder,

(i) The tangential stress at any radius, r

$$\sigma_t = \frac{(3-2\mu)\rho\omega^2}{8(1-\mu) \times 10^6}\left\{(R_i^2 + R_0^2) + \frac{R_i^2 R_0^2}{r^2} - \left(\frac{1+2\mu}{3-2\mu}\right)r^2\right\}$$

$$= C_3\left\{(R_i^2 + R_0^2) + \frac{R_i^2 R_0^2}{r^2} - \left(\frac{1+2\mu}{3-2\mu}\right)r^2\right\} \qquad 22.3(a)$$

(ii) The radial stress at any radius r

$$\sigma_r = \frac{(3-2\mu)\rho\omega^2}{8(1-\mu) \times 10^6}\left\{(R_i^2 + R_0^2) - \frac{R_i^2 R_0^2}{r^2}r^2\right\} = C_3\left\{(R_i^2 + R_0^2) - \frac{R_i^2 R_0^2}{r^2} - r^2\right\} \qquad 22.3(b)$$

Particular	Equation	Eqn. No.
(iii) The axial stress at any radius, r	$\sigma_a = \dfrac{\mu\rho\omega^2}{4(1-\mu)\times 10^6}\left\{(3-2\mu)\left(R_i^2+R_0^2\right)-2r_2\right\} = \left(\dfrac{2\mu}{3-2\mu}\right)C_3\left\{(3-2\mu)\left(R_i^2R_0^2\right)-2r^2\right\}$	22.3(c)

$$\text{where } C_3 = \frac{(3-2\mu)\rho\omega^2}{8(1-\mu)\times 10^6}$$

Particular	Equation	Eqn. No.
(iv) The maximum tangential stress at $r=R_t$	$\sigma_{t\,max} = C_3\left\{2R_0^2+R_i^2-\left(\dfrac{1+2\mu}{3-2\mu}\right)R_i^2\right\}$	22.3(d)
(v) The maximum radial stress at $r=\sqrt{R_iR_0}$	$\sigma_{r\,max} = C_3\left(R_0-R_i\right)^2$	22.3(e)
(vi) The maximum axial stress at $r=R_i$	$\sigma_{a\,max} = 2\mu C_3\left\{R_0^2+r_2\left(\dfrac{1-2\mu}{3-2\mu}\right)R_i^2\right\}$	22.3(f)
(vii) The maximum tangential stress when R_i^2/R_0^2 is very small (i.e. pinhole at the centre)	$\sigma_{t\,max} \approx 2C_3R_0^2$	22.3(g)
(viii) The maximum radial stress when R_i^2/R_0^2 is very small (i.e. pinhole at the centre)	$\sigma_{r\,max} \approx C_3R_0^2$	22.3(h)
(ix) The maximum axial stress when R_i^2/R_0^2 is very small (i.e. pinhole at the centre)	$\sigma_{a\,max} \approx \mu C_3R_0^2$	22.3(i)

(b) *Solid Cylinder:*

In the case of a uniformly rotating long solid circular cylinder (i.e. $R_i = 0$)

(i) The tangential stress at any radius r

$$\sigma_t = \frac{(3-2\mu)\rho\omega^2}{8(1-\mu)\times 10^6}\left\{R_0^2-\left(\frac{1+2\mu}{3-2\mu}\right)r^2\right\} = C_3\left\{R_0^2-\left(\frac{1+2\mu}{3-2\mu}\right)r^2\right\} \qquad \text{22.4(a)}$$

(ii) The radial stress at any radius r

$$\sigma_r = \frac{(3-2\mu)\rho\omega^2}{8(1-\mu)\times 10^6}\left\{R_0^2-r^2\right\} = C_3(R_0^2-r^2) \qquad \text{22.4(b)}$$

(iii) The axial stress at any radius r

$$\sigma_a = \frac{\mu\rho\omega^2}{4(1-\mu)\times 10^6}\left\{(3-2\mu)R_0^2-2r^2\right\} = \frac{2\mu C_3}{(3-2\mu)}\left\{(3-2\mu)R_0^2-2r^2\right\} \qquad \text{22.4(c)}$$

Particular	Equation	Eqn. No.
(iv) The maximum tangential stress (at $r=0$)	$\sigma_{t\,max} = C_3R_0^2$	22.4(d)
(v) The maximum radial stress (at $r=0$)	$\sigma_{r\,max} = C_3R_0^2$	22.4(e)
(vi) The maximum axial stress (at $r=0$)	$\sigma_{a\,max} = 2\mu C_3R_0^2$	22.4(f)

23

Metal Fits and Tolerances

Table 23.1 *Fundamental Tolerances of Grades 1 to 16*

Values of Tolerances in Microns (1 Micron=0.001 mm)

Diameter steps in millimetres	Tolerance Grades															
	IT 1	IT 2	IT 3	IT 4	IT 5	IT 6	IT 7	IT 8	IT 9	IT 10	IT 11	IT 12	IT 13	IT 14	IT 15	IT 16
(1)	(2)	(3)	(4)	(5)	(6)	(7)	(8)	(9)	(10)	(11)	(12)	(13)	(14)	(15)	(16)	(17)
Over 1 / To and inc. 3	1.5	2	3	4	5	7	9	14	25	40	60	90	140	250	400	600
Over 3 / To and inc. 6	1.5	2	3	4	5	8	12	18	30	48	75	120	180	300	480	750
Over 6 / To and inc. 10	1.5	2	3	4	6	9	15	22	36	58	90	150	220	360	580	900
Over 10 / To and inc. 18	1.5	2	3	5	8	11	18	27	43	70	110	180	270	430	700	1100
Over 18 / To and inc. 30	1.5	2	4	6	9	13	21	33	52	84	130	210	330	520	840	1300
Over 30 / To and inc. 50	2	3	4	7	11	16	26	39	62	100	160	250	390	620	1000	1600
Over 50 / To and inc. 80	2	3	5	8	13	19	30	46	74	120	190	300	460	740	1200	1900
Over 80 / To and inc. 120	3	4	6	10	15	22	55	54	87	140	220	350	540	870	1400	2200
Over 120 / To and inc. 180	4	5	8	12	18	25	40	63	100	160	250	400	630	1000	1600	2500
Over 180 / To and inc. 250	5	7	10	14	20	29	48	72	115	185	290	460	720	1150	1850	2900
Over 250 / To and inc. 315	6	8	12	16	23	32	52	81	130	210	320	520	710	1300	2100	3200
Over 315 / To and inc. 400	7	9	13	18	25	36	57	89	140	230	360	570	890	1400	2300	3800
Over 400 / To and inc. 500	8	10	15	20	27	40	63	97	155	240	400	630	970	1550	2500	4000

IS:991–1959

445

Table 23.2 *Commonly Used Classification of Types of Fits*

Type of Fit	Class of Shaft	With Holes				Remarks
		H6	H7	H8	H11	
(1)	(2)	(3)	(4)	(5)	(6)	(7)
Clearance fit	Shaft a	—	—	—	*all	Large clearance fit-not widely used
	Shaft b	—	—	—	—	
	Shaft c	—	c8	*c9	*c11	Slack running fit-Agricultural machinery
	Shaft d	—	d8	*d8 d10	d11	Loose running fit-suitable for applications, such as gland seals and loose pulleys-turbines, ball mills, and heavy bending machines.
	Shaft e	e7	e8	*e9 e8	—	Easy running fit-IC engine main bearings, camshaft bearings rocker arm bearings
	Shaft f	*f6	*f7	*f8	—	Normal running fit-shaft bearings in gear boxes and gear trains, gears running on fixed shaf's pump driving shaft bearings
	Shaft g	*g5	*g6	*g7	—	Close running fit or sliding fit. Also spigot and location fit. Used as a precision sliding fit.
	Shaft h	*h5	*h6	h7 *h8	*h11	Precision sliding fit. Also fine spigot and location fit
Transition fit	Shaft j	*j5	*j6	*j7	—	Push fit for very accurate location with easy assembly and dismantling-coupling spigots and recesses, gear rings fitted to hubs
	Shaft k	*k5	*k6	k7	—	Light keying fit (true transition fit for keyed shaft, non-running locked pins etc.)
	Shaft m	*m5	*m6	m7	—	Medium keying fit-cam holder
	Shaft n	n5	*n6	n7	—	Heavy keying fit (for tight assembly of mating surfaces)
Interference fit	Shaft p	p5	*p6	—	—	Light press fit with easy dismantling for non-ferrous parts. Standard press fit with easy dismantling for ferrous and non-ferrous parts assembly
	Shaft r	r5	*r6	—	—	Medium drive fit with easy dismantling for ferrous parts assembly. Light drive fit with easy dismantling for nonferrous parts assembly
	Shaft s	s5	*s6	s7	—	Heavy drive fit for ferrous parts permanent or semipermanent assembly. Standard press fit for non-ferrous parts
	Shaft t	t5	t6	*t7	—	Force fit on ferrous parts for permanent assembly
	Shaft u	u5	u6	*u7	—	Heavy force fit for shrink fit
	Shaft v	—	—	—	—	Very large interference fit Not recommended for use
	Shaft x	—	—	—	—	
	Shaft y	—	—	—	—	
	Shaft z	—	—	—	—	

* Fits recommended for common use

Table 23.3 Fits and Tolerances

System of basic hole		Limits	Diameter steps, mm												
			1 to 3	3 to 6	6 to 10	10 to 18	18 to 30	30 to 50	50 to 80	80 to 120	120 to 180	180 to 250	250 to 315	315 to 400	400 to 500
(1)		(2)	(3)	(4)	(5)	(6)	(7)	(8)	(9)	(10)	(11)	(12)	(13)	(14)	(15)
With large minimum clearance	d8	G	−20	−30	−40	−50	−65	−80	−100	−120	−145	−170	−190	−210	−230
		N	−34	−48	−62	−77	−98	−119	−146	−174	−208	−242	−271	−299	−327
	d9	G	−20	−30	−40	−50	−65	−80	−100	−120	−145	−170	−190	−210	−230
		N	−45	−60	−76	−93	−117	−142	−174	−207	−245	−285	−320	−350	−385
	d10	G	−20	−30	−40	−50	−65	−80	−100	−120	−145	−170	−190	−210	−230
		N	−60	−78	−98	−120	−149	−180	−220	−260	−305	−355	−400	−440	−480
With medium minimum clearance	e6	G	−14	−20	−25	−32	−40	−50	−60	−72	−85	−100	−100	−125	−135
		N	−20	−28	−34	−43	−53	−66	−79	−94	−110	−129	−142	−161	−175
	e7	G	−14	−20	−25	−32	−40	−50	−60	−72	−85	−100	−110	−125	−135
		N	−24	−32	−40	−50	−61	−75	−90	−107	−125	−146	−162	−182	−198
	e8	G	−14	−20	−25	−32	−40	−50	−60	−72	−85	−100	−110	−125	−135
		N	−28	−38	−47	−59	−73	−89	−108	−126	−148	−172	−191	−214	−232
	e9	G	−14	−20	−25	−32	−40	−50	−60	−72	−85	−100	−110	−125	−135
		N	−39	−50	−61	−75	−92	−112	−134	−159	−185	−215	−240	−265	−290
With small minimum clearance	f6	G	−06	−10	−13	−16	−20	−25	−30	−36	−43	−50	−56	−62	−68
		N	−12	−18	−22	−27	−33	−41	−49	−58	−68	−79	−88	−98	−108
	f7	G	−06	−10	−13	−16	−20	−25	−30	−36	−43	−50	−56	−62	−68
		N	−16	−22	−28	−34	−41	−50	−60	−71	−83	−96	−108	−119	−181
	f8	G	−06	−10	−13	−16	−20	−25	−30	−36	−43	−50	−56	−62	−68
		N	−20	−28	−35	−43	−53	−64	−76	−90	−106	−122	−137	−151	−165
	g4	G	−02	−04	−05	−06	−07	−09	−10	−12	−14	−15	−17	−18	−20
		N	−05	−08	−90	−11	−13	−16	−18	−22	−26	−29	−33	−36	−40

Running fit shaft

Table 23.3 Fits and Tolerances (Contd.)

(1)		(2)	(3)	(4)	(5)	(6)	(7)	(8)	(9)	(10)	(11)	(12)	(13)	(14)	(15)
With smallest minimum clearance	g5	G	−02	−04	−05	−06	−07	−09	−10	−12	−14	−15	−17	−18	−20
		N	−06	−09	−11	−14	−18	−20	−23	−27	−32	−35	−40	−43	−47
	g6	G	−02	−04	−05	−06	−07	−09	−10	−12	−14	−15	−17	−18	−20
		N	−08	−12	−14	−17	−20	−25	−29	−34	−39	−44	−49	−54	−60
Ground between centres	h5	G	−00	−00	−00	−00	−00	−00	−00	−00	−00	−00	−00	−00	−00
		N	−04	−05	−06	−08	−09	−11	−13	−15	−18	−20	−23	−25	−27
	h6	G	−00	−00	−00	−00	−00	−00	−00	−00	−00	−00	−00	−00	−00
		N	−06	−08	−09	−11	−13	−16	−19	−22	−25	−29	−32	−36	−40
Centreless ground	h7	G	−00	−00	−00	−00	−00	−00	−00	−00	−00	−00	−00	−00	−00
		N	−10	−12	−15	−18	−21	−25	−30	−35	−40	−46	−52	−57	−63
	h8	G	−00	−00	−00	−00	−00	−00	−00	−00	−00	−00	−00	−00	−00
		N	−14	−18	−22	−27	−33	−39	−46	−54	−53	−72	−81	−89	−97
Cold drawn	g9	G	−00	−00	−00	−00	−00	−00	−00	−00	−00	−00	−00	−00	−00
		N	−25	−30	−36	−43	−52	−62	−74	−87	−100	−115	−130	−140	−155
	j5	G	+04	+04	+04	+05	+05	+06	+06	+06	+07	+07	+07	+07	+07
		N	−01	−01	−02	−03	−04	−05	−07	−09	−11	−13	−18	−18	−20
	j6	G	+06	+07	+07	+08	+09	+11	+12	+13	+14	+16	+16	+18	+20
		N	−01	−01	−02	−03	−04	−05	−07	−09	−11	−13	−16	−18	−20
(Secure against turning)	j7	G	+07	+09	+10	+12	+13	+15	+18	+20	+22	+25	+25	+29	+31
		N	−02	−03	−05	−06	−08	−10	−12	−15	−18	−21	−26	−28	−32
	k6	G	+06	+09	+10	+12	+15	+18	+21	+25	+28	+33	+36	+40	+45
		N	+00	+01	+01	+01	+02	+02	+02	+03	+03	+04	+04	+04	+05
	k7	G	+10	+13	+16	+19	+23	+27	+32	+38	+43	+50	+56	+61	+68
		N	+00	+01	+01	+01	+02	+02	+02	+03	+03	+04	+04	+04	+05
	m6	G	+08	+12	+15	+18	+21	+25	+30	+35	+40	+46	+52	+57	+63
		N	+02	+04	+06	+07	+08	+09	+11	+13	+15	+17	+20	+21	+23

Running fit shaft (g5–g9) · Transition fit shaft (j5–m6)

Table 23.3 Fits and Tolerances (Contd.)

(1)		(2)	(3)	(4)	(5)	(6)	(7)	(8)	(9)	(10)	(11)	(12)	(13)	(14)	(15)
Transition fit, shaft	m7	G	—	+16	+21	+25	+29	+34	+41	+48	+55	+63	+72	+78	+68
		N	—	+04	+06	+07	+08	+09	+11	+13	+15	+17	+20	+21	+23
Interference fit, shaft	n5	G	+08	+13	+16	+20	+24	+28	+33	+38	+45	+51	+57	+62	+67
		N	+04	+08	+10	+12	+15	+17	+20	+23	+27	+31	+34	+37	+40
	p5	G	+10	+17	+21	+28	+31	+37	+45	+52	+61	+70	+79	+87	+95
		N	+06	+12	+15	+18	+22	+26	+32	+37	+43	+50	+56	+62	+68
	p6	G	+12	+20	+24	+29	+35	+42	+51	+59	+68	+79	+88	+98	+108
		N	+06	+12	+15	+18	+22	+26	+32	+37	+43	+50	+56	+62	+68
	r6	G	+16	+23	+28	+34	+41	+50	+62	+76	+90	+109	+130	+150	+172
		N	+10	+15	+19	+23	+28	+34	+43	+54	+65	+80	+98	+144	+132
	r7	G	—	—	—	—	+62	+79	+105	+139	+174	+226	+292	+351	+423
		N	—	—	—	—	+41	+54	+75	+104	+134	+180	+250	+294	+360
	H5	N	+04	+05	+06	+08	+09	+11	+13	+15	+18	+20	+23	+25	+27
		G	+00	+00	+00	+00	+00	+00	+00	+00	+00	+00	+00	+00	+00
	H6	N	+06	+08	+09	+11	+13	+16	+19	+22	+25	+29	+32	+36	+40
		G	+00	+00	+00	+00	+00	+00	+00	+00	+00	+00	+00	+00	+00
	H7	N	+10	+12	+15	+18	+21	+25	+30	+35	+40	+46	+52	+57	+63
		G	+00	+00	+00	+00	+00	+00	+00	+00	+00	+00	+00	+00	+00
Basic hole	H8	G	+00	+00	+00	+00	+00	+00	+00	+00	+00	+00	+00	+00	+00
		N	+14	+18	+22	+27	+33	+39	+46	+54	+63	+72	+81	+89	+97
	H9	G	+00	+00	+00	+00	+00	+00	+00	+00	+00	+00	+00	+00	+00
		N	+25	+30	+36	+43	+52	+62	+74	+87	+100	+115	+130	+140	+156
	H10	N	+40	+48	-58	+70	+84	+100	+120	+140	+160	+185	+210	+230	+250
		G	+00	+00	+00	+00	+00	+00	+00	+00	+00	+00	+00	+00	+00

G–Go, N–No go, Tolerances in microns, μ 1 micron=0.001 mm = 1×10^{-6} m

24

Preferred Numbers

Table 24.1 *Basic Series of Preferred Numbers*

Preferred Numbers of Basic Series				Serial Number
R5 (1)	R10 (2)	R20 (3)	R40 (4)	(5)
1.00	1.00	1.00	1.00	0
			1.06	1
		1.12	1.12	2
			1.18	3
	1.25	1.25	1.25	4
			1.32	5
		1.40	1.40	6
			1.50	7
1.60	1.60	1.60	1.60	8
			1.70	9
		1.80	1.80	10
			1.90	11
	2.00	2.00	2.00	12
			2.12	13
		2.24	2.24	14
			2.36	15
2.50	2.50	2.50	2.50	16
			2.65	17
		2.80	2.80	18
			3.00	19
	3.15	3.15	3.15	20
			3.35	21
		3.55	3.55	22
			3.75	23
4.00	4.00	4.00	4.00	24
			4.25	25
		4.50	4.50	26
			4.75	27

Table 24.1 *Basic Series of Preferred Numbers (Contd.)*

	5.00	5.00	5.00	28
			5.30	29
		5.60	5.60	30
			6.00	31
6.30	6.30	6.30	6.30	32
			6.70	33
		7.10	7.10	34
			7.50	35
	8.00	8.00	8.00	36
			8.50	37
		9.00	9.00	38
			9.50	39
10.00	10.00	10.00	10.00	40

Table 24.2 *Preferred Numbers of R80 Series*

1.00	1.80	3.15	5.60
1.03	1.85	3.25	5.80
1.06	1.90	3.35	6.00
1.09	1.95	3.45	6.15
1.12	2.00	3.55	6.30
1.15	2.06	3.65	6.50
1.18	2.12	3.75	6.70
1.22	2.18	3.87	6.90
1.25	2.24	4.00	7.10
1.28	2.30	4.12	7.30
1.32	2.36	4.25	7.50
1.36	2.43	4.37	7.75
1.40	2.50	4.50	8.00
1.45	2.58	4.62	8.25
1.50	2.65	4.75	8.50
1.55	2.72	4.87	8.75
1.60	2.80	5.00	9.00
1.69	2.90	5.15	9.25
1.70	3.00	5.30	9.50
1.75	3.07	5.45	9.75

IS: 1076-1967

Appendix

I

Designation and Properties of Materials

(I) Designation of Steels Based on Letter Symbols:

The designation shall consist of the following in the order given.

(a) Symbol 'Fe' or 'FeE' depending on whether the steel has been specified on the basis of minimum tensile strength or yield stress.

(b) Figure indicating the minimum tensile strength or yield stress in, N/mm^2. If no minimum tensile or yield strength is guaranteed, the figure shall be 00.

(c) Chemical symbols for elements the presence of which characterize the steel.

(d) Symbol indicating special characteristics as listed below.

(i) Method of deoxidation:

    (i) *R* for rimming steel, and

    (ii) *K* for killed steel.

Note: If no symbol is used, it shall mean that the steel is of semi-killed type.

(ii) steel quality:

    Q. 1–Non-ageing quality,

    Q. 2–Freedom flakes,

    Q. 3–Grain size controlled,

    Q. 4–Inclusion controlled, and

    Q. 5–Internal homogeneity guaranteed.

(iii) Degree of purity:

P.25–(0.025% phosphorous and 0.025% sulphur)

P.35–(0.035% phosphorous and 0.035% sulphur)

P.50–(0.050% phosphorous and 0.050% sulphur)

P.70–(0.070% phosphorous and 0.070% sulphur)

No symbol will mean (0.055% phosphorous and 0.055% sulphur)

(iv) Weldability guarantee:

W–Fusion weldable.

W_1–Weldable by resistance welding but not fusion weldable.

(v) Resistance to brittle fracture: Symbol 'B', 'B0', 'B2', or 'B4', indicating resistance to brittle fracture based on the results of the V-notch Charpy impact test.

(vi) Surface condition:

S1–Deseamed or scarfed.

S2-Descaled;

S3–Picked (including washing and neutralizing);

S4–Shot, grit or sand blasted;

S5–Peeled (skinned);

S6–Bright drawn or cold rolled: and

S7–Ground.

Note If no symbol is used, it shall mean that the surface is in as rolled or as forged condition.

(vii) Formability (applicable to sheet only):
   D1–Drawing quality,
   D2–Deep drawing quality, and
   D3–Extra deep drawing quality.

Note: If no symbol is used, it shall mean that the steel is commercial quality.

(viii) Surface finish (applicable to sheet only):
   F1–General purpose finish,
   F2–Full finish.
   F3–Exposed,
   F4–Unexposed,
   F5–Matt finish,
   F6–Bright finish,
   F7–Plating finish,
   F8–Unpolished finish,
   F9–Polished finish,
   F10–Polished and coloured blue,
   F11–Polished and coloured yellow,
   F12–Mirror finish,
   F13–Vitreous enamel finish, and
   F14–Direct annealed finish.

(ix) Treatment:
   T1–Shot peened,
   T2–Hard drawn,
   T3–Normalized,
   T4–Controlled rolled,
   T5–Annealed,
   T6–Patented,
   T7–Solution treated,
   T8–Solution treated and aged,
   T9–Controlled cooled,
   T10–Bright annealed,
   T11–Spherodized,
   T12–Stress relieved,
   T13–Case hardened, and
   T14–Hardened and tempered.

Note: If no symbol is used, it means that the steel is hot rolled.

(x) Elevated temperature properties: For guarantee with regard to elevated temperature properties, the letter 'H' shall be used. However, in the designation only the room temperature properties shall be shown. Elevated temperature properties shall be intimated to the purchaser separately by the manufacturer.

(xi) Cryogenic quality: For guarantee with regard to low temperature properties, the letter 'L' shall be used.

(e) Symbol indicating applications, if necessary.

Examples:

Fe 410 Cu K Killed steel containing copper as alloying element with a minimum tensile strength of 410 N/mm^2

FeE 300 P 35 Semi-killed steel with a minimum yield strength of 300 N/mm^2 and degree of purity as follows:
   S & P=0.035% max.

FeE 550 S6 Bright drawn or cold rolled steel with a minimum yield strength of 550 N/mm^2

Fe 00 R Rimming quality steel with no guarantee of minimum tensile or yield strength.

FeE 590 F7 Sheet steel of plating finish and minimum yield strength of 590 N/mm^2

Fe 710 H Steel with guaranteed elevated temperature properties and a minimum room temperature tensile strength of 710 N/mm^2

Fe 410 Q1 Semi-killed non-ageing quality steel with S&P=0.055% Max. and minimum tensile=410 N/mm^2.

(B) Steels Designation on the Basis of Chemical Composition:

  (i) *Unalloyed steels:* The designation shall consist of the following in the order given:

    (a) Figure indicating 100 times the average percentage of carbon content.

    (b) Letter 'C', and

    (c) Figure indicating 10 times the average percentage of manganese content. The figure after multiplying shall be rounded off to the nearest integer.

    (d) Symbol indicating special characteristics including guaranteed hardenability for which symbol 'G' shall be used at the end of the designation.

Examples:

25C5BO Semi-killed steel with average 0.25 percent carbon and 0.5 percent manganese content and resistance to brittle fracture grade BO.

45C10G Steel with average 0.45% carbon, 1% manganese and guaranteed hardenability.

  (ii) *Unalloyed tool steels:* The designation shall consist of:

    (a) Figure indicating 100 times the average percentage of carbon;

    (b) Symbol 'T' for tool steel; and

    (c) Figure indicating 10 times the average percent manganese content.

Examples:

75T5 Unalloyed tool steel with average 0.75% carbon and 0.5% manganese

80T11 Unalloyed tool steel with average carbon content of 0.80% and 1.1% manganese.

  (iii) *Unalloyed free cutting steels:* The designation shall consist of;

    (a) Figure indicating 100 times the average percentage of carbon;

    (b) Letter 'C';

    (c) Figure indicating 10 times the average percentage of manganese;

    (d) Symbol 'S', 'Se', 'Te' or 'Pb' depending on the element present which makes the steel free cutting followed by the figure indicating 100 times the percentage content of the element. In the case of the phosphorized steels the symbol 'P' shall be included; and

    (e) Symbol indicating special characteristics covering the method of deoxidation, surface condition and heat treatment.

Examples:

35C10S14K Free cutting steel with average 0.35% carbon, 1% manganese and 0.14% sulphur, killed quality.

20C12Pb15T14 Free cutting steel with average 0.15% lead, 0.20% carbon and 1.2% manganese, hardened and tempered.

  (iv) *Alloy steels:*

  (a) *Low and medium alloy steels* (total alloying elements not exceeding 10%)– The designation of steels shall consist of:

    (1) Figure indicating 100 times the average percentage carbon.

    (2) Chemical symbol for alloying elements each followed by the figure for its average percentage content multiplied by a factor as given below:

Element	Multiplying Factor
Cr, Co, Ni, Mn, Si and W	4
Al, Be, V, Pb, Cu, Nb, Ti, Ta, Zr and Mo	10
P, S, N	100

Note 1– The figure after multiplying shall be rounded off to the nearest integer.

Note 2– Symbol 'Mn' for manganese shall be included in case manganese content is equal to or greater than 1 percent.

Note 3– The chemical symbols and their figures shall be listed in the designation in the order of decreasing content.

(3) Symbol indicating special characteristics covering degree of purity hardenability, weldability guarantee, elevated temperature properties, surface condition, surface finish and heat treatment.

Examples:

25Cr4Mo2G Steel with guaranteed hardenability and having average 0.25% carbon, 1% chromium and 0.20% molybdenum

40Ni8Cr8V2 Hot rolled steel with average 0.40% carbon, 2% chromium 2% nickel and 0.2% vanadium.

(b) *High alloy steels* (total alloying elements more than 10%)–The designation shall consist of:

(1) Letter 'X'.

(2) Figure indicating 100 times the percentage carbon content.

(3) Chemical symbol for alloying elements each followed by the figure for its average percentage content rounded off to the nearest integer.

(4) Chemical symbol to indicate specially added element to attain the desired properties.

(5) Symbol indicating specific characteristics covering hardenability, weldability guarantee, elevated temperature properties, surface condition, surface finish and heat treatment.

Examples:

X10Cr18Ni9S3 Steel in pickled condition with average carbon 0.10%, chromium 18% and nickel 9%.

X15Cr25Ni12 Steel with 0.15% carbon, 25% chromium and 12% nickel.

(c) Alloy tool steels–The steel designation shall be as for low, medium and high alloy steels as given under (a) and (b) above except that the symbol 'T' will be included in the beginning of the designation of low alloy and medium alloy tool steel and 'XT' instead of 'X' in the case of high alloy tool steels.

Examples:

XT75W18Cr4V1

High alloy tool steel with average carbon 0.75%, tungsten 18%, chromium 4% and vanadium 1%.

XT98W6Mo5Cr4V1

High alloy steel with average carbon 0.98%, tungsten 6%, molybdenum 5%, chromium 4% and vanadium 1%.

(d) *Free cutting alloy steels:* The steel designation shall be as for low, medium and high alloy steals as given under (a) and (b) above except that depending on the percentage of *S*, *Se*, *Te* and *Zr* present, the designation shall also consist of the chemical symbol of the element present followed by the figure indicating 100 times its content.

Examples:

X15Cr25Ni15S40

Alloy free cutting steel with carbon 0.15%, chromium 25%, nickel 15% and sulphur 0.40%.

X12Cr18Ni3S25

Alloy free cutting steel with 18% chromium, nickel 3% and sulphur 0.25%

Designation of Ferrous Castings:

(II) (a) Based on mechanical properties: *300
*Any of the symbols listed below

FG – Grey Iron castings

BM – Black-heart (Malleable Iron)

PM – Pearlitic (Malleable Iron)

WM – White-heart (Malleable Iron)

SG – Spheroidal or nodular graphite iron

AFG – Austenitic flake graphite iron

AFG – Austenitic spheroidal or nodular graphite iron

ABR – Abrasion resistant iron

CS – Steel castings

CSH – Heat-resistant steel castings

CSC – Corrosion-resistant steel castings.

300 – Minimum tensile strength in N/mm^2

(σ_u = 300 N/mm^2)

(b) Based on chemical composition: *33Ni4Cr2

*Any of the above listed symbols

33 – Total carbon 3.3%

Ni4 – 4% Nickel (average)

Cr2 – 2% chromium (average),

(III) Designation of pig Iron: PG 12 Mn3P15

PG – Designation for Pig Iron

12 – Indicates silicon as four times its average percentage content rounded off to the nearest integer without its chemical symbol (Si). (i.e. in the case silicon content is about 3%).

Mn3 – indicates manganese as four times average percentage rounded off to the nearest integer i.e. 1% manganese).

P15 – indicate phosphorous as hundred times the average percentage (i.e. 0.15% phosphorous).

PG 12 Mn3P15K

$\left.\begin{array}{l} PG \\ 12 \\ Mn3 \\ P15 \end{array}\right\}$ same as listed above.

K – where the maximum limit of sulphur content is restricted below 0.04%, the symbol 'K' shall be used.

PG12Mn3P15KC35

$\left.\begin{array}{l} PG \\ 12 \\ Mn_3 \\ P15 \\ K \end{array}\right\}$ same as listed above.

C35 – indicates carbon as ten times the minimum limit (i.e. total carbon=3.5%).

Properties of Materials

Table I.1 *Mechanical Properties of Carbon Steel Castings for General Engg. Purposes*

*Grade designation (1)	Yield stress Min. (MN/m^2) (2)	Tensile strength Min. (MN/m^2) (3)	Elongation% Min. Gauge length 5.65 $\sqrt{S_0}$ (4)	Reduction of area percent Min. (5)	Impact strength Min. J/cm^2 (6)	Angle of bend Min. (7)
20-40	200	400	25	40	30	90°
23-45	230	450	22	31	25	90°
26-52	260	520	18	25	22	60
27-54	270	540	16	23	20	60
30-57	300	570	15	21	18	60

*On the basis of minimum yield stress and tensile strength values respectively expressed in 10 MN/m^2.

IS:1030-1982

Table I.2 *Mechanical Properties of Iron Castings with Spheroidal or Nodular Graphite*

Grade Designation (1)	Tensile Strength Min. N/mm^2 (2)	Elongation percent Min (3)	Typical Brinall Hardness Range (HB) (4)	Predominant Structural constituent and applications (5)
SG 800/2	800	2	248-352	Pearlite or tempered structure-High tensile strength and less ductility.
SG 700/2	700	2	229-302	Pearlite-High tensile strength and less ductility
SG 600/3	600	3	192-269	Pearlite and Ferrite-High tensile strength and less ductility
SG 500/7	500	7	170-241	Ferrite and pearlite-Medium strength with reasonable ductility
SG 400/12	400	12	201, Max	Ferrite-Medium tensile strength with substantial ductility and toughness
SG 370/17	370	17	179, Max	Ferrite-High resistance to impact.

IS: 1865-1975

Table I.3 *Typical Properties of Grey Cast Iron*

Properties	Unit	Grade						
		FG 150	FG 200	FG 220	FG 260	FG 300	FG 350	FG 400
Tensile strength	(N/mm²)	150	200	220	260	300	350	400
0.01 percent proof stress	(N/mm²)	42	56	62	73	84	98	112
0.1 percent proof stress	(N/mm²)	98	130	143	169	195	228	260
Total strain at failure	Percent	0.60-0.75*	0.48-0.67*	0.39-0.63*	0.57	0.50	0.50	0.50
Elastic strain at failure	..	0.15	0.17	0.18	0.20	0.22	0.25	0.28
Total minus elastic strain at failure	..	0.45-0.60*	0.31-0.50*	0.21-0.45*	0.37	0.28	0.25	0.22
Notched tensile strength (See Note 2)								
Circumferential 45° V-notch, root radius 0.25 mm (Notch depth 2.5 mm, notch dia 20 mm or notch depth 3.3 mm. notch diameter 7.6 mm)	(N/mm²)	120	160	176	208	240	280	320
Circumferential notch. Radius 9.5 mm (Notch depth 2.5 mm, notch diameter 20 mm)	(N/mm²)	150	200	220	260	300	350	400
Compressive strength	(N/mm²)	600	720	768	864	960	1080	1200
0.01 percent proof stress	(N/mm²)	84	112	123	146	168	196	224
0.1 percent proof stress	(N/mm²)	195	260	286	338	390	455	520
Shear strength	(N/mm²)	173	230	253	299	345	403	460
Torsional strength	(N/mm²)	173	230	253	299	345	403	460
Shear strain at failure	Percent	> 4	> 4	> 4	4	Up to 4	Up to 4	Up to 4
Modulus of elasticity	GN/mm²	100	114	120	128	135	140	145

Table I.3 Typical Properties of Grey Cast Iron (Contd.)

Properties	Unit	Grade						
		FG 150	FG 200	FG 220	FG 260	FG 300	FG 350	FG 400
Tension								
Compression	GN/mm²	100	114	120	128	135	140	145
Modulus of rigidity	GN/mm²	40	46	48	51	54	56	58
Poisson's ratio	–			0.26				
Fatigue limit (Wöhler)								
Unnotched (8.4 mm dia)	(N/mm²)	68	90	99	117	135	149	152
V-notched (Circumferential 45°V-notch with 0.25 mm root radius. Diameter at notch 8.4 mm, depth of notch 3.4 mm)	(N/mm²)	68	87	94	108	122	129	127
Relative density		7.05	7.10	7.15	7.20	7.25	7.30	7.30
Hardness								

Hardness is not simply related to tensile strength and varies with casting section thickness and material composition.

Note: 1 – The typical properties given in this appendix are the properties in a 30-mm diameter separately cast test bar or in casting section correctly represented by this size of test bar. Where the tensile strength does not correspond to that given, other properties may differ slightly from those given.

Note: 2 – Notched tensile strengths increases slightly as notch severity ratio, notch radius; notch diameter, increases above 0.47.

*Value depends on the composition of iron.

IS: 210-1978

Table I.4 *Mechanical Properties of Grey Iron Castings*

Grade (See IS: 4843-1968)*	Tensile strength Min (N/mm²)	Brinell Hardness (HB)
FG 150	150	130 to 180
FG 200	200	160 to 220
FG 220	220	180 to 220
FG 260	260	180 to 230
FG 300	300	180 to 230
FG 350	350	207 to 241
FG 400	400	207 to 270

*Code for designation of ferrous Castings.

IS: 210-1978

Table I.5 *Mechanical Properties of High Tensile Steel Castings*

Grade	Designa-tion	Tensile strength Min (MN/m²)	Yield stress (0.5 percent) (Proof stress), Min. (MN/m²)	Reduction in area, Min. Percent	Elongation of gauge length $= 5.65\sqrt{S_0}$ Min. Percent	Brinell Hardness, Min. HB	Izod Impact strength, Min. J†
(1)	(2)	(3)	(4)	(5)	(6)	(7)	(8)
1	CS 640	640	390	35	15	190	30
2	CS 700	700	560	30	14	207	30
3	CS 840	840	700	28	12	248	28
4	CS 1030	1030	850	20	8	305	20
5	CS 1230	1230	1000	12	5	355	–

IS: 2644-1979.

Table I.6 *Tensile Properties and Hardness of Carbon Steel Forgings for General Engg. Purposes*

Class	Designa-tion	Tensile strength. Min. N/mm²	Yield strength Min. N/mm²	Elongation percent, Min. Gauge Length $= 5.65\sqrt{S_0}$	Brinell Hardness, Min BHN	Normalizing Temperature C
(1)	(2)	(3)	(4)	(5)	(6)	(7)
1A	15 C 8	410	220	25	110	880-910
2	20 C 8	430	230	24	120	880-910
2A	25 C 8	460	250	22	130	880-910
3	30 C 8	490	270	21	140	860-890
3A	35 C 8	540	280	20	155	850-880
4	45 C 8	620	320	15	175	830-860
5	55 C 8	710	350	13	200	810-840
6	65 C 6	740	370	10	210	800-830

Note: The properties given in the table refer to 100 mm ruling section in the forged and normalized condition and are applicable to test samples taken along the direction of grain flow.

IS: 2004-1978

Table I.7 *Tensile and Yield Properties of Standard Wrought Steels*

Designation	Tensile strength (N/mm²)	Yield stress Min. (N/mm²)	Elongation, percent, Min. (Gauge length 5.65 √A)
(1)	(2)	(3)	(4)
Fe 290	290	170	27
FeE 220	290	220	27
Fe 310	310	180	26
FeE 230	310	230	26
Fe 330	330	200	26
FeE 250	300	250	26
Fe 360	360	220	25
FeE 270	360	270	25
Fe 410	410	250	23
FeE 310	410	310	23
Fe 490	490	290	21
FeE 370	490	370	21
Fe 540	540	320	20
FeE 400	540	400	20
Fe 620	620	380	15
FeE 460	620	460	15
Fe 690	690	410	12
FeE 520	690	520	12
Fe 770	770	460	10
FeE 580	770	580	10
Fe 870	870	520	8
FeE 650	870	650	8

Table I.8 *Properties and Uses of Corbon Steels*

Designation (ISI Grade)	%C	%Mn	Tensile strength† N/mm²	Yield stress† N/mm²	Minimum elongation percentage (gauge length $5.65\sqrt{A}$* round test piece)	Brinell hardness (HB)No.	Suggested uses
(1)	(2)	(3)	(4)	(5)	(6)	(7)	(8)
C 07	0.12 max	0.50 max	314-392	196	27	—	Cold forming and deep drawing Rimming quality used for automobile bodies and rivets, killed quality used for forgings
C 10	0.15 max	0.30-0.60	333-412	206	26	—	–do–
C 14	0.10-0.18	0.40-0.70	363-441	216	26	137	Cam shafts, cams, light duty gears, worms, gudgeon pins, spindles, ratchets chain wheels tappets, etc.
C 15	0.20 max	0.30-0.60	363-481	235	25	137	Cold worked-rivets
C 15 Mn 75	0.10-0.20	0.60-0.90	412-490	245	25	163	General purpose-low stressed components
C 20	0.15-0.25	0.60-0.90	432-510	245	24	156	-do-
C 25	0.20-0.30	0.30-0.60	432-520	275	27	170	-do-
C 25 Mn 75	0.20-0.30	0.60-0.90	461-560	275	22	207	-do-
C 30	0.25-0.35	0.60-0.90	490-588	294	21	179	Cold formed levers, Hardened and tempered tie rods, cables, sprockets, hubs and bushes, steel tubes etc.
C 35	0.30-0.40	0.30-0.60	510-608	304	20	187	Low stressed components, automobile tubes and fasteners
C35 Mn 75	1.30-0.40	0.60-0.90	540-637	314	20	223	Low stressed parts, cycle and motor cycle frame tubes, fish plates for rails and fasteners.

Table I.8 *Properties and Uses of Corbon Steels (Contd.)*

(1)	(2)	(3)	(4)	(5)	(6)	(7)	(8)
C 40	0.35-0.45	0.60-0.90	570-667	324	18	217	Crank shafts, shafts, spindles, axle beams, push rods, connecting rods, studs, bolts, gears, etc.
C 45	0.40-0.50	0.60-0.90	618-696	353	15	229	Shafts, bolts, gears and spindles of machine tools
C 50	0.45-0.55	0.60-0.90	647-765	373	13	241	Shafts, keys cylinders, hardened stock for worms and worm gears
C 50 Min.	0.45-0.55	1.00-1.10	706 (min)	392	11	255	Rail steel, bolts, gear shafts, rocking levers and cylinder liners.
C 55 Mn 75	0.50-0.60	0.60-0.90	706 (min)	392	13	265	Keys, crank shafts, cylinders, cams, gears, sprockets, parts requiring moderate wear resistance.
C 60	0.55-0.65	0.50-0.80	736 (min)	412	11	255	Hardened screws and nuts, Crank shafts, axles, couplings, gears and spindles for machine tools.
C 65	0.60-0.07	0.50-0.80	736 (min)	422	10	255	Locomotive carriage and wagon tyres, engine valve springs, washers and thin stamped parts.

*a, area of cross section.

†To obtain the values in metric units, i.e., kgf/mm^2, divide the value given in columns (5) and (6) with 9.80665.

Table I.9 *Properties and Uses of Alloy Steels (Other than Stainless and Heat Resisting Steels)*

Designation (ISI Grade)	Tensile strength MN/m²*	Yield strength MN/m²*	Minimum Elongation ($e = 6.55\sqrt{a^{**}}$)	Minimum Izod Impact value, Nm*	Brinell Hardness No. HB	Suggested uses
(1)	(2)	(3)	(4)	(5)	(6)	(7)
20 Mn 2	588-736	432	18	47.07	170-217	Welded structures, crank shafts, steering, shafting and spindles.
	687-834	490	16	47.07	201-248	
27 Mn 2	588-736	432	18	47.07	170-217	Welded structures, crank shafts, shafts, spindles and steering.
	687-834	490	16	47.07	201-248	
37 Mn 2	588-736	432	18	47.07	170-217	Crank shafts, shafts, axles and connecting rods
	687-834	530	18	47.07	201-248	
	785-932	588	16	47.07	229-277	
	882-1030	687	15	40.21	255-311	
35 Mn 2 Mo 28	687-834	530	18	54.00	201-248	Crank shafts, levers, bolts and connecting rods
	785-932	588	16	54.00	229-277	
	882-1030	687	15	54.00	255-311	
	981-1128	785	13	47.07	285-341	
35 Mn 2 Mo 45	785-932	588	16	54.00	229-277	Crank shafts, connecting rods, bolts, and levers.
	882-1030	687	15	54.00	225-311	
	981-1128	785	13	47.07	285-341	
40 Cr 1	687-834	530	18	54.00	201-248	Connecting rods, gears, wear resisting plates, etc.
	785-932	588	16	54.00	229-277	
	882-1030	687	15	54.00	255-311	
40 Cr 1 Mo 28	687-834	530	18	54.00	201-248	Shafts, gears, bolts and studs.
	785-932	588	16	54.00	229-277	
	882-1030	687	15	54.00	255-311	
	981-1128	785	13	47.07	255-341	
15 Cr 3 Mo 55 and	687-834	530	18	54.00	201-248	Parts requiring high surface hardness and wear resistance.
25 Cr 3 Mo 55	785-932	588	16	54.00	229-277	
	882-1030	687	15	54.00	255-311	
	981-1128	785	13	47.07	285-341	
	1080-1226	863	12	40.21	311-363	
	1520 min	1275	8	13.73	444 Min	

Table 1.9 Properties and Uses of Alloy Steels (Other than Stainless and Heat Resisting Steels) (Contd.)

(1)	(2)	(3)	(4)	(5)	(6)	(7)
40 Cr 3 Mo 1 V 20	1324 min	1098	8	20.60	363 Min	Components requiring high tensile strength.
	1520 Min	1275	8	13.73	444 Min	
40 Cr 2 Al 1 Mo 18	687-834	530	18	54.00	201-248	Components requiring high surface hardness and core strength.
	785-932	588	16	54.00	229-277	
	822-1030	687	15	37.27	255-311	
40 Ni 3	785-932	588	16	54.00	229-277	Heavy forgings, turbine blades, high stressed screws, bolts and nuts, cold though steel-used at low temperature (refrigerators and compressors).
	822-1030	687	15	54.00	255-311	
35 Ni 1 Cr 60	687-834	530	18	54.00	201-248	Aircrafts and heavy vehicle components
	785-932	588	16	54.00	229-277	
	882-1030	687	15	54.00	255-311	
30 Ni 4 Cr 1	1520 Min	1275	8	13.73	444 Min	Highly stressed gears.
40 Ni Cr 1 Mo 15	785-932	588	16	54.00	229-277	Gears, bolts, etc.
	882-1030	687	15	54.00	225-311	
	981-1128	785	13	47.07	285-431	
	1080-1226	863	11	40.21	311-363	
41 Ni 2 Cr 1 Mo 28	785-932	588	16	54.00	229-277	High strength machine parts like gears, bolts, spindles, collects, etc.
	882-1030	687	15	54.00	255-311	
	1080-1128	785	13	47.07	255-341	
	1080-1226	863	11	40.21	311-363	
	1180-1324	981	10	29.42	341-401	
	1520 min	1275	6	10.79	444 min	
40 Ni 2 Cr 65 Mo 55	981-1128	785	12	47.07	285-341	Highly stressed bolts, gears, shafts, mandrels, etc.
	1080-1226	863	11	40.21	311-363	
	1180-1324	981	10	34.32	341-401	
	1520 min	1275	8	13.73	444 min	

**a, area of cross-section.

*To obtain the values in metric units divide the given values in columns (2), (3) and (5) with 9.80665.

Table I.10 *Tensile Properties and uses of Corrosion Resistant Alloy Steel and Nickel Based Casting For General Applications*

Grade	Tensile Strength Min N/mm²	Yield Stress Min N/mm²	Elongation on Lo = 5.65 √So, Min Percent	Typical Uses
(1)	(2)	(3)	(4)	(5)
1	450	190	31	General service; pumps, values, etc, for chemical processing, oil refineries, textile dyeing, food machinery, architectural trim, fueljets, fuel values, engine supports.
2	480	190	31	General service, pumps, values, mixers, piping and fitting, etc.
3	480	210	26	Similar to Grade 1, but for less severe service.
4 & 4A	480	210	26	Pumps, values, fittings, etc. in reducing acids, paper mill equipment process industries, sea water service.
5	480	210	26	Similar to Grade 1, but especially useful where parts cannot be heat treated after welding.
6 & 6A	480	210	22	Improved Machinability-useful in service similar to Grade 3 or Grade 4 where finished product requires extensive drilling or threading.
7 & 7A	480	210	26	Paper pulp service, digester fittings, pumps, impellers, strainers, values, ornaments, fire wall fittings, hand rail fittings, grills.
8	450	190	26	Sulphite liquor, cold dilute sulphuric acid, agitators, fittings
9	550	280	9	Digester fittings, pumps, values for sulphite pulp service.
10 & 11	620	450	16	Valves and valve trim, pump parts for power plant and oil refining equipment, sliding or wearing parts, for parts in turbines.
12	450	210	—	Food processing, nitric acid and rayon manufacture, rabble blades in ore roasting furnace, nitrogen production, pumps, values, impellers
13	780	—	—	Nitrocellulose production, alkaline liquors, oxidizing acids, pumps for dilute sulphuric acid in mine water.

Table 1.10 *Tensile Properties and uses of Corrosion Resistant Alloy Steel and Nickel Based Casting (Contd.) For General Applications*

(1)	(2)	(3)	(4)	(5)
14	690	480	14	Value trim, abrasion and erosion resistance applications
15	650	190	31	Similar to Grade 1, but also resistant to intergranular corrosion.
16	480	210	26	Similar to Grade 4, but also resistant to intergranular corrosion.
17	520	240	22	Similar to Grade 4 where chance of pitting corrosion is more severe
18	430	170	31	Applications requiring resistance to hot sulphuric acid. For pump impellers used in naval boiler feed pumps
19	500	320	4	Resistance to highly corrosive chemicals (Hypochlorite solutions, ferric chloride and cupric chloride)
20	480	190	26	This is used in handling corrosive vapours above 400° C. It is mainly used in dairy, chemical, aeronautical, nuclear, petroleum and food processing industries
21	350	120	9	It is used for handling caustics processes where low iron and copper content in the equipment is important
22	450	210	22	It is highly resistant to salt water corrosion, erosion and abrasion and is used for impellers, for pumping salt cooling water and in chemical pumps
23	500	320	6	These alloys have resistance to corrosion by hot concentrated hydrochloride acid solutions and wet hydrogen chloride
24	760	550	14	This alloy has good corrosion resistance and resistance to abrasion.

IS: 3444-1978

Table I.11 *Mechanical Properties of Austenitic Stainless Steel Bars, Flats, Plates, Sheets and Strips in the Softened Condition*

Steel designation	HB Max	0.2% Proof stress Min	Tensile strength	Percentage Elongation		Percentage Elongation	
				Bars from	Flats from	Plates, sheets and strips	
				5 to 100 mm	3 to 30 mm	From 0.5 to 3 mm	From 3 to 30 mm
(1)	(2)	(3)	(4)	(5)	(6)	(7)	(8)
02Cr18Ni11	192	180	440 to 650	40	40	38	40
04Cr18Ni10	192	200	490 to 690	40	40	38	40
07Cr18Ni9	192	210	490 to 690	40	40	38	40
10Cr17Ni7	212	220	590 to 780	—	40	38	40
04Cr18Ni10Ti20	192	210	490 to 690	35	35	33	35
04Cr18Ni10Nb40	192	210	490 to 690	35	35	33	35
04Cr17Ni12Mo20	192	210	490 to 690	40	40	38	40
02Cr17Ni12Mo2	192	200	440 to 640	40	40	38	40
04Cr17Ni12Mo2Ti20	192	220	490 to 690	35	35	33	35
10Cr17Mn6N14	217	300	640 to 830	40	40	38	40
15Cr24Ni13	—	210	490 to 690	40	40	—	—
20Cr25Ni20	—	210	490 to 690	40	40	—	—

IS: 1570 (Part V)-1972

Table I.12 *Mechanical Properties of Stainless Steel Bars and Flats in the Hardened and Tempered Condition*

Steel designation	Annealed HB Max	0.2% proof stress Min N/mm^2	Tensile strength N/mm^2	Percentage Elongation Min		KCU* Min J/cm^2
				Bars from 5 to 100 mm	Flats from 3 to 30 mm	
(1)	(2)	(3)	(4)	(5)	(6)	(7)
12Cr13	212	410	590 to 780	16	16	6
20Cr13	229	490	690 to 880	14	14	4
30Cr13	235	590	780 to 980	11	11	—
15 Cr 16 Ni2	262	640	830 to 1030	10	10	3

*Values applicable on bars from 15 to 63 mm diameter.

IS: 1570 (Part V)-1972.

Table I.13 *Tensile Strength of Structural Steels*

Grade	Tensile Strength (N/mm^2)	Grade	Tensile Strength (N/mm^2)
St 30	300 to 380	St 47	470 to 570
St 32	320 to 440	St 50	500 to 600
St 34	340 to 460	St 52	520 to 620
St 37	370 to 490	St 55	550 to 650
St 39	390 to 510	St 58	580 to 680
St 42	420 to 540	St 63	630 to 710
St 44	440 to 540	St 88	880 to 1000

Table I.14 *Properties of Brasses of Different Chemical Compositions*

Chemical Composition			Tensile strength, MN/m^2†	% Elongation*	Brinell Hardness
%Cu	%Pb	%Zn			
54-47	upto 2.5	Rest	441	10	110
57-59.5	1.0-3.0	Rest	363-667	2 to 25	90-170
59.5-62	upto 0.3	Rest	333-580	3 to 30	80-170
62-65	upto 0.2	Rest	294-687	5 to 45	70-160
66-69	upto 0.1	Rest	284-530	5 to 45	70-160
69.5-73	upto 0.07	Rest	275-520	5 to 44	70-155

* Gauge Length

  5.8 $\sqrt{a}$ Round test piece;

  a, Area of cross-section

†MN/m^2 = (1/9.80665) kgf/mm^2

Table I.15 *Chemical Composition and Properties of Tin Bronze*

Chemical Composition					Mechanical Properties		
%Cu	%Sn	%Zn	%Pb	%P	Tensile Strength, MN/m²†	%elonga-tion Gauge length 5.8 √a*	Brinell Hardness HB
96	4	—	—	less than 0.4	314-440	10-55	65-120
94	6	—	—	0.4	343-490	12-60	70-130
92	8	—	—	0.4	392-540	20-60	80-150
91	8.5	—	—	0.3	540	5	150
90	10	—	—	—	216	15	60
88	12	—	—	—	235-275	8	80-95
86	14	—	—	—	196	3	85
85	5	7	3	—	147-245	10-12	60-75
86	10	4	—	—	196	10	65

*a area of cross-section, round

†$1 \text{ MN/m}^2 = (1/9.80665) \text{ kgf/mm}^2$

Table I.16 *Chemical Composition and Hardness Values of Bearing Materials (Lead and Tin Bases)*

Chemical Composition						Brinell Hardness HB	Use
%Su	%Pb	%Sb	%Cu	%Cd	%As		
—	86	12	1	—	1	18	for normal pressures
5	78.5	15.5	1	—	—	22	} for higher pressures
10	73.5	15.5	1	—	—	23	
6	76.5	15	1	0.8	0.7	26	} for the highest pressures
9	75	14	1	0.5	0.5	28	
80	2	12	6	—	—	27	} for shock loading
80	—	11	9	—	—	28	

Table I.17 *Properties of Typical Cast Irons*

Material	Ultimate strength, MN/m²† Tension σu^*	Compression σu^*	Endurance limit in reversed bending, MN/m²† σen^*	Brinell hardness number	Modulus of elasticity Tension and Compression GN/m²†	Shear G† GN/m²	Elongation in 50 mm %	Remarks and suggested uses
Gray, ordinary	124	557	62	100-150	69-82	28	0-1	General industrial casting
Gray, good	166	690	82	100-150	82	33	0-1	Pump cylinders, etc.
Gray, high grade	207	828	103	100-150	96	38	0-1	Important castings
Malleable, S.A.E. 32510	345	828	173	100-145	160	64	10	Substitute for unimport ant forgings
Nickel alloys: Ni-0.75, C-3.40, Si-1.75, Mn-0.55,	{ 221 166	828	110	{ 200 175	103	41	1-2	Light machine frames
Ni-2.00, C-3.00, Si-1.10, Mn-0.80.	{ 276 214	1080	138	{ 220 200	138	55	1-2	Heavy diesel cylinders pump, and valve bodies
Nickel-chromium alloys: Ni-0.75, Cr-0.30, C-3.40, Si-1.90, Mn-0.65	221	862	110	200	103	41	1-2	Light machine-tool tables, light engine cylinders
Ni-2.75, Cr-0.80, C-3.00, Si-1.25, Mn-0.60.	310	1103	152	300	138	55	1-2	Heavy forming dies

*Upper figures refer to arbitration test bars. Lower figures refer to the center of 100 mm round specimens

Flexure: For cast irons in bending the modulus of rupture may be taken as $1.75\sigma_u$ (tension) for circular section, $1.50\,\sigma_u$ for rectangular section and $1.25\,\sigma_u$ for I and T sections

Shear: The strength of cast iron in shear may be taken as $1.10\,\sigma_u$ (tension)

†1 MN/m² = (1/9.80665) kgf/mm²

†GN/m² = (1000/9.80665) kgf/mm²

Table I.18 Properties of Typical Carbon and Alloy Steels

Material	Ultimate strength		Yield stress, MN/m²†		Endurance limit inreversed bending, MN/m²† σen^*	Brinell hardness number	Modulus of elasticity		Elongation in 50 mm %	Remarks and suggested uses
	Tension σ_u† MN/m²	Shear τ_u† MN/m²	Tension and compression σ_{yp}	Shear τ_{yp}			Tension and compression E† GN/m²	Shear G GN/m²†		
(1)	(2)	(3)	(4)	(5)	(6)	(7)	(8)	(9)	(10)	(11)
Carbon Steels										
Wrought iron	332	345	186	110	173	100	193	77.5	30–40	
Cast steel, soft	414	290	186	110	180	110	207	82.0	22	
medium	483	338	218	131	207	120	207	82.0	18	General-purpose castings
hard	552	386	248	145	234	130	207	82.0	15	
S.A.E. 10.25, annealed	462	282	234	138	200	120	207	82.0	26	Machinery and general purpose steel
Water quenched	538	380	282	166	296	159			35	
	621	435	400	234	345	180	207	82.0	27	
S.A.E. 1045, annealed	586	414	310	180	289	140	207	82.0	20	Large forgings, axles, shafts
water quenched	655	462	414	241	365	197			28	
	828	580	621	360	462	248	207	82.0	15	
oil quenched	662	462	428	241	365	192			22	
	793	552	552	310	448	235	207	82.0	16	
S.A.E. 1095, annealed	760	520	380	228	360	200	207	82.0	20	Springs, cutting instruments
	896	586	455	270	470	300	207	82.0	16	
oil quenched	1300	828	896	520	690	380	207	79.4	10	

Table 1.18 Properties of Typical Carbon and Alloy Steels – (Contd...)

(1)	(2)	(3)	(4)	(5)	(6)	(7)	(8)	(9)	(10)	(11)
Alloy Steels										
Nickel: S.A.E. 2320, water quenched	504 / 965	380 / 676	345 / 758	207 / 448	338 / 470	143 / 277	207	82	30 / 18	Casehardening stock for heavy parts.
Oil quenched	527 / 896	373 / 621	332 / 690	200 / 414	318 / 345	140 / 262	207	82	30 / 18	Not desirable for, thin sections. Gears
S.A.E. 2340 water quenched	655 / 1206	414 / 758	448 / 1035	262 / 600	365 / 517	183 / 340	207	89	30 / 16	Forging, axles
oil quenched	641 / 1138	407 / 724	428 / 1020	248 / 586	380 / 517	183 / 330	207	82	17 / 14	Gears
Nickel-chromium: S.A.E. 3120, water quenched	593 / 965	414 / 676	393 / 792	234 / 470	380 / 400	174 / 269	207	82	34 / 15	Heavy sections requiring medium depth casehardening
Oil quenched	504 / 828	380 / 565	331 / 662	200 / 393	317 / 331	163 / 241	207	82	30 / 18	
S.A.E. 3220, water quenched	600 / 1138	414 / 792	414 / 986	248 / 573	400 / 496	187 / 331	207	82	23 / 16	Massive sections requiring deep casehardening
Oil quenched	552 / 380	386 / 738	364 / 896	214 / 655	352 / 448	174 / 311	207	82	30 / 20	
S.A.E. 3240, Oil quenched	758 / 1380	503 / 896	600 / 1240	360 / 724	580 / 621	229 / 388	207	82	23 / 14	Rollers, sprockets, gears
Chromium-molybednum S.A.E. 4140, oil quenched	828 / 1310	621 / 1035	690 / 1138	380 / 628	414 / 655	240 / 380	207	82	25 / 12	

Table 1.18 Properties of Typical Carbon and Alloy Steels – (Contd...)

(1)	(2)	(3)	(4)	(5)	(6)	(7)	(8)	(9)	(10)	(11)
Chromium-vanadium: S.A.E 6145, oil quenched	724 / 1586	517 / 1242	676 / 1448	373 / 792	654 / 724	220 / 425	207	82	25 / 12	Springs, Gears
Silicon-manganese: S.A.E. 9260, oil quenched	1090	828	690	414	428	240	207	82	16	
Stainless steel, 0.12C, 18.0 cr, 8.0 Ni	621 / 1380	414 / 1035	241 / 1206	138 / 690	276 / 621	135 / 380	207	82	60 / 5	Hot-rolled / Cold worked

The endurance limit for reversed shear may be taken as 55 percent of the endurance limit in reversed bending. Tabulated values are minimum values to be excepted with round bars up to 37 mm diameter. Smaller sections and careful heat-treatment will show higher values.

Upper figures : steel quenched and drawn to 700°C

Lower figures : steel quenched and drawn to 425°C

†1 MN/m² = (1/9.80665) kgf/mm²

†1 GN/m² = (1000/9.80665) kgf/mm²

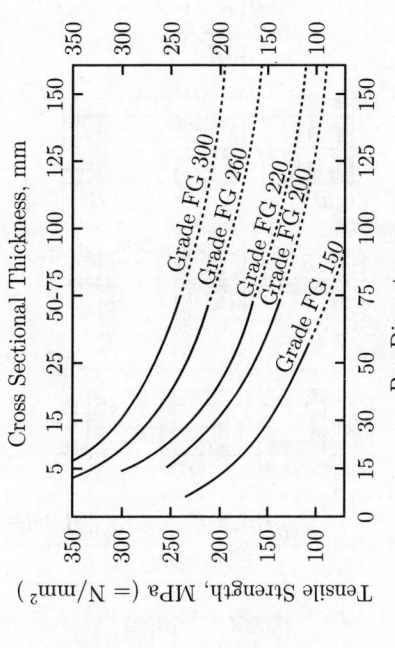

Fig. I.1: *Variation of Tensile Strength with Cross-Sectional Thickness of Grey Iron Castings.*

II

Appendix

Moments of inertia and moduli of various sections
(Refer table 1.3, Page 8 and 9)

(a)

Area, $A = \dfrac{\pi}{4}(BD - bd)$

Moment of inertia, $I = \dfrac{\pi}{64}(BD^3 - bd^3)$

Section modlus $Z = \dfrac{\pi}{32}\left(\dfrac{BD^3 - bd^3}{D}\right)$

(b)

$A = BD - bd; \quad I = \dfrac{1}{12}(BD^3 - bd^3); \quad Z = \dfrac{BD^3 - bd^3}{6D}$

(c)

$A = bD + Bd; \quad I = \dfrac{1}{12}(bD^3 + Bd^3); \quad Z = \dfrac{bD^3 + Bd^3}{6D}$

(d)

$A = BD - bd; \quad y_1 = \dfrac{BD^2 - bd^2}{2(BD - bd)}; \quad y_2 = \dfrac{BD^2 - bdD + bd^2}{2(BD - bd)}$

$I = \dfrac{(BD^2 - bd^2)^2 - 4B\, Dbd(D - d^2)}{12(BD - bd)}$

$Z_1 = \dfrac{I}{y_1} = \dfrac{(BD^2bd^2)^2 - 4B\, Dbd(D - d)^2}{6(BD^2 - bd^2)}$

$Z_2 = \dfrac{I}{y_2} = \dfrac{(BD^2 - bd^2 - 4B\, Dbd(D - d)^2)}{6(BD^2 - 2bd\, D + bd^2)}$

(e)

a_1 = area of top flange

a_2 = area of bottom flange

a = area of web

$y_1 = \dfrac{a_2(2D - t_2) + a_1t_1 + a(d + 2t_1)}{2(a_1 + a_2 + a)}$

$y_2 = \dfrac{a_1(2D - t_1) + a_2t_2 + a(d + 2t_2)}{(a_1 + a_2 + a)}$

$I = \dfrac{a_1t_1^2 + a_2t_2^2 + ad^2}{12} + \dfrac{a_1a_2(D + d)^2 + a_1a(t_1 + d)^2 + a_2a(t_2 + d)^2}{4(a_1 + a_2 + a)}$

$Z_1 = \dfrac{I}{y_1}$ $\qquad$ $Z_2 = \dfrac{I}{y_2}$

Note:– In actual practice it is often sufficiently accurate to take $Z_1 = a_1h$ and $Z_2 = a_2h$, where h is the perpendicular distance between the centres of the flanges.

III

Appendix

Table III-1 *Recommended values of Factor of Safety*

Material	for steady load	For varying load	For shock load
Cast Iron	5 to 6	8 to 12	16 to 20
Wrought Iron	4	7	10 to 50
Steel	4	8	12 to 60
Soft Metals and Alloys	6	9	15
Leather	9	12	15
Timber	7	10 to 15	20

Design stress or allowable stress, MN/m² (kgf/mm²) $\sigma_d = \dfrac{\sigma_u}{n}$.

Where σ_u is the ultimate strength of the material, MN/m² (kgf/mm²)

n is the factor of safety

The factor of safety $n = a \times b \times c$

Where a = elastic ratio

$$= \frac{\sigma_u}{\sigma_y} \text{ for static loads}$$

$$= \frac{\sigma_u}{\sigma_{e_n}} \text{ for variable loads}$$

b = shock or service factor

= 1, for steady or gradually applied loads

= 2, for suddenly applied loads

= 1.25 to 1.50 for light shocks

= 2 to 3 for heavy shocks

= 5 extreme cases

c = real margin of safety

= 1.5 to 2.0 for ductile materials of uniform

structure (Iron & Steel)

= 2.5 to 3.0 for CI & brittle materials

= 3 to 4 for timber

477

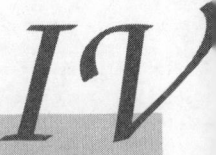

Appendix

International System (SI) Units

Table IV.1 *System International (SI)-Basic Units*

Physical quantity	Name of unit	Symbol
1. Length	metre	*m*
2. Mass	kilogram	*kg*
3. Time	second	*s*
4. Electric current	ampere	*A*
5. Thermedynamic temperature	degree Kelvin	*K*
6. Luminous itensity	candela	*cd*

Symbols for units do not take a plural form; the symbol 'K' now supersedes both °K and deg K.

Table IV.2 *System International (SI)–Dimensionless Supplementary Units*

Physical quantity	Name of unit	Symbol
1. Plane angle	radian	*rad*
2. Solid angle	steradian	*sr*
3. Activity of radio nuclides	curic	*Ci*
4. Amount of substance	mole	*mol*

Table IV.3 *System Internation (SI)–derived Units with special names*

Physical quantity	Name of unit	Symbol
Force	newton	$N = kg\,m/s^2$
Work, energy, quantity of heat	joule	$J = Nm$
Power	watt	$W = J/s = Nm/s$
Electrical charges	Coulomb	$C = As$
Electric potential	volt	$V = W/A$
Electric capacitance	farad	$F = As/V$
Electric resistance	ohm	$\Omega = V/A$
Inductance	henry	$H = Vs/A$
Luminous flux	lumen	$lm = cd\,sr$
Illumination	lux	$lx = lm/m$
Frequency	hertz	$Hz = s^{-1}$
Flux of magnetic induction, Magnetic flux	weber	$Wb = Vs$
Magnetic flux density, magnetic induction	tesla	$T = Wb/m^2$
Customary temperature	degree Celsius	$°C$

N.B.: The centigrade scale has been renamed the Celsius scale to fall in line with international practice. If the Celsius scale is used the symbol must remain °C to distinguish it from C, the Coulmob

Table IV.4 *System International (SI)–Some derived units with complex names*

Physical quantity	Name of unit	Symbol
Area	square metre	m^2
Volume	cubic metre	m^3
Density	kilogram per cubic metre	kg/m^3
Velocity	metre per second	m/s
Angular velocity	radian per second	rad/s
Acceleration	metre per second squared	m/s^2
Angular acceleration	radian per second squared	rad/s^2
Pressure or stress	newton per square metre	N/m^2
Dynamic viscosity	newton second per square meter	Ns/m^2
Kinematic viscosity	Square metre per second	m^2/s
Entropy	joule per Kelvin	J/K
Specific heat	Joule per kilogram Kelvin	$J/kg\,K$
Thermal conductivity	watt per metre Kelvin	$W/m\,K$

Table IV.5 *System International (SI)–Some Units to be allowed in conjunction with SI*

Physical quantity	Name	Symbol	Definition of unit
Length	parsec	*pc*	$30.87 \times 10^{15} m$
Area	barn	*b*	$10^{-28} m^2$
	hectare	*ha*	$10^4 m^2$
Volume	litre	*l*	$10^{-3} m^3 = dm^3$
Pressure	bar	*bar*	$10^5 N/m^2$
Mass	tonne	*t*	$10^3 kg = Mg$
Kinematic viscosity diffusion			
Coefficient	stokes	*st*	$10^{-4} m^2/s$
Dynamic viscosity	poise	*p*	$10^{-1} kg/ms$

Table IV.6 *System International (SI)–Multiple and Sub-multiple factors*

Multiplier	Prefix	Symbol
$1\ 000\ 000\ 000\ 000 = 10^{12}$	**tera**†	**T**
$1\ 000\ 000\ 000 = 10^9$	**giga**	**G**
$1\ 000\ 000 = 10^6$	**mega**	**M**
$1\ 000 = 10^3$	**kilo**	**k**
$100 = 10^{2*}$	hecto	*h*
$10 = 10^{1*}$	deca	*da*
$0.1 = 10^{-1*}$	**deci**	**d**
$0.01 = 10^{-2*}$	centi	*c*
$0.001 = 10^{-3}$	**milli**	**m**
$0.000\ 001 = 10^{-6}$	**micro**	**μ**
$0.000\ 000\ 001 = 10^{-9}$	**nano**	**n**
$0.000\ 000\ 000\ 001 = 10^{-12}$	**pico**	**p**
$0.000\ 000\ 000\ 000\ 001 = 10^{-15}$	femto	*f*
$0.000\ 000\ 000\ 000\ 000\ 001 = 10^{-18}$	atto	a

*To be restricted to instances where there is a strongly felt need, such as may be experienced in the case of centimetre as the unit of length in certain biological measurements

†Bold face has been used for prefixes most widely used

N.B.: Multiples of the fundamental unit should be chosen in powers of $\pm 3n$, where *n* is an integer

Table IV.7 *Some common physical quantities in mechanical and thermal sciences with SI units, some recommended multiples and submultiples of SI units, some other units permissible in SI and remarks*

Sl. No.	Quantity	SI units	Some recommended multiples and submultiples of SI units	Other permissible units	Remarks
(1)	(2)	(3)	(4)	(5)	(6)
1.	length (wave length)	m(metre)	km, mm, μm, nm	cm(limited use only)	'μm' is sometimes called 'micron'
2.	mass	kg(kilogram)	Mg, g, mg, μg	tonne(t)$=10^3 kg$ quintal (q) $=10^2 kg$	the metric carat $= 2 \times 10^{-4}$ kg, for precious materials
3.	time (period)	s(second)	ks, ms, μs, ns	day(d), hour(h), minute (min)	Other units like week, month and year are in common use
4.	Plane angle (angular displacement)	rad (radian)	m rad, μ rad	degree$°$ = $\pi/180$ rad minute' $= 1°/60$ second'' $= 1'/60$ grade(g) $= \pi/200$ rad	—
5.	Solid angle	sr(steradian)	—	—	
6.	area	m^2	km^2, mm^2	hectare(ha)$=10^4 m^2$ are(a)$=10^2 m^2$	cm^2 for limited use only
7.	Volume	m^3	mm^3	hectolitre(hl) litre(l)$=dm^3$ millilitre(ml)	litre and its multiples for limited use
8.	frequency	Hz(hertz)	THz, GHz, MHz, kHz	—	$1\ Hz = 1\ c/s$

Table IV.7 (Contd.)

(1)	(2)	(3)	(4)	(5)	(6)
9.	rotational frequency	s^{-1}	—	revolutions per minute or per second	—
10.	Velocity	m/s	—	$km/h = (1/3.6)\ m/s$	—
11.	Acceleration	m/s^2	—	—	—
12.	Angular acceleration	rad/s^2	—	—	—
13.	density	kg/m^3	Mg/m^3	$t/m^3,\ kg/l,\ g/l,\ g/ml$	$1\ g/l = 1\ kg/m^3$; $1\ kg/l = 1\ kg/dm^3$; $1\ g/ml = 1\ g/cm^3$
14.	Momentum	$kg\ m/s$	—	—	—
15.	Moment of momentum	$kg\ m^2/s$	—	—	—
16.	moment of inertia	$kg\ m^2$	—	—	—
17.	force	N(newton)	$MN,\ kn,\ mN$	—	—
18.	moment of force	Nm	$MNm,\ kNm,\ \mu Nm$	Nmm	—
19.	pressure (normal stress)	N/m^2	$GN/m^2 = kN/mm^2,$ $MN/m^2,\ kN/m^2,$ $mN/m^2,\ \mu N/m^2$	$1\ h\ bar = 10^7 N/m^2$, $1\ bar = 10^5 N/m^2$, $1\ mbar = 10^2 N/m^2$, $1\ \mu bar = 10^{-1} N/m^2$	the special name 'pascal' for N/m^2 is under consideration
20.	dynamic viscosity	Ns/m^2	mNs/m^2	$poise(P)=10^{-1}\ Ns/m^2$ Centipoise$(cP)=10^{-3}$ Ns/m^2	Poise(P)=dyne/cm^2 (cgs unit) Poisecuille(Pl)=Ns/m^2 (MKS) (SI)

Table IV.7 (Contd.)

(1)	(2)	(3)	(4)	(5)	(6)
21. Kinematic viscosity		m^2/s	—	stokes$(St)=10^{-4}m^2/s$ centistokes$(cSt)=10^{-6} m^2/s$	—
22. power		W(watt)	$GW,\ MW,\ kW,\ mW,\ \mu W$	—	$W = J/s = Nm/s$
23. impact strength		J/m^2	kJ/m^2	—	—
24. temperature		K(kelvin)	—	—	—
25. Customery temperature		°C	—	—	°C=degree Celsius
26. temperature interval		$K,\ °C$	—	—	$1°C = 1K$
27. linear coefficient of expansion		$K^{-1},\ °C^{-1}$	—	—	—
28. heat		J	$TJ,\ GJ,\ MJ,\ kJ,\ mJ$	—	—
29. thermal conductivity		$W/mK,\ W/m°C$	—	—	—
30. heat capacity		$J/K,\ J/°C$	$kJ/K,\ kJ/°C$	—	—
31. internal energy		J	—	—	—
32. Entropy		J/K	—	—	—

Conversion Factors and Conversion Tables

I. Conversion Factors

(a) Length

1 in = 25.4 mm

1 ft = 0.3048 m

1 yard = 0.9144 m

1 mile = 1.609 344 km

1 mm = 0.039 3701 in

1 m = 39.37 in

1 m = 1.093 613 yards

1 km = 0.621 371 mile

(b) Area

$1 \text{ in}^2 = 645.16 \text{ mm}^2$

$1 \text{ ft}^2 = 0.092 \ 903 \text{ m}^2$

$1 \text{ sq. yard} = 0.836 \ 13 \text{ m}^2$

$1 \text{ sq. mil} = 2.589 \ 99 \text{ km}^2$

1 acr = 0.404 686 hectare

$1 \text{ mm}^2 = 0.001 \ 55 \text{ in}^2$

$1 \text{ m}^2 = 1550 \text{ in}^2$

$1 \text{ m}^2 = 1.195 \ 99 \text{ sq. yard}$

$1 \text{ km}^2 = 0.386 \ 102 \text{ sq. mil}$

1 hectare = 2.47105 acres

(c) Volume and Capacity

$1 \text{ in}^3 = 16 \ 387 \text{ mm}^3$

$1 \text{ ft}^3 = 0.028 \ 317 \text{ m}^3$

1 pint = 0.568 24 litre

1 quart = 1.136 49 litres

1 gallon (UK) = 4.545 96 litres

1 gallon (US) = 3.785 33 litres

$1 \text{ mm}^3 = 0.000 \ 061 \text{ in}^3$

$1 \text{ m}^3 = 61 \ 023 \text{ in}^3$

1 litre = 1.759 80 pints

1 litre = 0.879 90 quart

1 litre = 0.219 976 gallon (UK)

1 litre = 0.264 178 gallon (US)

(d) Moment of Inertia

$1 \text{ in}^4 = 416 \ 231 \text{ mm}^4$

$1 \text{ ft}^4 = 0.008 \ 631 \text{ m}^4$

$1 \text{ mm}^4 = 0.000 \ 002 \ 403 \text{ in}^4$

$1 \text{ m}^4 = 2.402 \ 490 \text{ in}^4$

(e) Force

1 lbf = 0.453 59 kgf

1 lbf = 4.448 22 N

1 tonf = 1 016 kgf

1 tonf = 9 964.012 N

1 kgf = 2.205 lbf

1 kgf = 9.806 65 N

1 tonnef = 2 205 lbf

1 tonnef = 9 806.65 N

1 newton = 0.102 kgf

1 newton = 0.224 81 lbf

1 newton = 1000 000 dynes

(f) Force Per Unit Length

1 lbf/ft = 1.488 16 kg/fm

1 lbf/ft = 14.59 N/m

1 tonf/ft = 3 333.478 4 kgf/m

1 tonf/ft = 32690 N/m

1 kgf/m = 0.671 97 lbf/ft

1 kgf/m = 9.806 65 N/m

1 tonnef/m = 671.970 lbf/ft

1 tonnef/m = 9806.65 N/m

1 N/m = 0.102 kgf/m

1 N/m = 0.224 8 lbf/m

1 N/m = 0.068 5 lbf/ft

(g) Bending Moment

1 lbf in = 11.521 2kgf mm

1 lbf in = 112.9 Nmm

1 lbf ft = 0.138 254 kgf m

1 lbf ft = 1.355 81 N m

1 tonf in = 25.807 45 kgf m

1 tonf ft = 3037 N m

1 tonf in = 253 084 N mm

1 tonf ft = 309.688 kgf m

1 kgf mm = 0.007 234 lbf ft

1 kgf mm = 0.086 811 lbf in

1 kgf mm = 9.806 650 N mm

1 kgf m = 7.234 25 lbf ft

1 kgf m = 86.811 07 lbf in

1 kgf m = 9.806 65 N m

1 tonnef mm = 7.234 3 lbf ft

1 tonnef mm = 86.811 07 lbf in

1 tonnef mm = 9 806.65 N mm

1 tonnef m = 7 234.255 8 lbf ft

1 tonnef m = 86 811.07 lbf in

1 tonnef m = 9 806.65 N m

1 N m = 0.109 72 kgf m

1 N m = 8.850 39 lbf in

1 N m = 0.737 533 lbf ft

(h) Pressure and Stress

1 lbf/in^2 = 0.000 703 kgf/mm^2

1 lbf/in^2 = 0.006 895 N/mm^2

1 tonf/in^3 = 1.575 kgf/mm^2

1 tonf/in^2 = 15.444 N/mm^2

1 tonf/it^2 = 10.936.6 kgf/m^2

1 kgf/mm^2 = 1 422.33 lbf/in^2

1 kgf/mm^2 = 9.806 65 N/mm^2

1 tonnef/m^2 = 204.8 lbf/ft^2

1 tonnef/m^2 = 9 806.65 N/m^2

1 tonf/ft^2 = 107 251 N/m^2

1 N/m^2 = 0.102 kgf/m^2

1 N/m^2 = 0.000 145 lbf/in^2

1 N/m^2 = 0.020 87 lbf/ft^2

(i) Density

1 lb/in^3 = 0.000 027 68 kg/mm^3

1 lb/ft^3 = 16.018 5 kg/m^3

1 kg/mm^2 = 36 127.30 lb/in^2

1 kg/m^3 = 0.000 036 127 3 lb/in^3

(j) Miscellaneous Conversion Factors

1 atm = 1.013 3bar

1 atm = 1.033 kgf/cm^2

1 atm = 14.700 lbf/in^2

1 atm = 760 mm of Hg

1 atm = 101 330 N/m^3

1 bar = 0.986 875 atm

1 bar = 1 000 000 dynes/cm^2

1 bar = 1.020 kgf/cm^2

1 bar = 14.500 lbf/in^2

1 bar = 100 000 N/m^2

1 Btu = 1 055.100 J

1 Btu = 0.252 kcal

1 Btu = 0.000 293 1 kWh

1 Btu = 1 055 N m

1 Btu/ft h F = 1.730 8 J/m sK

1 Btu/ft h F = 1.488 kcal/m h C

1 Btu/ft^{2}h = 0.003 154 6 kW/m^2

1 Btu/ft^{2}h = 2.712 kcal/m^{2}h

1 Btu/ft^{2}h F = 5.678 4 W/m^2 C

1 Btu/ft^3 = 37 260 J/m^3

1 Btu/hr = 0.000 293 08 kW

1 Btu/lb = 2 326 J/kg

1 Btu/lb F = 4 186.800 J/kg K

1 Btu/s = 1.415 hp (FPS)

1 Btu/s = 1.435 hp (metric)

1 Btu/s = 1.055 1 kW

1 cal = 4.186 8 J

1 cal/s = 0.004 186 8 kW

1 Chu = 1.899 1 kJ

1 Chu/ft^3 = 0.067 067 MJ/m^3

1 Chu/hr = 0.000 527 54 kW

1 Chu/h ft°C = 1.730 8 W/m C

1 Chu/h ft^2 = 0.005 678 4 kW/m^2

1 Chu/lb = 4.186 8 kJ/kg

1 deg (angle) = 0.017 45 rad

1 deg/s = 0.002 778 rev/s

1 dyne = 0.010 mN

1 dyne/cm^2 = 0.100 N/m^2

1 erg = 1.000 dyne-cm

1 erg = 0.000 1 mJ

1 erg/s = 0.000 000 000 1 kW

1 ft candle = 10.760 lux

1 ft lbf = 1.355 8 J

1 ft lbf = 0.000 324 1 kcal

1 ft lbf = 0.138 3 kgf m

1 ft lbf/mm = 0.022 597 W

1 ft lbf/s = 0.077 17 Btu/min

1 ft lbf/ = 0.001 843 hP (metric)

1 ft lbf/s = 0.019 45 kcal/min

1 ft lbf/s = 1.355 8 W

1 ft/min = 0.018 29 km/h

1 ft/min = 0.005 08 m/s

1 ft/s = 1.097 km/h

1 ft/s = 18.290 m/min

1 ft/s^2 = 0.304 8 m/s^2

1 ft^2/h = 25.806 mm^2/s

1 ft^2/s = 0.092 903 m^2/s

1 ft^3/h = 0.028 317 m^3/h

1 ft^3/h = 0.062 428 m^2/kg

1 ft pdl = 0.042 139 J

1 ft pfl/s = 0.042 139 W

1 ft water = 0.029 5 atm

1 ft water = 2.989.100 N/m^2

1 furlong = 201.200 m

1 hemisphere (solid angle) = 6.283 Steradians

1 hemisphere (sold angle) = 4.000

                         Spherical right angles

1 hp (boiler) = 55.870 But/min

1 hp (boiler) = 980.400 W

1 hp (FPS) = 33 000 ft lbf/min

1 hp (FPS) = 1.014 hp (metric)

1 hp (FPS) = 10.700 kcal/min

1 hp (FPS) = 0.745 7 kW

1 hp-hr (FPS) = 2.684 5 MJ

1 hp (metric) = 75.000 kgf m/s

1 hp (metric) = 0.735 48 kW

1 hp-hr (metric) = 2.647 7 MJ

1 hundred weight (cwt) = 50.800 kg

1 hundred weight/cu. yard = 66.450 kg/m^3

1 J = 0.000 239 kcal

1 J = 0.102 kgf m

1 J = 0.000 277 8 W-hr

1 kcal = 4.186 8 kJ

1 kcal/h = 0.001 163 kW

1 kcal/h ft C = 3.815 6 W/m C

1 kcal/h ft^2 = 0.012 518 kW/m^2

1 kcal/s = 4.186 8 kW

1 kgf/m = 9.806 65 J

1 kg/ft h = 0.911 34 cP

1 kg/m h = 0.277 78 cP

1 kip = 1000 lb

1 lbf = 444.822 dynes

1 lb/ft = 1.488 kg/m

1 lbf/ft^2 = 47.880 N/m^2

1 lb/ft^3 = 16.018 kg/m^3

1 lb/ft^3°F = 28833 kg/m^3°C

1 lb/ft h = 0.413 38 cP

1 lb/ft s = 1.488 2 Ns/m^2

1 lb/in = 17.860 kg/m

1 lb/in^3 = 27 680 kg/m^3

1 lumen/ft^2 = 1.000 ft-candle

1 lux = 1.000 lumen/m^2

1 manud = 37.320 kg

1 maund = 40.000 seers

1 megaline = 1 000 000 maxwells

1 micron = 0.000 001 m

1 mile/h = 0.447 04 m/s

1 mil = 0.002 540 cm

1 minute(angle) = 0.000 290 9 rad

1 nautical mile = 1.853 km

1 N/m^2 = 0.01 mbar

1 Poise = 0.0102 kgf/s/m^2

1 Poise = 0.002 088 lbfs/ft^2

1 Poise = 0 100 Ns/m^2

1 poundal = 13.830 dynes

1 poundal = 14.100 gmf

1 quintal = 100 kg

1 quire = 25 sheets

1 rad/s = 0.159 2 rev/s

1 revolution = 6.283 rad

1 rod = 5.029 m

1 Stoke = 100 mm^2/s

1 tola = 10.660 gm

1 toone-cal/h = 1.163 kW

1 ton refrigeration = 3.516 9 kW

1 torr (mm Hg) = 133.333 N/m^2

(k) **Conversion of Thermometric Scales:**

F = temperature on the Fahrenheit scale

C = Equivalent temperature on the centigrade scale

K = equivalent temperature on the Kelvin scale

$$C = \frac{5}{9}(F-32)$$

$$C = K - 273.15$$

$$F = \frac{9}{5}C+32$$

$$F = \frac{9}{5}K-459.67$$

$$K = C+273.15$$

$$K = \frac{5}{9}F+255.372\ 22$$

(l) **Temperature Difference**

$$1°C = \frac{9}{5}°F$$

$$1°C = 1K$$

$$1°F = \frac{5}{9}°C$$

$$1°F = \frac{5}{9}K$$

$$1K = 1°C$$

$$1K = \frac{9}{5}°F$$

II. Conversion Tables

Table V.1 *Equivalent of Kilogram forces in Newtons*

kgf	0	1	2	3	4	5	6	7	8	9
0	0	9.80665	19.61330	29.41995	39.22660	49.03325	58.83990	68.64655	78.45320	88.25985
10	98.06650	107.87315	117.67980	127.48645	137.29310	147.09975	156.90640	166.71305	176.51970	186.32635
20	196.13300	205.93965	215.74630	225.55295	235.35960	245.16625	254.97290	264.77955	274.58620	284.39285
30	294.19950	304.00615	313.81280	323.61945	333.42610	343.23275	353.03940	362.84605	372.65270	382.45935
40	392.26600	402.07265	411.87930	421.68595	431.49260	441.29925	451.10590	460.91255	470.71920	480.52585
50	490.33250	500.13915	509.94580	519.75245	529.55910	539.36575	549.17240	558.97905	568.78570	578.59235
60	588.39900	598.20565	608.01230	617.81895	627.62560	637.43225	647.23890	657.04555	666.85220	676.65885
70	686.46550	696.27215	706.07880	715.88545	725.69210	735.49875	745.30540	755.11205	764.91870	774.72535
80	784.53200	794.33865	804.14530	813.95195	823.75860	833.56255	843.37190	853.17855	862.98520	872.79185
90	882.59850	892.50415	902.21180	912.01845	921.82510	931.63175	941.43840	951.24505	961.05170	970.85835

Table V.2 *Equivalents of Newtons in Kilogram forces (kgf)*

Newtons	0	1	2	3	4	5	6	7	8	9
0	0	0.1020	0.2039	0.3059	0.4079	0.5099	0.6118	0.7138	0.8158	0.9178
10	1.0197	1.1217	1.2237	1.3256	1.4276	1.5296	1.6316	1.7335	1.8355	1.9375
20	2.0394	2.1414	2.2434	2.3454	2.4473	2.5493	2.6513	2.7532	2.8552	2.9572
30	3.0592	3.1611	3.2631	3.3651	3.4670	3.5690	3.6710	3.7730	3.8749	3.9769
40	4.0789	4.1808	4.2828	4.3848	4.4868	4.5887	4.6907	4.7927	4.8946	4.9966
50	5.0986	5.2006	5.3025	5.4045	5.5065	5.6084	5.7104	5.8124	5.9144	6.0163
60	6.1183	6.2203	6.3222	6.4242	6.5262	6.6282	6.7301	6.8321	6.9341	7.0360
70	7.1380	7.2400	7.3420	7.4439	7.5459	7.6479	7.7498	7.8518	7.9538	8.0558
80	8.1577	8.2597	8.3617	8.4637	8.5656	8.6676	8.7696	8.8715	8.9735	9.0755
90	9.1775	9.2794	9.3814	9.4834	9.5853	9.6873	9.7893	9.8913	9.9932	10.0952

Table V.3 Equivalents of inches in mm

Inches	0	1	2	3	4	5	6	7	8	9
0	0	25.4	50.8	76.2	101.6	127.0	152.4	177.8	203.2	228.6
10	254.0	279.4	304.8	330.2	355.6	381.0	406.4	431.8	457.2	482.6
20	508.0	533.4	558.8	584.2	609.6	635.0	660.4	685.8	711.2	736.6
30	762.0	787.4	812.8	838.2	863.6	889.0	914.4	939.8	965.2	990.6
40	1016.0	1041.4	1066.8	1092.2	1117.6	1143.0	1168.4	1193.8	1219.2	1244.6
50	1270.0	1295.4	1320.8	1346.2	1371.6	1397.0	1422.4	1447.8	1473.2	1498.6
60	1524.0	1549.4	1574.8	1600.2	1625.6	1651.0	1676.4	1701.8	1727.2	1752.6
70	1778.0	1803.4	1828.8	1854.2	1879.6	1905.0	1930.4	1955.8	1981.2	2006.6
80	2032.0	2057.4	2082.8	2108.2	2133.6	2159.0	2184.4	2209.8	2235.2	2260.6
90.	2286.0	2311.4	2336.8	2362.2	2387.6	2413.0	2438.4	2463.8	2489.2	2514.6

Table V.4 Equivalents of mm in inches

mm	0	1	2	3	4	5	6	7	8	9
0	0	0.039370	0.078740	0.118110	0.157480	0.196850	0.236221	0.275591	0.314961	0.354331
10	0.393701	0.433071	0.472441	0.511811	0.551181	0.590551	0.629921	0.669291	0.708661	0.748032
20	0.787402	0.826772	0.866142	0.905512	0.944882	0.984252	1.023622	1.062992	1.102362	1.141732
30	1.181102	1.220472	1.259843	1.299213	1.338583	1.377953	1.417323	1.456693	1.496063	1.535433
40	1.574803	1.614173	1.653543	1.692913	1.732284	1.771654	1.811024	1.850394	1.889764	1.929134
50	1.968504	2.007874	2.047244	2.086614	2.125984	2.165354	2.204724	2.244095	2.283465	2.322835
60	2.362205	2.401575	2.440945	2.480315	2.519685	2.559055	2.598425	2.637795	2.677165	2.716535
70	2.755906	2.795276	2.834646	2.874016	2.913386	2.952756	2.992126	3.031496	3.070866	3.110236
80	3.149606	3.188976	3.228347	3.267717	3.307087	3.346457	3.385827	3.425197	3.464567	3.503937
90	3.543307	3.582677	3.622047	3.661417	3.700787	3.740158	3.779528	3.818898	3.858268	3.897638

Table V.5 Equivalents of lbf in Newtons

lbf	0	1	2	3	4	5	6	7	8	9
0	0	4.44822	8.89644	13.34466	17.79288	22.24110	26.68932	31.13754	35.58576	40.03398
10	44.48220	48.93042	53.37864	57.82686	62.27508	66.72330	71.17152	75.61974	80.06796	84.51618
20	88.96440	93.41262	98.86084	102.30906	106.75728	111.20550	115.65372	120.10194	124.55016	128.99838
30	133.44660	137.89482	142.34304	146.79126	151.23948	155.68770	160.13592	164.58414	169.03236	173.48058
40	177.92880	182.37702	186.82524	191.27346	195.72168	200.16990	204.61812	209.06634	213.51456	217.96278
50	222.41100	226.85922	231.30744	235.75566	240.20388	244.65210	249.10032	253.54854	257.99676	262.44498
60	266.89320	271.34142	275.78964	280.23786	284.68608	289.13430	293.58252	298.03074	302.47896	306.92718
70	311.37540	315.82362	320.27184	324.72006	329.16828	333.61650	338.06472	342.51294	346.96116	351.40938
80	355.85760	360.30582	364.75404	369.20226	373.65048	378.09870	382.54692	386.99514	391.44336	395.89158
90	400.33980	404.78802	409.23624	413.68446	418.13268	422.58090	427.02912	431.47734	435.92556	440.37378

Table V.6 Equivalents of Newtons in lbf

Newtons	0	1	2	3	4	5	6	7	8	9
0	0	0.22481	0.44962	0.67443	0.89924	1.12405	1.34886	1.57367	1.79848	2.02329
10	2.24810	2.47291	2.69772	2.92253	3.14734	3.37215	3.59696	3.82177	4.04658	4.27139
20	4.49620	4.72101	4.94582	5.17063	5.39544	5.62025	5.84506	6.06987	6.29468	6.51949
30	6.74430	6.96911	7.19392	7.41873	7.64354	7.86835	8.09316	8.31797	8.54278	8.76759
40	8.99240	9.21721	9.44202	9.66683	9.89164	10.11645	10.34126	10.56607	10.79088	11.01569
50	11.24050	11.46531	11.69012	11.91493	12.13974	12.36455	12.58936	12.81417	13.03898	13.26379
60	13.48860	13.71341	13.93822	14.16303	14.38784	14.61265	14.83746	15.06227	15.28708	15.51189
70	15.73670	15.96151	16.18632	16.41113	16.63594	16.86075	17.08556	17.31037	17.53518	17.75999
80	17.98480	18.20961	18.43442	18.65923	18.88404	19.10885	19.33366	19.55847	19.78328	20.22809
90	20.23290	20.45771	20.68252	20.90733	21.13214	32.35695	21.58176	21.80657	22.03138	22.25619

Table V.7 Equivalents of lbf/in² kN/m²

lbf in²	0	1	2	3	4	5	6	7	8	9
0	0	6.8948	13.7896	20.6844	27.5792	34.4740	41.3688	48.2636	55.1584	62.0532
10	68.9480	75.8428	82.7376	89.6324	96.5272	103.4220	110.3168	117.2116	124.1064	131.0012
20	137.8960	144.7908	151.6856	158.5804	165.4752	172.3700	179.2648	186.1596	193.0544	199.9492
30	206.8440	213.7388	220.6336	227.5284	234.4232	241.3180	248.2128	255.1076	262.0024	268.8972
40	275.7920	282.6868	289.5816	296.4764	303.3712	310.2660	317.1608	324.0556	330.9504	337.8452
50	344.7400	351.6348	358.5296	365.4244	372.3192	379.2140	386.1088	393.0036	399.8984	406.7923
60	413.6880	420.5828	427.4776	434.3724	441.2672	448.1620	455.0568	461.9516	468.8464	475.7412
70	482.6360	489.5308	496.4256	503.3204	510.2152	517.1100	524.0048	530.8996	537.7944	544.6892
80	551.5840	558.4788	565.3736	572.2684	579.1632	586.0580	592.9528	599.8476	606.7424	613.6372
90	620.5320	627.4268	634.3216	641.2164	648.1112	655.0060	661.9008	668.7956	675.6904	682.5852

Table V.8 Equivalents of kN/m² in lbf/in²

kN/m²	0	1	2	3	4	5	6	7	8	9
0	0	0.14504	0.29008	0.43512	0.58016	0.72520	0.87024	1.01528	1.16032	1.30536
10	1.45040	1.59544	1.74048	1.88552	2.03056	2.17560	2.32064	2.46568	2.61072	2.75576
20	2.90080	3.04584	3.19088	3.33592	3.48096	3.62600	3.77104	3.91608	4.06112	4.20616
30	4.35120	4.49624	4.64128	4.78632	4.93136	4.07640	5.22154	5.36648	5.51152	5.65656
40	5.80160	5.94664	6.09168	6.23672	6.38176	6.52680	6.67184	6.81688	6.96192	7.10696
50	7.25200	7.39704	7.54208	7.68712	7.83216	7.97720	8.12224	8.26728	8.41232	8.55736
60	8.70240	8.84744	8.99248	9.13752	9.28256	9.42760	9.57264	9.71768	9.86272	10.00776
70	10.15280	10.29784	10.44288	10.58792	10.73296	10.87800	11.02304	11.16808	11.31312	11.45816
80	11.60320	11.74824	11.89328	12.03832	12.18336	12.32840	12.47344	12.61848	12.76352	12.90856
90	13.05360	13.19864	13.34368	13.48872	13.63376	13.77880	13.92384	14.06888	14.21392	14.35896

Table V.9 Equivalents of horse-power (metric) in kilowatts (kW)

hp (metric)	0	1	2	3	4	5	6	7	8	9
0	0	0.73548	1.47096	2.20644	2.94192	3.67740	4.41288	5.14836	5.88384	6.61932
10	7.35480	8.09028	8.82576	9.56124	10.29672	11.03220	11.76768	12.50316	13.23864	13.97412
20	14.70960	15.44508	16.18056	16.91604	17.65152	18.38700	19.12248	19.85796	20.59344	21.32892
30	22.06440	22.79988	23.53536	24.27084	25.00632	25.74180	26.47728	27.21276	27.94824	28.68372
40	29.41920	30.15468	30.89016	31.62564	32.36112	33.09660	33.83208	34.56756	35.30304	36.03852
50	36.77400	37.50948	38.24496	38.98044	39.71592	40.45140	41.18688	41.92236	42.65784	43.39332
60	44.12880	44.86428	45.59976	46.33524	47.07072	47.80620	48.54168	49.27716	50.01264	50.74812
70	51.48360	52.21908	52.95456	53.69004	54.42552	55.16100	55.89648	56.63196	57.36744	58.10292
80	58.83840	59.57388	60.30936	61.04484	61.78032	62.51580	63.25128	63.98676	64.72224	65.45772
90	66.19320	66.92868	67.66416	68.39964	69.13512	69.87060	70.60608	71.34156	72.07704	72.81252

Table V.10 Equivalents of kilowatts (kW) in horse-power (metric)

kW	0	1	2	3	4	5	6	7	8	9
0	0	1.35966	2.71931	4.07897	5.43863	6.79828	8.15794	9.51759	10.87725	12.23691
10	13.59656	14.95622	16.31587	17.67553	19.03519	20.39484	21.75450	23.11416	24.47381	25.83347
20	27.19312	28.55278	29.91244	31.27209	32.63175	33.99141	35.35106	36.71072	38.07037	39.43003
30	40.78969	42.14934	43.50900	44.86865	46.22831	47.58797	48.94762	50.30728	51.66694	53.02659
40	54.38625	55.74590	57.10556	58.46522	59.82487	61.18453	62.54419	63.90384	65.26350	66.62315
50	67.98281	69.34247	70.70212	72.06178	73.42143	74.78109	76.14075	77.50040	78.86006	80.21972
60	81.57937	82.93903	84.29868	85.65834	87.01800	88.37765	89.73731	91.09697	92.45662	93.81628
70	95.17593	96.53559	97.89525	99.25490	100.61455	101.97421	103.33387	104.69352	106.05318	107.41283
80	108.77249	110.13215	111.49180	112.85146	114.21112	115.57077	116.93043	118.29008	119.64974	121.00940
90	122.36905	123.72871	125.08837	126.44802	127.80768	129.16733	130.52699	131.88665	133.24631	134.60596

Index

Suggested Corrections

Reads Now (Existing)	Should be (Corrected)	E.No / T.No and Page No
$T = \frac{1}{2}p_1 dl - \frac{dl^2}{r} tan\alpha$	$T = \frac{1}{2}p_1 dl - \frac{dl^2}{4} tan\alpha$	E4.4(a) Page 62
$G = 316d$ to $\frac{1}{4}d$	$G = 0.25d$	Fig.4.5 Page 68
$f = 31.5\sqrt{F_0/W}$	$f = 44.6\sqrt{F_0/W}$	E11.22(b) Page 177
$F_g = \frac{2i_g F_f}{2i_f}$	$F_g = \frac{2i_g F_f}{3i_f}$	E11.29(b) Page 181
$c = \frac{Fl^3}{i'h^3 E}$	$c = \frac{Fl^3}{ib'h^3 E}$	E11.32(a) Page 182
(b) Laminated semielliptic leaf spring Fig 11.12 Laminated Life Springs	(b) Laminated semielliptic leaf spring Fig 11.12 Laminated Life Springs	Fig 11.11(b) Page 182
$F_t = \frac{\sigma_d C_v bY}{P_{dn} C_w}$	$F_t = \frac{\sigma_d C_v bY}{P_{dn} C_w}$	E12.24(a) Page 214
$Q = 2d_2/(d_2 + 1)$	$Q = 2d_2/(d_2 + d_1)$	E12.26(c) Page 214
$tan\delta_1 = \frac{d_1 sin\theta}{d_1 + d_1 cos\theta}$	$tan\delta_1 = \frac{d_1 sin\theta}{d_2 + d_1 cos\theta}$	E12.29(a) Page 215
$tan\theta_d = \frac{2h_{f1} sin\delta_1}{d_1}$	$tan\delta_d = \frac{2h_{f1} sin\delta_1}{d_1}$	E12.29(d) Page 215
$F_{te} = \frac{F_t l}{l - 0.5b}$	$F_{te} = \frac{F_t L}{L - 0.5b}$	E12.45(a) Page 219
$r_0 = r\left(\frac{l - 0.5b}{l}\right)$	$r_0 = r\left(\frac{L - 0.5b}{L}\right)$	E12.45(a) Page 219
$F_c = F_{te} tan\alpha$	$F_c = F_{te} tan\alpha$	E12.45(c) Page 219
The permissible tooth load $F_t = \frac{2M_{te}}{d_2}$	The actual tooth load $F_{te} = \frac{2M_{te}}{d_2}$	E12.53(d) Page 223
The normal pressure angle, α_n Maximum $\alpha_n = 40^0 30'$	The normal pressure angle, α_n Maximum $\alpha_n = 18^0 15'$	T12.20 Page 241
The normal pressure angle, α_n Minimum $\alpha_n = 18^0 15'$	The normal pressure angle, α_n Minimum $\alpha_n = 14^0 30'$	T12.20 Page 241
Table 12.30 Load stress factor for worm gears for use in E12.53(d)	Table 12.30 Load stress factor for worm gears for use in E12.62(a)	T12.30 Page 246
$B = \left[\frac{D-d}{8}\right]^2$	$B = \frac{[D-d]^2}{8}$	E14.15(a) Page 295
$Z = \rho\left\{022S' - \frac{180}{S'}\right\} \times 10^{-6}$	$Z = \rho\left\{022S' - \frac{180}{S'}\right\} \times 10^{-3}$	E15.1(e) Page 350
The initial tensile load in a bolt (According to experimnets conducted at cornell University, N)	The initial tensile load in a bolt when there is metal to metal contact (According to experimnets conducted at cornell University, N)	E9.1(c) Page 127
The initial tensile load in a bolt (According to experimnets conducted at cornell University, N) $F_t = 2805d$	The initial tensile load in a bolted joint with flexible gasket (According to experimnets conducted at cornell University, N) $F_t = 1402d$	E9.1(c) Page 127